Determinants of Health

SETTINGS AND ISSUES

CANADA HEALTH ACTION: BUILDING ON THE LEGACY
PAPERS COMMISSIONED BY THE NATIONAL FORUM ON HEALTH

Determinants of Health

SETTINGS AND ISSUES

ÉDITIONS
MULTIMONDES

FORUM NATIONAL   NATIONAL FORUM
SUR LA SANTÉ   ON HEALTH

Canadian Cataloguing in Publication Data

Main entry under title:

Canada Health Action: Building on the Legacy

Issued also in French under title: La santé au Canada: un héritage à faire fructifier
To be complete in 5 v.
Includes bibliographical references.
Contents: v. 1 Childen and Youth – v. 2. Adults and Seniors – v. 3. Settings and Issues.

ISBN 2-921146-62-2 (set)
ISBN 2-921146-49-5 (v. 3)

1. Public health – Canada. 2. Medicine, Preventive – Canada. 3. Children – Health and hygiene – Canada. 4. Adulthood – Health and hygiene – Canada. 5. Aged – Health and hygiene – Canada. I. National Forum on Health (Canada).

RA449.C28 1998   362.1'0971   C97-941659-0

Linguistic Revision: Traduction Tandem
Proofreading: Traduction Tandem and Robert Paré
Cover Design: Gérard Beaudry
Graphics: Emmanuel Gagnon

Volume 3: Settings and Issues
ISBN 2-921146-49-5   Cat. No.: H21-126/6-3-1997E
Legal Deposit– Bibliothèque nationale du Québec, 1998
Legal Deposit – National Library of Canada, 1998
© Her Majesty the Queen in Right of Canada, 1998

The series The National Forum on Health can be ordered at this address:
Éditions MultiMondes
930, rue Pouliot
Sainte-Foy (Québec)
G1V 3N9 CANADA
Telephone: (418) 651-3885; toll free in North America: 1 800 840-3029
Fax: (418) 651 6822; toll free in North America: 1 888 303-5931
E-mail: multimondes@multim.com
Internet: http://www.multim.com

Published by Éditions MultiMondes in co-operation with the National Forum on Health, Health Canada, and Canadian Government Publishing, Public Works and Government Services Canada.

FOREWORD

In October 1994, the Prime Minister of Canada, The Right Honourable Jean Chrétien, launched the National Forum on Health to involve and inform Canadians and to advise the federal government on innovative ways to improve the health system and the health of Canada's people. The Forum was set up as an advisory body with the Prime Minister as Chair, the federal Minister of Health as Vice Chair, and 24 volunteer members who contributed a wide range of knowledge founded on involvement in the health system as professionals, consumers and volunteers.

To fulfil their mandate, the Forum focused on long-term and systemic issues. They saw their task as formulating advice appropriate to the development of national policies, and divided the work into four key areas – Values, Striking a Balance, Determinants of Health, and Evidence-Based Decision Making.

The complete report of the National Forum on Health consists of two volumes:

> *Canada Health Action: Building on the Legacy*
>> The Final Report of the National Forum on Health

and

> *Canada Health Action: Building on the Legacy*
>> Synthesis Reports and Issues Papers

Copies available from: Publications Distribution Centre, Health Canada Communications, PL. 090124C, Brooke Claxton Building, Tunney's Pasture, Ottawa, Ontario K1A 0K9. Telephone: (613) 954-5995. Fax: (613) 941-5366. *(Aussi disponible en français.)*

The Forum based its recommendations on 42 research papers written by the most eminent specialists in the field. The papers are brought together in a five-volume series:

VOLUME 1 – CHILDREN AND YOUTH
VOLUME 2 – ADULTS AND SENIORS
VOLUME 3 – SETTINGS AND ISSUES
VOLUME 4 – HEALTH CARE SYSTEMS IN CANADA AND ELSEWHERE
VOLUME 5 – EVIDENCE AND INFORMATION

Individual volumes or the complete series can be ordered from: Editions MultiMondes, 930, rue Pouliot, Sainte-Foy (Québec) G1V 3N9. Telephone: 1 800 840-3029. Fax: 1 888 303-5931. *(Aussi disponible en français.)*

Values

The Values working group sought to understand the values and principles that Canadians hold about health and health care, so that the system continues to reflect and respond to these values. To explore Canadian core values that are connected to the health care system and to understand the implications for decision making, the group conducted some original public opinion research, using scenarios or short stories which addressed many of the issues being investigated by the other working groups of the Forum. The scenarios were tested in focus groups. Quantitative research supplemented the focus groups making the findings more generalizable. The group also contributed to a review of public opinion research on health and social policy. Finally, a review of Canadian and international experience with ethics bodies was commissioned to identify the contribution that such groups can make to continuing the discusssion of values in decision making.

Striking a Balance

The Striking a Balance working group considered how to allocate society's limited resources to best protect, restore and promote the health of Canadians. Attention was given to the balance of resources within the health sector and other sectors of the economy. The group commissioned a series of papers to assist in their deliberations. They conducted a thorough review of international trends in health expenditures, use of resources, and outcomes. They paid considerable attention to public and private financing issues, health system oganization and federal-provicial transfers. The group produced a separate discussion paper on public and private financing, and a position paper on the Canada Health and Social Transfer.

Determinants of Health

The Determinants of Health working group sought to answer the question: In these times of economic and social hardship, what actions must be taken to allow Canadians to continue to enjoy a long life and, if possible, to increase their health status? The group consulted specialists to assist in identifying appropriate actions on the non-medical determinants of health. Specialists were asked to prepare papers on issues of concern to the health of the population related to the macro-economic environment, the contexts in which people live (i.e. families, schools, work and communities), as well as on issues of concern to people's health at different life stages. Each paper presents a review of the literature, examples of success stories or failures, and relevant policy implications.

Evidence-Based Decision Making

The working group on Evidence-Based Decision Making considered how individually practioners and policy makers can have access to, and utilize the best available evidence in making decisions. The group held two workshops with leading authorities to discuss how health information can be used to support and encourage a culture of evicence-based decision making, and to consider what information Canadians need to be better health care consumers and how to get that information to them. The group commissioned papers to: examine the meaning and concepts of evidence and evidence-based decision making as well as cases that illustrate opportunities for improvement; identify the health information infrastructure needed to support evidence-based decision making; examine tools which support more effective health care decision making; and identify strategies for assisting and increasing the role of Canadians in decision making in health and health care.

Members

William R.C. Blundell, B.A.Sc. (Ont.)
Richard Cashin, LL.B. (Nfld.)
André-Pierre Contandriopoulos, Ph.D. (Que.)
Randy Dickinson (N.B.)
Madeleine Dion Stout, M.A. (Ont.)
Robert G. Evans, Ph.D. (B.C.)
Karen Gainer, LL.B. (Alta.)
Debbie L. Good, C.A. (PEI)
Nuala Kenny, M.D. (N.S.)
Richard Lessard, M.D. (Que.)
Steven Lewis (Sask.)
Gerry M. Lougheed Jr. (Ont.)

Margaret McDonald, R.N. (NWT)
Eric M. Maldoff, LL.B. (Que.)
Louise Nadeau, Ph.D. (Que.)
Tom W. Noseworthy, M.D. (Alta.)
Shanthi Radcliffe, M.A. (Ont.)
Marc Renaud, Ph.D. (Que.)
Judith A. Ritchie, Ph.D. (N.S.)
Noralou P. Roos, Ph.D. (Man.)
Duncan Sinclair, Ph.D. (Ont.)
Lynn Smith, LL.B., Q.C. (B.C.)
Mamoru Watanabe, M.D. (Alta.)
Roberta Way-Clark, M.A. (N.S.)

Secretary and Deputy Minister, Health Canada

Michèle S. Jean

Secretariat Staff

Executive Director
Marie E. Fortier

Joyce Adubofuor
Lori Alma
Rachel Bénard
Kathy Bunka
Barbara Campbell
Marlene Campeau
Carmen Connolly
Lise Corbett
John Dossetor
Kayla Estrin
Rhonda Ferderber
Annie Gauvin
Patricia Giesler
Sylvie Guilbault
Janice Hopkins

Lucie Lacombe
Johanne LeBel
Elizabeth Lynam
Krista Locke
John Marriott
Maryse Pesant
Marcel Saulnier
Liliane Sauvé
Linda St-Amour
Judith St-Pierre
Nancy Swainson
Catherine Swift
Josée Villeneuve
Tim Weir
Lynn Westaff

We extend our sincere thanks to all those who participated in the various production stages of this series of publications.

TABLE OF CONTENTS – VOLUME 3

ISSUES

Settings

Toward Healthy Families

SUSAN A. MCDANIEL, PH.D., FRSC

Department of Sociology
University of Alberta

SUMMARY

This paper is intended to highlight strategic areas in which policy action towards healthy families is important, without specifying the level of jurisdiction or the areas of policy responsibility involved. Conceptualized as a policy background paper, examples rather than complete literature are cited but the paper rests on the most recent and best available research evidence and new ways of thinking about healthy families.

Highly diverse evidence, in both research and theory, and increasing numbers of Canadian and international policy initiatives have spotlighted the importance of social and economic well-being to the health of individuals, families and populations. This is a new awareness and policy application of what has long been known. For example, researchers have said for a long time that improvements in life expectancy would come more from nutritional and environmental changes (population-based interventions) than from advances in medicine (individual health care) (McKeown 1976). The ways in which societies create and distribute social resources determine the health and well-being of populations. More egalitarian societies demonstrate better population health and well-being than those with large gaps between rich and poor.

Family is the closest and most vital social determinant of health and well-being, and therefore key to population health. Families distribute social and economic rewards from work and social transfers (e.g., social assistance, pensions). Families provide essential social supports crucial to health and well-being. A "triple helix" of healthy families exists, in which the following three features are interwoven:

1. *Family status and family relations are key determinants of individual and population health and well-being.*
2. *Families are health givers, health promoters, health providers, health guardians and health educators, crucially important in child development but also vital in caregiving throughout life.*
3. *Family health and healthy families reveal the interconnections of health policies, social policies and economic policies.*

Analysis of Canadian and international success stories reveals that nonmedical interventions have profound implications for family health and well-being. Numerous studies and projects have confirmed the beneficial effects on health of social contacts and relationships. Families are the closest sources of social support for most people. Families in countries with narrower income distributions cope better with child rearing, even with different family forms (such as in Sweden and Japan), than families in countries with wider income disparities, such as the United States. Educational and employment opportunities matter greatly to healthy families.

The following principles may help guide government actions:

- *Health and socioeconomic well-being are not separate or separable, which is evident in family context.*
- *Acceptance of family cultural and social diversity is essential to designing successful policies to promote healthy families.*
- *Government action must take into account the health effects of increasing family insecurity in Canada.*
- *Supporting and enabling families to carry on their crucial health-enhancing roles is a basic building block of a healthy families policy.*

  Government policy faces these challenges:

1. *to acknowledge that healthy families involve social and economic conditions and approaches;*
2. *to find new means of achieving desired population health outcomes that acknowledge the vital contributions families make to healthy populations; and*
3. *to work toward new ways to support families in all the ways they live, to enhance their caring capacities.*

   The paper concludes with a list of policy targets that require action.

TABLE OF CONTENTS

LIST OF TABLES

HEALTHY FAMILIES AND HEALTH DETERMINANTS:
KEY CONCLUSIONS FROM THE RESEARCH LITERATURE

Families are the key to health and health determination for a number of intersecting reasons. Families give us our genetic inheritance, a crucial health determinant in terms of hereditary diseases and propensities and inherited vulnerabilities and invulnerabilities. Family is the central determinant of both life expectancy and socioeconomic chances. Families are the main means of distribution and redistribution of social resources, particularly to children and elders, although the means by which allocation and distribution occurs, or even if it occurs, is not understood. Families are often the first or last recourse for social support, now known as the one essential health determinant. Families provide social environments in which health behaviours are learned, and in which individual and family health can be enhanced or harmed. Families also provide access to health care, including medical care, health promotion and well-being. And, perhaps most importantly, families position us to cope with social pressures and opportunities.

In this paper, research, theoretical and policy literatures in highly diverse areas are mined for key conclusions and lessons about what does and does not encourage healthy families. The literature review draws on family theory, the history of health and ideas about health, family history, sociology of health and health care, clinical sciences, philosophy, health services, health promotion, health policy, family and social policy. It was impossible to make the review comprehensive. Principles to guide government action, specific policy recommendations, and strategic targets conclude the paper.

Definitional Conundrums and Old Reruns

The concept of health has been evolving in Canada by great leaps and strides, interspersed with long plateaus. The evolution of the health concept matters to the discussion of healthy families. The "health field" concept and framework, introduced by the Lalonde White Paper (Canada 1974), turned the previous conceptualization of health care as a "furnace/ thermostat" (Evans and Stoddart 1994, 34) on its head. Under the previous models, the health care system interpreted the environment of an individual (the thermostat), determined the appropriate response, and responded with treatment or medical intervention (like a furnace). Familial, social, economic and environmental needs were defined as nonneeds because the thermostat could not interpret them and the furnace could not respond. According to this model, those with health needs took themselves to a health care provider and became "patients," whose needs could be served by the health care system. If individuals did not have a perceived medical problem, no care or intervention occurred.

The Lalonde framework rethought health as a field with four categories: lifestyles, environment, human biology and health care organization. The health concept included the notion that health might be improved by means other than health care expansion or individual-level medical interventions. A second, extremely important, idea demoted health care from the "only health game in town," replacing it with several policy approaches to achieving health.

Evans and Stoddart (1994) advanced the conceptualization of health by incorporating research evidence from the years since the Lalonde report. Evans and Stoddart developed a model of linkages among health, health care, wealth production and population well-being. Family was included only implicitly.

Consistent with the Evans and Stoddart framework is the population health approach adopted by the ministers of Health in their 1994 Halifax meeting:

A population health approach differs from traditional medical and health care thinking in two main ways:

- Population health strategies address the entire range of factors that determine health. Traditional health care focuses on risks and clinical factors related to particular diseases.
- Population health strategies are designed to affect the entire population. Health care deals with individuals one at a time, usually individuals who already have a health problem or are at significant risk of developing one (Federal, Provincial and Territorial Advisory Committee on Population Health 1994, 7).

The population health concept includes the social, the collective and the nonmedical. Wilkinson (1994, 75) argues, based on international health analysis, that "the quality of the social fabric, rather than increases in average wealth, may now be the primary determinant of the real subjective quality of life." According to Frank and Mustard (1994, 14), "it is not the level of wealth a country has that improves the health of its population, but its commitment to allocate resources to key sectors, such as mothers and children, education and adequate nutrition." Syme, in discussing coronary heart disease, concludes that:

It is, therefore, clearly evident that despite the efforts of such programs as MRFIT, the distribution of disease in the population remains unchanged. This is not surprising considering that nothing is being done to alter the societal forces that caused the problem in the first place (1994, 80).

From the conceptual, through the empirical and into the policy realm, the population health concept has come into its own, revealing important new policy possibilities (Angus et al. 1995).

In the social realm, no system is more vital to well-being nor more proximate than family, however defined. Yet the term "family" is not clearly defined. Phillipps (1995) comments on this problem: "Our tax system cannot achieve the modern social welfare and equity goals claimed for it so long as we continue to base policy decisions on an image of family that belongs to old reruns" (31).

Old reruns seem to define family all too often, and can have profound and far-reaching implications for healthy family policies, implications that go well beyond the tax system examined by Phillipps. Bala (1995) notes: "One of the most controversial issues in the family policy field is a funda-mental definitional question: what types of relationships constitute 'a family,' and hence will be endowed with special rights, privileges and obligations?" (3). If healthy families are defined by form (such as two-parent families, or families with children, or young families), other kinds of families might be overlooked or underestimated as healthy—a wasteful and counterproductive policy approach (Eichler 1995).

The most common research approach is to define family by the functions it serves rather than by the form it takes (Bala 1995; Eichler 1995; McDaniel 1995b; United Nations 1993; Vanier Institute of the Family 1993). Elkind (1994) discusses family in terms of its child-rearing function:

> Although some contend that the classic nuclear family, consisting of two married parents and their biological offspring, is the best environment for rearing children, the evidence to support this contention has not been overwhelming... What appears to be crucial to effective childrearing is not so much the particular kinship structure as the emotional climate of the family (31).

In policy, however, definitions of family by form are more common (Baker 1995, 9–10; Vanier Institute 1993, xi–xii), so traditional families may be privileged and other types of families omitted from benefits. Worse are policies that attempt to strengthen families by imposing, either directly or indirectly, some structural family ideal. Policies like this are largely ineffective, and can hinder families (Baker 1995; Vanier Institute of the Family 1993, introduction).

Despite research evidence and strong agreement among family theorists and researchers that family should be defined by function rather than form, policies that impinge on families (and most of these have health implications) still tend to resist the functional approach. Any policy approach to healthy families must recognize the need to revise the typical policy definition of family from an outmoded postwar, gender-specialized, two-parent family with children, to include today's family diversity.

The Triple Helix Framework of Healthy Families

Families and health are interwoven in a triple helix:

1. Family status and family relations are key determinants of individual and population health and well-being.
2. Families are health givers, health promoters, health providers, health guardians and health educators. (The flip side is that families can also be health inhibitors, resulting in lifelong health and social problems.)
3. More than in any other area, family health and healthy families reveal the interconnection of health policies, social policies, and economic policies.

The triple helix offers a framework to organize and highlight the key conclusions from the research literature on healthy families, and frame lessons about what does and does not encourage, nurture and support healthy families.

Genetic Inheritance/Predisposition and Family

Genetic inheritance has been over- and underestimated as a component of family health and healthy families. Genetics can be crucial to well-being for single-gene diseases, inherited vulnerabilities, and propensities. Baird (1994, 134) tells us: "Genes set the limits of our possible responses, not only to physical and biological environments, but also to our psychological and social environments." Baird uses the example of early heart attacks due to high cholesterol. At one extreme are people whose biological makeup is such that changes to diet and lifestyle make negligible difference. At the other extreme are those who can reduce their risk of heart attack with family support and lifestyle changes. A significant factor is the individual's coping ability and the psychological likelihood of controlling diet and changing lifestyle, both of which may be related to family environments.

Inherited vulnerabilities and propensities may be even more important for populations than single-disease genetic predispositions. Evans and Stoddart (1994, 51–52) suggest:

> progress in genetics is... extending the older picture of a fixed genetic endowment, in which well-defined genetic diseases follow from single-gene defects. It now appears that particular combinations of genes may lead to predispositions, or resistances, to a wide variety of diseases, not themselves normally thought of as 'genetic.'

Baird (1994, 138) adds, "Treating a population as if all members were at uniform risk, and then attempting to improve their environment, cannot eliminate all disease and will certainly have diminishing returns."

Profound and so far relatively poorly understood interactions exist between genetic inheritance and predispositions and population well-being. Baird (1994, 159) cautions, "The simplistic model of disease causation that is currently prevalent in our culture... puts us at risk of foolish and precipitate action."

Popular literature's focus on genetics as a panacea to health is inappropriate, premature and ideological:

> Genetic predisposition needs to be understood in a larger social context. The Human Genome Project... does raise questions about the breadth (and depth) of consideration underlying this type of decision to make resources unavailable for any other use. We need to develop ways of allocating resources so as to better people's lives in the long run (Baird 1994, 158).

By acknowledging the powerful potential of social interventions, including policies that promote healthy families,

> we may eventually be able to apply our increasing genetic knowledge to the enhancement of people's opportunities for healthy lives. This will require interventions to change the environmental factors leading to the common disease outcomes rather than the genetic predispositions. Such interventions must be based on a more complete picture that also contains the social, economic, physical and cultural factors that interact with our biological make-up to determine health (Baird 1994, 159).

Life Chances: Surviving and Thriving

The importance of economic security and relative economic advantage to population health is now understood (Marmot 1994; Sagan 1987). Families are pivotal in this because economic resources are distributed through families. How societies create and distribute their wealth determines the health and well-being of the population (Sen 1993, 40–47). The clear relation of health to socioeconomic status is apparent in the Whitehall study of British public servants, who, though they work in similar conditions, have life and health expectancies correlated to their socioeconomic status (Frank and Mustard 1994, 8). Frank and Mustard (1994, 14) find in Manitoba, that it is not access to health care that determines health and well-being, but the underlying socioeconomic factors (employment, income and education). In a study of health changes over time in different societies, McKeown (1976) found that nutrition and social environmental changes have more positive effects on life and health expectancies than advances in medicine.

Wilkinson (1994) found that mortality rates in the developed world depend more on the degree of income inequality in the society than per capita economic growth or income. He finds that "in the twelve member states of the European Economic Community, average life expectancy between 1975 and 1985 has grown fastest in those countries where relative poverty decreased fastest (or increased slowest)" (Wilkinson 1994, 68). In particular, Wilkinson found that "In terms of family structures, Japan and Sweden are at opposite ends of the spectrum. Yet these two countries do almost equally well in terms of child welfare and health. What these two countries have in common (or had until recently) is a narrow income distribution" (1994, 73).

What factors are involved here and are they related to healthy families?

The importance of relative income to health suggests that psychological factors related to deprivation and disadvantage are involved. That is to say, it is less a matter of the immediate physical effects of inferior material conditions than of the social meanings attached to those conditions and how people feel about their circumstances and about themselves (Wilkinson 1994, 70).

The meaning of deprivation is usually learned in the family. Labels of and feelings about relative deprivation affect health, and are a family matter. "The protective sense of self-esteem or coping ability may well be a collective as well as an individual possession" (Evans and Stoddart 1994, 52).

Although deprivation and family health in early family life determine later well-being, early family deprivation or trauma and abuse does not cause later problems for all children (Keating and Mustard 1993). According to Scarf (1995, 373), this is because the child may have a stable affectional relationship with someone and a sense of success and achievement.

About stable relationships, Scarf (1995, 379) tells us "A secure relationship with someone seems to inspire a kind of inner optimism and trust, the deep belief that something good will happen if only one persists long and hard enough." Based on the Kauai birth cohort study that family status can affect well-being, Hertzman (1994, 170) adds that "[high class status] can actually help reverse the long-term consequences of birth stresses." There are large untapped pools of vigour and resilience in Canada, ways in which all kinds of relationships could sustain children and reverse negative effects to some extent. We could join together in communities and associations to give children a sense of security, trust, success and accomplishment, if we move beyond the belief that only family can provide for children.

Social Resources and Healthy Families

Families that share and mediate with other social institutions thrive best and are healthiest. Urie Bronfenbrenner at the White House Conference on Families, tells us that, "The future of the family lies in the relations between family and other institutions. That is where our attention must be" (in Curran 1983, 27).

Healthy families are not characterized by form. Experts on family dysfunction or troubled families seldom have the opportunity to deal with families that are not troubled or dysfunctional, but they most often define what a healthy family is (Beavers and Hampson 1990; Stinnett 1992). One of these "hands-on" family experts, Dolores Curran, has developed a set of 15 traits that she considers to define a healthy family:

> I have never worked with a family that exhibits all fifteen of the traits presented in this book, including mine. I doubt if I ever will… I hope readers model the man who told me after a talk on these traits that he felt pretty good about his family, 'Four out of fifteen isn't all bad,' he said.
>
> I laughed and agreed with him, but the woman behind him gasped. Actually, I have more hope for him than for her. A sense of humour is one of the healthy traits. Gasping isn't. (Curran 1983, introduction)

The 15 traits are all micro level, such as humour, communication, supporting privacy of family members, and sharing leisure. Traditional schemes to evaluate family competence, family health or well-being (see Beavers and Hampson 1993 for the most widely used assessment model) tend to focus only on the micro-level aspects of family life, such as inter-personal communications and individual coping skills. The social, economic and cultural contexts in which families live are largely ignored.

Families position us to cope, excel or fail. Control over one's life and a sense of social integration have been found to affect population health outcomes. Healthy families can provide both, but a sense of control depends on whether an individual has sufficient resources to make choices about his life. As a character in George Bernard Shaw's 1906 play *Major Barbara* says, "Security, the chief pretense of civilization, cannot exist where the worst of dangers, the danger of poverty hangs over everyone's head." Resources include money, education, power, literacy, housing, and health. Efficacy and self-esteem often depend on a family member's sense of contribution to and control over the circumstances of family life. Middle-class women who took jobs during the Great Depression to contribute to their families financially, for example, were healthier and more capable 40 years later than those who did not (Elder and Liker 1982).

Time use can reflect quality of life, with leisure time an important component of well-being (Frederick 1995). Wilkinson notes that there are three health factors that comprise health and well-being in work: control over work, pressures of work and support from colleagues. The primary infringements on leisure time are work, school and family demands, particularly for women (1994, 71). Based on 1992 Statistics Canada data, Canadians spend as much time on unpaid work (such as housework and child care, caring for older relatives, doing volunteer work, etc.) as on "paid" work (Frederick 1995, 7).

A persistent theme in Frederick's analysis is the lack of time. Work demands are increasing role responsibilities for both men and women, but "higher proportions of women were often stressed from lack of time than men over much of the life cycle" (1994, 53). Postsecondary students experience extreme time stress, as do mothers with young children at home. Almost one half of baby boom mothers saw themselves as extremely restricted in the amount of time they had to do what they had to do (Frederick 1995, 58). Most women now work outside the home, whether or not they have small children at home (Menaghan and Parcel 1990), so the time pressure is not surprising. Leisure, an essential component of well-being, is being increasingly compromised, and individual and family well-being are suffering. The lack of time also has serious implications for stress levels and sleeping time, which are vital to well-being. Perhaps most important for healthy families, there is less time to talk, and when social resources become stressed, there is an increased likelihood of miscommunication, abuse and violence.

A number of European countries have legislated support programs that alleviate some of the time stress parents experience (Baker 1995). Swedish work-family policies, for example, long recognized as among the most enlightened in the world, have developed parental leaves with pay following childbirth or adoption (Moen and Firebaugh 1994). This reduces parental stress in two ways: parents can spend time with their infant and not feel as time stressed, and they do not have the anxiety of lost wages during their time at home with the baby.

Social Support: The BIG Effect

Since the 1970s, the concept of social support as key to individual and population well-being has spawned a vast literature. "A Friend a Day Keeps the Doctor Away," a chapter in Oakley's book on social support (1992a, 21–43), sums up the research. Social support is known to be, on average, beneficial to health. The healing support of friends and family is not a new insight. As noted sixteenth-century philosopher Francis Bacon stated, "this communicating of a man's self to his friend works two contrary effects; for it redoubleth joys and cutteth griefs in half. For there is no man that imparteth joys to his friend, but he joyeth them more, and no man that imparteth his griefs to his friend but he grieveth the less" (in Oakley 1992a,

122). More recently, Berkman (1984) said: "The message is that social support is both good preventive and curative medicine. Like chicken soup, its powers are believed to be pervasive, the reason for its effects are unknown" (p. 413). New views of health and well-being accommodate social support, with a strong focus on families. This represents a sharp departure from the medical approach to health.

Social support has been found to alleviate stress, reduce mortality and decrease the likelihood of everything from cancer and cardiological problems to infections (Adams and Blieszner 1995; Evans and Stoddart 1994; Gottlieb 1981; Oakley 1992a; Syme 1994). Oakley (1992b) comments: "Of the random-allocated interventions that have been carried out in the general health field, almost without exception people assigned to receive support have fared better mentally and physically than have those in control groups" (52). Social support is, in sum, the big social effect on health and well-being.

The presumption that interpersonal and family relationships are uniformly supportive has led to substantial methodological and policy problems when studying the effects of families on well-being (Adams and Blieszner 1995, 209). As Gottlieb (1981) says, "… family members and friends do not always merit the appellation 'support system'" (30). Samples are often inadequate and do not represent the diversity of possible social relationships and supports. Research questions may presume that relatives are supportive, willing and available to help, which can have deleterious policy consequences when this has no empirical basis. Social support research is usually descriptive and atheoretical, which decontextualizes human relationships. For example, a strong social network may be presumed to replace cumulative life disadvantages among women, but may not compensate for lack of pension. Family commitments can also be simultaneously fulfilling and stressful. Too many people in one's social network can be as daunting and stressful as social isolation. McDaniel (1993a, 1995a) has shown that middle-aged women often have too many family members and friends calling on them in a crisis, which creates not well-being, but immense stress.

Access to Health through Family

Families provide several doors to health. They educate, provide role models, advocate, care for sick members, and, if they can afford it, pay for dental care, prescriptions, eyeglasses and fitness equipment. They also teach us how to seek health for ourselves, and offer the means by which that can be accomplished.

However, health through family is more available to some than others. For example, women are now known to play central roles as family health guardians (Heller 1986). The health guardian role comprises the primary physical, psychological and social activities of home-based family care, whether or not there is illness or disease in the family. It is the cliché, "Wear your boots and toque" and "Eat your carrots" advice of mothers that promotes health and serves the good of society. Yet, "many of the women report no one looks after them when they are sick" (Heller 1986, 17). Women may assign a different level of importance to their own care than to that of their families, which can have serious long-term implications for women's health. This is exemplified by one woman, Greta, interviewed by Heller (1986, 36):

> The nuclear family is too exhausting; it means I do everything. There is no way I can take care of all my children's needs and earn a living and be supportive to my friends. I can't be three people!... You don't get any credit so you have low self-esteem and then you're back on the job market...

Another woman, Teresa (age 45) puts it like this:

> Who else would do it [be responsible for the family's physical health]? My husband doesn't have time, or patience, both of these things go together.

Not surprisingly, women who give care at home (and most caregivers at home are women), commonly express a need for better access to professional, paraprofessional, or institutional health services, improved access to services closer to home (including home care), and more accessible health information. Those caring for the chronically ill, the elderly, disabled adults or children express strong interest in respite care so they can take much-needed breaks from unrelenting and, at times, debilitating day-in, day-out care (Neysmith 1989; Osterbusch et al. 1987).

Female caregivers also face the issue of choice and lost opportunities. Osterbusch and colleagues (1987, 217) suggest:

> The femininized structure of family caregiving raises issues of equity because, in order to fulfil what can be viewed as both a private and public responsibility, women must often forgo other opportunities and the freedom to make choices that may be critical to their well-being.

Neysmith and Chappell expand on the point that families, especially women in families, do not constitute an "informal sector of health care" (Neysmith 1989) or "community care" (Chappell 1994). Neysmith adds, "To refer to this person as a sector whose services are to be interweaved with those of the formal sector renders invisible the disparities of power, control, and resources available to the respective parties" (1989, 47).

Chains, Effects, and Amplification

A family affects the health of its members in numerous ways. The complexity of the relationships between family and health has yet to be fully explained in the research literature. One model, suggested by Wheaton (1985), focuses on the health implications of various social roles, including family. Causal chains explain the possible relationships of family and health. For example, early trauma and deprivation often lead to health and social problems. Conditional effects may modify or amplify the impact of various forces. Hence, the effects of early trauma and deprivation can be modified by positive relationships, a sense of early achievement, improved economic circumstances, social support and enhanced coping capabilities, or amplified by a lack of these effects. Causal chains and conditional effects together can produce "structural amplifications" that can help or hinder health outcomes either by diminishing harmful barriers or aggravating existing conditions. Two examples from the research literature show how this model might be applied to policy.

Married people are typically healthier than those who never married, are divorced, separated or widowed (Waite 1995), but it is not known how marriage works as health determinant. Marriage has more beneficial health effects for men than for women (Ross, Mirowsky, and Goldensteen 1990). There are three reasons for this: the perceived benefits of living with someone (the health guardian, health caregiver effect), the positive effects of social support that marriage can offer, and the higher socioeconomic status of married couples compared with unmarried, which can benefit health. Living with someone without being married to them seems to have more limited health effects than living with a spouse. Waite (1995, 498) suggests that "marriage assumes sharing of economic and social resources and what we can think of as co-insurance. Spouses act as a sort of small insurance pool against life's uncertainties, reducing their need to protect themselves *by themselves* from unexpected events" (emphasis in original).

The supportive effects of marriage depend on the quality of the marriage (Ross, Mirowsky, and Goldensteen 1990, 1063). On the whole, marriage seems to provide a net health benefit, but this is based on averages and does not imply that promoting marriage is good health policy. Higher socio-economic status may weigh differently for married men than for women, since women more often fall into poverty after divorce than men do (Popay and Jones 1991; Ross, Mirowsky, and Goldensteen 1990, 1064). Marriage may economically benefit women and emotionally benefit men. This has very different healthy family policy implications. After losing a spouse, for example, men might benefit more from being given emotional support, but women might benefit more from being given financial support.

Surprisingly little research has examined the health effects of lone parenthood. Popay and Jones (1991), in a British study, find that lone parents are in poorer health on all health indicators than married couples. Surprisingly, lone fathers have poorer long-term health than lone mothers, but lone fathers tend to be older and are more often widowed than are lone mothers (Popay and Jones 1991, 85). On all other health measures, however, lone mothers have less good health than lone fathers. The children of lone mothers have poorer health than those of either lone fathers or couples.

Poverty and marital disadvantage combine to contribute to the poorer health of lone mothers and their children. Kamerman links economic policy implications to family well-being for lone-parent families headed by women:

> The relative economic deprivation experienced by mother-only families will be alleviated, but not eliminated, when women's wages reach closer to parity with men's wages, and/or when low earnings are supplemented with transfer payments (1995, 254).

McLanahan and Garfinkel (1995) have two concerns about how one policy approach addressing the poverty of lone mothers may affect the well-being of their children:

> Reducing economic insecurity without increasing dependence on government means placing a greater burden on parents. It means requiring nonresident fathers to pay more child support and mothers to work more hours outside the home... Will placing a greater burden on parents increase or reduce child well-being... ?... two concerns. The first... some analysts fear that forcing fathers to pay more support will increase parental conflict and thereby reduce child well-being. The second... some analysts fear that encouraging (or forcing) mothers to work outside the home will increase family stress and undermine parental supervision (1995, 381).

The conditional effects of marriage combined with the causal chains of socioeconomic status and preselection factors provide structural amplifications that fend off negative health effects, particularly for men. Women, even if they experience structural health benefits from family status, experience them in different ways and for shorter amounts of time. Women are widowed more often than men, and usually in diminished circumstances. This can negatively affect a widow's long-term well-being (Adams and Blieszner 1995; Elder and Liker 1982; McDaniel 1993a, 1995b; McDaniel and Gee 1993).

Research in Third World countries reveals that the effects of lone parenthood on poverty among women are not consistent. For example, women family heads (single parents) in many parts of Africa and Asia (see United Nations 1993, for examples) are far from disadvantaged. In fact, they are microentrepreneurs who pay back loans at a good rate and invest in both businesses and their families. Women who are independent of men and independent economically in less-developed countries, are also more likely to invest money, time and resources in their children, particularly their female children, even if they have little to invest (McDaniel 1996). This has two positive outcomes, which might have implications for Canada. First, educating girls and women is one of the best worldwide predictors of overall improved health for families and family members (McDaniel 1993b, 1995b; Moen and Firebaugh 1994). Second, women who receive more of society's resources as girls are more capable of establishing their own families, having the desired number of children, and becoming better family health guardians (United Nations 1995).

POLICIES, PROGRAMS, PROJECTS, AND NATURAL EXPERIMENTS: LESSONS ON WHAT WORKS AND WHAT DOES NOT

> *Institutions learn from data; people learn from stories. 'The first time I heard that statement was in Canada—in Toronto, in 1984.'*
>
> Ilona Kickbusch, Director of Lifestyles and Health, WHO Regional Office in Europe (in Pederson, O'Neill, and Rootman 1994, 8).

Canada and its stories of health successes have left a clear and lasting impression on the leading expert in the World Health Organization on lifestyles and health. Stories of successful family health actions must cast nets widely, to influence policy. Stories that are directly interventionist, deterministic in their endings or in monitoring of outcomes, or narrow in design or orientation, can mislead policy. They may suggest that all that is to be learned can be learned by knowing (or predicting) likely outcomes at the outset. Success stories that occur by chance, without monitored outcomes or intended intervention, can teach vital lessons and applicable concepts that must not be overlooked. Considering only projects with direct interventions and planned evaluations, expenditures and outcomes could mean overlooking important policy insights.

Successful actions on nonmedical determinants of family health include:
- actions that work to improve or better assess social health or family health;
- actions that have the effect, intended or not, of facilitating healthful behaviours/well-being among family members and/or families; and
- actions that solve or contribute to a solution to perceived family health problems.

Two examples illustrate how naturally occurring actions affect health outcomes and assessments.

Salonica is a natural experiment, with results that would not have occurred in a controlled experiment (Oakley 1992b, 44–45). In a prisoner-of-war camp in 1941 in Salonica, Greece, epidemiologist Archie Cochrane accidently discovered that yeast cures leg oedema. Cochrane later said:

> On reflection, it was not a good trial. I was testing the wrong hypothesis... the numbers were too small and the time too short, and the outcome measurements poor. Yet the treatment worked. I still do not know why... I can take little credit as the design of the trial was largely fortuitous. The German doctor's remark, when I asked for more help, was ... 'doctors are superfluous.' This was probably correct, but it was amazing what a little bit of science and a little bit of luck achieved (Oakley 1992b, 44–45).

Lesson 1: Be attentive and alert to potentially significant, applicable policy findings even if they are not anticipated or sought.

Lesson 2: Be wary of looking for policy answers only under laboratory, project-based or controlled experimental conditions.

The second example of an accidental success comes from Antonovsky (1993), originator of the Sense of Coherence scale used in the 1994 Canadian Health Promotion Survey. Instead of focusing on factors leading to disease and illness, Antonovsky asked how people survived and thrived in adverse conditions, and who survived and thrived, and why. The Sense of Coherence scale grew out of Antonovsky's observations of concentration camp survivors, and comprises three components: (1) comprehensibility of one's situation, (2) manageability of life, and (3) life's meaningfulness. All three components are linked to family connections, which enhance well-being even when family members are separated. The sense of coherence is an orientation to living that encourages survival and well-being; the more one has, the better one's chances of health and survival.

Lesson 3: Profoundly useful measures of thriving and well-being are being used to assess social well-being in Canada. Policies to promote healthy families can benefit from further analyses of the 1994 Canada Health Promotion Survey.

Lesson 4: Healthy families are better assessed by indicators that rely on *thriving* and *surviving*, rather than indicators that rely on mortality, illness, or disease. These indicators are also better bases for healthy public policy.

SUMMARY OF SUCCESS STORIES

Criteria for success: improvements in family health, defined as:

- families are better enabled to develop and maintain their capacity to care for each other and to promote opportunities for each family member; and
- the capacity of families to facilitate individual health and healthful behaviours and practices among family members is enhanced.

Each example is examined along seven dimensions (to the extent these can be assessed):
- actions on nonmedical determinants of health,
- reasons for the initiative,
- actors,
- analysis of the results,
- replicability of the initiative,
- funding,
- evaluation.

Families as Actors as Well as Subjects: Lessons from History

Lessons from History

Actions on nonmedical determinants of health – Social change similar to the Industrial Revolution is currently happening. Families protect each other, to prevent negative health outcomes.

Reasons for the initiative – Large-scale socioeconomic changes occur periodically.

Actors – Family units are actors, and are also acted on by large-scale socioeconomic changes.

Analysis of the results – Social historical analyses of the ways families shaped and coped with change are relevant to families today, who face similar challenges.

Replicability of the initiative – Massive social changes are occurring in Canada at present, so although this is not a replication of the Industrial Revolution, there are parallels.

Funding – Not applicable.

Evaluation – Even in "naturally occurring" changes, impacts and benefits can be evaluated. Key conclusions about the adaptive powers of families are relevant to achieving healthy families in the future.

These times of rapid social change are being compared with other times of change in their implications for families, such as Canada's mid-nineteenth century. Family health is said to be negatively affected by social change. Elkind, among others, suggests that family is a retreat from a demanding world (1994, 2). Eichler (1995) critiques this view, arguing that families interact with changes and are often sources of stress rather than retreats. By examining families in different change contexts, family historians such as Hareven have discovered that "multilayered family patterns" (1991, 103) and family dynamism have always existed, and that families are seldom passive when faced with social change.

> How the family both initiates and adapts to change and how it translates the impact of the larger structural changes to its own sphere are questions governing the richest area of inter-section between the family and the process of social change... The important principle underlying these questions is a view of family as an active agent. The family planned, initiated, or resisted change; it did not just respond blindly (Hareven 1991, 111).

Lesson 5: Families actively shape and determine their own well-being and health-enhancing possibilities, and policies can assist families in this.

Lesson 6: Families, as both custodians of tradition and agents of change, can provide their members with a sense of continuity which Hareven sees as "a resource to draw on when [needed]... " (1991, 115).

Lesson 7: Families during the Industrial Revolution charted strategies involving calculated collective trade-offs, to preserve the family and enhance the well-being of family members (Hareven 1991).

Lesson 8: Families in Canada today might also be engaging in adaptive strategies to share resources and protect each other, thereby preventing the negative consequences of workplace restructuring, shrinking government programs and social change on family health (McDaniel 1995c).

These lessons suggest that families, by both adapting to and initiating change, may be resources that can be used to promote good population health outcomes. However, families may be severely stressed by their unheralded efforts to insulate people from the strains of change. Public policy could acknowledge families as societal resources, and support them more in creating health and well-being, and lessening the effects of the stresses of social change on individuals and on families.

Families and Children "at Promise"

The next three programs are examples of trying to help families and children at risk become families and children "at promise."

Single Mothers of Colour in the United States

Actions on nonmedical determinants of health – Reframing at-risk families so isolated and oppressed minority groups can "take back" pride and responsibility, and making the "homeplace" a place of strength.

Reasons for the initiative – Existing "at risk" approaches to health of families are inadequate, and isolate and label families.

Actors – Communities and families that are disadvantaged and most likely to experience health and social problems as a consequence.

Replicability of the initiative – Replication is possible with immigrant groups in urban centres in Canada, with Aboriginal people and with single mothers on social assistance.

Funding – Not applicable—not a funded initiative.

Evaluation – Evaluative analyses have shown that the "at promise" approach improves family well-being outcomes.

Campaign 2000 and the National Anti-Poverty Organization (NAPO)

Actions on nonmedical determinants of health – A public campaign to educate and inform the Canadian public and the poor about child poverty in Canada. Campaign 2000 reframes "poverty talk" to make poverty real and question myths and assumptions about poverty.

Reasons for the initiative – Concerns about recent government cutbacks to social assistance and other benefits, and about public poverty rhetoric.

Actors – Social services organizations in collaboration with poor people themselves.

Replicability of the initiative – Possibilities for replication and greater breadth of coverage exist.

Funding – Campaigns are funded by Family Services Canada, the funders of NAPO and public donations.

Evaluation – It is not clear what effect these campaigns have had, but "taking back" poverty talk and questioning definitions catch the attention of all who hear it.

William Charles Band and Its Community Health Centre

Actions on nonmedical determinants of health – A reserve taking charge of its health care through the establishment of a community health centre.

Reasons for the initiative – A different approach to health care was needed, judging from the very poor health conditions of the reserve.

Actors: Reserve leaders and the federal government worked together to set up the health centre.

Replicability of the initiative – Other reserves have taken similar initiatives, which could be broadly applied, with adjustments to local conditions and needs.

Funding – Grant support and support in kind was provided by the federal government. Funds were also provided for a feasibility study early in the project.

Evaluation – Follow-up analyses of the health centre reveal that the band members feel more secure about their health, more health education, and better home management of health problems.

Health care in Canada in the 1990s is marked by limited resources, but families are characterized by strength and renewal in the face of adversity.

The concept of "children and families at risk" implies that families are somehow deficit in whatever resources it takes to be healthy and functioning. These scarcity images contrast with the increasingly popular (and less expensive) synergistic, renewing, supportive, health-enhancing approaches to health (Katz and Seth 1987). "Synergy is said to exist in all communities. But a basic shift in perspective and understanding is needed to transform a community from one characterized by scarcity to one characterized by synergy" (Katz and Seth 1987, 123).

Significant critiques of the at-risk approach have been made by African Americans and other cultural groups in the United States, as they have tried alternative approaches and found them useful.

Lesson 9: "Oppressed groups have reframed home and community as sources of strength and the dominant society as a source of barriers to advancement" (Swadener and Lubeck 1995, ix).

Swadener and Lubeck suggest that "homeplace" helps resist the "colonizing power of the dominant society."

Similar arguments have been advanced in Canada by First Nations peoples.

Lesson 10: "The best chance for improved health in the Aboriginal population of Canada rests in the continuation and acceleration of the process of self-determination" (Waldram, Herring and Young 1995, 271).

Swadener and Lubeck note that the at-risk label evokes the language of pathology, even as it supposedly works toward health promotion. They reveal how "poverty talk" about poor single mothers of colour constructs the health and well-being problems faced by these families as of their own making, whereas "at promise" language defines mother and children as working for mutual benefit and family health. Cook and Fine describe low-income mothers' pride in helping their children to find creative solutions to the conditions in which they live (1995, 136). These mothers no longer see themselves as the problem but instead the problems are the shots outside the windows of the child's school, the rats in the apartment hallway, and the oppressive poverty in which they live.

Lesson 11: Positive well-being outcomes have been shown for minority and low-income mothers and children who learn to reconceptualize their situations as being "at promise," thus taking back from the dominant society the power to label and define.

Canada has undertaken a similar effort, with the Campaign 2000 project launched by the Family Services Association. Campaign 2000 seeks to educate the public and the poor about child poverty in Canada and its implications. The National Anti-Poverty Organization also reverses "poverty talk" by asking: Would the wealthy have more self-esteem if they had to work? Is there a culture of wealth? Is greed generational? If tax loopholes ended, would the wealthy lose their incentive to work? (Swanson 1995).

The William Charles Band on Montreal Lake in Saskatchewan is the first Aborginal band to control its own health care (Waldram, Herring, and Young 1995, 239). It is a well-documented, although not fully evaluated, success story that was funded by the federal government. When a feasibility study was launched in 1984, living conditions on the reserve (where 800 of the 1,800 in the band lived) were very poor—only five houses had running water and proper sewage disposal, and housing conditions were crowded. Health problems from skin conditions to respiratory disease, and high rates of addiction, were common. After prolonged negotiations, a new health centre run by the Montreal Lake reserve was opened in 1987. The centre offered school-based immunizations, alcohol education, and prenatal care and education. Band members now feel more secure about their health and, with health education, there is more home management of minor illnesses, particularly children's illnesses. Centre staff speak Cree, so more people have become involved and there is more preventive health care. The most important effect, however, was social.

> Before the health centre, the community fabric was disintegrating. Residents lived in considerable fear, isolation and despair… It is perhaps this element of spirit that causes the health centre to be seen as a 'community centre'… People have a greater sense of 'belonging'—an element that had been missing (Waldram, Herring, and Young 1995, 242).

Lesson 12: Aboriginal self-determination initiatives can cause improved health outcomes.

Lesson 13: The renewal of community spirit through local control of health can change "families at risk" into "families at promise."

The sense of belonging to a community extends family caring and sharing beyond a narrow view into community as care provider. In the success of the William Charles Band, all three aspects of the triple helix of healthy families are apparent and interconnected: family health is linked to socioeconomic health; families are encouraged to act as health givers, promoters and providers; and better family relations are encouraged.

Family Matters and the Family Matters Program

Family Matters Program

Actions on nonmedical determinants of health – Combined research and social action program undertaken by U.S. university-based researchers to establish and evaluate a mutual family support system.

Reasons for the initiative – Curiosity about the social impacts of family support and interest in enhancing parenting skills, reinforcing and encouraging parent-child activities, building informal social supports, facilitating parental efforts on behalf of their children, and encouraging parental information exchanges.

Actors – Researchers set up the networks and centres, and parents and families shaped the networks to enhance their well-being, and parents and children interacted.

Analysis – This is a much analyzed project with many, many published findings on outcomes.

Replicability of the initiative – The project is infinitely replicable.

Funding: It was funded by funding sources for research in the United States.

Evaluation – Because this was a research-based intervention, ongoing evaluation has been part of the process since 1979.

Of all the healthy family success stories, the largest and best known is the Family Matters Program (Cochran 1991). The program started in 1979 as a Cornell University research project, using change in personal networks to measure the impacts of a family support program. It was the first study of its kind anywhere. The study was initiated by some earlier, accidental findings, underlining again the importance of chance and astute observation to successful interventions. A previous, small-scale study hinted at the possibility of a relationship between enhanced parenting skills and involvement with outside family activities. The Family Matters Program provided a deliberate social program aimed at enhancing the informal relationships of parents with other parents.

The Family Matters Project set out five major goals:
– to find ways to recognize parents as experts;
– to exchange information with family members;
– to reinforce and encourage parent-child activities;
– to build social exchange of informal resources such as babysitting, child-rearing advice and emotional support; and
– to facilitate concerted effort by parents on behalf of their children, where parents thought such actions appropriate (Cochran 1991, 57).

With an initial sample of 160 families in 10 urban neighbourhoods, a home-visiting program was set up, with a cluster-building initiative to connect the Family Matters families to their neighbourhoods. Child care was provided at all cluster group occasions, which included socializing and finding common solutions to neighbourhood and family problems. The program ran for three years. Evaluation compared the sample group with 128 families living in other neighbourhoods in the same cities, who provided regular information on stresses, supports, child-parent relations and activities, and child performance at school (Cochran 1991, 58).

What lessons can be drawn from this success story? "Our evaluation of the Family Matters program indicates that affirmative steps can be taken by agencies operating at the community level to activate such informal supports on behalf of healthy family functioning" (Cochran 1991, 61).

The most important lesson is social:

Our model indicates that many of the policies likely to contribute to the expansion and enrichment of personal networks involve freeing the developing individual from social constraints. Policies that increase the availability of postsecondary education would seem to have highest priority because those parents who had acquired such schooling were much richer in network resources than those who did not… Policies that stimulate job creation and continuation would also deserve high priority… The neighbourhood represents another point of public policy access… , especially through assistance in home ownership, but also through basic safety and maintenance efforts like lighting, street repairs and active police and fire services (Cochran 1991, 62–63).

Lastly, Cochran found:

Public policies must give first priority to freeing parents and those who will become parents, from the constraints of inequality and oppression, by insuring the provision of adequate and sufficient education, employment and humane housing conditions. Our findings suggest that freedom to grow, through schooling, work and leisure activities, will lead in turn to the social network connections that form the basis of healthy productive communities (1991, 64).

Lesson 14: "The greatest pay-off would seem to come from loosening the restrictions experienced by the disadvantaged individuals and families in our society" (Cochran 1991, 63).

Three recent Canadian studies have found strong links between health and education, and health and work (Studies Link Health to Education 1996). A University of Manitoba study of 48,000 Manitobans found that health improves or declines depending on income and education. Another study, by Statistics Canada, of 38,000 Ontarians aged 25 and over, found that "education was the strongest marker of health status," (Studies Link Health to Education 1996, 15), while other indicators of good health are a good job, above-average income and a spouse. A third study by Shah, Jin and Savaboda of the University of Toronto, found that levels of national unemployment in several industrialized countries correlated strongly with higher mortality levels and greater rates of suicide and cardiovascular disease (Studies Link Health to Education 1996, 15). They also found that those without jobs are more likely to visit doctors, take drugs or be admitted to hospitals. Shah, Jin and Savaboda estimate the excess use of medical care by the unemployed in Canada in 1993 at $850 million to $1.2 million.

Lesson 15: Education and employment matter to the health status of individuals and of families.

Brighter Futures and Running in Place

Brighter Futures: Nobody's Perfect Program/Better Beginnings Program

Actions on nonmedical determinants of health – To support parents in caring for children, improve access to information on parenting, improve the living conditions of children in low-income families, and reduce family poverty.

Reasons for the initiative – International initiatives were undertaken, to show Canada's commitment to children's well-being.

Actors – The federal government, particularly the prime minister, who was co-chair of the World Summit for Children.

Analysis – Not much analysis has been done, but achievements have not matched the intent. Family poverty and poverty among children have, in fact, increased since Brighter Futures was initiated.

Replicability of the initiative – Brighter Futures' ideas are laudable, its actual success less so; if the initiative were replicated, more action would be needed.

Funding – Limited.

Evaluation – Outcome evaluation is needed.

Running in Place

Actions on nonmedical determinants of health – To assess how U.S. families are faring in a changing economy and society.

Reasons for the initiative – Concern about the increasing economic and social pressures on U.S. families, and interest in assessing how to combat negative impact for families.

Actors – Researchers who make their assessment accessible to the public, the media and policymakers.

Analysis – The project revealed the importance to healthy families of economic security, parental involvement in schools, education, job creation, job training, and child care to familial well-being.

Replicability of the initiative – An assessment in Canada would help chart the future direction of social policies to promote healthy families. With excellent Statistics Canada data on families available, such a report would be easily prepared.

Funding – Funded by private foundations in the United States.

Evaluation – The Zill and Nord (1994) report evaluates current trends in social and economic context. The impact of the report has yet to be determined.

The federal government undertook the Brighter Futures initiative in response to agreements made at the September 1990 World Summit for Children and Canada's 1991 ratification of the *United Nations Convention on the Rights of the Child* (Canada 1992a). (Alberta has not yet ratified the U.N. Convention.) Brighter Futures was launched in 1992 with a statement on the importance of healthy children: "Ultimately, our strength as a nation is reflected in our care for those who are most vulnerable. It is up to us to create brighter futures for children" (Canada 1992a, 7).

The initiative was followed later in 1992 by *Brighter Futures: Canada's Action Plan for Children* (Canada 1992b), which emphasizes government partnerships with nongovernmental organizations (NGOs) and parents and children (Canada 1992b, 25).

Canadians are challenged to:
- support parents in caring for their children by updating child and family support policies and programs... (26);
- improve access for all parents to the information, resources and community supports they need to help them care for their children (26);
- improve the living conditions of children in low-income families (27); and
- develop measures to reduce the number of families living on low incomes (27).

The Brighter Futures action plan was less developed than the challenges, but some small-scale projects showed promising results. The Nobody's Perfect programs in the Atlantic Provinces are educational programs aimed at parents of young children who may experience difficulties because of low income, young age, being single, or being culturally or geographically isolated. The program involves sharing experiences and advice, and offers information about child rearing and parenting (Canada 1992b, 11). In Ontario, the Better Beginnings: Better Futures program promotes healthy child development, prevents developmental problems, and strengthens communities (Canada 1992b, 14). Several Ontario communities and Indian reserves are participating in this program.

Lesson 16: Partnerships of various levels of government with communities and families can benefit family health, but the political will must consistently promote family resilience and well-being.

Lesson 17: The more that can be done before troubles and lack of well-being set in, the better.

Running in Place is a U.S. report (Zill and Nord 1994) assessing how U.S. families are faring in a changing economy and society, but it also applies to the Canadian situation of the ground lost for families during the late 1980s and 1990s. The Zill and Nord report focuses on three challenges faced by U.S. families that parallel challenges faced by Canadian families: (1) making ends meet, (2) combating negative peer influences on children, and (3) maintaining parental control as children get older (Zill and Nord 1994, 1–2). Zill and Nord note four lessons that can help promote healthy families in Canada:

Lesson 18: Families with limited resources risk long-term health and social problems. Some means to eradicate or reduce long-term poverty is vital to healthy families.

Lesson 19: More parental involvement in schools is necessary, and schools must actively seek the involvement of "the forgotten half" of the population (Zill and Nord 1994, 84): the poor, less educated, more isolated parents whose children might not attend university.

Lesson 20: Family well-being and children's achievement would be enhanced if schools were more "family friendly"; if teacher-student ratios were reduced and serious attempts were made to know students, family problems might be detected early and appropriate interventions made.

Lesson 21: Policymakers must move beyond ideological discord over the definition of a family and make progress on areas of agreement, such as job creation, realistic job training, and child care, that would enable families to become self-sufficient.

In Canada, "running in place" might be more appropriately termed "running behind," if family incomes and child poverty are examined since the 1990 World Summit. Maxwell (1996), relying on Statistics Canada data, shows that incomes of young families dropped in the 1981–1993 period, low income and poverty have increased, and government transfers to alleviate family poverty have declined. Campaign 2000 (1995) notes the following changes since 1989:

- numbers of poor children increased 55 percent;
- two-parent families in poverty increased 48 percent;
- single-parent families in poverty increased 13 percent;
- children in families with long-term unemployment increased 54 percent;
- children in families needing social assistance increased 69 percent;
- children in working poor families increased 37 percent;
- median family income decreased $5,000; and
- families with income less than $40,000 increased 26 percent.

Lesson 22: "If investment in health means investment in the health of future generations, then there are two priority areas for public policy with regard to health: (1) investments in child and daycare, because most societies now need women in the economic sector, and a majority of women now needs to work outside the home to make ends meet; (2) investments in education" (Kickbusch 1994b, 85).

Miracle at Duke and Water

Miracle at Duke and Water/The Working Centre of Kitchener-Waterloo, Ontario

Actions on nonmedical determinants of health – The development of a centre to meet the needs of those without work in the economic restructuring Ontario has experienced since the 1980s.

Reasons for the initiative – Community needs for intervention are growing, and existing services are not well suited to meet them.

Actors – Coalitions of churches, academics and volunteers.

Analysis – The goals and objectives of the initial project have broadened to reflect the changing needs of the community, and in response to ongoing evaluation of the funding arrangements and the successes and failures of the endeavour.

Replicability of the initiative – With a similar spirit and comparable driving personalities, the project could be replicated elsewhere. Seed granting is necessary.

Funding – Funding initially came from a coalition of churches, and there were grants from federal and provincial agencies.

Evaluation – Documented (Westhues 1995) evaluation of The Working Centre reveals that it has been remarkably successful in achieving its goals.

Another successful intervention toward healthy families comes from Kitchener, Ontario. The Working Centre (Westhues 1995, 40) is "an original institution" that can trace its roots to earlier innovative approaches such as Hull House, which was founded in Chicago by sociologist Jane Addams in 1899. The Working Centre combines intellectual commitment with social action. It was started in 1983, with a $6,000 start-up grant from a joint initiative of five churches (Presbyterian, Lutheran, United, Roman Catholic and Anglican) and a one-year grant from the Canadian Community Development Program. The Working Centre now has core funding from Ontario, some labour organizations and some churches. Initially, it had three stated purposes:

1. encouraging employment opportunities in the community through a self-help employment centre;
2. bringing unemployed people together to share and discuss their experiences, to learn to analyze their experiences in a societal framework... to propose and design action-oriented responses which bring about solutions;
3. understanding, exploring and developing a system of support, decision making, and participation that reflects in a creative way the needs of the unemployed in the Kitchener-Waterloo community (Westhues 1995, 17).

Lesson 23: Start-up and seed grants for projects can mean successful outcomes in family healthy and community well-being.

The Working Centre is an unemployment help centre, but it has spawned a drop-in centre and a soup kitchen. The Working Centre ethic favours "producerism," acquiring the skills and seizing opportunities to produce life's essentials alone or in small groups, instead of dwelling on deprivation, loss of hope or dependency. The grassroots and educational component of the centre contributes to its success, with support in kind coming from all parts of the community, including the local universities, which offer courses at the centre.

Dave Conzani, one of the soup kitchen's patrons, reveals the effectiveness of the Working Centre in promoting health and restoring responsible citizenship and family living through love, encouragement and self-esteem:

> When we are put down and shamed and blamed and vilified, it is hard to find any incentive to try to get back up again one more time. No, where shame and blame have never worked, love, encouragement and self-esteem have worked wonders (1995, 85).

Conzani says he is a "recovering alcoholic" with a son from whom he had been estranged for years during his life on the streets. He admits to turning to the bottle in despair over the breakup of his marriage when his son was two years old. His story of living on the streets in alcoholic oblivion is the story of too many in Canada. By the time he arrived at the Working Centre's soup kitchen, he had been through "the gamut" of treatment facilities, hostels, detoxification centres and food lines. At the centre's soup kitchen, he found he was treated differently for the first time—with respect as a human being, he says. He relates how one time when he was too drunk to carry his own tray, a centre worker helped him with it. He reports receiving constant positive encouragement from the people at the Working Centre until he finally gave up alcohol, was reunited with his son, and returned to school and made the Honours list. He is now self-sufficient, has his own apartment, and has a job. The Working Centre's success is a familial model of health and self-sufficiency worth emulating elsewhere.

Lesson 24: Family health can stem from genuine caring, and moving those in crisis to self-sufficiency through encouragement and connection.

Lesson 25: With small investments of funds and the right attitudes and structures, healthy families can be achieved without paying for far more expensive medical interventions.

Beyond Health Promotion: Is Family and Community Action Enough?

Beyond Health Promotion

Actions on nonmedical determinants of health – To assess the future of health promotion and health production, the successes achieved, and what has been and is to be learned.

Reasons for the initiative – The original intents of health promotion have been challenged by population health changes and advances in thinking on what produces health.

Actors – Canadian and international academics and health policymakers, who pose important questions about the conceptual base for health promotion in Canada and ask where we might proceed.

Analysis – Although health promotion approaches have been successful in Canada, globalization requires that the wider forces affecting healthy populations and families, such as environmental impacts, global workforces and international capitalism, be rethought.

Funding – A collaborative effort by the Centre for Health Promotion at the University of Toronto and the Groupe de recherche et d'intervention en promotion de la santé at Laval University, and by individual academics.

Evaluation – This effort evaluates health promotion in Canada since the Lalonde report of 1974.

Kickbusch takes a broad view of health promotion. "The health promotion questions are not simply, 'How do I get X to change her behaviour?' but 'How do we make the school/workplace/city a healthier place in order to change her behaviour?' Setting better health as a goal (possibly translating it into quantifiable targets) and managing the process of change toward that goal are crucial elements" (1994a, 13). Health promotion has helped shift the health policy agenda from consumption of medical services to production of health (Kickbusch 1994a, 8). However, it is being challenged in the 1990s by:

- the reemergence of infectious illnesses thought not long ago to have been conquered, such as tuberculosis, and the emergence of new ones, such as AIDS;
- new health paradigms, which move health production thinking away from lifestyles, individual responsibility, and healthy communities toward population well-being in socioeconomic contexts, such as the Evans and Stoddart approach discussed earlier; and
- the globalization of markets and labour, as well as social inequities across societies, making the challenges of health production loom larger, so that for example, the health and well-being of families in Canada may be challenged by the Chernobyl disaster, by the sex trade in a distant

country, or by rampant economic growth in a developing country without concern for environmental degradation.

Hancock questions how successfully health promotion has developed healthy public policies in Canada (1994, 368–369) for three reasons:

- federal inaction on developing the policies, mechanisms or structures needed to reorient health care, despite the government's initial leadership in developing health promotion;
- international inaction despite "much talk" (Hancock's term, 369) about sustainable development, democracy, and citizen empowerment, where Canada has not taken a genuine lead; and
- the growing struggle against the health-impairing and -impeding aspects of industrial capitalism, including pollution, environmental degradation, cultural conquest, the valuing of competition and individualism, and growing inequalities in Canada and elsewhere. "Certainly the greatest threat to health now comes from a consumption-oriented, growth-oriented ideology—industrialized capitalism—that accepts the necessity of inequality and that seeks control over the earth's resources, including its human resources" (Hancock 1994, 369).

Lesson 26: Local and community action matters, but federal leadership is still needed in promoting healthy families.

Lesson 27: A federal presence internationally on health issues matters in achieving healthy families in Canada.

Hancock's concerns place Canada's current efforts toward healthy policies in a global and historic context. Healthy families are a key component in a shift from individual to global connections. Healthy families can be the springboard for international competitiveness and national and international innovation.

Lesson 28: Healthy family values of renewal and resourcefulness can counter the global tilt toward marketism, unsustainability and inequity.

Lesson 29: Healthy families can enhance Canada's global competitiveness; promoting healthy families is good economic policy.

POLICY IMPLICATIONS—PRINCIPLES TO GUIDE GOVERNMENT ACTION

Three questions (Kickbusch 1994a, 15) are useful when examining priorities for government action on health:

- Where is health created?
- Which investment creates the largest health gain?
- Does this investment reduce inequities in health and respect human rights?

These questions frame this concluding section on policy implications and principles to guide government action on healthy families.

Policy Implications

Health policy is inseparable from social and economic policies. Health is connected to work, leisure, postsecondary education, housing, family security, and environment. These "social goods" are created more by social and economic policies and investments than by health care policy per se. Policy actions that contribute to healthy families and population health are more likely to be social and economic policies rather than health care policies. Social policy interventions are not as expensive as health care interventions at the individual level. Yet, the political will toward "the social" seems to be lessening, although that may be changing (see Peters 1995).

O'Neill (1994) argues that recasting public debate about family and family security is essential to Canadian nationhood. He favours a "covenant of care," which draws on our traditional senses of obligation to one another, obligations that are bigger than contracts in a market economy. Without these connections among generations, argues O'Neill, there can be no continuity of nation-states, or sustenance of our collective being. Market forces that privatize family caring can doom nations.

Although research shows that health care availability contributes less to population health than social and economic policies, the availability of health care is psychologically vital (Peters 1995, 15). Further, universal public health care in Canada is social security for families.

> For four decades, our investment in health services [in Canada] has been dedicated to protecting the citizens of this country against the single major cause of impoverishment that appeared at the time to be modifiable, serious illness. Social security procurement rather than health enhancement was thus the rationale (Turcotte 1994, 161).

Families are the central determinants of well-being. Children who live in poverty or are homeless may suffer permanent long-term health damage. Prenatal, postnatal and early childhood experiences can have major, lifelong influence on physical and mental development, as well as on coping abilities and social, educational, and familial skills. Concerns are mounting about the growing number of families with young children relying on food banks across Canada. Adequate nutrition is essential to children's development and subsequent well-being. Any sincere effort at promoting healthy families must centre on children, particularly children who are deprived.

The best approach to promoting healthy families is to prevent health and social problems before they occur. Hertzman (1994) call this "the vaccination approach," and it is consistent with a nonmedical approach to health policy and promoting healthy families.

From the point of view of both society and families, optimal social [and health] policies should support family commitments and caring, reducing the strains on family members and strengthening the abilities of families and their kinship networks to manage for themselves and to help one another (Moen and Firebaugh 1995, 43).

Principles to Guide Government Action for Healthy Families

Policies for healthy families should take existing research evidence and the analytical frameworks and bring them to action. Key actors will be the "usual suspects," but with a key difference: the partnerships may have different leadership and may have to give up old habits and adopt new ones. According to Judith Maxwell (1996), attitudes have changed more among citizens in Canada than among policymakers or employers. Maxwell argues that citizens have already experienced dramatic changes, and have adjusted their thinking to reallocate resources in and for families, engage in voluntary action and democratic dialogue, and accept mutual obligations and responsibilities. Employers and policymakers need similar "reality check" adjustments. Perhaps the largest changes are needed at the corporate level, according to Maxwell, to give up state subsidies and protections and make a "true commitment" to supporting a lifelong learning culture. Corporations must also step up contributions to social capital, through community membership, shared values, a sense of common enterprise, and trust and reciprocity.

Government and public policies also need to rethink the self-reliance and resilience of individuals, families, communities and Canada, and provide more "one window" connections between people and government services and policies.

The responses to Kickbusch's guiding questions are clear.
- Health (or illness) is created mostly in families.
- Investments in children and families reap the greatest health gains.
- Investments in families, particularly poor, isolated, less-educated families, reduce inequities and respect human rights.

Families are the gateways to the future of healthy public policies. Research evidence and the lessons from the applications are clear. We now need the political will to take action on what we know.

Table 1 summarizes the essential principles that should guide government action on healthy families. In table 2, the basic challenges and policy are outlined.

Table 1

Principles to guide government action on healthy families

- Value the role and work of families in caring.
- Acknowledge families as health-promoting, health-providing and health-giving units.
- Support alternative means of care for those families who cannot provide healthy caring.
- Conscientiously nurture families in their caring, thus nurturing social capital.
- Maintain secure and continuing investments in children and child care.
- Maintain an effective resource redistribution system to ensure provision of housing, health care, education and work to those in need, and prevent widening income gaps (a key factor in population health).
- Invest in education at all levels.

Table 2

Essential challenges to policy in moving toward healthy families

- To acknowledge that healthy families involve social and economic conditions, social and economic approaches to health, as well as individual, family and social well-being;
- To find new ways of approaching population health outcomes that go beyond individual responsibility for lifestyle choices to acknowledge the vital contributions families make to health; and
- To work toward new means to support different family lifestyles, to enhance their caring capacities and not add further burdens.

Strategic Targets That Require Policy Action

Redefine health to include socioeconomic and family health by example.

Although Canada has been a world leader on social frameworks for health and on health promotion, Canada has not been a world leader in actions on social health. Canada should:

- Sponsor joint research initiatives on family and health, so that the determinants of family health can be fully and accurately assessed;
- Involve at least two social scientists in the newly established Advisory Council on Science and Technology, and encourage a broad focus on health as part of the science and technology approach, as advocated by the report of the National Advisory Board on Science and Technology (1995);

- Adopt new health policies that recognize that secure, safe, well-fed, well-educated families are the first step to preventing societal health and social problems;
- Integrate health care with social services and preventive actions at the community, municipal, provincial and federal levels;
- Rely on technology (e.g., telemedicine or telediagnosis, as well as on-line technologies) as an efficient entry point to both social and medical services, enable families to use services more efficiently and spend more time caring for each other;
- Intervene in health risk groups as identified by Statistics Canada's national longitudinal survey of children, the survey of income and labour dynamics, and other ongoing research, such as the survey of aging and health; and
- Adopt public policies that acknowledge that family health is key to productivity and to national health and well-being.

Accept and use a broad functional definition of "family" that includes all the ways in which caring occurs.

The Vanier Institute of the Family (1993, xii) and the Canada Committee for the International Year of the Family effectively use such definitions. The federal government should:
- Rely on a broad definition of family to accommodate policy support groups struggling to survive on the edge of survival of society and thus enhance the health of more families;
- Pass legislation giving rights to gays and lesbians, many of whom are raising children; and
- Encourage all provinces to become signatories to the *United Nations' Convention on the Rights of the Child.* Canada is one of the few jurisdictions in the industrial world where, in some jurisdictions, children are not seen to have rights.

Prevent further erosion of family incomes, since low income is the single largest cause of inadequate family health and well-being.

Since lone mothers have the lowest incomes, and their family and individual health are often impaired by poverty, public policy should address gender inequities to promote healthy families. Three steps are recommended:
- Pass the Employment Equity Act, tabled in Parliament on 12 December 1994;
- Clearly and unequivocally support gender equity legislation and policies; and
- Enforce pay equity laws and comparable worth policies. Although women and men have comparable wages when they graduate from

university, the wage gap widens after children are born and families are established.

Prevent the gap between the lowest and highest family income groups from widening further.

There are several ways to do this. Among them, prevention of further erosion of incomes among the poorest is key and can be accomplished by:

- Maintaining national poverty cap standards, below which Canadians should not live (these standards disappeared with the beginning of the Canada Health and Social Transfer, but there were promises to maintain future national standards);
- Raising the minimum wage to alleviate poverty and improve family well-being, particularly for single mothers and young families;
- Extending benefits to part-time work; and
- Redistributing work and benefits so that year-round, full-time work does not take priority over other meaningful and contributing types of work.

Value, by tax credits and other means, family members' roles as health givers, health guardians and caregivers.

This can be done by:

- Allowing primary family caregivers (of young, of disabled, of those in crisis, of elderly relatives) the option of deducting their services from income taxes; or
- Paying family caregivers for the services they perform, as has been done experimentally in Nova Scotia.

Support the poorest families most, particularly the children in these families.

At a national level there are several concerns:

- With delisting of health services and many prescription drugs in a number of provinces, all children have access to health care, including medical checkups and preventive dental care;
- Protective care must be ensured for children in abusive families, children who are addicted or have addicted parents, and children whose basic needs are not being met;
- Long-term effects of cutbacks on poor children must be considered— deprived children are more likely to become unproductive and irresponsible as adults;

- Income security programs must be maintained for the promotion of healthy families (see Vanier Institute of the Family 1993, for examples); and
- Since income security is essential for family health and well-being, job creation must be a component of promoting healthy families.

Promote family-friendly workplace policies, recognizing that most people in Canada work and also have families.

Public policy should:
- Bring about legislation on family leaves—it is insufficient to leave it to private employers, because the majority of Canadians do not work in large companies with family-friendly policies;
- Act on child care;
- Develop partnerships among private and public sectors, and among jurisdictions, since 77 percent of Canadians support the development of a national subsidized child care service, and 73 percent would be willing to pay additional taxes to fund a national child care service (Angus Reid Group 1994, 52–53); and
- Acknowledge, by appropriate workplace encouragements, that balancing work and family is not only a women's issue, but an issue for Canadian society. According to a 1983 UNICEF report, "The critical business of building strong families can no longer be considered a private endeavour, least of all a private female endeavour (as quoted in Friendly 1994, 270).

Support flexible and responsible roles for men and women in families, while giving priority to children's opportunities and protections.

All levels of government can contribute to this by:
- Undertaking media educational campaigns, through the mass media such as the very successful ParticipAction campaign, to promote healthy families—for example, an Egyptian advertising campaign encourages "real men prove themselves not by big talk but by how they take care of their families" (Bruce, Lloyd, and Leonard 1995, 108), while a U.S. advertisement suggests: "Teach boys what makes a man: caring about your partner and your future is what makes a man" (Bruce, Lloyd, and Leonard 1995, 108);
- Acknowledging that paid work by women, including mothers of young children, is often necessary for family well-being and to keep families out of poverty—Bruce and colleagues found from a study of eight industrialized countries that "the only mothers who have a better than average chance of staying out of poverty are those who combine parenthood with work and marriage" (1995, 113);
- Investing in the next generation of parents, since parenthood can have economically negative consequences, particularly for women (poverty,

increased vulnerability and insecurity, and increased exposure to spousal violence)—ongoing support for new parents—can range from home-visiting programs for newborns and mothers, to facilitating reentry to the workforce and (or) education for new mothers and fathers;

- Acknowledging that parents who experience crises can regain their autonomy and reassume parental roles, with community supports—such as the Working Centre in Kitchener-Waterloo, and the Family Matters Program in the United States;
- Adopting the community support model that reinvigorates vital institutional supports for families, such as health centres, churches, after-school programs, culture and arts, libraries, sporting activities, and drop-in centres, which can help foster communication, affiliation and community and family pride—examples include the William Charles Band community health project, the "children/families at-promise" approach, the Working Centre, several of the Brighter Futures initiatives, and the Families Matter Program; and
- Not cutting back on family violence prevention initiatives so that families experiencing violence have the victims protected, and the public aware-ness campaign on family violence continues.

Remove impediments to parents in fulfilling responsibilities as parents and spouses.

Broadening the responsibility for children from individual parents to society at large has become an international rallying cry in the world, particularly following 1994, the International Year of the Family. Specifically,

- Family policies must encourage the vital, health-promoting aspects of connection, and focus on individual rights and responsibilities within families;
- A family-centred data collection system with the lifelong parent-child link at its core should be developed on questions about impediments to successful parenthood—the answers would lead policy development on healthy families (Statistics Canada could collaborate on this initiative);
- Given that increasing numbers of children in Canada are living their lives in poverty, partnerships must be developed immediately between public and private resources, to nourish opportunities for the next generation;
- Reproductive choices must be maintained for healthy families to thrive;
- That family support in Canada may come from family members who live outside of Canada, and must be acknowledged and encouraged; and
- Policies should encourage more involvement of men in families as caregivers, and as full family members.

Susan A. McDaniel, *Ph.D., FRSC, professor of sociology, University of Alberta, does research in social and health policy, family, gender, aging, and demography. She is the author of many research articles and book chapters. Frequently cited publications include:* Canada's Aging Population *(1986),* Family and Friends, 1990 *(1994), "Demographic Aging as the Guiding Paradigm of Canada's Welfare State,"* Canadian Public Policy *(1987). Editor of the* Canadian Journal of Sociology *(1994–1997), she is Editor of* Current Sociology *(1997–2001), official journal of the International Sociological Association, and the oldest and most widely cited sociology journal in the world.*

Acknowledgements

Helpful suggestions by Marc Renaud, Carmen Connolly and the many other reviewers on an earlier version are appreciated. Particular thanks to Martin Wilk (Statistics Canada and the Canadian Institute for Advanced Research Population Health Program), who offered crucial suggestions on principles to guide policy, to Bob Glossop (Vanier Institute of the Family), who pointed me in the direction of some of the success stories, and to Susan Hutton and Kerri Calvert, who provided help in tracking down references.

BIBLIOGRAPHY

ADAMS, R. G., and R. BLIESZNER. 1995. Aging well with friends and family. *American Behavioral Scientist* 39(2): 209–224.

ANGUS, D. E., L. AUER, J. E. CLOUTIER, and T. ALBERT. 1995. *Sustainable Health Care for Canada*. Ottawa (ON): Queen's–University of Ottawa Economic Projects.

ANGUS REID GROUP. 1994. *The State of the Family in Canada*. Toronto (ON): Angus Reid Group and Canada Committee for the International Year of the Family.

ANTONOVSKY, Aaron. 1993. The structure and properties of the sense of coherence scale. *Social Science and Medicine* 36(6): 725–735.

BAIRD, P. A. 1994. The role of genetics in population health. In *Why Are Some People Healthy and Others Not? The Determinants of Health of Populations*, eds. R. G. EVANS, M. L. BARER and T. R. MARMOR. New York (NY): Aldine de Gruyter. pp. 133–160.

BAKER, M. 1995. *Canadian Family Policies: Cross-National Comparisons*. Toronto (ON): University of Toronto Press.

BALA, N. 1995. The evolving definition of the family. *Policy Options/Options Politiques* 16(10): 3–7.

BEAVERS, W. R., and R. B. HAMPSON. 1990. *Successful Families: Assessment and Intervention*. New York (NY): W. W. Norton.

———. 1993. Measuring family competence: The beavers system model. In *Normal Family Processes*, 2nd ed., ed. F. WALSH. New York (NY): Guilford. pp. 73–95.

BERKMAN, L. F. 1984. Assessing the physical health effects of social networks and social support. *American Review of Public Health* 5: 413–432.

BRUCE, J., C. B. LLOYD, and A. LEONARD. 1995. *Families in Focus: New Perspectives on Mothers, Fathers, and Children*. New York (NY): The Population Council.

CAMPAIGN 2000. 1995. *Report Card on Child Poverty in Canada 1995*. Toronto (ON): Family Service Association.

CANADA. 1974. *A New Perspective on the Health of Canadians (Lalonde Report)*. Ottawa (ON): Department of National Health and Welfare.

———. 1992a. *Brighter Futures: Canada's Action Plan for Children*. Ottawa (ON): Minister of Supply and Services.

———. 1992b. *Brighter Futures: Children Matter*. Ottawa (ON): Government of Canada.

CANADA. STATISTICS CANADA. 1996. Hospital annual statistics and indicators 1992–1993. *The Daily*, 19 March.

CHAPPELL, N. L. 1994. Health care reform: Will it be better or worse for families? Opening plenary address, Canadian Association on Gerontology, Winnipeg (MB), October 1994.

COCHRAN, M. 1991. Personal social networks as a focus of support. In *Families as Nurturing Systems: Support across the Life Span*, eds. D. G. UNGER and D. R. POWELL. New York (NY): Haworth. pp. 45–67.

CONZANI, D. 1995. Miracle at Duke and Water. In *The Working Centre: Experiment in Social Change*, ed. K. WESTHUES. Kitchener (ON): Working Centre Publications. pp. 79–85.

COOK, D. A., and M. FINE. 1995. Motherwit: Childrearing lessons from African American mothers of low income. In *Children and Families "at Promise": Deconstructing the Discourse of Risk*, eds. B. B. SWADENER, and S. LUBECK. Albany (NY): State University of New York Press. pp. 118–142.

CURRAN, D. 1983. *Traits of a Healthy Family: Fifteen Traits Commonly Found in Healthy Families by Those Who Work with Them*. Minneapolis (MN): Winston Press.

EICHLER, M. 1995. Three approaches to family policy. *Policy Options/Options Politiques* 16(10): 33–37.

ELDER, G. H., and J. K. LIKER. 1982. Hard times in women's lives: Historical influences across forty years. *American Journal of Sociology* 88: 871–879.

ELKIND, D. 1994. *Ties That Stress: The New Family Imbalance.* Cambridge (MA): Harvard University Press.

EVANS, R. G., and G. L. STODDART. 1994. Producing health, consuming health care. In *Why Are Some People Healthy and Others Not? The Determinants of Health of Populations,* eds. R. G. EVANS, M. L. BARER and T. R. MARMOR. New York (NY): Aldine de Gruyter. pp. 27–64.

FEDERAL, PROVINCIAL AND TERRITORIAL ADVISORY COMMITTEE ON POPULATION HEALTH. 1994. *Strategies for Population Health: Investing in the Health of Canadians.* Paper prepared for the meeting of Ministers of Health, Nova Scotia, 14–15 September 1994. Ottawa (ON): Health Canada.

FRANK, J. W., and J. F. MUSTARD. 1994. The determinants of health from a historical perspective. *Daedalus: Journal of the American Academy of Arts and Sciences* 123(4): 1–19.

FREDERICK, J. A. 1995. *As Time Goes By... Time Use of Canadians, General Social Survey.* Statistics Canada Catalogue no. 89–544E. Ottawa (ON): Minister of Supply and Services.

FRIENDLY, M. 1994. *Child Care Policy in Canada: Putting the Pieces Together.* Don Mills (ON): Addison-Wesley.

GOTTLIEB, B. H. 1981. Social networks and social support. In *Social Networks and Social Support,* ed. B. H. GOTTLIEB. Beverly Hills (CA): Sage.

HANCOCK, T. 1994. Health promotion in Canada: Did we win the battle and lose the war? In *Health Promotion in Canada: Provincial, National and International Perspectives,* eds. A. PEDERSON, M. O'NEILL, and I. ROOTMAN. Toronto (ON): W. B. Saunders. pp. 350–373.

HAREVEN, T. K. 1991. The history of the family and the complexity of social change. *American Historical Review* 96(1): 95–124.

HELLER, A. F. 1986. *Health and Home: Women as Health Guardians.* Ottawa (ON): Canadian Advisory Council on the Status of Women.

HERTZMAN, C. 1994. The lifelong impact of childhood experiences: A population health perspective. *Daedalus: Journal of the American Academy of Arts and Sciences* 123(4): 167–180.

KAMERMAN, S. B. 1995. Gender role and family structure changes in the advanced industrialized West: Implications for social policy. In *Poverty, Inequality and the Future of Social Policy: Western States in the New World Order,* eds. K. MCFATE, R. LAWSON, and W. J. WILSON. New York (NY): Russell Sage Foundation. pp. 231–256.

KATZ, R., and N.SETH. 1987. Synergy and healing: A perspective on Western health care. In *Prevention and Health: Directions for Policy and Practice,* eds. A. H. KATZ, J. A. HERMALIN, and R. E. HESS. New York (NY): Haworth. pp. 109–136.

KEATING, D. P., and J. F. MUSTARD. 1993. Social economic factors and human development. In *Family Security in Insecure Times,* ed. The National Forum on Family Security. Ottawa (ON): National Forum on Family Security. pp. 87–105.

KICKBUSCH, I. 1994a. Introduction: Tell me a story. In *Health Promotion in Canada: Provincial, National and International Perspectives,* eds. A. PEDERSON, M. O'NEILL, and I. ROOTMAN. Toronto (ON): W. B. Saunders. pp. 8–17.

———. 1994b. Principles and strategies of interventions. *Innovation* 7(1): 83–88.

MARMOT, M. G. 1994. Social differentials in health within and between populations. *Daedalus: Journal of the American Academy of Arts and Sciences* 123(4): 197–216.

MAXWELL, J. 1996. *The Social Dimensions of Economic Growth.* Edmonton (AB): University of Alberta, Eric J. Hanson Memorial Lecture, January 1996.

———. 1993a. Emotional support and family contacts of older Canadians. *Canadian Social Trends* 28 (spring): 30–33.

———. 1993b. Half the sky: Women's status and fertility. *Ecodecision: Environment and Policy Journal* 10: 66.

———. 1995a. *Family and Friends 1990: General Social Survey Analysis Series.* Ottawa (ON): Statistics Canada, Catalogue no. 11–612E, no. 9.

————. 1995b. *Families Function: Family Bridges from Past to Future.* Vienna: International Year of the Family Secretariat.

————. 1995c. Serial employment and skinny government: Reforming caring and sharing in Canada at the millennium. Paper invited for the Federation of Canadian Demographers Symposium, "Toward the XXIst Century: Emerging Socio-Demographic Trends and Issues in Canada". Ottawa (ON), October 1995.

————. 1996. Towards a synthesis of feminist and demographic perspectives on fertility. *The Sociological Quarterly* 37(1): 601–622.

MCDANIEL, S, A., and E. M. GEE. 1993. Social policies regarding caregiving to elders: Canadian contradictions. *Journal of Aging and Social Policy* 5(1/2): 57–72.

MCKEOWN, T. 1976. *The Role of Medicine.* London (ON): Nufeld Provincial Hospitals.

MCLANAHAN, S., and I. GARFINKEL. 1995. Single-mother families and social policy: Lessons for the United States from Canada, France, and Sweden. In *Poverty, Inequality and the Future of Social Policy: Western States in the New World Order,* eds. K. MCFATE, R. LAWSON, and W. J. WILSON. New York (NY): Russell Sage Foundation. pp. 367–383.

MENAGHAN, E. G., and T. L. PARCEL. 1990. Parental employment and family life: Research in the 1980s. *Journal of Marriage and Family* 52: 1079–1098.

MOEN, P., and F. M. FIREBAUGH. 1995. Family policies and effective families: A life course perspective. *International Journal of Sociology and Social Policy* 14 (1/2): 29–52.

NATIONAL ADVISORY BOARD ON SCIENCE AND TECHNOLOGY. 1995. *Healthy, Wealthy and Wise: A Framework for an Integrated Federal Science and Technology Policy.* Ottawa (ON): National Advisory Board on Science and Technology.

NEYSMITH, S. 1989. Closing the gap between health policy and the home-care needs of tomorrow's elderly. *Canadian Journal of Community Mental Health* 8(2): 141–150.

OAKLEY, A. 1992a. "A friend a day keeps the doctor away": Social support and health. In *Social Support and Motherhood,* ed. A. OAKLEY. Oxford (U.K): Blackwell. pp. 21-43.

————. 1992b. Sickness in Salonica and other stories. In *Social Support and Motherhood,* ed. A. OAKLEY. Oxford (U.K): Blackwell. pp. 44–75.

O'NEILL, J. 1994. *The Missing Child in Liberal Theory: Towards a Covenant Theory of Family, Community, Welfare and the Civic State.* Toronto (ON): University of Toronto Press.

OSTERBUSCH, S. E., S. M. KEIGHER, B. MILLER, and N. L. LINSK. 1987. Community care policies and gender justice. *International Journal of Health Services* 17(2): 217–232.

PEDERSON, A., M. O'NEILL, and I. ROOTMAN. 1994. *Health Promotion in Canada: Provincial, National and International Perspectives.* Toronto (ON): W. B. Saunders.

PETERS, S. 1995. *Exploring Canadian Values, A Synthesis Report.* Ottawa (ON): Canadian Policy Research Networks, Inc.

PHILLIPPS, L. 1995. "The family" in income tax policy. *Policy Options/Options Politiques* 16(10): 30–32.

POPAY, J., and G. JONES. 1991. Patterns of health and illness amongst lone-parent families. In *Lone Parenthood: Coping with Constraints and Making Opportunities in Single-Parent Families,* eds. M. HARDEY, and G. CROW. Toronto (ON): University of Toronto Press. pp. 66–87.

Report of the National Advisory Board on Science and Technology. Ottawa.

ROSS, C. E., J. MIROWSKY, and K. GOLDENSTEEN. 1990. The impact of the family on health: The decade in review. *Journal of Marriage and the Family* 52: 1059–1078.

SAGAN, L. A. 1987. *The Health of Nations: True Causes of Sickness and Well-Being.* New York (NY): Basic.

SCARF, M. 1995. *Intimate Worlds: Life Inside the Family.* New York (NY): Random House.

SEN, A. 1993. The economics of life and death. *Scientific American* (May): 40–47.

STINNETT, N. 1992. Strong families. In *Marriage and Family in a Changing Society,* eds. J. HEMSLIN et al. New York (NY): The Free Press. pp. 496–506.

STUDIES LINK HEALTH TO EDUCATION. 1996. *University Affairs* (February): 15.

SWADENER, B. B., and S. LUBECK . Eds. 1995. *Children and Families "at Promise": Deconstructing the Discourse of Risk.* Albany (NY): State University of New York Press.

SWANSON, J. 1995. *Impacts on People Panel: Remaking Canadian Social Policy: Staking Claims and Forging Change.* University of British Columbia, Vancouver (BC), June.

SYME, S. L. 1994. The social environment of health. *Daedelus: Journal of the American Academy of Arts and Sciences* 123(4): 79–86.

TURCOTTE, F. 1994. Review of Evans, Barer and Marmor, Why Are Some People Healthy and Others Not? The Determinants of Health of Populations. *Health and Canadian Society* 2(1): 159–162.

UNITED NATIONS. 1993. *Family Enrichment: Programmes to Foster Healthy Family Development.* Occasional Paper Series, no. 8. Vienna: International Year of the Family Secretariat.

———. 1995. *Platform for Action. Fourth World Conference on Women.* Beijing, China, September 4–15, 1995.

VANIER INSTITUTE OF THE FAMILY. 1993. *Inventory of Family-Supportive Policies and Programs in Federal, Provincial and Territorial Jurisdictions.* Ottawa (ON): The Vanier Institute of the Family.

WAITE, L. J. 1995. "Does marriage matter?" Population Association of America presidential address. *Demography* 32(4): 483–507.

WALDRAM, J. B., D. A. HERRING, and T. K. YOUNG. Eds. 1995. *Aboriginal Health in Canada: Historical, Cultural and Epidemiological Perspectives.* Toronto (ON): University of Toronto Press.

WESTHUES, K. Eds. 1995. *The Working Centre: Experiment in Social Change.* Kitchener (ON): Working Centre Publications.

WHEATON, B. 1985. Models for the stress-buffering functions of coping resources. *Journal of Health and Social Behaviour* 26: 352–364.

WILKINSON, R. G. 1994. From material scarcity to social disadvantage. *Daedalus: Journal of the American Academy of Arts and Sciences* 123(4): 61–77.

ZILL, N., and C. WINQUIST NORD. 1994. *Running in Place: How American Families are Faring in a Changing Economy and an Individualistic Society.* Washington (DC): Child Trends, Inc.

Schools, Mental Health and Life Quality

Kathryn J. Bennett, M.Sc.

Assistant Professor, Department of Clinical Epidemiology and Biostatistics
Centre for Studies of Children at Risk
McMaster University

David R. Offord, M.D.

Professor, Department of Psychiatry
Director, Centre for Studies of Children at Risk
Chedoke-McMaster Hospitals and
McMaster University

SUMMARY

School attendance is a social policy that affects every child and every family. This paper asks whether schools influence the mental health and life quality of children and adolescents and, if so, how. It also derives principles from the available evidence to guide government action. Mental health and life quality are defined in terms of specific dimensions of cognitive and noncognitive development, namely academic achievement and behavioral, emotional and social functioning. Early school problems, school failure and dropout are associated with maladaptive behavioral, emotional and social functioning and with psychiatric disorders such as conduct disorder and substance abuse (Hinshaw 1992).

This paper addresses three objectives. The first is to review the known effects of schools on cognitive and noncognitive functioning and to relate key conclusions of the literature to the broad determinants of health. The second objective is to set out stories and lessons learned. The third objective is to identify the policy implications of the available evidence.

The following are conclusions from the literature and their relation to the broad determinants of health. First, there is a serious lack of experimental evidence on the relationship between specific school characteristics and student outcomes.

Such evidence is needed to demonstrate that changes in specific schoolwide or classroom-level policies or practices actually improve academic achievement and behavioral, emotional and social functioning.

Second, the available studies consistently show that student cognitive and noncognitive outcomes differ from school to school. Examination scores, school attendance, classroom behaviour and delinquency have been shown to vary from one inner-city secondary school to another. At the primary school level, academic outcomes show pronounced between-school differences with smaller variations between schools in behaviour and attitude.

Third, although student characteristics at school entry and school exit outcomes are strongly related, studies consistently show that variations from school to school cannot be explained from student intake characteristics alone.

Fourth, school-to-school variations in student outcomes cannot be explained by differences in teacher-to-pupil ratios, instructional resources, quality of physical facilities or other circumstances. Therefore, interventions that focus on these school features will not significantly affect student outcomes.

Fifth, school and classroom processes are related to differences in the cognitive and noncognitive outcomes of students; for example, superior student performance is associated with schoolwide expectations for academic achievement and appropriate conduct, and instructional practices such as time spent on lessons, record keeping and giving feedback. Therefore, interventions that focus on these school and classroom processes may improve results in student outcomes.

Finally, evidence suggests that school and classroom processes can mitigate the effects of risk factors associated with nonmedical determinants of health. Good school and classroom practices can favourably influence children at risk of academic underachievement and maladaptive behavioral, emotional and social functioning caused by physical, social, economic, cultural and psychological factors. On the other hand, poor school and classroom practices can worsen the effects of risk factors associated with the physical, social, economic, cultural and psychological determinants of health. For example, schools that are characterized by programs or processes that have been associated with superior student outcomes may lower risk by buffering the effects of poverty or low motivation to learn. Schools without these processes may add to the effects of poverty or low motivation to learn, thus increasing the risk of school failure and other negative outcomes.

This paper's stories and lessons learned concern school improvement strategies that include evaluation. The first lesson is that no single approach guarantees improvement. Process-oriented approaches (for example, school management systems and teacher professional development) are designed to support the development of change. In contrast, prespecified interventions define changes to be made in school and classroom practices, such as interventions that ease the transition to primary school or secondary school.

The second lesson is that intervention design and evaluation requires a multidisciplinary approach that recognizes cognitive and noncognitive school goals and unites educators, mental health professionals and researchers. Studies of approaches that include such collaborative partnerships have yielded the most useful evidence on the relationship between school and classroom practices and the student's behavioral, emotional and social functioning.

The third lesson concerns the feasibility and replicability of the intervention. Interventions should be able to operate without the enthusiasm or special expertise of the original developers. Simple, low-resource strategies that fit the school routine are more likely to be sustainable and become integrated than are expensive approaches requiring radical changes to school philosophy and routines.

The fourth lesson concerns taking a participatory approach to school improvement, involving the individuals who will implement changes in decisions about intervention design and implementation. This permits a mutual adaptation in which participants can develop an understanding of the intervention, and the proposed changes are harmonized with local conditions, beliefs and values.

The fifth lesson concerns the role of evaluation in policy and practice. Our current knowledge of school improvement is limited. Promising interventions need to be systematically implemented and evaluated in collaborative experimental studies to avoid promoting changes that have no beneficial effects.

Principles to guide the actions of governments consist of the following nine "elements of best practice." The first principle, prevention, is that interventions to prevent the onset of problems should be given high priority. Second, interventions need to be designed to address both cognitive and noncognitive outcomes. Third, intervention content must be multi-disciplinary and based on a collaborative partnership between educators, mental health professionals and researchers. Fourth, interventions that are under the daily control of the principal and teachers promise school improvement. For example, interventions that focus on schoolwide expectations for academic achievement, appropriate conduct (including teacher consensus on curriculum and values), instructional practices (such as time on lesson, record keeping and feedback), and student responsibility in class and in school are promising methods for improving students' academic achievement and behavioral, emotional and social functioning.

Fifth, school improvement interventions must be sensitive to local needs and interests. Improvement strategies will vary from school to school and district to district according to the needs of the student population, the schools and the teachers. The sixth principle is that school improvement strategies are more successful when all the actors are involved in design and intervention decisions. Seventh, school improvement interventions must be able to run without the skills, expertise and enthusiasm of their developers. This will minimize the risk of failure and increase long-term sustainability. Eighth, ideal interventions operate with the system's own resources.

Finally policy changes must be evaluated. Educators, mental health professionals and researchers must collaborate on rigorous and timely evaluations of school improvement interventions. A coordinated approach to school improvement is probably more effective than applying many different approaches of uncertain effectiveness and cost with little exchange of ideas, experience and data.

The available evidence provides principles to inform action at the local, regional and national level. These principles will be most useful if they are applied in the context of: local needs assessment and intervention design, intervention implementation and evaluation (including multisite collaboration when appropriate), and systems that monitor student outcomes and meet the information needs of schools.

TABLE OF CONTENTS

FIGURE

LIST OF TABLES

INTRODUCTION

This position paper analyzes the effects of school on the mental health and life quality of children and adolescents. Mental health and life quality are defined in terms of specific dimensions of cognitive and noncognitive development, namely academic achievement and behavioral, emotional and social functioning. Early school problems, school failure and dropout are associated with maladaptive behavioral, emotional and social functioning and with psychiatric disorders such as conduct disorder and substance abuse (Hinshaw 1992).

Over the past 20 years, tremendous progress has been made in our understanding of school effects on child and adolescent development. This progress arose primarily from two well-known studies, Coleman and colleagues (1966) and Jencks and colleagues (1973), which concluded that schools exert very little effect on student achievement and are only marginally significant in comparison with the influence of child characteristics and family background.

Consequently, new studies on the effects of school and classroom practices on student achievement and other noncognitive outcomes have proliferated. Studies conducted in both elementary and secondary schools show that students vary significantly from school to school in academic achievement and behavioral, emotional and social functioning, and that these variations cannot be accounted for by variations in student characteristics at school entry (Rutter 1983; Purkey and Smith 1983; Maughan 1988; Willms 1992; Sylva 1994). However, much less is understood about whether and how specific features of schools cause between-school differences in student outcomes.

OBJECTIVES

The discussion that follows addresses three objectives. The first is to provide a critical review of the known effects of school on academic achievement and behavioral, emotional and social functioning. The second is to set out stories and lessons learned from evaluations of school improvement interventions. The third is to identify policy implications to guide government actions.

The literature on school effects is vast and includes work in such fields as education, psychology, child psychiatry, pediatrics, social policy and organizational theory. Therefore, the current review is selective and designed to summarize current knowledge based on the best available empirical evidence. The review covers only studies of elementary and secondary schools. Many studies cover the immediate and long-term gains of preschool (Lazar et al. 1982; Berrueta-Clement et al. 1984; Sylva 1994). However, to maintain both focus and control the task, we have not included the literature on the effects of preschool in the review.

The section entitled "School Effects on Student Outcomes" defines school effects. The section "Research Design Issues" presents the research design issues relevant to interpreting studies of school effects. The section "School Effects Studies" presents a critical review of the literature on school effects, including key conclusions and their relationship "to the broad context of the determinants of health." The section "Stories and Lessons Learned" sets out five stories and the lessons to be learned from them. The final section, "Policy Implications," discusses principles to guide government actions. These principles are expressed as the "elements of best practice."

SCHOOL EFFECTS ON STUDENT OUTCOMES

Definitions—Cognitive and Noncognitive Domains of Child Functioning

We define school effects in terms of both cognitive and noncognitive outcomes. Cognitive outcomes concern academic achievement and comprise two types: the acquisition of basic cognitive skills related to literacy, numeracy and problem solving, and academic success in the curriculum-related aspects of school, usually indicated by passing examinations and completing school. Noncognitive outcomes concern behavioral, emotional and social functioning, and can be seen in such aspects as attitudes toward school and self, interpersonal relationships, employment, and the presence (or absence) of psychiatric disorders such as antisocial behaviours, substance abuse, depression and anxiety.

Relationship between Cognitive and Noncognitive Outcomes

Children develop both the cognitive and noncognitive planes simultaneously. For example, epidemiological follow-up studies have observed a strong association between academic underachievement and externalizing behavioral disorders. Twenty-five percent of the children in the Isle of Wight Study who had specific reading delays were rated above the cut-off for antisocial behaviour compared to five percent in the general population (Rutter 1974; Rutter et al. 1976). Specific reading delays were observed in more than one-third of antisocial children (Rutter, Tizard, and Whitmore 1970). Numerous other investigations have linked academic underachievement and externalizing behaviour problems (Stevenson et al. 1985; McGee et al. 1988; Patterson 1986; Rutter 1989; Schonfield et al. 1988). However, the nature of the relationship is unclear (Hinshaw 1992). The causal relationship probably operates in both directions: for example, academic problems may give rise to behavioral problems, and behavioral problems may contribute to academic underachievement. As well, socio-economic status, family adversity, low IQ, language deficits and neuro-developmental delay may also contribute to both problems through complex pathways.

The Importance of Prevention

Intensified prevention efforts are justified for a number of reasons. First, effective prevention strategies could reduce the burden of suffering, costs and consequences experienced by children, families, school professionals and society due to academic, behavioral, emotional and social problems (Offord 1987). Second, evidence that established academic and behavioral disorders can be effectively treated is extremely limited (Offord and Bennett 1994). Prevention strategies are designed to reduce the incidence and severity of these disorders. Third, few children who need treatment receive it. In the Ontario Child Health Survey, only one in six children who needed care had contacted an appropriate mental health or social service in the previous six months (Offord et al. 1987). Recent data also show that children who receive treatment are not always the ones most in need (Boyle et al. 1987). Offering prevention programs through schools could eliminate some barriers to use of services by children in need. Fourth, even if effective treatments were available, the clinic resources available would never stretch to provide individual treatment to children in need. Schools are an attractive prevention venue because children and families can be targeted in groups, rather than as individuals.

RESEARCH DESIGN ISSUES

Four research design issues are central to drawing conclusions from school effects studies: a) the strengths and limitations of the study design chosen; b) the choice of student outcomes and school variables studied; c) the sample of schools studied; and d) the assessment of school effects in terms of student progress over time.

Study Design

School effects studies are designed to establish the existence and direction of causal relationships between school characteristics and student outcomes. Experimental studies provide the strongest research evidence for addressing causal questions because they separate the effects of school variables from the influence of nonschool variables (such as student characteristics and family background at school entry, community and environmental factors). However, it is impossible to assign students randomly to schools, so most of what we know about school effects comes from observational studies, particularly cross-sectional surveys that use routinely collected standardized achievement test scores. In a few exemplary observational studies, longitudinal designs were used to allow investigators to control for student characteristics at school entry and to compare student functioning before and after exposure to school. These studies evaluated cognitive and noncognitive student outcomes and assessed school and classroom characteristics using special questionnaires and observational methods. The longitudinal designs also allowed the investigators to examine natural changes in school variables to determine their influence on student outcomes.

The validity of observational studies depends upon the strategies for controlling for variations in student intake from school to school (Maughan 1988). School effects researchers must either use statistical techniques in the analysis to control for variations from school to school in student ability and background or attempt to match schools by student characteristics and then examine how various outcomes can be attributed to various school characteristics and processes.

Very few experimental and controlled studies of school improvement interventions are available. Most do not include a control group and limit outcome assessment to academic achievement. Most studies do not note changes in school process variables or relate these changes to changes in student outcomes. Without such evidence, it is impossible to determine whether improvements in academic achievement and behavioral, emotional and social functioning can be attributed to changes in school processes.

School effects studies focus on between-school differences in student outcomes. They do not address whether school affects student outcomes compared to "no school." As Rutter (1983) states, a study conducted without a "no treatment" group could erroneously conclude that schools have no effect because no variations are observed from school to school. For example, if all schools in a study taught a particular skill equally well, student achievement in that skill would be the same in all schools, and no variation would be observed. Researchers would falsely conclude that schools do not influence acquisition of the skill when, in fact, without exposure to school, students would not learn the skill. Therefore, in the absence of a "no treatment" comparison group, the finding of no variation from school to school can be interpreted in two ways: equal effectiveness or no effectiveness.

Choice of Student Outcomes and School Variables

The second research design issue concerns the choice of student outcomes and school variables to be studied. The choice of student outcomes must be sensitive to the goals of schools and the various student functions that may be affected by the school experience (Madaus et al. 1979; Rutter 1983; Good and Weinstein 1986; Maughan 1988). The most common weakness in the available studies is an exclusive focus on academic achievement and the use of standardized achievement tests of basic skills (Madaus et al. 1979; Rutter 1983; Good and Weinstein 1986). A comprehensive assessment of school outcomes is needed that is sensitive to curriculum goals and content, not just to the narrow range of basic skills assessed on standardized achievement tests. Measures should also be sensitive to the age and developmental level of the target population. Noncognitive outcomes should cover student behavioral, emotional and social functioning; attitudes and self-concept; and vocational outcomes (Rutter 1983; Good and Weinstein 1986; Maughan 1988; Willms 1992).

Many specific school variables that determine student outcomes have been discussed in the literature. There is no accepted scheme for classifying and defining the variables identified, but they generally fall into two categories—school inputs and school processes. School inputs are structural or administrative school features that tend to be outside the direct daily control of schools and teachers. (Examples include teacher-to-pupil ratio, instructional resources and quality of the physical facilities.) School processes are generally within the daily control of schools and teachers and can, therefore, be modified. School ethos, the instructional leadership of the principal, academic demands, expectations regarding conduct, teaching style and methods (time spent on lessons, record keeping and feedback) are all school and classroom processes.

Table 1, adapted from Willms (1992), shows a useful way to organize school input and school process variables. It distinguishes four levels at which school variables operate—the student, the classroom, the school and the external environments—and includes a method for identifying potential improvements. The remainder of this review uses Willms' structure.

Willms' four levels highlight the "nested" nature of the student in the classroom, the school, and the external environment. Very few investigators have designed their research in light of this hierarchical relationship. Appropriate statistical techniques such as hierarchical linear modelling are available and investi-gators are beginning to apply them.

Sample of Schools Studied

Results can be generalized depending on the type of schools included in the study. Schools can be randomly selected from a district or region, or selected according to characteristics such as grade range, location, proportion of disadvantaged or ethnic minority students served, private or public, co-educational or single sex, effective or ineffective as defined by the investigator.

The number of schools studied affects the precision of results. This is of particular concern with schoolwide variables because each school provides a single data point for such characteristics.

Most of the best studies were done in secondary schools and included relatively small numbers of schools in disadvantaged, inner-city areas.

Table 1

School inputs and school processes

Level	School Inputs	School Processes
Student	Sex Race and ethnicity Attitudes toward school Cognitive ability Parents' occupations Parents' education Number of siblings Family composition	Quality of school life Sense of efficacy Attitudes toward school
Classroom	Class size Intake composition Curriculum quality Instructional resources Teacher characteristics Classroom appearance	Working conditions Teacher sense of efficacy Teacher commitment and morale Disciplinary climate Ability grouping Academic press
School	School size Intake Per-pupil expenditures Principal characteristics Teacher turnover Building age and appearance Access to community resources	Principal's instructional leadership Disciplinary climate Tracking or streaming Parent-school relations
Environment	District size Community SES Per-pupil expenditures Opportunities for employment	Between-school segregation Community-school relations

Source: Adapted from J. D. Willms. 1992. *Monitoring School Performance: A Guide to Educators.* Washington (DC): The Falmer Press, p. 33.

School Effects Defined as Progress over Time

School effects should be defined in terms of student progress over time, and this change should be related to specific school features or processes. The cross-sectional studies of school effects by Coleman and colleagues (1966) and Jencks and colleagues (1973) looked at the student-to-student variation in scores on an achievement test taken at one point in time. Less than 5 percent of the variance in student outcomes could be attributed to between-school variations, while more than 50 percent could be attributed to family background. Because these studies were cross sectional, they could not examine students' progress over time and whether the school-to-school variation in rates of progress depended on variations in specific school and classroom features.

Improvement in the average level of achievement concerns the increase in average student achievement for a particular school. Schools are compared to determine whether some achieve larger average increases than others. Important between-school differences in average progress can occur without any change in the overall width of the distribution of outcomes. These different average rates of progress can reflect the ability of some schools to keep their students above the threshold of achievement that protects them from subsequent school failure and dysfunction in other domains. This distinction is sometimes discussed with respect to the tension between the competing schooling objectives of excellence and equity (Willms 1992).

SCHOOL EFFECTS STUDIES

Overview

As noted in the section "Research Design Issues," most knowledge of school effects comes from observational studies, particularly correlational, cross-sectional studies. Moreover, in most studies, the only student outcomes covered are standardized achievement test scores.

The next section is a critical review of the effective schools model. This is followed by a review of three studies that produced the best evidence to date of the effects of school on students' academic achievement and behavioral, emotional and social functioning. Key conclusions from the literature are then presented including the relationship between school effects and nonmedical determinants of health.

Effective Schools Model

The effective schools model proposed by Edmonds (1979) lists five characteristics of an effective school: strong administrative leadership; high expectations for students' achievement; orderly atmosphere conducive to learning; emphasis on acquisition of basic skills; and frequent monitoring of students' progress. Several variations of this list exist but, overall, various authors propose remarkably consistent lists of key elements of effective schools (Purkey and Smith 1983; Ralph and Fennessey 1983; Good and Brophy 1986; Reynolds, Davie, and Philips 1989; Willms 1992).

The effective schools model has been challenged vigorously because there is little empirical evidence to support it (Ralph and Fennessey 1983; Purkey and Smith 1983; Maughan 1988). Several excellent, comprehensive review papers are available (Gray 1981; Gray, McPherson, and Raffe 1982; Purkey and Smith 1983; Rutter 1983; Ralph and Fennessey 1983; Reynolds 1985; Austin and Garber 1985; Good and Weinstein 1986; Good and Brophy 1986; Maughan, 1988; Scheerens and Creemers 1989; Sylva 1994) and, therefore, a detailed review of individual studies is not justified here.

Many features of the model, including school ethos, could depend on the characteristics of the student population rather than principal or teacher action. For example, a highly motivated, well-behaved, academically able school population may be the source of high teacher expectations for academic achievement and an orderly atmosphere conducive to learning. The available studies do not allow the direction of the relationship to be determined. The authors call for further experimental studies to determine whether interventions derived from the effective schools model actually improve student outcomes.

Review of Exemplary Studies

Despite the gaps noted above, it is possible to guide action with a number of conclusions from the existing studies. This section reviews three exemplary observational studies that meet the following methodological criteria: i) they controlled for student intake characteristics; ii) they assessed school processes, not just school inputs, and related them to student outcomes; and iii) they included measures of behavioral, emotional and social functioning and academic achievements other than scores of standardized achievement tests.

Tables 2, 3 and 4 summarize the methods and findings of each study. The first study was conducted in secondary schools (Rutter et al. 1979; table 2) over six years, from entry to, to exit from secondary school. The second study was conducted in primary schools (grades 4 and 5) over one year (Brookover et al. 1979; table 3). The third study was conducted in primary schools over four years (Mortimore et al. 1988; table 4). Table 5 summarizes the methodology and results of the studies by Coleman and colleagues and Jencks and colleagues, which can be contrasted with these exemplary studies.

Rutter's study of 12 London inner-city secondary schools is prospective and longitudinal. Students were assessed before entry to secondary school at age 10 and then yearly to age 14; further assessment of examination passes was conducted at age 16 (Rutter et al. 1979; see table 2). This study showed school-to-school variations on four outcomes: public examination passes, attendance, classroom behaviour and delinquency. The variations could not be accounted for by variations in student intake characteristics. School and classroom inputs such as resources and physical plant, school and class size and organizational structure (ability grouping, sex composition) were not associated with variations in outcomes. This finding confirms the findings of Coleman and colleagues and Jencks and colleagues: that physical

Table 2

School effects studies: Rutter et al. 1979

Authors	Rutter, M., B. Maughan, P. Mortimore, J. Ouston and A. Smith 1979
Design	Longitudinal study Baseline = 10 years (conclusion of primary school) Follow-up 1 = 14 years Follow-up 2 = 16 years
Sample	12 inner-city London secondary schools

Outcomes
- cognitive   • public examination passes (age 16)
- noncognitive   • attendance, classroom behaviour, delinquency

Explanatory Variables
- school inputs
  - students   • achievement testing (nonverbal intelligence, reading ability)
                   • behaviour
                   • primary school attended
                   • parents' occupations, place of birth

  - classroom and school   • sex composition, church school or not, school size and space, age of building and number of sites, teacher-pupil ratio, overall school staffing, pastoral care, ability grouping vs. mixed ability

  - environment   • area differences, balance of student intake (ability, parent occupation, ethnic, child behaviour)

- school processes
  - school and classroom level   • academic emphasis, teacher actions in lessons, discipline, pupil conditions, student responsibilities and participation, teacher continuity, stability of peer groups, staff organization and monitoring of teachers, teacher skills, overall process

Findings
- schools differ on all four outcome measures
- outcome differences cannot be explained by differences in intake
- variation in outcome is not associated with classroom- and school-level inputs
- variation in outcome is associated with classroom- and school-level processes
- of the four outcomes, behaviour in the classroom and on school grounds had the strongest relationship with school processes

features and school resources do not explain variation in student achievement. Individual school and classroom processes (degree of academic emphasis, teacher actions in lessons, the availability of incentives and rewards, good conditions for pupils, and student responsibilities and participation) affected all four outcomes. Of the four outcomes studied, behaviour was the most strongly related to school processes.

A composite measure comprised of the individual measures of school process and interpreted to reflect school ethos affected outcomes more than any of the individual process measures. A schoolwide balance in intellectually able students was related to outcomes, but ethnic balance and social class balance were not.

The second study by Brookover and colleagues looked at fourth and fifth graders from a representative sample of Michigan schools (Brookover et al. 1979; table 3). Student achievement, self-perceptions of academic ability and reliance (motivation to complete tasks and solve problems on their own) were studied. School-to-school variations on three outcomes could not be explained by student intake characteristics. This study showed a relationship between school processes (classroom organization methods, time spent on lessons and staff satisfaction) and student achievement and showed that schools with comparable resources could have different school ethos.

Table 4 summarizes the results of Mortimore's primary school study, which is one of the few studies conducted at the primary level. School outcomes in 2,000 children attending 50 randomly selected inner-city London primary schools were followed over four years beginning at age 7 (Mortimore et al. 1988, 1989). Rates of progress on cognitive outcomes varied markedly from school to school. A similar but less pronounced pattern was found for three of the noncognitive outcomes studied (behaviour in school, attitude toward school and teachers' and peers' attitudes toward self). Variations in student intake did not explain school-to-school variations. School attendance did not vary, and this was interpreted to reflect a lack of autonomy of primary school students over attendance compared with older, secondary school students.

Contrary to other studies, Mortimore concluded that small schools with good physical environment contribute to student outcomes. However, the influence of these school inputs seemed to depend on the presence of important school processes. Both school and classroom processes were shown to vary in relation to student outcomes. Mortimore and colleagues concluded that the influential school processes included purposeful leadership by the head teacher, teacher involvement of the deputy head and teachers in decision making, consistency between teachers, parent involvement, and a positive atmosphere. Classroom processes included structured lessons, intellectually challenging teaching, a work-centred environment, limited focus on sessions, good communication between teachers and students, and record keeping.

Table 3

School effects studies: Brookover et al. 1979

Author	Brookover, W. B., D. Beady, P. Flood, J. Schweitzer and J. Wisenbaker 1979
Design	Cross-sectional survey
Sample	Random sample of students from grades 4 and 5 in Michigan (drawn from 68 schools)
Outcome Measures	
• cognitive	• achievement (Michigan School Assessment Test—proportion of students who mastered 40 reading and mathematics achievement objectives)
	• self-concept of academic ability (perception of self as a student
• noncognitive	• self-reliance (perception of extent to which students could and wanted to complete tasks or solve problems on their own)
Explanatory variables	
• school inputs	
– students	• social composition of student body (SES and percent white)
– school and classroom	• school size, average daily attendance, staff-student ratio, teacher characteristics (training and experience)
• school processes	• ability grouping, openness of classroom organization, time allocation, staff satisfactions
	• school climate (perception of norms, expectations and beliefs about school social system)
Findings	• student outcomes cannot be completely explained by student characteristics or other school inputs
	• school processes predict student outcomes
	• schools with comparable resources can have different climates

Subgroup analyses to determine whether school effects varied for different types of students showed that, in generally effective schools, student outcomes did not vary by sex, social class or ethnicity. The same result was found for ineffective schools.

Table 4

School effects studies: Mortimore et al. 1988

Author	Mortimore, P., P. Sammons, L. Stoll, D. Lewis and R. Ecob 1988
Design	Longitudinal study Baseline = age 7 Yearly follow-up to age 11
Sample	50 randomly selected London inner-city elementary schools (2,000 pupils)
Outcomes	
• cognitive	• yearly standardized tests of reading and mathematics, • practical mathematics, creative writing, oral skills • London Reading Test: reading and verbal reasoning in 4th year
• noncognitive	• behaviour in school • attitudes toward school • self-perceptions of how seen by teacher, peer and self
Explanatory variables	
• school inputs	
– student/family	• age, SES, sex, race, family background, attainment at entry to primary school (reading, math and viseo-spatial), preschool experiences
– classroom and school	• defined by investigators as all features of school and classroom outside the control of the head teacher and staff: condition of building and classroom, quantity and quality of instructional materials, staff-to-student ratios
• school processes	• defined by investigators as all organization and policy under the control of the head teacher and staff: curriculum, grouping and allocation of students and teachers to classes, teacher involvement in decision making, promotion of equal opportunity, involvement of parents
Findings	• student cognitive outcomes (reading, math, writing and oracy) varied markedly between schools • noncognitive outcomes (behaviour, self-concept, attitudes toward schools) varied between schools, but the effect was not as large as for cognitive outcomes

- the effect of school on attendance was small
- differences could not be explained by student intake differences
- 12 school- and classroom-level policies were concluded to be related to outcomes: purposeful leadership of head teacher; involvement of deputy head; involvement of teachers; consistency among teachers; structured lessons; intellectually challenging teaching; work-centred environment; limited focus in sessions; maximum communication between teachers and students; record keeping; parental involvement; positive climate

Table 5

School effects studies: Coleman et al. 1966 and Jencks et al. 1973

Design	Cross-sectional survey
Sample	4,000 elementary and secondary schools in the United States (645,000 students)
Outcomes	
• cognitive	Standardized tests of verbal ability
• noncognitive	None included
Explanatory Variables	
• school inputs	
– students	• student family background
– classroom	• class size, teacher qualifications
• school processes	• not studied
Findings	• school differences in student achievement on tests of verbal ability explained under 5% of the total variance in test scores; family background variables explained 50% of the variance

Key Conclusions

The available studies consistently show that student outcomes vary from school to school in both cognitive and noncognitive functions. First, examination passes, school attendance, classroom behaviour and delinquency vary among inner-city secondary schools. Academic outcomes vary the most between primary schools, with smaller between-school differences in behaviour and attitudes.

Second, although student characteristics at school entry are strongly related to school exit outcomes, the available studies consistently show that school-to-school variations cannot be explained from student intake characteristics alone.

Third, school-to-school variations in student outcomes cannot be explained by variations in teacher-to-pupil ratios, instructional resources, quality of physical facilities or other resource inputs. Therefore, interventions that focus on these features will not affect student outcomes significantly.

Fourth, school and classroom processes are related to variations in both cognitive and noncognitive outcomes. For example, student performance reflects schoolwide expectations for academic achievement and conduct, and instructional practices such as time on lesson, record keeping and giving feedback. Therefore, interventions that focus on school and classroom processes may improve student outcomes.

Finally, the available evidence suggests that school and classroom processes can mitigate the effects of risk factors associated with nonmedical determinants of health. Good school and classroom practices can help children at risk of poor academic, behavioral, emotional and social functioning due to physical, social, economic, cultural and psychological factors. On the other hand, poor school and classroom practices can aggravate the effects of risk factors associated with physical, social, economic, cultural and psychological determinants of health. For example, schools characterized by school and classroom processes associated with superior student outcomes may lower risk by buffering the effects of adverse factors, such as poverty and low motivation to learn.

The existing studies raise many issues: a) the stability of school effects over time; b) the consistency within schools of school effects on cognitive and noncognitive outcomes; c) the consistency of school effects across a student body; d) the effects of school inputs on outcomes; e) the elements of school and classroom processes that affect outcomes; f) the causal role of school ethos; g) the magnitude of school effects; h) the effect of schools on dropouts; i) the relationship between school and classroom processes; j) the mechanisms behind observed relationships; k) the measures of school processes and school outcomes; and l) the need for experimental studies of the effect of school and classroom processes on student outcomes.

There is some evidence that school effects are stable over time. That is, an effective school continues to be effective, but an ineffective school tends to continue to produce student outcomes below that expected (Rutter 1983).

The consistency of within-school effects on cognitive and noncognitive outcomes, and the consistency of school effects for subgroups of students, are important issues in the effective schools debate. Rutter and colleagues showed that cognitive and noncognitive outcomes were related (1979). However, Brookover and colleagues (1979) showed that achievement and student self-concepts and self-reliance were only weakly correlated. Mortimore and colleagues (1988, 1989) concluded that, for primary school children, cognitive and noncognitive outcomes appeared independent in the overall analysis, although they were related in some schools.

A key point in the effective schools debate is that several authors challenge the usefulness of the term "effective schools" and the validity of generalizing about school performance. These authors argue for a more thoughtful analysis that recognizes that schools affect a range of outcomes, not just academic achievement, and that a specific school will produce a variety of student outcomes, which will depend on the school's strengths and on the priorities and characteristics of the student population and the surrounding community (Ralph and Fennessey 1983; Good and Weinstein 1986; Maughan 1988). Assessing local needs and the implementation of school monitoring systems could expand our understanding of performance consistency within schools and the factors that determine it (Willms 1992). Local needs assessment and school monitoring are discussed in the section "Policy Implications."

The studies consistently show that school inputs, such as physical facilities and instructional resources, are not related to student outcomes. However, the results are limited to the range of variation studied. For example, reducing class size beyond the range that is currently realistic might improve outcomes.

A key outstanding question concerns the individual elements of school and classroom processes that effect outcomes. Promising elements of schoolwide processes include: leadership from the principal, strong emphasis on academics, expectations for good conduct and orderly discipline, and consistency between teachers in curriculum and values. Rutter et al. (1979) showed that the intellectual capabilities of students were related to improved overall school performance, and that ethnicity and social class did not influence overall school performance. Classroom processes include teacher-pupil communication, time spent on lessons, limits to curricular focus, instructional style, student monitoring, record keeping and feedback. Grouping students by ability does not appear to affect overall achievement levels (Rutter 1983; Slavin 1987).

The causal role of school ethos remains uncertain (Anderson 1985; Gottfredson et al. 1986). Raudenbush (1990) points out that student characteristics alone cannot create a positive school ethos. For example, teacher practices, such as whole class communication, limited curricular focus and good record keeping, are independent of student characteristics. The best evidence that a positive ethos improves outcomes comes from the Rutter et al. 1979 finding that the correlation between school ethos and student characteristics was much lower at school entry than at school exit. Brookover (1979) also showed that schools with similar inputs could vary in ethos. A recent study by Kasen (1990) showed that school ethos was related to changes in eight behavioral and emotional syndrome scores over a two-year period.

The magnitude of school effects cannot be determined from available studies (Rutter 1983; Mortimore et al. 1988). A better understanding of the significance of school effects depends on resolution of two issues. First, to obtain a better estimate of the size of an effect, researchers need methodologies that include longitudinal studies of student progress, sensitive measures of what schools teach, controls for student intake characteristics and new statistical techniques (Bryk and Raudenbush 1988; Raudenbush 1990). Second, the magnitude of school effects must be broadly defined so as to account for the sequelae of school success or failure, not just outcomes at the completion of formal schooling.

This review of school effects studies provides very few insights into the relationship between school processes and school dropout (Wehlage et al. 1989). Low grades, high absentee rates and behavioral problems have been shown to predict school failure and school dropout (U.S. Department of Health, Education and Welfare 1975). Nonschool variables that are risk factors for school dropout include behavioral and emotional disorders, family background and peer group influences (Racine et al. 1995). Very little is known about effective strategies to prevent school dropout, and this area needs increased research attention (Morris, Pawlovich, and McCall 1988; Wright and Offord 1992).

The relationship between school and classroom processes is not well understood. Most research about school processes has focused on the classroom. The definition and measurement of school variables and how school processes may modify or interact with classroom processes need more attention (Willms 1992).

The mechanisms behind the observed relationships are not well understood. For example, how does the school ethos influence cognitive and noncognitive outcomes? Possible models include cumulative effects of long-term exposure, causal chains of linked events, and acute responses mitigated by developmental milestones or transitions (Maughan 1988).

The last two issues concern the limitations of the research methodology used to date, particularly the measures of school processes and school outcomes and the need for experimental studies of the effects of school and classroom processes on student outcomes. Both these issues are discussed in detail in the section "Research Design Issues."

STORIES AND LESSONS LEARNED

This section summarizes initiatives that designed, implemented and evaluated interventions to improve the effectiveness of schools and classrooms on student outcomes. First, the criteria used to select the stories are presented. Second, the application of story descriptors provided in the instructions to authors are discussed. The stories are described in detail under the heading "Five Stories" and in tables 6–11. Lessons learned are then summarized in "Lessons Learned."

Criteria for Selection of Stories

Stories were selected according to five criteria derived from the key conclusions in the literature. First, the intervention must include school and classroom processes. Second, the intervention should target cognitive and noncognitive outcomes. Third, the setting must be field based and represent as closely as possible the real-life context for a school improvement intervention. Fourth, intervention elements must be described in sufficient detail to allow replication. Fifth, intervention implementation and student outcomes must be evaluated to assess the process, outcomes and costs.

As discussed in the section "School Effects Studies," there are very few studies of school improvement strategies that attribute changes in student outcomes to changes in school processes. There is even less information about approaches that meet the above five criteria.

Story Descriptors

Five stories are set out in the following terms:

Actions on the nonmedical determinants of health – Schools promote human development by teaching specific knowledge, skills, attitudes and values. Schools can act on and interact with the physical, social, economic, cultural and psychological determinants of health, thus increasing or decreasing risk for poor mental health outcomes and life quality.

Each story notes the content of the intervention, the setting where it was applied and the values reflected in the actions taken. Four values are highlighted: prevention, schoolwide actions, participatory intervention design and decision making, and multidisciplinary intervention and evaluation.

Reasons for undertaking change – School improvement strategies must be linked to documented needs and weaknesses of the school, the classroom and the student.

Actors involved – Top-down approaches to school improvement are unlikely to succeed because intervention implementation requires participation by many individuals operating at different levels, including teachers, parents, education and mental health specialists, and administrators. The stories note how the relevant actors were included in decisions about intervention design, implementation and evaluation.

Replicability – Replicability includes feasibility, cost, the extent to which intervention success depends on the skills and enthusiasm of its developers, and the extent to which the intervention harmonizes with the social routines and philosophies of the school. The long-term sustainability of an intervention and its capacity to become systematized depend on these factors.

Funding – Intervention descriptions note the need for additional funding and the source of support for the evaluation.

Evaluation and analysis of results – Descriptions use the available evidence to support the intervention's effectiveness in improving school processes and student outcomes.

Five Stories

The Comer approach (see table 6) is a schoolwide improvement approach that creates a mechanism to support change, rather than implementing predefined changes or actions. The Comer approach focuses on school organization and management, and the participation of teachers, parents and mental health professionals in identifying problems and developing solutions through a School Action Committee (Comer 1980, 1985, 1988; Cauce, Comer, and Schwartz 1987). The approach has many strengths. Its intent is to change school systems, it focuses on prevention, it uses a participatory approach that includes teachers, parents and mental health professionals, and it recognizes the relationship between academic outcomes and behavioral, emotional and social functioning. The Comer approach is prominent in the United States, and the Rockefeller Foundation is funding its dissemination. The program was very successful in the extremely disadvantaged New Haven primary schools with predominantly black student populations, where it was developed. There is some evidence that both cognitive and noncognitive outcomes are influenced by the program, but these results are from a nonexperimental study that used a sample size of only 48 subjects (24 in the program group and 24 in the control group).

The generalizability of the Comer approach to less-disadvantaged settings where the original team is not involved is yet to be reported. A challenge to programs such as the Comer approach is whether they can be replicated. Many good projects depend on the special talents and motivation of their developers (Offord and Jones 1993); the challenge is to identify the elements of successful dissemination and to develop programs that can be disseminated easily and with fidelity to the original.

The Felner program (see table 7) focuses on interventions to support school transitions and seeks to implement a specific set of changes. The program changes the role of the Grade 9 homeroom teacher and classroom organization (Felner, Ginter, and Primavera 1982). The homeroom teacher becomes a student mentor, and the social group of each student is stabilized through administrative changes to class scheduling. This approach aims to buffer the stressful transition to high school, and thereby, decreases students' potential to begin a downward spiral. The approach used is simple,

Table 6

Story 1: The Comer approach

1. Actions
- content
  - multidisciplinary, systemwide approach to school change
  - intervention targeted dysfunctional elements of school social environment consisted of:
    - establishment of a School Advisory Council made up of teachers, parents and staff responsible for identifying school problems, allocating school resources, development and evaluation of programs to address needs and problems
    - multidisciplinary mental health team provided consultation to staff on management of student behaviour problems
    - establishment of a social calendar integrating academic and athletic events
    - encouragement of parent participation in school events
- setting
  - poor, black elementary school in New Haven (grades 5 to 7)
- values
  - prevention
  - schoolwide, ecological perspective (i.e., dysfunction is due to interactional factors rather than intra-personal factors)
  - participatory (teachers, mental health professionals and parents)
  - multidisciplinary (mental health focus rather than exclusively educational principles)

2. Reasons
- extremely poor achievement scores
- frequent and severe behavioral problems

3. Actors
- participants
  - teachers, parents, mental health professionals
- implementors
  - same

4. Replicability
- reproducible
  - intervention is a process, not an easily defined package of materials and discrete acts
  - replicability likely dependent on the qualities of the teachers, parents and mental health professionals
- feasible
  - yes, but intensive
  - establishment of mental health team may involve additional costs

Table 6 (cont.)

5. Funding	• school-university partnership • funding of mental health team not clear • School Advisory Council low cost
6. Evaluation	
• process	• ?
• outcome	• comparison of 24 students who received the intervention with 24 matched controls showed that 3 years after receiving the program, program recipients were functioning at a higher level than controls on GPA, school grades and self-perceptions about self-confidence and school competence • before-after comparisons of attendance, achievement scores and parent attendance at school functions shows dramatic increases over a 10-year period
• cost	• ?

inexpensive and less dependent on the characteristics of the program designers for its success.

Evidence from nonexperimental controlled studies suggests that, in both the short and the long term, the Felner program affects cognitive and noncognitive outcomes, including attendance and dropouts (Felner, Ginter, and Primavera 1982; Felner and Adan 1988). However, these results should be interpreted with caution because they may arise partly from unblinded evaluation.

The Ottawa Board of Education's School Readiness Program (see table 8) focuses on the transition to school during the kindergarten to Grade 1 period. The intervention is currently being developed. The objective is to offer early literacy, behavioral and social skills training to children in kindergarten and Grade 1. The intervention seeks to link current scientific knowledge about effective literacy and behaviour enhancement with natural school routines, existing programs, and philosophies of Ottawa Board of Education kindergarten and Grade 1 teachers.

Program strengths include schoolwide actions, a focus on prevention, a program that targets cognitive and noncognitive outcomes, a participatory approach using a multidisciplinary project team to design and implement the program, and a reliance on existing resources. An evaluation that includes intervention process, student outcomes and costs will be implemented in the fall of 1997.

The Tri-Ministry Helping Children Adjust Project (see table 9) illustrates a universal strategy to prevent academic failure and behavioral maladjustment in elementary school pupils. Universal programs (Institute of Medicine 1994)

Table 7

Story 2: Transition to secondary school, Felner et al. 1982

1. Actions
- content
  - program to maximize continuity of teachers and peer groups during first year of secondary school and thereby reduce the effect of transition
  - program consisted of
    - homeroom teacher was primary contact for all student counselling needs
    - class composition the same for four classes per day
    - movement of students within school reduced to one part of the building
- setting
  - large urban high school, predominately nonwhite, lower income
- values
  - prevention
  - multidisciplinary

2. Reasons
- to address the perceived needs of first-year secondary students

3. Actors
- participants
  - teachers, students, mental health professionals
- implementors
  - same

4. Replicability
- reproducible
  - school organizational change easily replicable
  - teacher counsellor role not well defined
- feasible
  - yes, uses existing resources

5. Funding
- uses existing resources

6. Evaluation
- process
  - ?
- outcome
  - program students were compared with matched controls at the end of Grade 9 and four years later
  - at the end of Grade 9, control students had lower GPAs than program students and scored lower on self-concept; absenteeism was higher among controls; program students gave higher ratings of the social environment
  - four years later program students were found to have higher grades and lower rates of absence and dropout
- cost
  - a low-cost intervention but no systematic cost information found

Table 8

Story 2: Transition to primary school, Ottawa Board of Education School Readiness Project

1. Actions
- content
  - early literacy skills, social and behavioral skills
- setting
  - disadvantaged and general population kindergarten and Grade 1 classes in the Ottawa Board of Education
- values
  - prevention
  - schoolwide, ecological approach
  - participatory
  - multidisciplinary

2. Reasons
- school readiness identified as a problem

3. Actors
- participants
  - teachers, early childhood educators, mental health professionals, epidemiologists, volunteers
- implementors
  - early literacy program consists of private story time for each student conducted by volunteer parent/grandparent
  - early literacy program designed by kindergarten teachers and early childhood educators within the Board
  - social and behavioral skills program conducted by school mental health workers (Children Learning for Living Project)

4. Replicability
- reproducible
  - literacy program includes manual, book with crib sheets for the reader, and video
  - program uses existing resources
- feasible
  - dependent on Board leadership

5. Funding
- external funding supports the evaluation component of the program

6. Evaluation
- process
- outcome
- cost
  - the pilot phase of this project under way since September 1995; a full-scale evaluation is in the planning stages with pilot work to begin in May 1996
  - the evaluation will address process, outcomes and costs

are delivered to all children and do not target children at risk or children with problem symptoms. The Tri-Ministry project offers a school and classroom social skills intervention and a reading partners program to

Table 9

Story 3: Tri-Ministry Helping Children Adjust Project, Boyle 1994

1. Actions	
• content	• social skills training and reading partners program
• setting	• kindergarten to Grade 3 in 11 school boards across Ontario
• values	• prevention • multidisciplinary • schoolwide
2. Reasons	• to implement and evaluate promising school-based strategies to promote academic achievement and prevent behavioral maladjustment
3. Actors	
• participants	• teachers, mental health professionals, epidemiologists
• implementors	• same
4. Replicability	
• reproducible	• manuals and standardized materials available for both programs
• feasible	• depends on leadership at the level of the school board and school
5. Funding	• additional personnel costs for program facilitators
6. Evaluation	
• process	• qualitative study was completed during year 4 of program implementation to investigate factors related to the acceptance of the social skills program
• outcome	• impact of the program on academic achievement, behavioral, emotional and social functioning is being evaluated in an experimental study
• cost	• costs are being measured

children in kindergarten to Grade 3 (Boyle et al. 1990; Boyle 1994). The social skills program lasts 18 months, from September and until the Christmas break of the following year; the reading partners program begins in September and ends in June of the same school year.

The strengths of the program include a focus on prevention, schoolwide and classroom-level actions, a program that targets cognitive and non-cognitive outcomes, a universal focus and a strong evaluation component.

The social skills and reading partners programs are standardized and delivered in schools by expert program designers. The advantage of this approach is that the intervention uses known effective strategies to enhance social skills and reading. The content and administration methods are standardized and are, thus, easily reproduced across sites. However, these programs require expert facilitators to visit each participating class. This may make the program too expensive for some school boards. Also, if the program is not introduced in a manner that is sensitive to the conditions and attitudes of the school, it can seem to be a top-down imposition.

The project's evaluation component employs qualitative and quantitative approaches to assess the implementation process and program effects. For example, a qualitative study investigated the acceptance of the social skills program (Lohfeld et al. 1994). The findings suggest that rejection was associated with feasibility problems or perceived lack of involvement in program design. The effect of the full program on a broad range of student outcomes is currently being evaluated in a five-year experimental study involving 59 schools in 11 school boards across Ontario.

The Families and Schools Together (FAST) Track program (see table 10) is included to contrast universal and targeted approaches to intervention in the primary grades (Conduct Problems Prevention Research Group 1992). The FAST Track program identifies children at risk of conduct disorder and offers them a five-pronged, intensive intervention program. Children are identified as high risk in kindergarten. The full program is offered throughout elementary school, beginning in Grade 1. The intervention includes strategies to improve disciplinary practices and to alter peer and teacher responses to disruptive behaviour. All children participate in this aspect of the program, but only high-risk children receive the other four components of the program, which include academic tutoring and social skills training.

The FAST Track program has many of the strengths of the universal approach seen in the Tri-Ministry project: a focus on prevention; schoolwide and classroom-level actions; targeting cognitive and noncognitive outcomes; and a rigorous evaluation component. However, the overall effectiveness of the FAST Track program's targeted approach depends on whether the children who need the program are correctly identified as high risk on entry to primary school. Preliminary evidence suggests that only 40 percent of the children identified as high risk on entry to kindergarten have behavioral problems when assessed again at the end of Grade 1, and that 45 percent of children with problems at the end of Grade 1 are missed by kindergarten high-risk screening (Lochman 1995). This level of predictive accuracy is consistent with other studies and highlights the limitations of a targeted approach in this age group (Bennett 1996).

The Cardiff School Improvement Program (see table 11) shows how professional development of teachers affects school improvement. This program establishes a process, rather than implementing specific changes at the school and classroom level. Reynolds, Davie and Philips (1989) developed a two-year course for teachers that focused on the findings of effective schools research. During the course, teachers studied the relationship

Table 10

Story 4: The FAST (Families and Schools Together) Track Program, Conduct Problems Prevention Research Group 1992

1. Actions	
• content	• class discipline, behavioral and social skills training that aims to alter teacher and peer responding to child conduct problems: self-control, positive peer climate, emotional awareness, interpersonal problem-solving skills
	• schoolwide reinforcement strategies
• setting	• throughout elementary school starting in Grade 1
• values	• prevention
	• multidisciplinary
	• focused on the needs of high-risk populations (defined in terms of behavioral symptoms) rather than all children
2. Reasons	• prevention of conduct disorder
3. Actors	
• participants	• teachers, mental health professionals, parents of high-risk children
• implementors	• same
4. Replicability	
• reproducible	• manuals and materials available
• feasible	• resource intensive
5. Funding	• heavily supported by outside funding
6. Evaluation	
• process	• being evaluated as part of an experimental
• outcome	study of the effects of a five-part prevention program
• cost	on outcomes for children at high risk of behaviour problems on entry to kindergarten
	• other four components (offered to high-risk children only) are: parent training, home visiting, social skills training, academic tutoring

in their own schools between school processes and pupil outcomes. Graduates were followed up to assess whether they applied what they learned to change school processes and whether these changes benefitted students. The authors were able to show that many teachers who took the course made apparently enduring changes in their schools. Reynolds, Davie and Philips also provide evidence that student outcomes in program schools were superior to student outcomes in nonprogram schools. These results are suggestive, but it is important to note that the study design was

Table 11

Story 5: The Cardiff School Improvement Program, Reynolds, Davie, and Philips 1989

1. Actions	
• content	• teachers invited to take a school improvement course that taught them: what was known about effective school practices; how to evaluate their own school; how to implement change
• setting	• Cardiff, Wales, secondary schools
• values	• prevention
	• new forms of teacher professional development
	• participatory
	• multidisciplinary
2. Reasons	• creative way to address the lack of application and evaluation of knowledge from effective schools research
	• potential to reverse resistance created by top-down approaches
3. Actors	
• participants	• teachers and educators/researchers
• implementors	• teachers who completed the course
4. Replicability	
• reproducible	• yes
• feasible	• ?
	teachers spent one day per week at the course for two years
5. Funding	• supported by external funding that became available to address the lack of attention to effective schools research
6. Evaluation	
• process	• ?
	• more than half the participants generated institutional and organizational change in their schools
• outcome	• based on a before-after comparison of student outcomes in program and control schools attendance, high academic achievement and basic academic achievement were all better in schools where teachers had participated in the program
• cost	• ?

nonexperimental and that variations in student outcomes were small. However, the study does suggest that influencing the behaviour of the teachers has a lasting effect on their schools. Unfortunately, very little information is available about the content of the course and its effectiveness in improving teacher knowledge and skills. Also, the course requires teachers to attend a weekly university class for two years, which may not be feasible in many settings. However, enhancing teachers' skills with information about effective school practices and teaching them to conduct needs assessments in their own school warrants further attention and evaluation.

Lessons Learned

Five lessons emerge from these stories. The first lesson is that no single approach guarantees school improvement. It is better to use a range of approaches, including strategies to support development of changes and strategies that prespecify the changes to be made in school and classroom practices. Process-oriented approaches include school management systems and professional development for teachers. Prespecified interventions focus on specific age groups or milestones and, therefore, their content depends on the timing of intervention.

The second lesson is that a multidisciplinary approach to intervention design and evaluation is needed to recognize cognitive and noncognitive school goals and bring together educators, mental health professionals and researchers. One of the main reasons that there are so few studies that meet the needs of this position paper is that collaboration between educators, mental health professionals and researchers has been the exception rather than the rule. The studies that included these types of collaborative partnerships have yielded the most useful evidence on the relationship between school and classroom practices and academic achievement, and behavioral, emotional and social functioning.

The third lesson concerns the feasibility and replicability of the interventions. Interventions that do not depend on the enthusiasm or special expertise of the original developers are needed to avoid intervention failure in the developers' absence. Moreover, in the long term, simple, inexpensive strategies that fit into school routines are more likely to be sustainable and become systematized than expensive approaches that require radical changes to school routines and philosophies.

The fourth lesson is that it is better to use a participatory approach to school improvement. The individuals who will implement the changes should be involved in decisions about intervention design and implementation. This permits a process of mutual adaptation in which individuals learn how the intervention works and how to fit the proposed changes into local conditions, beliefs and values.

The fifth lesson concerns the role of evaluation in policy and practice. Our current knowledge of school improvement is limited. To avoid promoting changes that will not improve the school, a promising intervention should be systematically implemented and evaluated in collaborative experimental studies.

POLICY IMPLICATIONS

Principles to Guide the Actions of Governments— "Elements of Best Practice"

Analysis of the studies produces nine principles or "elements of best practice."

The first principle, prevention, means that a high priority should be given to interventions designed to prevent problems.

The second principle is that, because cognitive and noncognitive outcomes are linked, interventions should target both cognitive and noncognitive functioning of children.

The third principle is that interventions must be multidisciplinary, that is, based on collaboration between educators, mental health professionals and researchers.

Fourth, interventions that target school and classroom processes that are under the daily control of the principal and teachers are promising targets for school improvement. For example, interventions that focus on schoolwide expectations for academic achievement and conduct, including teacher consensus on curriculum and values; improved instruction practices, such as time spent on lessons, record keeping and feedback; and enhanced opportunities for student responsibility. These are promising methods to improve student academic, behavioral, emotional and social outcomes.

The fifth principle is that school improvement interventions must be sensitive to local needs and interests. School improvement strategies will vary according to the documented needs of students, schools and teachers.

The sixth principle is that school improvement strategies are more successful when participants are involved in decisions regarding intervention design and implementation.

The seventh principle is that interventions must not require the skills, expertise and enthusiasm of their developers. This will minimize the risk of intervention failure and increase long-term sustainability.

The eighth principle is that ideal interventions are systematized and do not require extra or external resources.

The ninth and final principle is that policy changes should be evaluated. Coordination of effort and collaboration between educators, mental health professionals and researchers is needed for rigorous and timely evaluations of school improvement interventions.

The available knowledge provides principles to inform action at the local, regional and national level. These principles will be most useful if they are applied in the following sequence: local needs assessment and intervention design; implementation; evaluation, including multisite collaboration when appropriate; and establishment of systems that monitor student outcomes and meet the information needs of schools.

The School Improvement Cycle

The School Improvement Cycle, shown in figure 1, identifies five school improvement steps that can be applied at the local, regional or national level.

Figure 1

The school improvement cycle

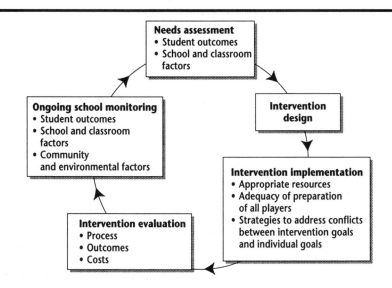

Needs assessment – School improvement interventions should be based on needs assessment conducted at the school level. Information on cognitive and noncognitive student outcomes is necessary. Subgroup differences in student outcomes should be examined. The relationship between school priorities and student outcomes should also be assessed.

Intervention design – Each school board and each school can use what is known about school and classroom processes to identify the procedures required in their situation. Schools can then develop strategies that meet local needs and conditions, and are financially feasible.

Intervention implementation – To be successful, programs must have appropriate resources. The individuals involved in the intervention must be adequately prepared and the strategies must be applied effectively to address conflicts between individual goals and intervention goals.

Evaluation – Evaluations of intervention processes, student outcomes and costs should be developed and carried out along with the intervention. Evaluation needs will vary according to the type of intervention and local issues. However, given the current lack of knowledge about what works to improve schools, collaborative efforts to evaluate the most promising school improvement strategies are necessary.

Ongoing school and student monitoring – Student outcomes, school and classroom processes, and community and environmental factors should be monitored. Methods are available to inform the development and implementation of these monitoring systems (Willms 1992).

Facilitating Factors and Barriers to Change

School improvement strategies depend on facilitating factors and barriers to change among individuals and organizations. In the process of self-analysis and change, top-down approaches should be balanced by efforts to build commitment among players at all levels (Reynolds, Davie, and Philips 1989; Scheerens and Creemers 1989; Roger 1990). As Creemers and Scheerens (1989) and Peck and colleagues (1993) point out, more attention to initiation and maintenance of the change process is needed.

The Role of Evaluation in Policy and Practice

Changes to policy and practice must be evaluated. The widespread adoption of new ideas, such as the change from phonics to whole language in the teaching of reading, must be accompanied by appropriate evaluation to determine whether expectations for program effectiveness are reflected in student outcomes (Lewington 1996).

The coordinated efforts of educators, mental health professionals and researchers are now needed to gather evidence about what works. For example, the most promising school improvement approaches could be implemented and evaluated in sites with a demonstrated need and desire for school improvement. The identification of research-oriented schools would permit partnerships between educators, mental health professionals and researchers, and would demonstrate the leadership that can be provided by the education and mental health professions. A coordinated, multi-disciplinary approach that builds leadership and knowledge will be more effective than many programs of uncertain effectiveness and cost being applied with little communication or exchange of ideas, experience and data.

Incentives to develop such partnerships should be provided by the appropriate levels of government. Schools and school boards probably cannot implement the steps of the School Improvement Cycle with their existing resources. However, forming partnerships and supporting the development of simple methods or "templates" that are universally applicable are attainable goals, if the necessary incentives and resources are made available.

CONCLUSION

School attendance affects every child. Evidence suggests that schools can be a force for good and reduce the risk to children of mental health problems and poor life quality. However, schools can also diminish potential and increase risk through poor school and classroom practices. There is tremendous opportunity to build on current knowledge and strengthen the capacity of schools to exert a positive influence on the development of children and youth. Progress toward this goal requires the coordinated efforts of educators, mental health professionals and researchers in the design and implementation of new programs, and a recognition of the fundamental role of research and evaluation in policy and programming decisions.

Kathryn J. Bennett, *M.Sc., is an assistant professor in the Department of Clinical Epidemiology and Biostatistics at McMaster University. She is a core member of the Centre for Studies of Children at Risk, Hamilton Health Sciences Corporation and McMaster University, and director of the McMaster International Clinical Epidemiology Training Program. Her research interests focus on school readiness and the design and evaluation of programs to prevent emotional and behavioral problems in elementary school children. She is funded by an Ontario Mental Health Foundation research training award.*

BIBLIOGRAPHY

ANDERSON, C. S. 1985. The investigation of school climate. In *Research on Exemplary Schools*, eds. G. R. AUSTIN and H. GARBER. London: Academic Press. pp. 97–126.

AUSTIN, G. R., and H. GARBER. Eds. 1985. *Research on Exemplary Schools*. London: Academic Press.

BENNETT, K. J. 1996. The predictive accuracy of preschool predictors of externalizing behaviour disorders in young children: Symptoms and contextual variables. Manuscript in preparation.

BERRUETA-CLEMENT, J. R., L. J. SCHWEINHART, W. S. BARNETT, A. S. EPSTEIN, and D. P. WEIKART. 1984. *Changed Lives: The Effects of the Perry Preschool Programs on Youths through Age 19.* Yipsilanti (MI): High/Scope.

BOYLE, M. H. 1994. The prevention of maladjustment among young children: Helping Children Adjust—A Tri-Ministry Study. Working paper, Inaugural Symposium, Centre for Studies of Children at Risk, McMaster University, May 1994.

BOYLE, M. H., D. R. OFFORD, Y. RACINE, C. CUNNINGHAM, and J. HUNDERT. 1990. Helping Children Adjust: A Tri-Ministry (Education, Health and Community and Social Services) Project. (Grant proposal available from the author.)

BOYLE, M. H, D. R. OFFORD, H. G. HOFFMANN, G. P. CATLIN, J. A. BYLES, D. T. CADMAN, J. W. CRAWFORD, P. S. LINKS, N. I. RAE-GRANT, and P. SZATMARI. 1987. Ontario child health study: I—Methodology. *Arch. Gen. Psychiatry* 44: 826–831.

BROOKOVER, W. B., C. BEADY, P. FLOOD, J. SCHWEITZER, and J. WISENBAKER. 1979. *Social Systems and Student Achievement: Schools Can Make a Difference.* New York (NY): Praeger.

BRYK, A. S., and S. W. RAUDENBUSH. 1988. Toward a more appropriate conceptualization of research on school effects: A three-level hierarchical linear model. *Am. J. Educ.* 11: 65–108.

CAUCE, A. M., J. P. COMER, and D. SCHWARTZ. 1987. Long-term effects of a systems-oriented school prevention program. *Am. J. Orthopsychiatry* 57: 127–131.

COLEMAN, J. S., E. Q. CAMPBELL, C. J. HOBSON, J. MCPARTLAND, A. M. MOOD, F. WEINFELD, and R. L. YORK. 1966. *Equality of Educational Opportunity.* Washington (DC): U.S. Government Printing Office.

COMER, J. P. 1980. *School Power.* New York (NY): Free Press.

_____. 1985. The Yale–New Haven Primary Prevention Project: A follow-up study. *J. Am. Acad. Child Adolesc. Psychiatry* 24: 154–160.

_____. 1988. Educating poor minority children. *Scientific American* 259: 42–48.

CONDUCT PROBLEMS PREVENTION RESEARCH GROUP. 1992. A developmental and clinical model for the prevention of conduct disorder: The FAST Track Program. *Dev. Psychopath.* 4: 509–527.

EDMONDS R. 1979. Effective schools for the urban poor. *Educational Leadership* 37: 15–24.

FELNER, R. D., and A. M. ADAN. 1988. The school transitional environment project: An ecological intervention and evaluation. In *Fourteen Ounces of Prevention*, eds. R. H. PRICE, E. L. COWEN, R. P. LORION, and J. RAMOS-MCKAY. Maryland (MD): American Psychological Association. pp. 111–122.

FELNER, R. D., M. A. GINTER, and J. PRIMAVERA. 1982. Primary prevention during school transitions: Social support and environmental structure. *Am. J. Comm. Psychol.* 10: 227–240.

GOOD, T. L., and J. BROPHY. 1986. School effects. In *Handbook of Research on Teaching*, ed. M. WITTROCK. New York (NY): MacMillan. pp. 570–602.

GOOD, T. L., and R. S. WEINSTEIN. 1986. Schools make a difference: Evidence, criticisms and new directions. *Am. Psychologist* 41: 1090–1097.

GOTTFREDSON, D. C., L. G. HYBL, G. D. GOTTREDSON, and R. P. CASTENEDA. 1986. *School Climate Assessment Instruments: A Review.* Boston (MA): Centre for Social Organization of Schools, Johns Hopkins University.

GRAY, J. 1981. Towards effective schools: Problems and progress in British research. *Br. Educ. Res. J.* 7: 59–69.

GRAY, J., A. F. MCPHERSON, and D. RAFFE. 1982. *Reconstructions of Secondary Education: Theory, Myth and Practice Since the War.* London: Routledge and Kegan Paul.

HINSHAW, S. P. 1992. Externalizing behaviour problems and academic underachievement in childhood and adolescence: Causal relationships and underlying mechanisms. *Psychological Bull.* 111: 127–155.

INSTITUTE OF MEDICINE. 1994. *Reducing Risks for Mental Disorder: Frontiers for Preventive Intervention Research.* Washington (DC): National Academy Press.

KASEN, S., J. JOHNSON, and P. COHEN. 1990. The impact of school emotional climate on student psychopathology. *J. Ab. Child. Psych.* 18: 165–177.

JENCKS, C. S., M. SMITH, H. ACLAND, M. J. BANE, D. COHEN, H. GINTIS, B. HEYNS, and S. MICHELSON. 1973. *Inequality: A Reassessment of the Effects of Family and Schooling in America.* London: Allen Lane.

LAZAR, I., R. B. DARLINGTON, H. W. MURRAY, and A. S. SNIPPER. 1982. Lasting effects of early education: A report from the consortium for longitudinal studies. *Monog. Soc. Res. Child Dev.* 47, nos. 2–3.

LEWINGTON, J. 1996. Schools mix old, new for literacy. *Globe and Mail,* 22 February.

LOCHMAN, J. E., and CONDUCT DISORDERS PREVENTION RESEARCH GROUP. 1995. Screening of child behaviour problems for prevention programs at school entry. *J. Cons. Clin. Psychol.* 63: 549–559.

LOHFELD, L., Y. RACINE, B. BOYLE, and J. HUNDERT. 1994. Helping Children Adjust—A Tri-Ministry Project: Implementation and continuation of the Classwide Social Skills Program (CSSP). Available from the authors.

MADAUS, G. F., T. KELLGHAN, E. A. RAKOW, and D. J. KING. 1979. The sensitivity of measures of school effectiveness. *Harvard Ed. Rev.* 49: 207–230.

MAUGHAN, B. 1988. School experiences as risk/protective factors. In *Studies of Psychosocial Risk: The Power of Longitudinal Data,* ed. M. RUTTER. Cambridge: Cambridge University Press. pp. 200–220.

MCGEE, R., D. SHARE, T. E. MOFFITT, S. WILLIAMS, and P. A. SILVA. 1988. Reading disability, behaviour problems and juvenile delinquency. In *Individual Differences in Children and Adolescents: International Perspectives,* eds. D. H. and S. B. G. EYSENCK. London: Hodder and Stroughton. pp. 158–172.

MORRIS, S., W. PAWLOVICH, and D. MCCALL. 1988. *Evaluating the Effectiveness of School Drop-Out Pre-vention Strategies: Some Suggestions for Further Research.* Toronto (ON): Canadian Education Association.

MORTIMORE, P., P. SAMMONS, L. STOLL, D. LEWIS, and R. ECOB. 1988. *School Matters.* Berkeley (CA): University of California Press.

———. 1989. A study of effective junior schools. *Int. J. Educ. Res.* 13: 753–768.

OFFORD D. R. 1987. Prevention of behavioral and emotional disorders in children. *J. Child Psychol. Psychiat.* 28: 9–19.

OFFORD, D. R., and K. J. BENNETT. 1994. Outcome and intervention in conduct disorder. *J. Am. Acad. Child Adolesc. Psychiatry* 33: 1069–1078.

OFFORD, D. R., and M. JONES. 1993. After the demonstration project. Unpublished manuscript available from the author.

OFFORD, D. R., M. H. BOYLE, P. SZATMARI, N. I. RAE-GRANT, P. S. LINKS, J. A. BYLES, D. T. CADMAN, J. A. BYLES, J. W. CRAWFORD, H. MUNROE-BLUM, C. BYRNE, H. THOMAS, and C. A. WOODWARD. 1987. Ontario child health study. II. Six month prevalence of disorder and rates of service utilization. *Arch. Gen. Psychiatry* 44: 832–836.

PATTERSON, G. R. 1986. Performance models for antisocial boys. *Am. Psychologist* 41: 432–444.

PECK, C. A., G. C. FURMAN, and E. HELMSLETTER. 1993. Integrated early childhood programs: Research on the implementation of change in organizational contexts. In *Integrating Young Children with Disabilities into Community Programs*, eds. C. A. PECK, S. L. ODOM, and D. D. BRICKER. Baltimore (MD): PH Brookes. pp. 187–205.

PURKEY, S. C., and M. S. SMITH. 1983. Effective schools: A review. *Elem. School J.* 83: 427–452.

RACINE, Y., D. OFFORD, M. BOYLE, and I. BORDIN. 1995. *Teenage Dropout and Young Adult Unemployment: Findings from the Ontario Mental Health Supplement.* Centre for Studies of Children at Risk Working Paper.

RALPH, J. H., and J. FENNESSEY. 1983. Science or reform: Some questions about the effective schools model. *Phi Delta Kappan* 5: 689–694.

RAUDENBUSH, S. W. 1990. New evidence in the search for effective schools. *Am. J. Educ.* 7: 175–183.

REYNOLDS, D. 1985. *Studying Effective Schools.* London: Falmer.

REYNOLDS, D., R. DAVIE, and D. PHILIPS. 1989. The Cardiff Program: An effective school improvement project based upon school effectiveness research. *Int. J. Educ. Res.* 13: 801–813.

ROGERS, E. M. 1990. *The Diffusion of Innovations.* New York (NY): The Free Press.

RUTTER, M. 1974. Emotional disorder and educational underachievement. *Arch. Dis. Child* 49: 249–256.

———. 1983. School effects on pupil progress: Research findings and policy implications. *Child Dev.* 54: 1–29.

———. 1989. Isle of Wight revisited: Twenty-five years of child psychiatric epidemiology. *J. Am. Acad. Child Adolesc. Psychiatry* 28: 633–653.

RUTTER, M., J. TIZARD, and K. WHITMORE. 1970. *Education, Health and Behaviour.* London: Longmans.

RUTTER, M., A. COX, C. TUPLING, M. BERGER, and W. YULE. 1975. Attainment and adjustment in two geographical areas, I—The prevalence of psychiatric disorder. *Brit. J. Psychiatry* 126: 493–509.

RUTTER, M., J. TIZARD, W. YULE, P. GRAHAM, and K. WHITMORE. 1976. Isle of Wight studies, 1964–1974. *Psychological Medicine* 6: 313–332.

RUTTER, M., B. MAUGHAN, P. MORTIMORE, J. OUSTON, and A. SMITH. 1979. *Fifteen Thousand Hours: Secondary Schools and Their Effects on Children.* Cambridge (MA): Harvard University Press.

SCHEERENS, J., and B. P. M. CREEMERS. 1989. Conceptualizing school effectiveness. *Int. J. Educ. Res.* 13: 691–704.

SCHONFIELD, I. S., D. SHAFFER, P. O'CONNOR and S. PORTNOY. 1988. Conduct disorder and cognitive functioning: Testing three causal hypotheses. *Child Dev.* 59: 993–1007.

SLAVIN, R. 1987. Ability grouping and student achievement in elementary schools: A best evidence synthesis. *Rev. Ed. Res.* 57: 293–336.

STEVENSON, J., N. RICHMAN, and P. GRAHAM. 1985. Behavioral problems and language abilities at three years and behavioral deviance at eight years. *J. Child Psychol. Psychiat.* 26: 215–230.

SYLVA, K. 1994. School influences on children's development. *J. Child Psychol. Psychiat.* 35: 135–170.

U.S. DEPARTMENT OF HEALTH, EDUCATION AND WELFARE. 1975. *Dropout Prevention.* Washington (DC): Education Resources Information Centre. (ERIC Document Reproduction Service no. ED 105 354).

WEHLAGE, G. G., R. A. RUTTER, G. A. SMITH, N. LESKO, and R. R. FERNANDEZ. 1989. Dropping out: Can school be expected to prevent it? In *Reducing the Risk: Schools as Communities of Support.* London: Falmer Press. pp. 28–47.

WILLMS, J. D. 1992. *Monitoring School Performance: A Guide for Educators.* London: Falmer Press.

WRIGHT, R., and D. OFFORD. 1992. Secondary schools demonstration project: Literature review on dropping out. Manuscript available from the authors.

Creating Healthier Work Environments: A Critical Review of the Health Impacts of Workplace Change

MICHAEL F. D. POLANYI, M.A.

Institute for Work & Health

JOAN EAKIN, PH.D.

Department of Public Health Sciences
University of Toronto

JOHN W. FRANK, M.D., CCFP, M.SC., FRCP(C)

Institute for Work & Health
Department of Public Health Sciences
University of Toronto

HARRY S. SHANNON, PH.D.

Institute for Work & Health
Department of Clinical Epidemiology and Biostatics
McMaster University

TERRENCE SULLIVAN, PH.D.

Institute for Work & Health
Department of Sociology
York University

SUMMARY

Organizational change (OC) strategies can help to create healthier work environments. However, there are a number of barriers to OC. Therefore, much can be learned from both successful and unsuccessful workplace change initiatives. In this paper, we draw from a detailed examination of the health impacts of OC efforts at a number of companies and agencies and suggest opportunities for, and barriers to, improving the health of workers through OC.

Conventional forms of workplace health promotion (WHP), occupational health and safety (OHS), and OC interventions have made some gains in improving health in the workplace, yet each approach has limitations. WHP has focused on individual lifestyle factors while largely ignoring the ways working conditions contribute to such factors. OHS has traditionally emphasized the reduction of toxic exposure and physical demands and only recently started to deal with the effects of workplace organization and its psychological demands on health. OC has been primarily oriented toward improving productivity and has treated workers' health, if at all, as merely a means to that end.

In recent decades, the demands of work have been changing rapidly, and reductions to the burden of work-related illness and injury in Canada have stalled. New approaches may be required to make further improvements to workers' health. There is a need to integrate WHP, OHS and OC efforts to more fully address the organizational determinants of health.

In this paper, we a) outline various work-related determinants of health; b) describe and critically assess OC strategies implemented at a number of companies and organizations; c) discuss implications for future actions to improve workplace health; and d) suggest policies supportive of healthier work environments. Interventions examined include improving employee relations (through training, education and conflict resolution), redesigning and enlarging jobs, and changing organizational structures (e.g., increased participation).

The implications of the interventions are discussed, including the determinants of health, the desired health outcomes and the outcomes achieved, and the lessons learned. Despite some apparent mutual benefits of organizational changes for both management and labour, the attempts to improve workplace health through OC appear to have been limited. Likewise, some barriers to health-enhancing OC are discussed, including the collective bargaining environment, legislative framework, government policy, and market conditions.

We make a number of recommendations relevant to parties in the work-site, researchers, and government. In particular, we point to the importance of participative interventions that jointly address individual lifestyle, job and organizational factors. We suggest that researchers can play an important role in evaluating the effectiveness of interventions. And we recommend that governments promote joint action by the various constituencies that are working to improve workplace well-being (e.g., unions, business, and public health and social planning councils) and create conditions that encourage firm-level actions to improve workers' health.

TABLE OF CONTENTS

LIST OF TABLES

CONTEXT: THE CHANGING WORK ENVIRONMENT AND WORKERS' HEALTH[1]

Since the start of this century fatality rates in most industrialized workplaces have decreased substantially (Workplace Health and Safety Agency 1994), a result in part of occupational health efforts. However, in the United States, since about 1950 the gains in workplace health, as measured by injury rates, absenteeism, benefit use and mental health indicators, have been limited (Robinson 1988). Employers' Workers' Compensation (WC) costs as a percentage of payroll have more than doubled since 1960, totalling more than $57 billion in 1993 (Burton 1995). The situation in Canada is similar. Claim rates for lost time resulting from injury remained relatively constant between 1979 and 1987, and direct costs associated with injuries tripled in constant dollars (Labour Canada 1990). In 1994, there was one compensation claim for every 13 workers, amounting to direct medical costs of more than $250 per person (Association of Workers' Compensation Boards of Canada 1995) and perhaps twice as much again in indirect costs to society, associated with, for example, replacement, training, lost productivity, and indemnity benefits.

As the physical demands of heavy manual labour and the toxicity of work environments appear to be decreasing, we should expect to see continued improvements in workplace health indicators. Why is this not happening? Part of the answer may be that as the bulk of work shifts from the manufacturing to the service sectors, new physical and psychosocial demands of work are appearing, as a result, in part, of new technologies and the demands for higher productivity associated with increasingly intense global economic competition. More and more, it is recognized that the psychosocial conditions of work play a role in occupational health and safety (OHS).

New strategies are needed to reduce the heavy human and economic burden of workplace illness and injury. We believe that some organizational change (OC) strategies not usually explicitly linked to health outcomes, such as communication and problem-solving training, job enlargement and redesign, and participatory decision-making approaches, may offer a fruitful path to healthier workplaces. This belief is based on the idea that improving the health of individuals requires changing the social and economic conditions under which people live. This was the central message of the Ottawa Charter on Health Promotion (World Health Organization 1986). Recently, proponents of frameworks for health promotion and population health have called for greater attention to the underlying social determinants of health, such as income distribution, employment and social support

---

1. The sections "Workplace Determinants of Health," "The Impact of Efforts to Improve Workers' Health," and "Selection of Case Studies" draw extensively on Polanyi et al. (in press).

(Frank 1995; Labonte 1995). Likewise, further improvements to worker health may require addressing fundamental social and psychological determinants of physical and mental health at the job and firm levels.

There have been attempts to improve health through OC, but few such interventions have been rigorously evaluated. This suggests a number of questions: What are the various OC strategies to improve health? How successful have they been? What are the facilitating factors and the barriers to improving employee health through such approaches? What strategies are suited to what settings? By reviewing a selection of some of the better-documented studies of workplace intervention, we grapple with these and other questions, with the objective of recommending policies and practices to effectively improve workplace health.

WORKPLACE DETERMINANTS OF HEALTH[2]

A number of factors can cause workplace injuries and illness (see table 1). The physical work environment and the conditions and hazards of jobs remain relevant. However, many believe that the social and psychological conditions of work are becoming increasingly important as firms strive to cut costs and increase output. Social, psychological and physical conditions all typically stem from company-level decisions that are in turn constrained by the social, economic and policy environment. Therefore, strategies to improve these conditions need to address the determinants of health both inside and outside workplaces.

Individual Lifestyle Factors

Individual workers' characteristics, nonwork stressors, and personal resources seem to be related to injury and disability rates. Sometimes, however, studies of such factors fail to control adequately for the different levels of physical and psychological hazards of jobs in which workers of some types tend to be overrepresented. For example, a recent study of rates of soft tissue injury among Canadian construction workers showed only a slightly increased risk to younger workers (contrary to the findings of several previous studies), once the type of job on the construction site was controlled for (Rael 1992).

Events in outside life clearly generate stress among workers. For example, a 1992 survey of 5,000 Canadian employees found that 77 percent of workers have child care or elder care responsibilities and that these employees report more stress and higher absenteeism (Canadian Aging Research Network n.d.). Personal characteristics, the presence of various personal

---

2. See Polanyi et al. (in press) for a fuller discussion of workplace determinants of health.

Table 1

Determinants of health in the workplace

Level of determinant	Sub-level of determinant	Factors related to worker health
External/societal	Sectoral	Structure of business, technology
	National, global	Government labour and economic policies, economic competition, technological change
Organizational structure and environment	Terms of employment	Salary, hourly pay or pay by piecework (benefits, shift work), safety incentives for managers and employees, job security (and turnover)
	Decision making structures	Employee participation in decision making
	Approach to health and safety	Commitment to health and safety factors (structure, support of management)
	Physical environment	Lighting, noise level, toxic exposures, air quality, etc.
	On-site facilities	Fitness, daycare
Task requirements	Physical and psychosocial demands	Job content (lifting, turning, repetitive movements), equipment used, pace and load of work, job control, range of skills used, social support
Individual lifestyle	Basic characteristics	Age, gender, marital status, health and injury history, smoking, obesity, socioeconomic status, education, language ability
	Nonwork demands	Child care and elder care needs
	Personal resources	Education, coping skills, family and social support

resources, and supportive social or community programs can mediate these stresses and the absenteeism related to ill health (for further discussion of personal characteristics, see Ivancevich et al. 1990).

Job Factors

Karasek and Theorell (1990) developed a model of "job strain" by integrating job control and job demands. They summarized a number of studies, showing that "the most adverse reactions of psychological strain (fatigue, anxiety, depression, and physical illness) occur when psychological demands are high and the worker's decision latitude in the task is low" (Karasek and Theorell 1990, 32–33). In this way, the pace and volume of work, the repetitiveness of tasks and the range of skills used are all related to health outcomes. More recently, social support has been considered a buffer of psychological strain (Johnson and Hall 1988). Organizational factors, such as level and method of remuneration and quality of benefits, level of worker participation in decision making, management approach to OHS issues, and overall management philosophy concerning workers and their well-being, have all been found to be related to health and safety in the workplace (Karasek and Theorell 1990; Shannon et al. 1996; Shannon et al. 1997). However, it should be noted that the relationships established between organizational factors and health outcomes are correlations only, making it difficult to infer causality. As in all workplace research, it is difficult to control for all the factors at play or even to hold enough factors constant to assess the relative importance of various psychosocial variables. As well, most research is done on men, for whom perceived control may be a more important contributor to well-being than it is for women (Heaney 1993). Finally, the mechanisms through which psychological strain affects health remain largely unexplained, though numerous clues are now available from psychoneuroimmunology and -endocrinology (Evans et al. 1994).

Organizational Factors at Unit or Firm Level

In most past and present societies, health status has been related to wealth, income or social status (Hertzman et al. 1994). Because an individual's income is closely linked to his salary, the level of pay an employee receives is likely related to health status. As suggested above, the method of pay is also relevant. For example, the influence of piecework on rates of injury is frequently debated, and employees who work shifts may have higher accident rates (Karasek and Theorell 1990). From a set of detailed studies of British civil servants, it is also clear that being higher in the organization's hierarchy is associated with better health (Marmot and Theorell 1988; Evans et al. 1994). Stress levels also appear to increase with fears of income (or job) loss (Karasek and Theorell 1990).

Worker participation, both generally and in health and safety decision making, is evidently correlated with reduced WC lost time frequency rates (Shannon et al. 1996). Greater participation has also been found to be related to lower alienation, superior mental health (Rothschild and Russell 1986), and improved job satisfaction, morale, and level of performance (Rubenowitz et al. 1983). Miller and Monge's (1986) review of 47 studies found that participation has a positive effect on job satisfaction and, to a lesser extent, productivity. Again, determining the direction of causality in the studies reviewed, many of which are cross sectional, is problematic. Moreover, the link between job satisfaction and physical and mental health also remains unclear.

Senior management's involvement in health and safety and the ability of organizations to solve their occupational health conflicts internally, without outside party involvement, tend to be related to lower rates of lost time resulting from injury (Shannon et al. 1997). Companies that tie managers' appraisals and incentives to health and safety also have better safety records (Shannon et al. 1992).

Firms with older workers, longer seniority and lower turnover have been found to have lower accident rates (Shannon et al. 1992). And, in a recent review (Shannon et al. 1996), modified work provision and some physical environment variables—good housekeeping and safety controls on machinery—were also found to be significant factors.

External (Community, Regional, National, and Global) Influences

Over the past two decades, the international movement in capital and goods has expanded. Firms have been faced with increased competition and the need to increase productivity, flexibility and innovation. Some management theorists argue that worker satisfaction and autonomy are therefore increasingly crucial to the economic success of companies in industrialized countries (Levering 1988). Competitiveness is seen to be based on the creation of flexibility, skill and motivation in the workplace (Verma and Irvine 1992). A recent review found that employee participation and training, and a progressive management and organizational structure, increased productivity and profits (Mavrinac et al. 1995). Mainstream health promoters agree and often suggest that healthier workers are more productive.

However, some companies have ostensibly sought to increase worker control and recognition but have, if anything, increased job demands and further alienated workers (Robertson 1993). Critics of free trade and globalization argue that the drive for competitiveness is undermining worker rights and leading to a deterioration of working conditions. Firms seek to reduce costs and increase flexibility by cutting wages and laying off full-time staff (those who tend to be unionized and have better pay and benefit packages) and by contracting out work to workers who have less job security and less control over their working conditions and remuneration. In Canada between 1975 and 1993, the number of part time jobs expanded at three times the rate of full-time jobs (Roberts et al. 1995). In 1989, 35 percent of the workforce was made up by "contingent workers" (part time, seasonal or self-employed) who typically have less job security, lower pay and fewer fringe benefits (Roberts et al. 1995). Similarly, two out of three new private-sector jobs in the United States are temporary, and 25 percent of U.S. jobs are now temporary, part-time or contract jobs, at pay levels 20–40 percent less than those of full-time workers doing comparable work (Rifkin 1995, 191). While union rates in Canada have remained relatively stable (contrasting with declining rates in the United States, United Kingdom and Australia), the expansion of the largely nonunion service sector, as well as enduring high unemployment rates, is shifting the balance of power to employers. Increased government debts have resulted in cuts to income support and social programs, exacerbating workers' fears of job loss (another factor reducing workers' and unions' bargaining power). One-third of Canadian workers feel their jobs are insecure (Angus Reid Group, Inc. 1995), which probably causes widespread stress and the potential for adverse health effects.

Perhaps both these trends (firms investing in workers and the deterioration of work conditions) are taking place, and the question is which one is predominant. In any case, the good and bad effects on workers' health are becoming apparent. Policies to promote workforce health are needed to take into account these broad and fundamental transformations.

THE IMPACT OF EFFORTS TO IMPROVE WORKERS' HEALTH

Efforts to improve health in the workplace have traditionally fallen under the categories of OHS and workplace health promotion (WHP). There have also been many OC interventions, although the vast majority of these are focused on economic objectives and have not been used primarily (or even explicitly) to improve workers' health. We will briefly review the strategies, impacts, lessons and limitations for each of these three types of interventions (see table 2 for a summary).

Occupational Health and Safety

OHS has been primarily concerned with the protection of health: to reduce the physical and chemical hazards of the work environment and to reduce work-related injury, illness and disability resulting from hazardous job demands.

OHS involves a variety of preventive measures, such as improved personal protection, and the modification of machinery, equipment and work practices, as well as curative and rehabilitation services (Rantanen 1995). Over the past 25 years, OHS has achieved a number of things. Work-related fatalities have been significantly reduced, and exposure to toxic substances has been reduced through improved occupational hygiene, knowledge of hazardous materials, and legislation giving workers increased ability to control their work environment. The more flagrant occupational health hazards associated with heavy manufacturing, while not disappearing, are affecting fewer people. In Western industrialized countries, however, safety gains have levelled off. New technologies and possibly more insidious

Table 2

Strategies to improve health in the workplace

Strategy	Stimulus	Goals	Examples	Impact	Possible limitations
Conventional OHS[a]	Physical hazards of heavy industrial labour	Reduce toxicity of environment Reduce physical demands of work	Industrial hygiene Modification of equipment and practices Protection OHS legislation	Reduced exposure to unsafe work; decline in number of fatal accidents	Need to address psychosocial factors
Conventional WHP[b]	Management: high absenteeism and benefit costs Health professionals: attractions of workplace as site for health education	Reduce individual risk of illness through education, skills development, and support programs	Fitness programs Smoking cessation courses Counselling Weight-reduction programs	Short-term improvements in individual health-related behaviour for some workers in some workplaces	Need to address organizational-level factors
Conventional OC[c]	Desire to improve productivity	Reduce workplace inefficiency and promote the quality of working life Increase worker participation in decision making	Job redesign Job rotation Worker participation Supervisor training	Productivity gains in some sectors	Need to broaden goal to include health outcomes

[a]OHS, occupational health and safety; [b]WHP, workplace health promotion; [c]OC, organizational change.

health problems are arising, such as those associated with the use of video display terminals, violence in the workplace, and "sick building syndrome." Soft tissue injuries, many of which may be associated with computer keyboarding, now make up almost half of all workplace injuries in Canada (Statistics Canada 1994). Finally, psychological and psychosocial problems are playing a larger role as demands for worker productivity increase (Rantanen 1995). As argued in a recent World Health Organization document on occupational health, OHS must pay "more attention to the control of psychosocial aspects of work including the prevention of work stress" (Rantanen 1995, 51).

Workplace Health Promotion

The majority of WHP programs are designed to encourage healthier individual behaviour by providing support and information, and by developing skills. Programs commonly focus on fitness, cardiopulmonary resuscitation, nutrition, stress reduction, weight control, counselling for alcohol and drug abuse, and smoking cessation. Organizational interventions tend to be limited to establishing nonsmoking policies, improving nutrition in cafeteria food, and setting up fitness facilities (Polanyi et al. in press).

A number of studies show the effectiveness of WHP programs in smoking cessation and the control of blood pressure, although the effect on other lifestyle factors is less certain (Bertera 1990; Fielding 1990; Baker and Green 1991). Stress management programs have been found to have moderate effectiveness (Murphy 1988). Many corporate program evaluations are anecdotal, short term and cross-sectional, making it difficult to determine causality (Warner 1988). A review of recent interventions concluded that the weight of the evidence indicated that there are positive, if inconsistent, health effects of WHP programs but that "even the 'better' outcome studies have significant limitations that preclude conclusive statements about whether the health promotion program *caused* the observed changes" (Rush 1995, 39; emphasis in the original).

One of the few WHP models designed to integrate individual lifestyle, safety and organizational factors is Health Canada's Workplace Health System (WHS) (Health and Welfare Canada 1991), which is currently implemented through the Corporate, Small Business and Farm Business Health Models. The Corporate Health Model has been implemented by about 95 Canadian companies. The WHS takes the important step of broadening the focus of WHP by identifying and seeking to improve health practices and personal resources, as well as enhancing physical and psychosocial conditions in the workplace. Results from a nationwide process evaluation of the Corporate Health Model are expected soon (see Macdonald et al. 1994). Preliminary discussions suggest that the vast majority of WHS interventions have been focused on the individual lifestyle level and that there are a number of barriers to organizational-level change. For example, decision makers in many organizations do not believe that the psychological and social environment of the workplace affects employees' health or even productivity, morale and absenteeism (Preece and Weber 1995). Initiating and sustaining WHS interventions seems to be a major challenge because of widespread public sector cutbacks, the lack of the demonstrated effectiveness of the WHS program, and the belief that government should not subsidize employees' health programs, which are seen as the responsibility of employers.

While there is some evidence of short-term changes in individual behaviour and even improvements in economic performance as a result of WHP, the approach has a number of serious limitations. First, it hardly deals with the "roots" of human motivation and behaviour: the social and economic determinants of health emphasized in the Ottawa Charter on Health Promotion and elsewhere (see, for example, Gerstein et al. 1991). Second, even if individual lifestyles can be successfully changed, health outcomes may not necessarily be improved, as health status is powerfully influenced by factors other than lifestyle (Evans et al. 1994). Even after controlling for lifestyle differences, there is still a significant gradient in health outcomes across occupational hierarchy (Marmot and Theorell 1988). Third, behavioral changes tend to be short term, when not accompanied by changes to the social and cultural context that shapes individual behaviour. Fourth, WHP programs seem to be reaching only a limited and unrepresentative groups of workers. WHP programs have tended to focus on large, profitable, white-collar workplaces (Hollander and Lengermann 1988), largely ignoring small workplaces, which employ about one-third of the total workforce and tend to have higher rates of injury and ill health (Eakin and Weir 1995). Finally, a focus on individuals' lifestyles may be simply a self-serving effort of competitive companies to reduce the costs of health care benefits as much as possible, without addressing deeper, job-related and organizational factors influencing health.

Properly developed WHP programs, as discussed above, can have a short-term impact on individual health-related behaviour and status. However, OHS and WHP programs have only peripherally addressed the psychosocial impacts of job, organizational and social conditions. Indeed, this criticism is now acknowledged by many, and a number of writers have recommended that programs to change behaviour, such as stress management training, only be used when the causes of stress cannot be removed or reduced (Murphy 1988; Ganster 1995).

Finally, some have called for an integration of OHS and WHP, although this does not yet seem to be taking place in Canada (Eakin and Weir 1995).

Organizational Change

The broad field of OC developed in the 1940s and 1950s in response to mass automation and specialization (and alienation) of assembly line "Taylorism" (Landsbergis et al. 1992). OC is a mostly top-down approach focusing either on "human processes" or "technostructural change" (Neuman et al. 1989). Human processes OC seeks to improve human functioning by changing attitudes and perceptions, through training, goal setting, increased participation, team building, and feedback (Neuman et al. 1989). The U.S. Quality of Working Life movement initiated in the 1950s is an example of this approach. The "technostructural" approach aims to change structures by altering work content, methods and relationships through job redesign, job enrichment, "flextime" (e.g., working an extra hour the first four days of the week and getting Friday afternoons off), and other organizational changes (Neuman et al. 1989). Scandinavian work reform initiatives of the 1960s and 1970s, action research approaches to OC that grew out of the World War II work of Kurt Lewin, and "sociotechnical" systems are all in this school.

OC interventions have largely focused on improved productivity and employee job satisfaction and have generally not investigated the impact (direct or indirect) of such interventions on workers' health. Metanalyses have found that OC (Neuman et al. 1989) and job redesign (Kelly 1992) have moderate effects on job satisfaction, but job satisfaction is a contested and culturally dependent construct that has not been clearly linked to health outcomes (see, for example, Jackson 1983, Wall et al. 1986). Neuman et al. (1989) also found that initiatives to improve employee relations had a more positive effect on workers' attitudes than did structural OC. Macy et al.'s (1989) review revealed that interventions to increase employee participation improved the quality of work life and enhanced mental health by fostering employee autonomy, responsibility and material well-being. Schurman and Israel (1995) held that the OC interventions of the 1970s increased job satisfaction, but these interventions were focused mostly at the task level; diffusion to the whole organization often failed. Ganster (1995) suggested that the evidence that job control and job demands are related to health outcomes is mixed at best but that the impact of social support is potentially more important. A recent review showed that according to 17 of 25 studies there is a significant correlation between job control and cardiovascular disease but that only 8 of 23 found job demands to be a significant predictor (Schnall et al. 1994). Finally, a survey of 15 Canadian companies engaged in significant participatory OC suggested that substantial reductions in accidents, injuries and absenteeism resulted in most firms (Premier's Council on Economic Renewal 1993).

Some of the common barriers to successful OC mentioned in review articles include lack of management support, lack of participation in the process, employees' fear of job loss, and failure to create organizational-level reward systems and to delegate authority (Neuman et al. 1989; Karasek and Theorell 1990; Karasek 1992; Landsbergis et al. 1993; Premier's Council on Economic Renewal 1993; Schurman and Israel 1995). Some of these are discussed below in reference to our case studies.

In general, there is a lack of convincing, even partly controlled inter-vention studies of organizations (Ganster 1995), and few attempts have been made to integrate theoretical models with empirical evidence (Macy et al. 1989). This is partly explained by the difficulty of carrying out experimental research in complex workplace environments. Researchers need to move beyond the narrow range of dependent variables usually considered (job satisfaction, motivation, attendance) to include industrial relations, attitudes, grievances, stress, accidents and health (mental and physical) (Wall and Martin 1987). Some of these are intermediary outcomes: their links to actual health outcomes need to be better demonstrated. Clearly, there is a need to classify and assess the health impacts of well-evaluated OC initiatives. Also needed are qualitative studies to explicate the functioning mechanisms of the determinants of workplace health and to generate further hypotheses. While difficulties will always arise in reaching clear-cut conclusions in research in nonlaboratory (workplace) settings, some studies have been well evaluated and do hold lessons for improving health in the workplace. We turn to these studies below.

SELECTION OF CASE STUDIES

We have chosen to critically assess selected case studies for a number of reasons. Few reviews to date have pulled together and compared intervention studies from across the many relevant disciplines (occupational health, behavioral science, management studies, safety research, etc.). No matter how sound one's theoretical framework, OC is a challenging and unpredict-able process, so it is important that we try to learn from past efforts. Finally, such a review uncovers a number of barriers and aids to success, which we hope will hold lessons for practitioners and policymakers.

We have limited our selection of cases to interventions that were designed to change a) employee relations; b) job or task requirements; or c) organizational structures. We have excluded interventions primarily focused on changing individual behaviour because of our emphasis on creating healthier workplaces and because of the inherent limitations (discussed above) of interventions targeted to individual behaviour. We have excluded interventions intended to directly change the external or policy environment. We have limited our cases to industrialized countries to achieve greater applicability to the Canadian setting. We searched for interventions that deal with small and nontraditional workplaces (e.g., those involving work at home).

We chose not to include studies that measured only intermediate psychosocial outcomes (such as job demand, job control and social support) because of the lack of a clear causal relation between such indicators and employees' health (see above). Finally, because of the vastness of the productivity-oriented literature, we have not sought to systematically explore the effects of interventions on productivity, instead deciding to limit our efforts to providing some selected discussion.

To get the best access to case studies, we drew on our contacts working in fields related to organizational change and health. We received information from more than 60 researchers, health professionals, company and union representatives, and OC consultants (see appendix C). We searched a number of databases and libraries at the Institute for Work & Health, Canadian Centre for Occupational Health and Safety, Ontario Ministry of Labour, and the Labour databases.[3] We collected only reports in English.

We have categorized our examples in two groups (Groups A and B). Our primary group (Group A) includes descriptions of interventions that have a convincing evaluation component; that is, they

a) use pre- and postintervention tests and comparison groups to assess intervention outcomes;

b) analyze health outcomes, including one or more of the following:
   – rates of work-related injury;
   – absence resulting from sickness or injury;
   – mental health indicators (e.g., burnout, emotional strain, depression);
   – physical health indicators (e.g., gastrointestinal disorders, headaches); and
   – health-impacting behaviour (e.g., smoking, drinking); and

c) use study methods that are credible and clearly described, drawing on a number of cross-disciplinary theories.

We found 11 studies that met the criteria. Their outcomes and implications are discussed later.

Group B includes a number of studies that did not have clearly described or convincing evaluation designs but had thoughtful descriptions of the strengths and weakness of the intervention process. The insights of these 15 studies are also discussed later.

It should be noted that the majority of the studies were derived from the academic literature. While many company and organizational representatives were contacted, few could provide material that offered sufficient

---

3. ABI Inform, Employee Benefits Information, National News Index, Management Contents, Trade and Industry, Legal Resources Index, Newsearch, Labor Law, Public Opinion Online, Delphis, European Business, and BNA Daily.

insight into the process or outcomes of OC initiatives to be useful here.[4] We have included some discussion of two such reports (Dicken 1993; Premier's Council on Economic Renewal 1993), which concern changes at companies in the United Kingdom and Canada, respectively.

DESCRIPTION OF GROUP A CASE STUDIES

Drawing on Neuman et al. (1989) and Karasek (1992), we classified our cases according to three target levels of interventions: interpersonal relations, task requirements and organizational structure (see table 3). Karasek (1992) described the various levels as follows: interventions targeting interpersonal relations are intended to improve mutual support and reduce conflict between employees without necessarily changing organizational structures and processes of production; task-level interventions are intended to increase workers' skills and decision-making latitude within their jobs; and organizational structure interventions are intended to change the organizational, political and technical context of workers' tasks. Interventions are classified according to the broadest level addressed in a given project.

Table 3

Levels of intervention

	Intervention	Examples of strategies
Level I:	Interpersonal relations	Supervisor training, conflict resolution, communications training
Level II:	Task requirements	Job redesign, job enlargement
Level III:	Organizational structure	Job sharing, semiautonomous teams, gain sharing

Some of the characteristics of the cases are described in table 4. The majority of cases were from the United States. The manufacturing sector was best represented, although there were examples from the service sectors, as well as hospitals and government agencies. There was a good spread across levels of intervention. We discovered few Canadian studies evaluating the health impacts of OC. We also found that most published and readily accessible unpublished evaluations of interventions took place in large, unionized workplaces.

---

4. It was beyond the scope of this project to document oral stories of OC initiatives; however, we suggest the need to do this in the future

Table 4

Summary of case characteristics

Characteristic	Group A: accepted cases (*n*)	Group B: suggestive cases (*n*)
Country	United States, 7; United Kingdom, 3; Sweden, 1	United States, 8; Canada, Finland, Japan, Netherlands, South Africa, Sweden, United Kingdom, 1
Sector	Manufacturing, 6; hospitals, 1; governments, 1; mining, 1; service, 1; unspecified, 1	Manufacturing, 8; service, 2; governments, 2; hospitals, 1; mining, 1; unions, 1
Firm size	<100 employees, 0; 100–500 employees, 4; >500 employees, 1; "large" firms, 4; unspecified, 1	<100 employees, 1; 100–500 employees, 2; >500 employees, 5; "large" firms, 5; "small" firms, 1; unspecified, 2
Level of intervention[a]	Level I, 2; Level II, 1; Level III, 8	Level I, 3; Level II, 5; Level III, 7

[a]Level I, interpersonal relations; Level II, task requirements; Level III, organizational structure.

OUTCOMES OF GROUP A CASE STUDIES

The outcomes of the interventions are summarized in table 5. Further information is provided in tabular form in appendix A.

It is impossible to generalize about the quantifiable effectiveness of specific strategies from the small number of case studies above that met all our inclusion criteria. However, it is of use to describe briefly the nature of each intervention, the outcome achieved, and the implications. It should be noted that none of these studies represents a perfect experiment.

Engstrom et al. (1995)

Engstrom et al. assessed an attempt to combine "cost-effectiveness" and "better working conditions" through the development of a "parallel-flow" production process in the Uddevalla Volvo plant in Sweden. This initiative grew out of a "vaguely formulated agreement between management and unions" (Engstrom et al., 295). Under parallel-flow design, small autonomous teams work in parallel to build the whole automobile, thus reducing the amount of repetitive work found in traditional short-cycle, serial-flow assembly lines.

Table 5

Group A case outcomes

Author (year)	Level[a] and nature of intervention	Health outcome variables	Effects[b]
Engstrom et al. (1995)	Level III, production redesign	Psychological workload	+
Fiedler et al. (1984)	Level III, organizational development	Accident rate	–
	Level I, training	Accident rate	–
Frank and Hackman (1975)	Level II, job enrichment	Absenteeism	NC
Golembiewski et al. (1987)	Level III, organizational development	Burnout levels	–
Heaney et al. (1993)	Level III, PAR[c]	Worker stress	+
Jackson (1983)	Level III, participation in decision making	Emotional strain	–
		Absenteeism	+
Landsbergis and Vivona-Vaughan (1995)	Level III, organizational development and action research	Psychological and physical stress	NC
Pasmore and Friedlander (1982)	Level III, PAR[c]	Upper limb injuries	–
Wall and Clegg (1981)	Level III, autonomous work groups	Mental health	+
Wall et al. (1981)	Level II: job redesign	Strain	NC
Wall et al. (1986)	Level III: autonomous work groups	Mental health	NC

[a]Level I, interpersonal relations; Level II, task requirements; Level III, organizational structure.

[b]+, significant increase in particular health outcome variables; –, significant decrease; NC, no significant change.

[c]PAR, participatory action research.

The new production process was found to have better job control, stimulation and employee and supervisor relations than a more traditional and highly specialized assembly line at another Swedish Volvo plant.

However, compared with the traditional plant, the psychological workload at Uddevalla (measured in stress at work, fatigue after work, ability to take breaks, and mental strain) was higher. This unexpected result was attributed by the authors to the fact that in the new production method, the whole team fell behind if the assembly of a car encountered difficulty, thus requiring a subsequent increase in the pace of work to make up lost time. Engstrom et al. also noted that this higher load was "matched" by greater "influence on and control over work." Within the new Uddevalla plant, workers building both the subassembly and the body of the vehicle achieved the best productivity and quality output and worked under a better psychosocial climate.

The authors concluded that the new, parallel means of production illustrates the potential for creating more humane and productive working conditions. They argued that it may overcome some of the limitations of Japanese "lean production," which they saw as perpetuating many of the dehumanizing conditions (e.g., assembly line, short work cycles, standardized work methods, and hierarchical organization) associated with traditional mass production. They suggested that parallel production may also be beneficial in smaller plants that do not have the capital to develop "perfect design" processes and therefore need competency overlaps that allow workers to deal with minor design flaws.

This intervention raises the question of whether increasing productivity through greater worker control may also increase psychological strain. As control rises, so may responsibility, which in this case amounted to increased psychological demands.

Fiedler et al. (1984)

Fiedler et al. worked from a belief that management interventions to improve organizational climate and quality of working life are likely to impact positively on injury and accident rates. To assess this hypothesis, they initiated and studied the impact of interventions at two different mines in the United States. One intervention focused on supervisory training, the other on increasing the power of the safety manager and creating incentives for better safety performance. There were no formal control groups, and there were a number of potentially confounding factors (a new owner and changes to the management and production processes). Still, the potential is suggested for positive change through organizational development strategies targeting both individual relations and organizational structures. Supervisor training was less expensive than OC and had a greater effect on safety. The long-term sustainability of such efforts needs to be assessed.

Frank and Hackman (1975)

Frank and Hackman assessed the impact of a work redesign intervention in the stock transfer department of a large metropolitan bank. The intervention originated from the bank's corporate personnel department, which had detected signs of employee dissatisfaction and work inefficiency in the stock transfer department. A series of workshops were held for managers to divide the department into small teams, or "modules," that would be responsible for a full range of tasks. It was hoped that this would improve workers' identification with their jobs, strengthen their commitment to work, and increase the quality and quantity of output. Contrary to the expectations, employees whose jobs were supposedly enriched ended up having a smaller variety of skills, and poorer feedback from and interactions with other employees. Absenteeism rates were unchanged. However, although this is an example of a failed intervention, the jobs did not actually change. Work continued to be passed between modules, rather than completed within them, indicating a lack of autonomy of modules; the jobs were not given more significance (only reorganized); and work was not shared among all employees within each module, perhaps because of lack of training. Frank and Hackman suggested a number of underlying reasons why the job redesign was unsuccessful, including the time demands and lack of commitment from management and the failure to meet basic needs of employees (e.g., pay, supervision and job security). This case suggests that documenting the actual implementation of OC is important if one is to properly assess the outcomes of a given strategy.

Golembiewski et al. (1987)

Golembiewski et al. assessed the impact of "high-stimulus" organizational development (staff-management meetings and the introduction of a new career advancement plan) to deal with high levels of employee burnout in a human resources department. They found a 25 percent reduction in the number of employees at high burnout levels (based on the Maslach Burnout Inventory), as well as a 45 percent reduction in departmental employee turnover and some improvement in measures of satisfaction with the working environment. This suggests that facilitated processes of employee-supervisor interaction can be effective, although in this case this pertained only to particular employees, those with an "active mode of adapting." Interestingly, this is measured using a work environment scale that assesses the extent to which employees function independently of their supervisors. In this case, then, organizational-level factors (specifically, employee participation and control) moderated the success of more traditional organizational development interventions.

Heaney et al. (1993)

Heaney et al. described results from a five-year project in participatory action research (PAR) aimed at reducing the deleterious effects of occupational stress at an automotive manufacturing plant (different aspects of the project are discussed below as a Group B case study; see Israel et al. 1989; Israel et al. 1992a, 1992b; Schurman and Israel 1995). Israel et al. (1992a, 78) explained that they chose an action research approach because it emphasizes "establishing a coequal and interdependent relationship between researchers [and] its long-term intent is to transfer ownership and control of the process to employees themselves."

Heaney et al. (1993) compared the impact of the PAR intervention after the one plant at the project's start split into two plants with very different employee-management relations (one "cooperative," one "adversarial"), providing a natural experiment. Management and union selected 26 "key union and management decision makers," including "influential hourly and salaried representatives from the shop floor," to work with the university researchers on a Stress and Wellness Committee (SWC). Based on a plant-wide survey and their own insider knowledge, the SWC identified four priority problem areas: lack of information, communication and feedback; problems with supervisors; lack of influence in decision making; and conflicts between meeting quantity production demands and meeting quality production demands. Specific recommendations, including the development of a newsletter to improve communications, training in problem-solving techniques and enhanced performance evaluations, were submitted to management and union leaders. Many of the recommendations were accepted by the leaders, but few were implemented. Attempts were made to overcome this inaction by increasing management involvement, which proved difficult, according to the authors, perhaps as a result of management's lack of understanding of the SWC goals (and hence defensiveness on their part) and their preoccupation with production-related problems. Finally, it was decided that management and union leaders needed to go through a learning process similar to the one the SWC members had engaged in. At an all-day joint meeting, management and union leaders "observed that the problems SWC members had identified as creating stress and health problems were the same problems they (the leaders) had identified as causing quality and production problems" (Schurman and Israel 1995). After this meeting, management and the union agreed to take over leadership on the four problem areas identified by the SWC. Since then and after the research project ended, a corporate-wide quality program has been developed, based on many of the SWC recommendations (Schurman and Israel 1995).

Despite the significant actions taken to address the causes of stress in the workplace, Heaney et al. (1993) did not find a measurable change in the level of workplace depressive symptoms, and, surprisingly, employees involved in the project in the more cooperative plant had more depressive symptoms and those involved in the adversarial environment had fewer.

Jackson (1983)

Jackson's study is often cited as one of the few experimental assessments of the impact of increased participation. Six months after the introduction of more frequent staff meetings at a hospital outpatient facility, she found reduced role conflict and ambiguity, which in turn reduced emotional strain. Emotional strain was, surprisingly, inversely related to absenteeism. This outcome must lead us to question the use of absenteeism rates as a direct proxy for health and may be explained by the fact that those experiencing high strain may have felt less able to be absent (Jackson 1983, 16), perhaps as a result of their occupational status or fear of job loss. The fact that no effect was found after three months indicates that effects build over time and that excessively short studies may miss them.

Landsbergis and Vivona-Vaughan (1995)

Using a sophisticated design and data analysis, Landsbergis and Vivona-Vaughan provided a careful interpretation of the mixed effects of action research that were hinted at by the some of the other studies. In a large public health agency, physicians noted that many clinical symptoms seemed to be stress related. Management asked the authors to develop a program for individual stress management; however, researchers proposed a pilot PAR project, since the source of stress appeared, at least in part, to be organizational. In addition, it was felt that increased participation in the process of change would avoid the "pitfalls and limitations" of previous OC efforts at the agency, which relied on surveys and written recommendations to management. Management and the union members (representing the majority of employees at the agency) agreed to the proposal. Employee representatives were elected to "problem-solving committees" in two departments, which "identified and prioritized aspects of work organization and job design causing stress among their fellow employees" (Landsbergis and Vivona-Vaughan 1995, 35). The committees were aided by a workplace survey carried out by the consultants. The committees "developed proposals and action plans, provided feedback to other employees and encouraged and assisted management in implementing changes" (Landsbergis and Vivona-Vaughan 1995, 35). The top areas of concern included uneven and repetitive workload leading to underuse of skills; poor communication about policies and procedures; inadequate space, filing system, and computer data; and performance appraisals. Some of the changes implemented by management included drafting of a new policy and procedures manual; more even distribution of work and more task variety; more regular staff meetings;

changes in filing processes; and a quiet hour without phone calls for employees.

Despite all these actions, the intervention had only a mixed impact on the psychosocial work environment in one department, a negative impact in the other, and no direct health impact in either department. As noted by the authors, this outcome was disappointing, although the short duration of the intervention (less than a year), small sample sizes (limiting the ability to detect small changes), and the exclusion of a number of psychometric scales may have hindered the detection of an impact. Interestingly, despite the lack of measurable benefits, more than two-thirds of the employees in the two departments involved felt the program should be replicated in other departments. Perhaps some important perceived benefits were overlooked. The authors extensively discussed the obstacles to success: the lack of communication between committees and other departments; the limitation of the intervention to the department level (rather than its being agency-wide); the short duration of the intervention; and the negative impact of an agency reorganization without significant employee or union participation (Landsbergis and Vivona-Vaughan 1995). They also mentioned the lack of formal involvement of unions (such as through a collective agreement) and cutbacks in government support for occupational stress and health programs as other barriers.

Pasmore and Friedlander (1982)

Pasmore and Friedlander explored the role of action research in creating significant changes in labour-management relations in general and in reducing injuries in particular. They were asked by a manager at an electronics plant in the midwestern United States to explore the increasing prevalence of injuries in the arm and hand muscles of employees carrying out repetitive tasks. Based on suggestions from managers, researchers set up a Studies and Communications Group (SCG), made up of employees from each department with different attitudes to management (including some who had experienced the injury). The SCG carried out interviews and a survey. From the results, the SCG developed a list of 61 recommendations that emphasized continued biomechanical adjustments of equipment; the continuation of the SCG as a sounding board for management plans; a new employee-management methods redesign group; and foreperson training. The article was unclear about what actions actually took place in these areas. While limited data are presented in the article and a number of confounding factors were present (new technology, management turnover, change in biomechanical processes of work), there were very significant reductions in the levels of "soreness" and injury after the project started. This seems to suggest a strong potential of action research for reducing injuries at work.

Wall and Clegg (1981)

Wall and Clegg evaluated the introduction of semiautonomous work groups in a department of a partly unionized U.K. confectionery firm that was characterized (by both labour and management) as having "low morale," "poor shop floor–management relations," and "poor work attitudes." The intervention steps included meetings with management and shop floor employees to agree to a project framework, administration of a survey, recommendations for work redesign, establishment of a steering committee to carry out redesign, and two follow-up surveys to assess short- and long-term changes. Work redesign involved integrating production and packaging so that two permanent, leaderless teams participated in the full production process; increasing the autonomy of teams; and establishing group feedback. The authors found a link between group work redesign and enhanced group identity and autonomy, as well as improved work motivation, job satisfaction, performance, labour retention, and mental health (no traditional clinical outcomes were included in this measure). Interestingly, changes in job satisfaction and mental health were much slower to appear than changes in perceptions of job characteristics and performance, suggesting that long-term evaluations are required to capture the full range of effects of such interventions.

Wall et al. (1986)

Wall et al. sought to assess the long-term impact of autonomous work groups on employees' attitudes and behaviour. The authors wanted to see whether increased job control present in such work groups enhanced work motivation, job satisfaction, group performance, and mental health. Their setting was a large, nonunionized U.K. confectionery company whose management, being committed to increasing responsibility on the shop floor, wanted to try new methods of working that better capitalized on the skills of their workers in the design of a new factory. Small groups were given control of training, job allocation, supervision and production functions and charged with meeting quality and output requirements. When compared with nonequivalent control groups at another factory, those working in autonomous groups had higher perceived autonomy, job satisfaction and organizational commitment, yet there was no impact on job motivation or mental health.

Wall et al. (1990)

Wall et al. studied the effects of training operators at an electronics company to handle more technical problems themselves (at the same pay). There were improvements in productivity and job satisfaction, but there was no reduction in strain or improvement in psychological well-being. This reasserts that psychological outcomes are not a simple function of job or task attributes.

IMPLICATIONS OF GROUP A CASE STUDIES

As indicated, it is impossible to draw conclusions about which level of strategy or which specific strategy is most effective on the basis of our small and selective sample of written studies. Indeed, no one strategy is likely to work all the time, as the context of each workplace is so particular. Still, the 11 intervention studies described above provide a number of lessons for decision makers seeking to create healthier work environments (see table 6).

Inherent Barriers to Organizational Change

OC in workplaces is complex, slow and rather unpredictable in its effects. The case studies reviewed show the potential benefits of job changes and OC and also their risks (Frank and Hackman 1975; Engstrom et al. 1995). There will often be unpredictable factors that hinder (or sometimes support) change, such as turnover in management (Fiedler et al. 1984), the relocation (and thus curtailed participation) of key project participants (Landsbergis and Vivona-Vaughan 1995), or concurrent overall agency reorganization (Landsbergis and Vivona-Vaughan 1995). Hierarchical organizations in which employees carve out their own niches and territories can lack the flexibility to change (Pasmore and Friedlander 1982), and managers will often be resistant to flattening of their organization (Wall and Clegg 1981). This is one reason why implementing OC for improved health may be far easier in a new plant (Wall et al. 1986). In the end, OC can cause more harm than no action at all, by raising and dashing expectations and by exacerbating conflict and self-interest (Landsbergis and Vivona-Vaughan 1995).

The Context: Employee Characteristics, Workplace Culture, Industrial Relations and the Macroeconomy

Different approaches to change may work for different personalities, such as those using active or passive coping strategies (Golembiewski et al. 1987), and it may even be impossible to bring about change until basic employee needs are met (Frank and Hackman 1975).

OC needs to be tailored to the characteristics of specific workplaces (see Eakin 1992), such as the cultural background of employees, the size and structure of the workplace, and the relations between employees and management (e.g., Fiedler et al. 1984).

Finally, the macroeconomic situation is important: a climate of global competitiveness and economic rationalization, OC is often associated with the reengineering exercises of downsizing, which create employee resistance

Table 6
Issues Identified in Group A case studies

Case	Inherent barriers to OC[a]	Context	Individual-, task-, and firm-level interventions	Participation	Management support	Union-employee support	Role of research
Engstrom et al. (1995)	✓		✓				
Fiedler et al. (1984)			✓	✓			
Frank and Hackman (1975)	✓	✓	✓	✓	✓		✓
Golembiewski et al. (1987)		✓					
Heaney et al. (1993)	✓	✓	✓	✓	✓		✓
Jackson (1983)	✓						✓
Landsbergis and Vivona-Vaughan (1995)		✓	✓	✓		✓	
Pasmore and Friedlander (1982)	✓			✓			
Wall and Clegg (1981)	✓						✓
Wall et al. (1986)	✓	✓					
Wall et al. (1990)			✓		✓		

[a]OC, organizational change.

(Landsbergis and Vivona-Vaughan 1995; Engstrom et al. 1995). The drive for competitiveness may hinder companies' willingness to make changes not definitely related to health, reduce the resources they have to give to such changes, and limit the demands from employees for improvements to their working conditions. The lack of government funding for health-enhancing OC efforts in the private sector was also noted in a U.S. study of a public health agency (Landsbergis and Vivona-Vaughan 1995).

Individual-, Task-, and Organizational-Level Interventions

The limitations of change focusing on individual worker's lifestyles were discussed above, yet such interventions still have a role to play. Not every kind of stress can be removed at its source. If the approach is to be participatory, which is important if real OC is the goal (see below), then there needs to be an openness to the full range of interventions desired by parties in the workplace. Healthy individual lifestyle programs were, interestingly, an intervention desired by the workplace committee in an action research project at a U.S. automobile plant, despite the reservations of the researchers (Heaney et al. 1993). Action research projects with extensive worker participation may be a means to increase the effectiveness of programs to improve individual lifestyles by removing the "blame-the-victim" flavour. Still, at least five of the case studies presented here suggest that programs directed at changing lifestyles alone are insufficient to create a healthy work environment, as the success of training programs is linked to the active or passive nature of the work environment (Golembiewski et al. 1987), and the frequency of leadership turnover suggests the need for "the creation of new structures that can sustain processes of change after key managers or union leaders leave (Schurman and Israel 1995).

It seems generally agreed that helping workers manage stress is insufficient to create a healthy work environment. While effecting OC is seen as challenging and probably is more difficult than individual lifestyle interventions, there are benefits. Indeed, even supervisory training and conflict resolution may fail without OC (Golembiewski et al. 1987; Heaney et al. 1993).

All the implications of an OC cannot be known, such as the side effects on jobs adjacent to those targeted (Frank and Hackman 1975). Thus, the more substantive and lasting changes may be those implemented throughout the organization (Landsbergis and Vivona-Vaughan 1995).

Participation

A frequent refrain was the need for early, wide and significant employee and management participation in interventions. Communication between project participants and the broader workplace population is important

(Landsbergis and Vivona-Vaughan 1995). Participation is, by definition, key to action research projects (e.g., Heaney et al. 1993), but strong participation also often leads to sustainability (i.e., an organization's capacity to maintain changes over time on their own) (e.g., Landsbergis and Vivona-Vaughan 1995). Fiedler et al. (1984) mentioned the importance of training as many employees as possible.

Participation is important for the success of the interventions, but it is also beneficial in and of itself. Much learning takes place through participation (Frank and Hackman 1975; Heaney et al. 1993), and the cooperative problem-solving process helps to sustain long-term OC (Pasmore and Friedlander 1982). Participation is also related to lower stress levels, as stress is related to one's ability to deal with the demands of one's job (Pasmore and Friedlander 1982). OC seems to create less psychological strain among top management than among other workers, perhaps because many managers have a greater sense of control over the process of change.

There are a number of barriers to participation. Workers under increased stress may lack (or not make) the time to become involved in projects if they are not sure that they will have any effect, if they have competing demands, or if they lack buy-in to the change process (Heaney et al. 1993; Landsbergis and Vivona-Vaughan 1995).

Management Support

Projects need the involvement and commitment of top management. This can be difficult because change often means extra work for management (Frank and Hackman 1975) and may challenge the existing distribution of authority (Wall and Clegg 1981). Clearly, the support of those with power in any given workplace is important. That is why the need for participation of top management is so often mentioned. Landsbergis and Vivona-Vaughan (1995) suggested, for example, "responsibility mapping" by top management early in the change effort to institutionalize the process. The extent to which employee-employer relations are adversarial is also a factor mitigating against the successful implementation of projects (Heaney et al. 1993; also see below).

Union-Employee Support

Some argue that the presence of a union is a critical support to OC at work. The unions are important because they often keep the focus on organizational factors such as workplace stress and ill health (Landsbergis and Vivona-Vaughan 1995). In the automobile plant project, "plant-level union representatives provided the stability, support, and continuity that allowed the project to survive high levels of managerial turnover" and "discourage[d] any attempt by management to scuttle the effort" (Schurman and Israel 1995).

Role of Research and the Difficulty of Doing Scientifically Conclusive Workplace Research

It would be helpful if there were more truly experimental (controlled) studies of interventions to improve our understanding of what actions are likely to bring about healthier workers under what circumstances. Unfortunately, "completely convincing," rigorously controlled studies are virtually impossible and probably would reflect an unusual setting even if they were accomplished. The development of "healthy organization" indicators requires further work, as even seemingly straightforward indicators such as absenteeism and job satisfaction are not unambiguous indicators of health (for one attempt see National Institute for Occupational Safety and Health 1996). Indicators such as WC claim rates and requests for health information may relate to organizational factors but also obviously reflect the influence of many other factors.

Particular trade-offs are made between carrying out rigorous experimental research and facilitating work site led interventions, as clearly elucidated by Heaney et al. (1993, 508):

> An experimental or quasi-experimental design would allow for stronger, more certain causal inferences. However, it is virtually impossible to use designs that utilize comparison groups when evaluating PAR [participatory action research] projects. A PAR process unfolds according to the needs and values of employees and according to the organizational context. An appropriate comparison group would have to be a worksite with similar needs and values and context. Even if such a worksite could be found, it would be difficult to engage it in a protracted data collection agreement if there would be no payoff in terms of intervention. In addition, even if two worksites were well matched at the beginning of the study, it is unlikely they would experience the same organizational events and changes over time.

Even comparing departments within one firm is problematic (Heaney et al. 1993). Given the importance of general participation in interventions for OC, keeping some workers in the dark about an intervention may create distrust and opposition to future participation, especially if the pilot intervention is perceived as being successful (Trist et al. 1977).

Thorough qualitative research can provide rich and credible descriptions of the processes (and perceived health impacts) of OC in workplaces. These descriptions can complement and help overcome the limitations of quantitative workplace research (Steckler et al. 1992; Holman 1993).

A point on which observers disagree (depending in part on their disciplinary and scientific framework) is whether researchers should be closely involved in the workplace and the intervention or maintain a more distant "objectivity." Pasmore and Friedlander (1982) suggested that close interaction between researchers and workers can help the development of accurate hypotheses and build trust, a prerequisite of worker openness. Moreover, involved researchers can better describe the process of change, which is as important to planners of interventions as the outcomes are. Heaney et al. (1993) showed that researchers' involvement in the workplace does not preclude a thorough and self-critical evaluation of process and outcome. However, it is important that researchers resist playing so central a role that the sustainability of an intervention depends on their involvement, which is likely to be time limited. This points to the need to develop methods to create and evaluate change that does not rely on researchers.

Others argue that externally led evaluations are important to ensure that the research does not reflect vested interests of researchers in the success of interventions they have helped initiate. The institutional autonomy of university-based researchers can be important in this regard. Researchers have a special role to play in helping those involved in action research projects to be self-critical and in facilitating a process of planning and evaluation based on a theoretical framework (Frank and Hackman 1975).

Just as multilevel interventions seem to have the most impact on health, mixed-design research seems to be the most informative. Quantitative measures seem important for assessing the impact of interventions in a standard and comparable way, but qualitative research tells us much more about the nature and mechanism of the impacts achieved by interventions (Schurman and Israel 1995).

INSIGHTS FROM GROUP B CASE STUDIES

A number of lessons can also be drawn from the Group B case studies (see appendix B for a list of studies). OC is perceived as difficult, and thus some workplace actors prefer interventions more on the microlevel (Chihara et al. 1992). Inherent resistance to OC is acknowledged, as is the potential for unforeseen ill effects (Trist et al. 1977) that may cause management to return to old decision-making practices, thus undermining the change initiative (Hugman and Hadley 1993). Broad participation, consultation and the presence of champions are all believed to be needed to ensure the relevance and effectiveness of change (Trist et al. 1977; Hugman and Hadley 1993; Premier's Council on Economic Renewal 1993; Preece and Weber 1995; Schurman and Israel 1995). The process of cooperation in its own right is thought to have positive effects on workplace relations and health and safety (Israel et al. 1992a; Saari 1992). However, it is recognized that participation and involvement are not easily achieved, because of workers' scepticism and distrust about reorganization efforts that are perceived as (and may be!) management-led downsizing efforts that threaten workers' interests (Hazzard 1992; Hugman and Hadley 1993; Murphy and Olthuis 1995). Workers may be suspicious of being involved in a joint project with management (Hazzard 1992) and may be seen by coworkers as "brown-nosing" if they do get involved (e.g., Trist et al. 1977). Gaining union and employee participation and commitment to change requires a demonstration of a company's commitment to improving the work environment (Premier's Council on Economic Renewal 1993), as well as training, goal setting, team building and feedback to help staff make the change toward a more participative operation (Hugman and Hadley 1993). Even employee relations changes may require changes at the higher organizational level. The lack of free time and incentives can hinder worker involvement in change efforts (May 1992; Schurman and Israel 1995). Hackman et al.'s (1978) finding that job enrichment will only be positive for those satisfied with the work environment underlines the fact that changing jobs without changing other working conditions may not improve the overall well-being of employees.

Management-union relations, as well as the level of unionization, are often mentioned. Unionization can increase bargaining power to bring about health-enhancing OC if such change is successfully negotiated (Landsbergis et al. 1992). However, inflexibilities and adversarial relations can hinder change, such as job rotation, which may improve workers' health in some settings (Hazzard 1992). Union and management need opportunities to assess separately the potential effects of OC (Trist et al. 1977). A simultaneous top-down and bottom-up approach to job redesign can allow employees the opportunity to design low-stress jobs and employers the opportunity to develop efficient and flexible operations (Terra 1995).

DISCUSSION

Below we discuss some of the common issues that arise from the body of intervention studies we have reviewed.

Determinants of Health Addressed and Those Not Addressed

The literature on health-enhancing workplace OC seems, on the whole, to contain a very narrow conceptualization of the important aspects of OC.

Some aspects of organizational structures and processes are looked at in the studies, while others are ignored. For example, a number of the studies listed focused on increasing participation and job control (particularly through more frequent staff meetings), enlarging job skills (through job redesign), and improving interpersonal interactions (through supervisor training and enhanced performance evaluations).

On the other hand, we found few efforts to address other work-related determinants of health, such as reducing the work pace, implementing more flexible and supportive (family-friendly) terms of employment (work hours, level of pay, overtime, benefits), increasing employee ownership, enhancing job security, or increasing social support. While some stories have been told about such efforts (e.g., Ontario Women's Directorate 1991; B. Mateer, General Electric [Bromont], personal communication, 26 March 1996), few of these efforts have been formally evaluated. They may also be less easily implemented in the current socioeconomic environment of increasing international competition, high unemployment, and the weak bargaining power of unions. It is nevertheless important to determine the extent to which such changes have been carried out and to assess the ways a firm's socioeconomic context constrains its choice of intervention. These are important questions that are rarely discussed in quantitative, outcome-oriented studies. In this regard, it is important that we explore the impact of both the balance of power among parties in the workplace and the ways options are shaped and limited by the way that workplace health issues are defined. For example, the vast majority of workplace research on musculo-skeletal disorders has revolved around physical demands, leaving aside the psychosocial factors. This is not the result of neutral, scientific decision making but an indication that research on OC has political implications and that research and intervention agendas are struggled over and negotiated among parties with sometimes conflicting objectives (see "Barriers to the Creation of Healthier Workplaces" for further comment).

Health Outcomes

Many of the organizational interventions looked at above seem to centre around mental health, aiming at reducing psychological strain. Only two (Pasmore and Friedlander 1982; Fiedler et al. 1984) connect organizational factors with physical injuries (accidents, strains and sprains). This could reflect a general perception that organizational conditions are "soft" factors, related to less serious health issues. However, the increased prevalence of occupational musculoskeletal disorders (e.g., repetitive strain injuries) dis-cussed above and the increasing evidence that psychosocial factors are related to the incidence of such disorders (Bongers et al. 1993) make it particularly important that the organizational context be considered in attempts to reduce accidents and injuries at work, as well as in efforts to improve mental health.

It is important to recognize that the etiology of many modern occu-pational health problems (such as soft tissue injuries and sick building syndrome) is disputed. These are not just scientific disputes but political conflicts between various groups with vested interests, wherein notions of causation are rooted in either the worker or the work, rather than in the interaction between the two (Frank et al. 1995).

Methods of Evaluation

The studies reviewed point to a paradox of workplace intervention evaluations. They seem either to be quantitative (e.g., assessing outcomes through the use of predetermined questionnaire constructs) or qualitative and process oriented (often offering in-depth descriptions of the process of intervention and the worker's or manager's perceptions of such changes). Both approaches are limited. It is important to try to measure the actual physical demands of jobs. However, psychosocial demands, which depend on the perceptions, beliefs and needs of employees, are far more difficult to quantify, and therefore in-depth, open-ended qualitative investigation is needed to understand to what extent and how an organization's psychosocial environment is influencing the health of its workers.

Attention is lacking in this literature to the overall process of the redesign of work. In fact, our ability to interpret some studies' outcomes is contingent on our knowing whether the intervention was carried out as intended. This is rarely investigated (only in a few studies cited here) and is a serious issue in evaluation research. Any conclusions about the degree of success of a given type of intervention must be highly tentative if we know little about what actually was changed. Another "black-box" study is of no use. More studies such as that of Heaney et al. (1993), which details the nature and texture of changes, are needed.

It is not only difficult to aim for adequately controlled experimental designs in organizational analysis but unrealistic. Typically, some organizational units in a workplace have reasons to ask for interventions or to invite research involvement to evaluate them. Often the unit is focused on more pressing problems. "Control units" are almost always noncomparable at baseline. Thus, the design is open to criticism from the very start because the "secular trends" of the outcomes are not necessarily expected to be the same across intervention and control settings. In this respect, workplace intervention researchers are not in the position of "experimental investigators" because they cannot control the allocation of the subjects to intervention or control groups. Calling research "quasi-experimental" does little to overcome potential threats to validity. Given this reality, in-depth documentation and analysis of the process of change are needed so that logical linkages between interventions and outcomes can be better discerned.

Finally, any attempt to evaluate the impact of change in an often polarized environment such as a workplace is by necessity a political endeavour. Employers, employees, unions, health professionals, government, and researchers may have conflicting stakes in the success (or failure) of an intervention. The measures chosen, the way that *health* and *illness* are defined, the factors examined, the sources of data, the duration of the evaluation, and numerous other issues can affect the results of the evaluation and may be subtly or overtly struggled over by parties in the workplace. For example, managers may want to include consideration of nonwork factors influencing workers' health, whereas unions may resist, perceiving the inclusion of such factors as an attempt to deny the work-relatedness of an injury or illness. While attempts can be made to reduce bias in evaluations, such bias can never be fully removed; thus, it is important that researchers understand and describe the political context and interests of various groups involved and consider how these influence their evaluation of the impacts of OC. The role, perceived affiliations and identity of an evaluator will also influence the results of the research—naiveté in this regard is unhelpful.

Generalizability of Studies

As related above, serious limitations are attached to making generalizable and conclusive causal statements regarding the impacts of specific sorts of OC in complex social setting like a workplace. One of the lessons of the studies is that there are no off-the-shelf approaches guaranteed to improve workers' health in a wide range of settings. Indeed, workplaces are idiosyncratic, complex, dynamic, and socially and politically shaped. The studies reviewed above deal with only a small and likely unrepresentative subsection of workers, who appear to work mostly in unionized, large work-places. Understandably, researchers find it easier to liaise with such organized environments, and they may feel that workers' interests will be automatically protected in the project if a union is present. The applicability, therefore, of such interventions to sites with different social, physical and demographic conditions (such as small workplaces and those of people who work at home, those in the service sector, and self-employed consultants) is questionable. It is not at all clear that a) the organizational determinants of health are even the same in such settings and b) strategies for intervention and change would or could be the same in such settings (see, for the case of small workplaces, Eakin 1992). There is the need, therefore, for further research in these settings and thoughtful examination of the differences across them.

BARRIERS TO THE CREATION OF HEALTHIER WORKPLACES

Firms function in a global, national, regional and sectoral context and face political, cultural, economic and legislative constraints. We have focused on firm-level interventions in this paper because we believe it is still unclear what interventions are truly capable of improving health in the workplace. Little of the literature we examined explicitly addressed the broader context in which OC is effected. However, two examples, one from the workplace stress arena and one from the OHS area, deserve mention.

A recent report of the former Ontario-based Workplace Health and Safety Agency outlined the potential benefits of "best practices" in workplace health and safety (Ignatieff 1995). Ignatieff argued, somewhat in line with us, that success in workplace health and safety requires employee involvement, positive labour relations, strong and committed leadership, integration with quality and high performance, evaluation and benchmarking, rewards systems, and training. Ignatieff recommended that the Ontario government support leadership and education efforts by representatives of companies with success in health and safety, develop "creative" enforcement mechanisms (e.g., contracts and advisory services, and training of chief executive officers), support education and training, and develop information tools (costing accidents and injuries; benchmarking guidelines).

Sauter et al. (1990) suggested workplace health-enhancing policies for the United States. The authors argued that the psychosocial aspects of jobs, unlike the physical, have received little attention from government agencies and industrial organizations. While recognizing that the interventions needed will vary, depending on the sector and type of organization, Sauter et al. called for the U.S. government to develop positive healthy workplace principles to guide the design of jobs, with the aim of improving the mental health of workers (see table 7).

While the results of the studies we have assessed are mixed, at least four of the cases offer some support for three of the work principles in table 7: work pace, content and participation (Wall and Clegg 1981; Pasmore and Friedlander 1982; Jackson 1983; Engstrom et al. 1995).

Government can play an important role in promoting health in workplaces by creating conditions that allow and encourage firms to make health-enhancing OC (e.g., offering incentives for better workplace health) and by enforcing minimum standards of workplace health (psychosocial as well as physical). A full review of the impact of policy-level interventions on health in the workplace (and beyond) is beyond the scope of this paper (Sullivan et al. 1997 [this volume] take a step in this direction). We do make some preliminary recommendations regarding government interventions in the workplace that are deserving of further study.

Firms do not engage in OC initiatives in a vacuum. Rather, firms function under strict social, political and economic constraints. Most obviously, the firms must be economically viable, that is, profitable. While we have seen some evidence that OC to increase job task diversity, job control, participative and team-based decision making and mutual support may be conducive to improving workers' health, the relationship of such OC to firm-level productivity has not often been explored. Undoubtedly, the perceived impact on productivity of such changes influences firms' willingness to invest time and energy into such areas.

As indicated in the section "Workplace Determinants of Health," a number of studies have found that participation in decision making at work is related to high productivity and the improved health of workers. If this is the case, then the enhancement of workers' participation, teamwork, and job enlargement would seem to offer benefits to both workers and

Table 7

Summary of healthy workplace principles

Aspect of job or organizational design	Characteristics
Workload or work pace	Physical and mental demands commensurate with worker capabilities and resource Allowance for recovery from demanding tasks Increased control over pace of work
Work schedule	Compatibility with outside demands and responsibilities faced by workers (e.g., opportunities for flextime, reduced workweek, job sharing) Shift work that is predictable and set in a forward (day-to-night) direction
Work roles	Clearly defined roles and responsibilities
Job future	Reduce ambiguities in job security and career development
Social environment	Opportunities for personal interaction for emotional and technical support
Content	Jobs that are meaningful and stimulating and give workers the opportunity to use their skills (e.g., job rotation and job enlargement)
Participation and control	Opportunities for workers to have input into decisions that affect jobs and performance of tasks

Source: Sauter et al. (1990).

management. Why, then, have new organizational approaches not been implemented more broadly? Why have there not been visible improvements in employees' health? And why have management, unions and workers in general continued to resist such OC?

Apparently, reorganization to increase job control and teamwork are not perceived as being simple win-win situations by either unions or management, and even where they are, there may be serious barriers to change. To see how this is the case, we consider briefly how the collective bargaining environment, the legislative framework, government policy and market conditions support or hinder firm-level attempts to address a fuller range of workplace determinants of health.[5] The implications for the role of government will be addressed.

---

5. Thanks go to Doug Hyatt at the Institute for Work and Health for his suggestions on the framework and content of this section.

Collective Bargaining

Collective bargaining has led to numerous gains in employees' health through firm-level and, occasionally, sector-level clauses limiting, for example, hazardous work and institutionalizing compensating wage differentials (although these gains may be reversed, as argued below, by increased competition with jurisdictions with lower health and safety standards). Nonunionized workers and those with weak unions lack the power to raise health and safety concerns. This may be particularly true in highly competitive markets. In addition, unions may trade off health concerns for gains in other areas, such as pay, benefits and job security.

Some labour legislation places strong limitations on a company's ability to negotiate with individual workers. The National Labor Relations Board in the United States recently ruled that some provisions aimed at increasing workers' participation in day-to-day shop floor decision making were illegal because they abrogated the union's right to negotiate on behalf of workers.

Finally, management often resists acknowledging that injuries and illnesses are related to psychosocial conditions in the workplace, for fear of opening themselves up to increased liability for illness or injury compensation.

Legislative Environment

Legislation influences firm-level decision making through both regulations and incentives. In Canada, the responsibility for legislation can be taken at the provincial or federal levels, or it is shared between two levels of government. In Ontario, for example, regulations function through both the internal system of responsibility (mandatory OHS committees) and external regulations, such as the Occupational Health and Safety Act (which establishes the right to know about potential workplace hazards, the right to participate in decision making about health and safety, and the right to refuse unsafe work), employment standards legislation, and compensation standards in the Workers' Compensation Act. Incentives can operate through taxes and the experience-based rating systems, pegging workers' compensation rates to past-injury experiences.

There are clear indications that legislation has promoted health and safety in many workplaces. For example, health and safety committees have provided an opening for increased consultation, particularly in workplaces where workers are not represented. Recent research in Ontario suggests that mandatory joint health and safety committees have reduced workers' compensation claims by as much as 17 percent (Lewchuk et al. 1995).

Economic Policies

Current corporate-restructuring initiatives tend to be reactive, taking place when a company is on the brink of failure and there is little time to fully consider alternatives. Such restructuring is often poorly thought out and imposed with little involvement of workers. (One recent U.S. survey found that one-third of workers believe their employers "never" value their ideas [Smith 1995].) This has created the (understandable) perception among workers and unions that OC directed to expanding job control (and responsibility) of workers is just a way of transferring stress to workers, co-opting workers to the management agenda of increased productivity, and dividing and undermining the power of unions (Canadian AutoWorkers 1990). In general, reorganization efforts carried out in the middle of a crisis are less likely than at other times to succeed (Landsbergis and Vivona-Vaughan 1995).

Government policies are needed to encourage proactive OC. In higher value-added sectors, companies that rely on highly motivated employees may have more opportunity and reason to improve the health and well-being of their employees. These firms may be more likely to meet the pre-requisites for OC to meet their employees' basic needs (Frank and Hackman 1975). It is difficult (if not impossible) for Canadian firms to successfully compete in low-wage industries on the basis of anything but low wages (i.e., new technology, better customer service, etc., are unlikely to offset the competitive demand for low wages) (see Drache and Boyer 1996). At the macroeconomic level, therefore, the best way to improve standards of living is to be on the leading edge of new product development and to produce these products while the value added is high (that is, until cheaper production processes are developed and production is shifted to lower-cost production sites). Investments in human capital (education, health) and infrastructure (communications, transportation) play a central role in creating the environment and culture for high-performance economies. Government has an important role to play in fostering these conditions. Indeed, interventions at this broad level are perhaps less susceptible to failure than direct industrial policy interventions at the microlevel. Sectoral training and adjustment programs that increase the skills of the labour force are also needed (Sullivan et al. 1997).

Companies need incentives and supports to provide, to the greatest extent possible, employment security during processes of reorganization. Unemployment insurance work-sharing programs can provide the "carrots," while experience-based unemployment insurance should be explored as a possible "stick." Tax rates linked to health in the workplace may also encourage healthy firm-level policies, although there is the ever-present danger of employee selection (i.e., excluding all but very fit workers).

However, government policy is shaped not just by ideas but also (and perhaps more so) by its own political and economic agenda, such as maintaining a tax base and answering to powerful and organized interest groups. Federal governments may be unlikely to accept tax revenue losses (an immediate concern of the Treasury Board of Canada) that may be associated with providing incentives for healthier workplaces if the benefits (i.e., reduced health care expenditures) are to be reaped largely at the provincial level and perhaps only in the longer term.

There are also limits to what government legislation can accomplish. Legislation may be ignored for many reasons—such as lack of enforcement mechanisms, workplace resistance, and organizational culture (e.g., smoking restrictions in small workplaces; see Eakin et al. 1995)—and may bring about unintended effects (e.g., experience-based rating of unemployment and health benefits may discourage companies' hiring of older or disabled workers). If government interventions are to avoid inducing an undesired reaction, educational efforts targeted at companies, unions and the public are needed to raise awareness of the increasing evidence that employees' health status is strongly affected by workplace organization.

Market Framework

In theory, markets compensate for unhealthy or dangerous work by paying higher wages for such work. In practice, workers often have limited mobility (i.e., the option of leaving an unsafe or unhealthy job for a healthy job) and lack full information about the kinds of risks they are facing in the workplace (e.g., the long-term effects of exposures to potentially hazardous chemicals). Thus, there is no guarantee that the compensating wage received by the worker reflects the correct fully compensating wage differentials. In addition, individual workers often have little bargaining power to reduce hazardous or unhealthy workplace conditions, particularly if they are not unionized or belong to a union that is in a weak bargaining position. At any rate, compensating for hazardous work does little to reduce the prevalence of such work in the first place, particularly as the full costs of work-related injuries and illnesses are so rarely reflected in the prices of products. Finally, many would question, on grounds of moral principle, whether high pay is an appropriate exchange for unsafe work.

Most agree that there are indirect social costs (or externalities) that are ignored by the supply and demand functioning of markets, including labour markets. Whether such externalities are seen as "market imperfections" or inherent flaws in the market system, it is increasingly held that these externalities need to be included in market prices if marketplace decisions are to be compatible with the broader and longer-term social good (see, for example, Sullivan et al. 1997, this volume). Full-cost analysis of certain products could lead to a set of taxes and subsidies encouraging or deterring purchasing decisions (allocation of revenues from so-called sin taxes on tobacco or alcohol to subsidize health-enhancing activities such as recreation, continuing education, and job training and placement). There are certainly barriers to such an endeavour, such as the difficulty of pricing social goods and restrictions imposed by international trade agreements, not to mention public and corporate resistance. However, given the potential benefits of markets that reflect true social costs, this avenue merits attention in the field of occupational health.

Finally, the international context deserves mention. As we have seen, critics of free trade and globalization argue, with some evidence to back up their view, that the drive for competitiveness and labour market flexibility is undermining workers' rights and worsening working conditions. While free trade proponents argue that these changes encourage workforce flexibility and support innovation, critics hold that such changes only support competitiveness based on cheap labour (Myles 1988). Technological and economic change do seem to be encouraging a "dual economy," one with a small stratum of well-paid professionals and a large group of unskilled working with little job security. The current context of deep cuts in many public agencies makes OC interventions extremely difficult, given uncertainty about levels of funding and staffing. This is the context in which we try to improve health in the workplace and a context that must be considered by health policymakers trying to create healthier workplaces.

In a global market of hugely disparate working conditions, the common ground between health and wealth in workplaces may not naturally exist. Rather, by creating a judicious mix of incentives and regulation at the national and provincial levels and by working toward the creation of a more level playing field at the international level, governments and people may be able to balance the sometimes diverging objectives of economic growth and workers' (and society's) health and well-being. Governments should play a role of leadership, rather than resorting to claims of powerlessness in face of global economic and market forces, and find ways to ensure that workforce health is not compromised by concern for economic competitiveness.

RECOMMENDATIONS

Firm-Level Recommendations

1. Interventions to make OC for the benefit of workers' health should be based on the involvement of unions (or employee representatives), management and, if possible, outside researchers. Ample time should be given to allow the various parties involved at the worksite to discuss interventions and their possible implications with each other and with their groups' members.
2. Interventions to improve health should start with an assessment of employees' physical and psychosocial health status and concerns (see Health and Welfare Canada 1991; National Institute for Occupational Safety and Health 1996) and take into consideration a wide variety of factors that may be influencing health, including individual lifestyle, job, organizational and external factors. Interventions should recognize

the links between these various factors influencing health and should attempt to address all the relevant levels.

3. Large firms (over 300 employees) should undertake comparative, best practice demonstrations in different organizational units within their organizations (this is easily done for large firms like banks and large public sector organizations).

Government-Level Recommendations

4. Government has an important role to play in implementing policies to encourage healthier work environments and ensure that health hazards are adequately controlled in all workplaces. Government policies can encourage healthier workplaces by incorporating health consequences in policy decisions in other domains. The role of taxation measures in this regard should be a research priority. For example, government should create and study incentives using a set of demonstration programs. Provincial governments could provide rebates in the Employer Health Tax, and the federal Ministry of Finance could link corporate tax rates to significant improvements in workforce health.

5. Governments need to recognize the severity of the psychosocial demands of work and should support research to develop psychosocial health indicators. Governments should help to develop and promote systems for collecting data on employees' health status and on key risk factors, including organizational risk factors.

6. Governments should set an example in developing healthier workplaces by introducing, measuring and monitoring OC in their own workplaces (e.g., the civil service) and by ensuring that results, especially the success stories, are widely disseminated.

7. Provincial and federal labour and economic development ministries should officially sponsor and champion "model restructuring" efforts that focus on the positive consequences for employees' health. This could take the form of promoting model organizations, company health awards, and annual competitions with prestige value conferred by corporate leaders and politicians.[6] The current preoccupation with downsizing offers government an important opportunity to take the lead in showing how to minimize the harmful effects of such changes. As there is a need for the dissemination of stories of innovative health-enhancing OC, the federal government should sponsor a program to

---

6. We understand that Health Canada is exploring the creation of an awards program for initiatives to promote health. We encourage the inclusion of broad organizational health indicators in the criteria for awards.

interview and (or) videotape key participants in such endeavours which have not been documented and may never appear in the formal literature.

8. Government should facilitate discussion and joint action among occupational health professionals, health promoters, and OC consultants to try to build an integrated, widely shared approach to creating healthier work environments. The pending evaluation of the WHS program may provide the opportunity to bring together the three constituencies to develop interventions to improve health in the workplace. The WHS or an appropriately adapted alternative model should be marketed in nontraditional workplaces (the workplaces of the nonunionized service sector, home workers, etc.), with special emphasis on long-term sustainability.

9. Government should support the development of model collective agreements, in generic language, on workplace change and health.

Research Agency–Level Recommendations

10. National and provincial research agencies should explore the potential for action research as an approach to understanding and improving health in the workplace. By working directly with the people who make the changes, researchers can help ensure that new interventions are properly evaluated.

11. Process and outcome evaluations of workplace interventions that use both quantitative and qualitative methods are needed to understand and improve health in the workplace and to trace exactly how interventions achieve desired outcomes. More longitudinal intervention studies are needed to test theoretical models of health in the workplace.

12. The Natural Sciences and Engineering Research Council's research program on technological change and restructuring should be expanded to support specific studies or award research chairs that focus on the health consequences of restructuring and OC.

Michael F. D. Polanyi *is a research associate at the Institute for Work & Health and a doctoral student in environmental studies at York University. His research focuses on organizational change and its impact on health. He helped coordinate a major research project on musculoskeletal disorders among newspaper workers. He holds a master's degree in political science from the University of Toronto.*

BIBLIOGRAPHY

ANGUS REID GROUP, INC. 1995. *The Angus Reid/Southam News: Economic Outlook/Consumer Economic Confidence and the Generation's Perspective.* Toronto (ON): Angus Reid, November 30.

ASSOCIATION OF WORKERS' COMPENSATION BOARDS OF CANADA. 1995. *Canadian Workers' Compensation Basic Statistical and Financial Information 1990–1993.* Association of Workers' Compensation Boards of Canada, Edmonton (AB).

BAKER, F., and G. M. GREEN. 1991. Work, health and productivity: An overview. In *Work, Health, and Productivity,* eds. G. M. GREEN and F. BAKER. Oxford (U.K.): Oxford University Press.

BERTERA, R. L. 1990. Planning and implementing health promotion in the workplace: A case study of the Du Pont Company experience. *Health Education Quarterly* 17: 307–327.

BETCHERMAN, G. 1996. Globalization, labour markets and public policy. In *States against Markets: the Limits of Globalization,* eds. D. DRACHE, and P. BOYER. Londo (U.K.): Routledge.

BONGERS, P. M., C. R. DE WINTER, M. A. J. KOMPIER, and V. H. HILDEBRANDT. 1993. Psychosocial factors at work and musculoskeletal disease. *Scandinavian Journal of Work, Environment and Health* 19(5): 297–312.

BURTON, J. 1995. John Burton's workers' compensation monitor. *John Burton's Workers' Compensation Monitor* 8: 1–15.

CANADIAN AGING RESEARCH NETWORK. N.d. *Work and Family: Executive Summary.* Guelph (ON): University of Guelph.

CANADIAN AUTOWORKERS. 1990. *CAW Statement on the Reorganization of Work.* Toronto (ON): CAW Research Department.

CHIHARA, S., H. ASABA, T. SAKAI, J. KOH, and M. OKAWA. 1992. A stress reduction program for nurses at Osaka Medical College. *Conditions of Work Digest* 11: 239–243.

DICKEN, A. 1993. *The Strategic Importance of Innovative Work Systems at ICI Chemical and Polymers: The 1991 Staff Agreement.* Presented at Innovative Work Organization in Europe and North America, 3rd European Ecology of Work Conference, 2–5 Nov. 1993, Loughlinstown House Shankill, County Dublin, Ireland.

DRACHE, D., and R. BOYER. 1996. *States against Markets: The Limits of Globalization.* London: Routledge.

EAKIN, J. 1992. Leaving it up to the workers: Sociological perspectives on the management of health and safety in small workplaces. *International Journal of Health Services* 22: 689–704.

EAKIN, J., and N. WEIR. 1995. Canadian approaches to the promotion of health in small workplaces. *Canadian Journal of Public Health* 86: 109–113.

EAKIN, J., M. ASHLEY, S. BULL, and L. PEDERSON. 1995. *Legislated Workplace Smoking Restrictions in Ontario: A Report to the Ontario Workplace Health and Safety Agency.* Ontario: Workplace Health and Safety Agency, November 1995.

ENGSTROM, T., J. A. JOHANSSON, D. JONSSON, and L. MEDBO. 1995. Empirical evaluation of the reformed assembly work at the Volvo Uddevalla Plant: Psychosocial effects and performance aspects. *International Journal of Industrial Ergonomics* 16: 293–308.

EVANS, R. G., M. L. BARER, and T. R. MARMOR. Eds. 1994. *Why Are Some People Healthy and Others Not? The Determinants of Health of Populations.* New York (NY): Aldine de Gruyter.

FIEDLER, F. E., C. H. BELL, and D. PATRICK. 1984. Increasing mine productivity and safety through management training: A comparative study. *Basic and Applied Social Psychology* 5: 1–18.

FIELDING, J. E. 1990. Worksite health promotion programs in the United States: Progress, lessons and challenges. *Health Promotion International* 5: 75–84.

FRANK, J. W. 1995. Why "population health"? *Canadian Journal of Public Health* 86: 162–164.

FRANK, L. L., and J. R. HACKMAN. 1975. A failure of job enrichment: The case of the change that wasn't. *Journal of Applied Behavioral Science* 11: 413–436.

FRANK, J. W., I. R. PULCINS, M. S. KERR, H. S. SHANNON, and S. STANSFELD. 1995. Occupational back pain—an unhelpful polemic. *Scandinavian Journal of Work, Environment and Health* 21: 3–14.

GANSTER, D.C. 1995. Interventions for building healthy organizations: Suggestions from the stress research literature. In *Job Stress Interventions*, eds. L. R. MURPHY, J. J. HURELL, S. L. SAUTER, and K. G. KEITA.Washington (DC): American Psychological Association.

GERSTEIN, R., J. LABELLE, F. MUSTARD, R. SPASOFF, and J. WATSON. 1991. *Nurturing Health: A Framework for the Determinants of Health.* Toronto (ON): Premier's Council on Health Strategies and Queen's Printer.

GOLEMBIEWSKI, R. T., R. HILLES, and R. DALY. 1987. Some effects of multiple OD interventions on burnout and worksite features. *Journal of Applied Behavioral Science* 23: 295–313.

HACKMAN, J., J. PEARCE, and J. WOLFE. 1978. Effects of changes in job characteristics on job attitudes and behaviours: A naturally occurring quasi-experiment. *Organizational Behavior and Human Performance* 21: 289–304.

HAZZARD, L. 1992. Job rotation cuts cumulative trauma cases. *Personnel Journal* 71: 29–32.

HEALTH AND WELFARE CANADA. 1991. *Corporate Health Model.* Ottawa (ON): Supply and Services Canada, Cat. no. H39–225/1991E.

HEANEY, C. A. 1993. Perceived control and employed men and women. In *Women, Work and Coping: A Multidisciplinary Approach to Workplace Studies*, eds. B. C. LONG, and S. E. KAHN. Montreal (QC): McGill-Queen's University Press. pp. 193–213.

HEANEY, C. A., R. H. PRICE, and J. RAFFERTY. 1995. The caregiver support program: An intervention to increase employee coping resources and enhance mental health. In *Job Stress Interventions: Current Practices and New Directions*, eds. G. KEITER, J. HURRELL, and L. MURPHY. Washington (DC): American Psychological Association. pp. 93–108.

HEANEY, C. A., B.A. ISRAEL, S. J. SCHURMAN, E. A. BAKER, J. S. HOUSE, and M. HUGENTOBLER. 1993. Industrial relations, worksite stress reduction, and employee well-being: A participatory action research investigation. *Journal of Organizational Behavior* 14: 495–510.

HERTZMAN, C., J. W. FRANK, and R. G. EVANS. 1994. Heterogeneities in health status and the determinants of population health. In *Why Are Some People Healthy and Others Not? The Determinants of Health of Populations*, eds. R. G. EVANS, M. L. BARER, and T. R. MARMOR. New York (NY): Aldine de Gruyter. pp. 67–92.

HOLLANDER, R. B., and J. J. LENGERMANN. 1988. Corporate characteristics and worksite health promotion programs: Survey findings from Fortune 500 companies. *Social Science and Medicine* 26: 491–501.

HOLMAN, H. R. 1993. Qualitative inquiry in medical research. *Journal of Clinical Epidemiology* 46: 29–36.

HUGMAN, R. and R. HADLEY. 1993. Involvement, motivation, and reorganization in a social services department. *Human Relations* 46: 1319–1348.

IGNATIEFF, N. 1995. *Best Work Practices and Safety Outcomes.* Report to the Workplace Health and Safety Agency. Toronto, December 1995.

ISRAEL, B. A., S. A. SCHURMAN, and J. S. HOUSE. 1989. Action research on occupational stress: Involving workers as researchers. *International Journal of Health Services* 19: 135–155.

ISRAEL, B. A., S. J. SCHURMAN, and M. K. HUGENTOBLER. 1992a. Conducting action research: Relationships between organizational members and researchers. *Journal of Applied Behavioral Science* 28: 74–101.

ISRAEL, B. A., S. J. SCHURMAN, M. K. HUGENTOBLER, and J. S. HOUSE. 1992b. A participatory action research approach to reducing occupational stress in the United States. *Conditions of Work Digest* 11: 152–163.

IVANCEVICH, J. M. , M. T. MATTESON, S. M. FREEDMAN, and J. S. PHILLIPS. 1990. Worksite stress management interventions. *American Psychologist* 45: 252–261.

JACKSON, S. E. 1983. Participation in decision making as a strategy for reducing job-related strain. *Journal of Applied Psychology* 68: 3–19.

JOHNSON, J. V., and E. M. HALL. 1988. Job strain, work place social support, and cardiovascular disease: A cross-sectional study of a random sample of the Swedish population. *American Journal of Public Health* 78: 1336–1342.

KARASEK, R. 1992. Stress prevention through work reorganization: A summary of 19 international case studies. *Conditions of Work Digest* 11: 23–41.

KARASEK, R., and T. THEORELL. 1990. *Healthy Work: Stress, Productivity and the Reconstruction of Working Life.* New York (NY): Basic Books.

KELLY, J. 1992. Does job re-design theory explain job re-design outcomes? *Human Relations* 45: 753–774.

KVARNSTROM, S. 1992. Organizational approaches to reducing stress and health problems in an industrial setting in Sweden. *Conditions of Work Digest* 11: 227–232.

LABONTE, R. 1995. Population health and health promotion: What do they have to say to each other? *Canadian Journal of Public Health* 86: 165–168.

LABOUR CANADA. 1990. *Employment Injuries and Occupational Illnesses 1985–1987.* Ottawa (ON): Minister of Supply and Services.

LANDSBERGIS, P. A., and E. VIVONA-VAUGHAN. 1995. Evaluation of an occupational stress intervention in a public agency. *Journal of Organizational Behavior* 16: 29–48.

LANDSBERGIS, P. A., B. SILVERMAN, C. BARRETT, and P. L. SCHNALL. 1992. Union stress committees and stress reduction in blue- and white-collar workers in the United States. *Conditions of Work Digest* 11: 144–151.

LANDSBERGIS, P. A., S. J. SCHURMAN, B.A. ISRAEL, P. L. SCHNALL, M. K. HUGENTOBLER, J. CAHILL, and D. BAKER. 1993. Job stress and health disease: Evidence and strategies for prevention. *New Solutions* 3: 42–58.

LEVERING, R. 1988. *A Great Place to Work: What Makes Some Employers So Good (and Most So Bad).* New York (NY): Avon Books.

LEWCHUK, W., A. L. ROBB, and V. WALTERS. 1995. *The Effectiveness of Bill 70 and Joint Health and Safety Committees in Reducing Injuries and Illness in the Workplace: The Case of Ontario.* Hamilton (ON): McMaster University, April 1995.

MACDONALD, S., M. SHAIN, S. LOTHIAN, H. SUURVALI, and S. WELLS. 1994. An input and process evaluation of the Workplace Health System (corporate health model). Unpublished document.

MACY, B. A., M. F. PETERSON, and L. W. NORTON. 1989. A test of participation theory in a work re-design field setting: Degree of participation and comparison site contrasts. *Human Relations* 42: 1095–1165.

MARMOT, M. L., and T. THEORELL. 1988. Social class and cardiovascular disease: The contribution of work. *International Journal of Health Services* 18: 659–674.

MAVRINAC, S. C., N. R. JONES, and M. W. MEYER. 1995. *The Financial and Non-Financial Returns to Innovative Workplace Practices: A Critical Review.* Washington (DC): U.S. Department of Labor.

MAY, L. 1992. A union programme to reduce work and family stress factors in unskilled and semi-skilled workers on the east coast of the United States. *Conditions of Work Digest* 11: 164–171.

MILLER, K. I., and P. R. MONGE. 1986. Participation, satisfaction, and productivity: A meta-analytic review. *Academy of Management Journal* 29: 727–753.

MURPHY, L. R. 1988. Occupational stress management: A review and appraisal. *Journal of Occupational Psychology* 57: 1–15.

MURPHY, C., and D. OLTHUIS. 1995. The impact of work reorganization on employee attitudes toward work, the company and the union: Report of a survey at Walker Exhaust. In *Reshaping Work: Union Response to Technological Change,* eds. C. SCHENK, and J. ANDERSON. Toronto (ON): Ontario Federation of Labour. pp. 76–102.

MYLES, J. 1988. Decline or impasse? The current state of the welfare state. *Studies in Political Economy* 26: 73–107.

NATIONAL INSTITUTE FOR OCCUPATIONAL SAFETY AND HEALTH. 1996. In *Checklist of Work-Related Psychosocial Conditions*, eds. A. TEPPER, and J. HURRELL. Cincinnati (OH): NIOSH, Oct.

NEUMAN, G. A., J. E. EDWARDS, and N. S. RAJU. 1989. Organizational development interventions: A meta-analysis of their effects on satisfaction and other attitudes. *Personnel Psychology* 42: 461–489.

ONTARIO WOMEN'S DIRECTORATE. 1991. *Work and Family: The Crucial Balance.* Toronto (ON): Ontario Ministry of Community and Social Services.

ORPEN, C. 1979. The effects of job enrichment on employee satisfaction, motivation, involvement and performance. *Human Relations* 32: 189–217.

PASMORE, W., and F. FRIEDLANDER. 1982. An action-research program for increasing employee involvement in problem solving. *Administrative Science Quarterly* 27: 343–362.

POLANYI, M. F., J. W. FRANK, H. S. SHANNON, T. J. SULLIVAN, and J. LAVIS. In press. Promoting the determinants of good health in the workplace. In *Settings in Health Promotion: Linking Theory and Practice*, eds. B. POLAND, I. ROOTMAN, and L. GREEN. Newbury (MA): Sage.

PREECE, H., and D. WEBER.1995. *Accepting and Emplementing Change: The Workplace Health System and Organizational and Consultant Perspectives.* Toronto (ON): The University of Toronto, M.Sc. project.

PREMIER'S COUNCIL ON ECONOMIC RENEWAL. 1993. Meeting materials prepared by the Task Force on the Organization of Work. Toronto. Unpublished document.

RAEL, E. G. S. 1992. *An Epidemiological Study of the Incidence and Duration of Compensated Lost Time Occupational Injury for Construction Workmen, Ontario, 1989: An Assessment and Application of Workers' Compensation Board and Labour Force Data.* Downsview (ON): University of Toronto Press.

RANTANEN, J. 1995. *Division of Health Promotion, Education and Communication Workers' Health Working Document: Unit of Occupational Health.* Geneva, Switzerland: World Health Organization,

RIFKIN, J. 1995. *The End of Work: The Decline of the Global Labor Force and the Dawn of the Post-Market Era.* New York (NY): G.P. Putnam's Sons.

ROBERTS, K., D. HYATT, and P. DORMAN. 1995. The effect of free trade on contingent work in Michigan. Unpublished manuscript.

ROBERTSON, D., J. RINEHART, C. HUXLEY, J. WAREHAM, H. ROSENFELD, A. MCGOUGH, and S. BENEDICT. 1993. *The CAMI Report: Lean Production in a Unionized Auto Plant.* Willowdale (ON): CAW Canada Research Department.

ROBINSON, J. C. 1988. The rising long-term trend in occupational injury rates. *American Journal of Public Health* 78(3): 276–281.

ROTHSCHILD, J., and R. RUSSELL. 1986. Alternatives to bureaucracy: Democratic participation in the economy. *Annual Review of Sociology* 12: 307–328.

RUBENOWITZ, S., N. FLEMMING, and A. TANNENBAUM. 1983. Some social psychological effects of direct and indirect participation in ten Swedish companies. *Organization Studies* 4(3): 243–259.

RUSH, B. 1995. *Program Evaluation and the Workplace Health System: What Do Comprehensive Evaluations of Health Promotion Programs in the Workplace Tell Us about Program Effectiveness and Cost-Efficiency?* Report prepared for Workplace Health System, Work and Education Health Promotion Unit, Health Promotion Directorate, Health Canada. Ottawa (ON).

SAARI, J. 1992. Scientific housekeeping studies. In *Profits Are in Order*, ed. F. E. BIRD. Atlanta (GA): International Loss Control Institute. pp. 27–42.

SAUTER, S. L., L. R. MURPHY, and J. J. HURRELL. 1990. Prevention of work-related psychological disorders: A national strategy proposed by the National Institute for Occupational Safety and Health (NIOSH). *American Psychologist* 45: 1146–1158.

SCHNALL, P. L., P. A. LANDSBERGIS, and D. BAKER. 1994. Job strain and cardiovascular disease. *Annual Review of Public Health* 15: 381–411.

SCHURMAN, S. J., and B. A. ISRAEL. 1995. Redesigning work systems to reduce stress: A participatory action research approach to creating change. In *Job Stress Interventions: Current Practices and New Directions*, eds. G. KEITER, J. HURRELL, and L. MURPHY. Washington (DC): American Psychological Association. pp. 235–263.

SHANNON, H. S., J. MAYR, and T. HAINES. 1997. Overview of the relationship between organizational and workplace factors and injury rates. *Safety Science* 26: 201–217.

SHANNON, H. S., V. WALTERS, W. LEWCHUK, J. RICHARDSON, L. A. MORAN, T. HAINES, and D. VERMA. 1996. Workplace organizational correlates of lost time accident rates in manufacturing. *American Journal of Industrial Medicine* 29: 258–268.

SHANNON, H. S., V. WALTERS, W. LEWCHUK, R. J. RICHARDSON, D. K. VERMA, A. T. HAINES, and L. MORAN. 1992. *Health and Safety Approaches in the Workplace*. Hamilton (ON): McMaster University. Report for the International Accident Prevention Association.

SMITH, K. 1995. Empowerment a joke, employees say. *Globe and Mail*, 24 Nov, p. B5.

STATISTICS CANADA. 1994. *Work Injuries*. Ottawa (ON): Ministry of Supply and Services, Cat. no. 72–208 Annual.

STECKLER, A., K. R. MCLEROY, R. M. GOODMAN, S. T. BIRD, and L. MCCORMICK. 1992. Toward integrating challenges for research and policy. *Health Education Quarterly* 19: 1–8.

SULLIVAN, T., O. UNEKE, J. LAVIS, D. HYATT, and J. O'GRADY. 1997. Labour adjustment policy and health: Considerations for a changing world. Ottawa (ON): National Forum on Health. (This volume.)

TERRA, N. 1995. The prevention of job stress by redesigning jobs and implementing self-regulating teams. In *Job Stress Interventions: Current Practices and New Directions*, eds. G. KEITER, J. HURRELL, and L. MURPHY. Washington (DC): American Psychological Association. pp. 265–281.

TRIST, E. L., G. I. SUSMAN, and G. R. BROWN. 1977. An experiment in autonomous working in an American underground coal mine. *Human Relations* 30: 201–236.

VERMA, A., and D. IRVINE. 1992. *Investing in People: The Key to Canada's Prosperity and Growth*. Willowdale (ON): Information Technology Association of Canada.

WALL, T. D., and C. W. CLEGG. 1981. A longitudinal field study of group work redesign. *Journal of Occupational Behavior* 2: 31–49.

WALL, T. D., and R. MARTIN. 1987. Job and work redesign. *International Review of Industrial and Organizational Psychology* (1987): 61–91.

WALL, T. D., N. J. KEMP, P. R. JACKSON, and C. W. CLEGG. 1986. Outcomes of autonomous work groups: A long-term field experiment. *Academy of Management Journal* 29: 280–304.

WALL, T. D., J. M. CORBETT, R. MARTIN, and C. W. CLEGG. 1990. Advanced manufacturing technology, work design and performance: A change study. *Journal of Applied Psychology* 75: 691–697.

WARNER, K. E. 1988. Wellness at the worksite. *Health Affairs* 8: 64–79.

Workplace Health and Safety Agency. 1994. *Working together for Health and Safety: The Impact of Joint Health and Safety Committees on Health and Safety Trends in Ontario*. Ontario: Workplace Health and Safety Agency.

WORLD HEALTH ORGANIZATION. 1986. *The Ottawa Charter on Health Promotion*. Geneva, Switzerland: WHO.

APPENDICES

APPENDIX A

Descriptions of Group A case studies

Authors (year)	Country	Level and nature of intervention[a]	Reason for initiative	Setting	Funding	Nature of evaluation
Engstrom et al.	Sweden	III: Total redesign of assembly plant layout and process and supportive OC ("parallel-flow production")[b]	Management-unions agreement	New manufacturing plant (automobile assembly, Volvo [Uddevalla]; 367 line workers(2/3 men; mean age, 30;mean seniority, 2.5 years)	Volvo; Swedish public research foundations	One-time questionnaire; compared 2,394 blue-collar workers in (all sectors) with 33 Volvo plant workers
Fiedler et al. (1984)	United States	III: Organizational development I: Management-training program		4 metal and nonmetal mines	Perceptronics Inc.	2 case studies with comparison groups
Frank and Hackman (1975)	United States	III: Job enrichment–work modules	Employee dissatisfaction; work inefficiency	Stock transfer department of a metropolitan bank		Survey, company records, interviews
Golembiewski et al. (1987)	United States	I: High-stimulus organizational development	Strain and burnout among human resources staff; high turnover rates	Human resources staff of corporation		Survey administered 5 times
Heaney et al. (1993)	United States	III: PAR[c]	Researchers	UAW—General Motors[d]	NIH-NIAAA research grant[e]	3 plantwide surveys taken over 6 years;

Appendix A – Descriptions of Group A case studies (cont.)

Study	Country	Intervention	Reason/problem	Setting		Methodology
Jackson (1983)	United States	I: Participation in decision making (increased frequency of staff meetings)	Solomon 4-group design; 2 posttests; random allocation of units to groups	Hospital outpatient facility; 25 semi-autonomous specialty clinics; RNs (34%), clerical (46%), RNAs (16%), technicians (4%), all women; 126 of 163 employees participated		Pretest and post-test measures, complete data for 94 employees
Landsbergis and Vivona-Vaughan (1995)	United States	III: Organizational development and action research	Employee stress	Large public health agency	Management	Pre- and post-intervention surveys
Pasmore and Friedlander (1982)	United States	III: PAR[c]	Increased upper limb injuries	Electronics corporation; 335 employees; workers, 90% women; supervisors, 100% men	Company	Qualitative analysis and survey of symptoms ($n = 312$)
Wall and Clegg (1981)	United Kingdom	III: Group work redesign		Medium-sized confectionery company, partly unionized		
Wall (1986)	United Kingdom	III: Autonomous work groups in new plant	Management wanted changes to more fully use employee skills	New confectionery plant	Company	Experimental and nonequivalent control group in established plant (surveys after 6, 19 and 30 months).
Wall (1990)	United Kingdom	III: Work redesign		Department of electronics company (11 women, 8 men, 2 shifts)		$n = 35$ (24 men)

[a] Level I, interpersonal relations; Level II, task requirements; Level III, organizational structure; [b] OC, organizational change; [c] PAR, participatory action research; [d] UAW, United Auto Workers; [e] NIH-NIAAA, National Institute of Health–National Institute of Alcohol Abuse and Alcoholism.

APPENDIX B

Descriptions of Group B case studies

Authors (year)	Country	Level and nature of intervention[a]	Setting	Reason for exclusion	Lessons
Chihara et al. (1992)	Japan	I: Small group stress reduction	Hospital	No formal evaluation	Cultural context is important
Dicken (1993)	United Kingdom	III: Pay structure	Chemical	No formal evaluation	Changed pay structure can affect job satisfaction and employee relations
Hazard (1992)	United States	II: Job rotation	Electronics company	No formal evaluation	Distrust of OC effects in unionized environment[b]
Heaney (1995)	United States	I: Problem-solving training	Group homes	No health outcomes	
Hugman and Hadley (1993)	United States	III: PAR[c]	Government	No formal evaluation	Unpredictable events took place; need more training support for participation
Israel et al. (1989, 1992a, b); Schurman and Israel (1995)	United States	III: PAR[c]	Automotive sector	No formal evaluation	Labour-management relations are important; systemic change is needed; union has key supportive role to play; changes at industry and government levels are needed
Kvarnstrom (1992)	Sweden	II: Job enlargement and enrichment	Manufacturing firm	Weak evaluation	
Landsbergis et al. (1992)	United States	III: Union stress committees	Manufacturing plant	Weak evaluation	Effect of union in enhancing bargaining power to address health issues
May (1992)	United States	I: Work and family committees	Union	Anecdotal evidence	Need employee time for committees to function effectively
Murphy and Olthuis (1995)	Canada	II: Job enlargement, rotation, teamwork	Automobile parts plant	No health outcomes; subjective data only; many changes at once	Scepticism about TQM[d]; cultural context is important; need multilevel interventions for effective OC
Orpen (1979)		II: Job enrichment	Government clerical service		

Appendix B – Descriptions of Group B case studies (cont.)

Saari (1992)	Finland	III: Housekeeping feedback	Shipyard	Minimal discussion of research; no formal comparison groups	Process of cooperation is more important than actions taken
Terra (1995)	The Netherlands	III: Self-regulating design teams	Metal can company	Minimal description of evaluation	Top-down and bottom-up together; participation is key; win-win situation
Trist et al. (1977)	United States	III: Action research, formation of autonomous working groups	2 metal mines	No formal evaluation	Management-union need change to think through effects separately; participation is important; industrial relations; iatrogenesis; research-action conflict

[a]Level I, interpersonal relations; Level II, task requirements; Level III, organizational structure; [b]OC, organizational change; [c]PAR, participatory action research; [d]TQM, total quality management.

APPENDIX C

Author contacts who provided support

Ben Amick
New England Medical Centre, Boston MA

Marjorie Armstrong-Stasson
School of Business
University of Windsor
Windsor, Ont.

Julian Barling
Queen's University
Kingston, Ont.

Allen Bierbreyer
Northern Telecom Limited
Mississauga, Ont.

Angel Bilodeau
City of Montreal
Montreal, Que.

Sue Bogner
Food and Drug Administration
Rockville, MD

Chris Brand
North York Public Library
North York, Ont.

Sherry Castali
Safety Performance Solutions
Arlington, VA

Centre for Industrial Relations Library
University of Toronto
Toronto, Ont.

Lynn Chipman
Bayer Rubber Inc.
Sarnia, Ont.

Cordia Chu
Griffith University
Brisbane, Australia

Louis Clarke
University of Saskatoon
Saskatoon, Sask.

Cary Cooper
University of Manchester
Manchester, U.K.

Terence Dalton
Health Canada
Ottawa, Ont.

Joyce D'Arcy
Montel (formerly Shell)
Sarnia, Ont.

Ergonomic and Human Factor Society
Santa Monica, CA

Sara Farrell
North York Public Health
North York, Ont.

Suzanne Ferguson
Nordion International
Kanata, Ont.

Dominique Francoeur
Department of National Defence
Ottawa, Ont.

Birgit Greiner
University of California (Berkeley)
Berkely, CA

Rick Hackett
School of Business
McMaster University
Hamilton, Ont.

Cathy Heaney
Ohio State University
Columbus, OH

Mike Hersh
Ontario Institute for Studies in Education
Toronto, Ont.

Ole Ingstrup
Queen's University
Kingston, Ont.

Barbara Israel
University of Michigan
Ann Arbor, MI

Glen Ivison
Saskatoon Chemicals—CEP local 609
Saskatoon, Sask.

Catherine Johnson
Conference Board of Canada
Ottawa, Ont.

Kevin Kallaway
University of Guelph
Guelph, Ont.

Mike Knell
Nelco
Waterloo, Ont.

Brian Kohler
Communications Energy and Paperworkers Union
of Canada
Ottawa, Ont.

Paul Landsbergis
Cornell University Medical College
New York, NY

Appendix C – Author contacts who provided support (cont.)

Wayne Lewchuck
Labour Studies
McMaster University
Hamilton, Ont.

Shelley Lothian
Addiction Research Foundation
London, Ont.

Phyllis MacDougall
Health Canada
Ottawa, Ont.

Victor Marshall
Centre for Studies in Aging
University of Toronto
Toronto, Ont.

Bill Mateer
General Electric
Bromont, Que.

Scott McDonald
Addiction Research Foundation
London, Ont.

Lynn Mclean
Ottawa–Carleton Health Unit
Ottawa, Ont.

Chris Miller
W.T. Lynch Foods
Toronto, Ont.

Joe Montgomery
Pacific Northwest Laboratories

Collette Murphy
Steelworkers of America
Toronto, Ont.

Bruna Nota
Consultant
Toronto, Ont.

Bruce O'Hara
Shorter Work Week Coalition
Vancouver, B.C.

Jack Quarter
Ontario Institute for Studies in Education
Toronto, Ont.

Jorma Saari
Visiting Professor
University of Waterloo
Waterloo, Ont.

Martin Shain
Addiction Research Foundation
London, Ont.

Art St. Aubin
Canadian Centre for Occupational Health and
Safety
Hamilton, Ont.

Andy Suddons
ICI Manufacturing
United Kingdom

Lisa Sullivan
Ottawa-Carleton Health Unit
Ottawa, Ont.

Swedish Embassy
Ottawa, Ont.

Irene Swinson
North York Public Health Department
North York, Ont.

Marcel Sylvestre
Montreal, Que.

Elsie Taylor
Toronto, Ont.

Adrian Tetley
Ontario Federation of Labour
Toronto, Ont.

Tores Theorell
National Institute for Psychological Factors and
Health
Stockholm, Sweden

Anil Verma
Faculty of Management Studies
University of Toronto
Toronto, Ont.

Mike Wills
Workers Health Centre
Toronto, Ont.

Jackie Woodwark
Peel Memorial Hospital
Mississauga, Ont.

Balance as a Method to Promote Healthy Indigenous Communities

KIMBERLY A. SCOTT, M.SC.

Director of Population Health,
Medical Services Branch
Kishk Anaquot Health Research and
Program Development

SUMMARY

This document, prepared for the Determinants of Health Working Group of the National Forum on Health, examines the similarities between Indigenous notions of well-being and the determinants of health *framework. Various elements of the framework and their impact in the Indigenous context are analyzed. Recommendations are offered for the effective and culturally sensitive application of the framework which will lead to personal balance, balance between Canadians and Indigenous peoples, and balance in human service delivery. With respect to socioeconomic considerations, the following suggestions are offered: more equitable distribution of economic opportunity, more even participation in economic activity between the genders, greater sensitivity to the intimate relationship of Indigenous peoples to land, greater local availability of goods and services and emphasis on collective needs as well as removal of policy barriers to workaday life. With respect to physical factors, the policy climate must move toward improved access to adequate, culturally appropriate housing, removal of policy barriers to mortgages on-reserve, support for alternative energy and waste disposal systems, and reduction of environmental degradation, with a mind to increasing the availability and purity of country foods. When psychological forces are addressed, the framework is best applied if: equal or prominent investment is made in developing opportunities for efficacious action as an image enhancement strategy for both self and culture, rather than focusing on social comparison alone. The development of stress resistance involves accounting for the colonial history, celebrating successful individuals, communities and partnerships, and increasing opportunity for shared responsibility. Most importantly, cultural efforts must allow for greater moral independence in system design, reduce policy barriers to system integration, recognize that culturally sensitive systems are most powerful and preferred, and strengthen, guard and improve the image and integrity of Indigenous culture in the Canadian context.*

The success stories illustrate the impact of people on socioenvironmental contexts as well as their reciprocal relationship. Cultural celebration, and movement toward holistic human services and personal empowerment in Métis communities are highlighted. Flourishing urban institutions in Winnipeg show how the Indigenous community can develop in a policy environment which is sometimes harsh. The importance of internal group relations to early life experience is featured in the comparison of two systems of community human services. In the first example, the Hollow Water holistic healing circle, the development of internal moral authorities, culturally appropriate collective action and the even distribution of power show how caring communities can improve the lives of Indigenous children. As a poignant contrast, the devastating impact of external accountability, runaway individualism and power imbalance are analyzed in the sad life and death of Lester Desjarlais. The role and tenacity of Inuit women who, in partnership with daring health professionals and academics, struggled successfully against both provincial and medical establishments to reclaim ownership of birthing in the North illustrates how qualified partnership between Indigenous health authorities and external agents can promote healthy communities.

The most significant policy implications of the above illustrations surface as balance within communities and between communities. With respect to the relationship between Indigenous groups and Canadians generally, not only should there be situations where morally independent self-directing freedom exists, but Indigenous Canadians should expect and enjoy the same environmental conditions, services, institutionally guarded cultural integrity and opportunities as other Canadians. A rationale is offered for the development of balance within Indigenous groups as a necessary precondition for other politico-legal changes and healthy development. A central part of movement toward equitable distribution of control is the development of internal moral authorities which guarantee the safety of the weak and dependent.

TABLE OF CONTENTS

TABLE

PREFACE

This discussion paper was written primarily for the Health Determinants Working Group of the National Forum on Health, which will provide principled guidance to the federal government on how to promote healthy Indigenous communities. But external players have a limited role in the promotion of strong healthy Indigenous groups because, consistently, Indigenous individuals and communities desire and adhere to healing and direction from within. It is for this reason that both internal and external forces are recognized in balance as important variables to consider in the development of healthy Indigenous communities.

For further clarity, I would also like to explain my use of the terms *Indigenous, human services* and *development.* Indigenous peoples will refer collectively and individually to Métis, Inuit and First Nations groups because the term aboriginal is not only value laden (referring to those "often primitive in comparison with more advanced types" [Webster's Ninth New Collegiate Dictionary 1991]), but is used primarily to describe colonized people of colour. Indigenous, on the other hand, is a colourless word referring to the original inhabitants and more accurately reflects the collective and their descendants. *Human services* is used to refer to all that is commonly separated into health (medical services, health education and promotion) and social services (child and family, community development, welfare) in Euro-American terms. *Development* refers to the facilitation of morally independent self-directing freedom, and not the adoption of modified Western systems or the ability to embrace and win at capitalism.

Furthermore, some limitations of the descriptive data highlighted here should be described because health statistics are collected by the federal government from First Nations and Inuit communities only, therefore, a sizable portion of Indigenous peoples, namely the Métis, are not reflected in this profile unless specifically stated. Unfortunately, provinces, which are primarily responsible for health care, also do not have Métis profiles. Additionally, the First Nations and Inuit communities from which these data come are, for the most part, not located in or near urban centres, thereby limiting their generalizability to the urban context, where the majority of Indigenous people reside.

In addition, the reader must consider that Indigenous peoples are heterogeneous with extreme variability in politico-legal circumstance, Euro-Christian accommodation and resistance, community structure, language and culture. The challenge this represents to policymakers and governments would require a treatise to address and is beyond the scope of this work. Therefore, although some homogenization has occurred and salient themes are common, there is no one prescription for change.

Finally, I would like to thank Cheryl Sutherland for her research assistance with the Métis-specific portions of this paper and the kind participation of Métis key informants who contributed freely of their time to share their stories. I would also like to thank Wayne Helgason of the Winnipeg Social Planning Council and the Hollow Water community for their patient contributions to this work.

INTRODUCTION

The primary objective of this document is to illustrate how the health determinants framework can be most appropriately applied to promote healthy Canadian Indigenous communities. As part of this exercise, each element of the framework—physical, psychological, cultural and socioeconomic—and its impact in the Indigenous context is analyzed with attention to how the framework would work best if proactive efforts in these specific areas were undertaken. Success stories from Métis, First Nations, Inuit and urban contexts are presented which highlight the impact of various elements of the framework. The major thrust of this analysis advocates for balance at an individual level, between groups, within groups and in human service systems.

For the sake of clarity, "balance" will mean the absence of discord, disruption and dissonance. On a personal level, balance refers to equilibrium between the physical, mental (intellectual), emotional and spiritual needs of the self. It is best schematically represented as four points on a circle where all needs are equal in priority. In contrast, a hierarchy of needs assumes that before emotional or mental needs can be met, more basic physical needs like hunger and thirst must be satisfied. In the balanced equation, spiritual needs are every bit as important as hunger and thirst.

On a societal level, balance involves valuing the contributions of all members equally. Balanced divisions of labour distribute power in a way which guards the weak and infirm, and cultural diversity is supported, protected and celebrated with fair allocation of resources. This kind of balance is obvious when the work of both genders allows them to participate fully in political life. In balanced societies, parents can choose the language in which their children shall be educated, and the media's contemporary and historical portrayal of various groups is positive or negative in equal proportion.

With respect to human services, balance involves the equal distribution of resources to reactive (curative) and proactive (preventive) activity. Balanced human services should not only respond to crisis; they must put equal amounts of energy towards forging a positive path to prevent illness. Such balance is best represented by clear institutional, communal and familial efforts to guard health through the maintenance of healthy environments. Balance in human service efforts also requires the recognition that individuals are inextricably bound to complex social environments and the influence between them is reciprocal.

To balance literally means to match, offset or equalize. The success stories in this paper illustrate how individual balance, balance within and between groups and balanced human service efforts might best serve the healthy aspirations of Indigenous groups. But before discussing success, it is important to look at the context.

INDIGENOUS HEALTH ISSUES

Current Indigenous health issues really revolve around two things: an alarmingly poor health status and a healing movement characterized by increased control of health services and information as well as the resurrection of traditional health practices. The poor health of Indigenous peoples in Canada is not news: they are at significantly greater risk for all social and physical distress (with the exception of the cancers) when compared with their Canadian counterparts generally, and have been for some time (Canada, Department of Health and Welfare 1986, 1991; Canada, Department of Indian Affairs and Northern Development 1981, 1989; Assembly of First Nations 1988). The relative risk of certain health behaviours changes, however, when sociodemographic variables are controlled (Wallace and Bachman 1991; Diem et al. 1994), and it is likely that mortality and morbidity patterns would also change if matched group comparisons or confounding variables were systematically accounted for and controlled. Such evidence would have powerful implications for the application of a health determinants framework in Indigenous communities.

While positive trends are obvious with respect to some infectious diseases (Wherett 1977) and potential years of life lost (Layne 1984), many other infectious diseases and social problems such as addictions, suicide and family violence go unabated. Despite these grim odds, it would be a mistake to characterize all Indigenous communities as unhealthy places, because remarkable strength, creativity and tenacity can be found there. Just as communities are culturally, geographically and structurally heterogeneous, so too do they differ in health status. Even in those scenarios which seem despairing, many robust, balanced individuals survive and are usually at the forefront of community development. In fact, an increasing number of individuals in such contexts are finding the resolve to change their lives through personal empowerment. In the process, they are having an impact on their families and friends, or in some cases are leading community health endeavours. So widespread are the sparks of hope that their work has been labelled a *healing movement.*

This new wave comes with increasing control over human services. Many Indigenous health authorities (incorporated health and social service boards, band councils, and tribal governments) are taking charge and implementing a more comprehensive approach to health in both rural and urban communities. While the administrative transfer of human services is not the ideal as it is primarily through devolution, it does provide greater opportunity for political and cultural revitalization which will lead to socioenvironmental improvements and, subsequently, improved health status. The federal government and some provincial governments have an official administrative transfer policy guiding the shift in responsibility to Indigenous health authorities, but many provincial and municipal governments still lack such policies. Because Canadian human services for Indigenous groups are plagued by serious constitutional ambiguities, some provinces have refused to establish and provide human services for "Indians off-reserve" without federal cost-recuperating guarantees. This tangled jurisdictional web has inhibited urban or "off-reserve" service development.

A significant part of the Indigenous healing movement and its concomitant institutional developments is a strong resurgence of traditional health practices—some of which are recognized and supported by provincial health initiatives. Included among these practices are spiritual and cultural rejuvenation, use of natural medicines, midwifery and the resurrection of traditional social codes. Addiction treatment facilities, local community health care centres, private practitioners and even hospitals are using more traditional approaches to health and altering their environments structurally and linguistically to be more culturally hospitable. But much work needs to be done toward achieving balance at an individual level, and between and within groups, as well as toward more holistic and preventive strategies of guarding health. Current shifts in the way we think about determinants offer hope.

THE HEALTH DETERMINANTS FRAMEWORK

In recent popular discourse, a more comprehensive health paradigm has emerged which closely parallels traditional Indigenous notions of well-being. Both recognize the many synergistic and multifaceted contributors to health—namely economic, social, psychological, physical and cultural forces. Popular discourse is shifting attention to the role of genetics, nutrition, adequate housing, stress, core notions of self, social stratification, environmental integrity, social support and early life experience in determining health. Necessarily, the paradigm extends the influence upon individual health beyond a client/practitioner relationship to include more broad-based institutions such as corporations, media, a wider range of government departments, education systems and others not previously thought part of the health web. This new paradigm is known as the *health determinants framework* (subsequently referred to as the *paradigm* or *framework*) and is being advocated by leading economists, sociologists, psychologists and health practitioners. The following text analyzes the various elements of the framework, illustrating the impact of these forces and identifying the sensitivities that will yield the greatest results in the Indigenous context.

The focus has intentionally been shifted away from fact-filled discussion about relative risk and target groups because such surveillance is generally reductionist. In other words, it is philosophically incongruous with holism and the framework which advocates the reciprocal influence between environment and health. Rather, the analysis more generally addresses the sphere of influence and etiological relationship between the elements and group well-being.

Socioeconomic Forces

Power relationships and hierarchies can almost always be explained by economic forces. Within the health determinants framework, the link between health and socioeconomic stratification is strong (Syme 1994), not only within the community but also in the workplace (Frank and Mustard 1994; Wilkinson 1994; Renaud 1995). Rank in the social hierarchy appears to have important implications for health behaviour, with those higher up feeling more control over life and unhealthy habits (Renaud 1995). Participation in a cash economy has led to significant social stratification between Canadians generally and Indigenous groups, as well as within Indigenous communities. The history of economic change in Indigenous communities is long and complex, but in the most basic terms these changes have led to activity which encourages individual consumerism rather than collective wealth. This significantly compromises traditional social organization and creates stratification along monetary lines. Previously important and contributing members, including women, the young and the old, have been transformed from valued contributors in a subsistence economy to dependent consumers in a cash economy. This has reduced their inherent value and made them prime targets for abuse. The economic marginalization of women in the group has also strengthened patriarchal domination of political life.

With the shift from a subsistence to a cash economy, a longstanding, warmly intimate relationship to the land and a sense of pride-instilling self-sufficiency have also been eroded, leaving many communities largely dependent upon social assistance. Regular employment is a remote possibility for many. The significant association between unemployment and illness (Jin et al. 1995) argues strongly for gainful employment opportunities as safeguards. But economic opportunities have not been equitably distributed or supported in the Indigenous context, and current social assistance policies prohibit regular employment, even for able-bodied, eager recipients. Another unintended social repercussion of the welfare state is its ability to undermine internal authority. With guaranteed survival in a cash economy through welfare, the potence of internal moral authorities and social sanctions against violent and other unacceptable behaviours has been diluted or quashed entirely. For the sake of clarity, internal moral authority refers to any individual or group which is the accepted and acknowledged "law"-making body and holds collective interests at heart. Traditional examples include clan mothers and elders' councils who had significant decision-making power and could apply sanctions to those operating outside of commonly accepted ethical codes.

In short, economic changes have led to significant social stratification between Indigenous groups and Canadians generally as well as within Indigenous groups. Changes in economic policy must focus upon bringing those who have been marginalized by cash economies into the circle as active contributors and participants. In addition, income distribution policy (namely social assistance) has thwarted community and individual desires for workfare, where workfare means flexibility to offer meaningful employment to social assistance beneficiaries so they have a *choice* between being a paid contributor versus a dependent recipient. Most adults and community leaders prefer this option because they recognize the value of living a workaday life. Finally, economic activity should be conceived as something more than the ability to participate in and win at capitalism. Subsistence economies where demand is localized and traditional land connections are maintained may be the ideal for some groups. For the framework to be most effective, four economic goals must be prominent:

1. Within groups, the economic roles of women and children must be resurrected so that they can be integrated as active contributors and their rightful place in political life is reinstated.
2. Between groups, there must be equitable distribution of economic opportunities so that Indigenous groups are not marginalized in the nation's economy.
3. Social assistance policies must be flexible enough to allow for workfare where it is desired by individuals and communities.
4. Economic development must be conceived more broadly to include the support of subsistence-oriented activity which maintains and strengthens intimate relationships with the land.

Psychological Forces

Rank in the social hierarchy and the great socioeconomic disparity between Canadians generally, and Indigenous groups certainly, play a role in the development of self-image, but this is essentially a passive and conformist view of Indigenous peoples which may not best serve their health aspirations. Gecas and Schwalbe (1983) call the result of social comparison the "looking-glass self"—one that is primarily based upon the evaluations which come from others rather than from oneself. While the power of a self-fulfilling prophecy and the influence of others should not be overlooked, these factors must not overtake the importance of what can be drawn from experience:

Beyond the looking-glass self is a self that develops out of the autonomous and efficacious actions of the individual. It is a self that derives its experiential locus not primarily from the imagined perceptions of others, but from a sense of volition or causal agency and its consequences (Gecas and Schwalbe 1983, 79).

This perspective is most consistent with the traditional view that various conceptualizations loosely labelled self-image, respect, esteem, efficacy and internalized locus of control are derived from the ability to survive in harsh and sometimes hostile environments. In fact, in many Algonquian languages, the notion of *self-respect is drawn exclusively from industrious, efficacious interaction with the environment*: comparisons among people were relatively unimportant within the more egalitarian social organization afforded by a subsistence economy. The importance of personal industry is another area where Indigenous notions of health are compatible with the framework. For prominent Indigenous health authorities, "a healthy person is one who has achieved and is able to maintain a balanced outlook and response to her/his environment" (Aboriginal Health and Wellness Centre of Winnipeg [AHWCW] 1995, 5). For the elders, health is drawn mainly from efficacious environmental interaction. Syme has called this "control of destiny", which basically refers to how "people deal with forces that affect life or living circumstances" (Syme 1994, 84–85).

Evidence of individual resilience or stress resistance is clear in the fact that some health patterns are very divergent in Indigenous groups who endure the same socioeconomic and political conditions (Scott 1995). Theoretically, individual perceptions of the context, as well as the resources and resolve to deal with the situation, must be at work. Antonovsky, in attempting to determine what helps people manage stress and stay well, has called such coping ability a strong *sense of coherence,* or the perception that provides the personal ability deal with the enduring bombardment of life stressors (Antonovsky 1987). Very simply, it is stress resistance born from beliefs that the 'world' is predictable (*comprehensibility*), that there are internal (personal) and external (friends, community, institutions) resources to deal with the 'world' (*manageability*) and that "I can and should deal with it" (*meaningfulness*).

Suffering in the Indigenous psyche is represented by rates of addiction, suicide and family violence, all of which has been repeatedly traced to colonization. To understand this history is to make the world more *comprehensible.* The identification of internal resources (or personal ability) and external resources (or community agencies), as well as allies outside of the community, makes the world *manageable.* The best way to boost belief in personal ability is through personal accomplishment in a variety of situations and by watching others who are similar (Bandura 1977). In other words, a person would be more successful at changing community attitudes about Métis culture if he had already done so in local institutions, in conversation with individuals and in shaping federal policies which now support its celebration. Being repeatedly successful in a variety of situations means that occasional failure has less of an impact on beliefs about personal ability. Opportunities to act with some control (i.e., moral independence) support accomplishment. Moral independence is self-directing freedom based on philosophical tenets which are culturally appropriate (e.g., laws based on the primacy of collective rights vs. the primacy of individual rights in Western judiciary). Similarly, if an individual watches people lead a healing movement in a neighbouring community and believes he is like those people, then that individual is more likely to attempt healing in his own community. By identifying and celebrating role models and successful egalitarian partnerships, not only are internal resources (that is, beliefs about personal ability) strengthened, but external resources in the community and in the broader Canadian context are identified, making the world seem more manageable. Finally, shared ownership of the issue or the problem through opportunity to act in a culturally appropriate way (i.e., self-determination) not only strengthens beliefs in personal/group ability but also gives *meaning* to the endeavour.

With respect to psychological forces, the paradigm can be most effective if:

- Self-image enhancement strategies consider the impact of both social comparison and efficacious action, where efficacious action is most prominent not only because it is most consistent with traditional notions of self but also because it recognizes the *active* nature of Indigenous groups and individuals. Action, or performance accomplishment, is the best way to strengthen internal resources.
- Efforts to strengthen stress resistance or coping style (sense of coherence) must:
  - account for the colonial history to make the world understandable;
  - create opportunity for action as a way of strengthening internal resources and celebrate/share success to identify external resources to manage the world;
  - foster shared ownership of the problem through self-determination to give it meaning.

Any scrutiny of individual dispositions or characteristics, however, cannot be isolated from familial and communal contexts. Here balance means recognition that individual dynamics are very much related to social environment: one cannot be divorced from the other and the flow of influence is reciprocal. In other words, individuals impact social environments and vice versa.

Physical Forces

Within the health determinants framework, social and physical environments feature prominently as important factors contributing to health (Keating and Mustard 1993; Syme 1994). Having addressed social environment in the context of economy, it is important to look at the physical environment in more detail. Nutrition, water, air and housing must be clean and adequate for optimal health. The impact of these physical forces on Indigenous health is significant. Throughout an Indigenous person's life span, the risk of infectious disease is significantly greater due to poor housing conditions and a lack of clean water. Many homes inhabited by Indigenous people lack central heating systems, leading to greater risk of lower respiratory tract infections and chronic lung disease. Crowding, culturally insensitive housing design and community layout all create social stress and have been acknowledged as factors affecting family and community. Freezes on housing investment, the inability of on-reserve Status Indians to qualify for personal mortgages, and complications associated with sewage disposal and alternative energy sources are all factors which indicate the need for great change.

Environmental degradation resulting in the toxification or depletion of country foods has led to dramatic dietary and economic changes as well as poor health. Diabetes, obesity and severed connections to the land are the direct result of changes to the physical environment and shifting economies. For example, flooding in northern Manitoba and oil exploration in Alberta have disrupted vast trapping areas, significantly reducing participation in subsistence economies and causing commercially produced and processed foods to be substituted for traditional foods. In concrete terms, this shift has meant leaving a physically active lifestyle with a nutrient-dense, high- fibre and protein diet for a more sedentary existence and a diet that is high in carbohydrates and saturated fat. Other industrial developments have led to unacceptable levels of pesticide and metal contamination of Indigenous food sources. With respect to the physical environment, the framework would work best if it focused on:

– eliminating barriers to alternative forms of energy ;
– reinstating investment in accessible, adequate housing and clean water as basic priorities;
– recognizing important cultural considerations in housing design and community layout;
– recognizing the strong and qualitatively different relationship of Indigenous peoples to the land and the importance of country foods to social life, cultural expression and physical health.

Cultural Forces

Perhaps the most important element within the framework for Indigenous groups is the notion of cultural integrity. The demoralizing loss and denigration of culture has been cited repeatedly in the literature and clinical environments as a cause for a range of health disorders. Perhaps this is because culture is really an umbrella under which all the determinants fall. Community control features prominently here as a mechanism for safeguarding language and culture. It includes control of human service systems, and of those broader elements which affect health. Community control consistently allows for greater integration of health determinants, although some policies prohibit optimal integration. For example, the structure of most government contribution agreements do not allow community priorities to be established. Culturally appropriate healing in any circumstance—whether administered by the community or the province—is very powerful and preferred especially in the clinical setting. While external agents are important, sometimes even their best intentions have been misguided. In certain scenarios, especially where internal moral authorities are strong, it is best to have the opportunity for moral independence.

Of course, in some contexts it is clear that control must be shared, and mutually respectful partnerships are desirable, especially in sensitizing institutions which guard cultural integrity. In other words, mobilizing and securing the commitment and partnership of those institutions which help shape opinions, including schools and media, can be an incredibly potent tool in changing the image and strengthening the integrity of Indigenous cultures in the broader Canadian context. Again, balance means recognizing that strategic partnerships involving the broader social environment can have an important influence on Indigenous individuals: the individual cannot be divorced from his environment and the influence between them is reciprocal.

Therefore, equilibrium is established not only by convincing and moving external agents but also by harnessing and channelling Indigenous power from within. This power from within needs independence to flourish. This kind of interaction and integration of individual with environment is a basic Indigenous cultural tenet. It is a holistic view which is shared by the health determinants analysis. Its polar opposite, reductionism (a term borrowed from biology), refers to the isolation of individuals from all that is their socioenvironmental context and has limited ability to serve Indigenous health aspirations. The paradigm would be most effective if cultural endeavours focused on:

- allowing for moral independence when desired;
- removing policy barriers to greater system integration at the community level;

- encouraging the involvement of cultural insiders, or cultural sensitivity, in direct healing efforts;
- improving the image and integrity of Indigenous cultures in the broader Canadian context through strategic partnership.

Overview

Having examined each element of the framework, its impact on Indigenous health, and the best way to direct efforts in that area, it would be useful to have a bird's-eye view of the key conclusions from framework literature and a quick reference to the important considerations when applying it in the Indigenous context. From the literature base, the following points are clear:

- Health is the result of a broad array of determinants which include environmental, social, cultural, economic and psychological factors. This means that institutions beyond the health care system—including corporations, governments, education systems, media and other opinion-shaping institutions—play a role. Highly individualized foci of prevention and cure have limited value because they ignore these influences.
- Social stratification, determined largely by wealth in a cash economy and status in the Western view (e.g., institutional education), plays an important role in health status and behaviour. Those at the top of the hierarchy enjoy the highest level of well-being and sense of control. Those at the bottom experience psychosocial stress resulting from feelings of inferiority and relative deprivation, which may contribute to poor health habits and an overall depressed host response to a variety of infectious and chronic diseases. Accessibility of health care has not influenced relative risk gradients between the classes.
- Internal or psychological dynamics which influence coping style, host response and resilience seem to account for differences between individuals who share similar socioenvironmental conditions.
- A clean physical environment (both natural and constructed), which adequately meets peoples' needs, contributes to health.
- Imposed cultural incongruence in the form of ill-fitting world views and lifestyles have a greater impact upon societal and individual health than previously recognized.

The framework is best applied in the Indigenous context if it is sensitive to the needs and issues summarized in table 1.

Table 1

Health Determinants framework adaptation to the Indigenous context: Core considerations

Socioeconomic	Physical	Psychological	Cultural
• More equal participation between genders	• Improve access to adequate, culturally appropriate housing	• Equal or prominent investment in opportunity for effective action to foster enhanced images of self and culture	• Morally independent control over design of systems
• More equitable distribution of economic opportunity	• Remove policy barriers to mortgages on-reserve	• Account for colonial history (i.e., residential school, relocation)	• Cultural sensitivity in the forms most powerful and preferred
• Relationship to land	• Remove barriers to alternative energy forms	• Identify and celebrate successful individuals, communities and partnerships	• Remove policy barriers to greater system integration
• Remove policy barriers to living workaday life	• Reduce toxification, increase availability of country food		• Strengthen, guard and improve image and integrity of Indigenous culture in Canadian context
• Localization of goods and services with greater emphasis on collective needs			

While a success story highlighting progress in each of the core elements of the framework would have been ideal, there is little to celebrate with respect to housing developments or the integrity and availability of country foods. Similarly, while there have been economic developments which merit attention, their impact on health has not been well documented, probably because the marriage between economic, environmental and health goals is just budding. As Marmot points out, health in broader contexts is still only a priority of an isolated sector, namely health departments. The following stories were selected first and foremost to reflect the range of geographical and cultural diversity among Indigenous groups. Social, cultural and psychological elements are analyzed in current discussions of Indigenous health issues, where revitalization and increased control feature prominently. While great changes have been occurring with respect to these elements, changes in the economic and physical environment have been slow. These stories illustrate the power of internal forces such as community mobilization, increased control, and strategic partnership in promoting healthy communities and recognizing the important balance between reactive and proactive energies, as well as between holism and reductionism. In most cases presented here, actions to promote healthy community have been initiated from within the community by individuals who have assigned meaning to their task and deemed it worthy of their investment and commitment, sometimes in partnership with external players and sometimes in spite of them. In other cases, the support and flexibility of determined partners was necessary and critical to the success of the projects. Healing movement in Métis communities, urban health systems in Winnipeg and the development of internal moral authorities in First Nations communities are highlighted. The role and tenacity of Inuit women and their allies who successfully struggled against both provincial and medical establishments to reclaim ownership of birthing in the North is also discussed.

MÉTIS COMMUNITIES RECLAIMING HEALTH

For the most part, Métis people share the poor health status of other Indigenous groups and believe that their problems are rooted in socio-economic conditions which include inadequate housing, drinking water, food, employment and education (Kinnon 1994). They are culturally distinct from other Indigenous groups, and their unique role in Canadian history has been minimized or ignored. Painful anecdotes of how grand-mothers denied their Métis roots "to survive" are only now coming to light, and the effects of that racism have yet to be traced. The Métis also believe that their broken connection with the land has been a factor in many current mental health problems (Kinnon 1994).

As with other Indigenous groups, cultural identity features strongly in the health equation for the Métis. Resilience, they believe, can be increased if cultural awareness and acceptance can be enhanced. Many are reclaiming Métis cultural identity and sharing their rich traditions and contributions with Canadians generally. The following stories analyze the effect on Métis health of various elements of the framework, as well as the impact of balanced individuals on their environment and the essential role of environments in individual healing.

Cultural Vitalization and Sharing in Red Deer, Alberta

Before the Allard dance troupe existed, no one was reaching out to the general community to inform them about Métis culture, and racial tension fed by ignorance was strong. Because little guarded the integrity and endurance of Métis culture in Red Deer, Alberta, the Allard family, running on sheer determination and volunteer effort, decided to teach Métis children to dance. The Allards began by teaching their children. They then recruited from local schools to form a group of forty children and adults, who have been involved since the beginning of the program three years ago. Almost immediately there was a remarkable demand for public performances. There are now about 24 appearances per year. Motivated by their value of cultural identity, community involvement and self-reliance as well as by their desire to celebrate and share their heritage with a multicultural world, the Allards have transformed Red Deer into a more hospitable place for Métis people, while building self-esteem and cultural pride in the participants. Their efforts help children feel pride in their identity as Métis, giving them psychological strength. Community involvement, public speaking and leadership opportunities are part of dance troupe activities. While participation is stressed more than technique, there is an expectation that the group will act responsibly in the spirit of teamwork and that each member will try his best. Therefore, in addition to promoting a positive self-image through accomplishment, interpersonal skills are enhanced and connection to the larger community is nurtured. Children are encouraged to reach out and share Métis culture during performances by approaching members of the audience to teach and learn dance in cultural exchange.

Métis vitalization through dance in Red Deer is entirely self-financed: fundraising, personal donations and volunteers keep it going. The group was an immediate and popular local favourite, partially because many in Red Deer were anxious to learn about and celebrate Métis culture but had never had the opportunity. The fact that they did not charge for their performances added to their popularity, although it caused some tension and resistance from competing dance troupes.

The Allards' experience volunteering with children, working with committees and making their own journeys of personal growth facilitated their ability to initiate and lead the Métis dance troupe. Although no formal evaluation has been done, the impact of their activities is clear at both an individual and community level. As cultural identity is strengthened, the children seem to respond more positively to conflict and report feeling more accepted by their peers. They are proud to be Métis, and entire families—in fact the broader Métis community—have reclaimed their roots as a result. The focus on community connection and sharing has also given the children a greater ability to manoeuvre in the broader community. This is probably the result of their enhanced image of their abilities, themselves and their culture, as well as the inevitable changes in the community. Racial tensions have eased, and Métis culture is publicly recognized and appreciated. Even local institutions, which might not otherwise have had such a cultural resource, refer inquiries on Métis history and culture to the Allards. Enduring individual participation and community response are a testimony to the dance troupe's success at solidifying the Métis community, celebrating a rich culture and building a bridge to the general community.

To initiate similar efforts in other communities, a strong volunteer ethos, cultural pride and sense of social responsibility must exist. Broader community responsiveness is also a plus. The National Aboriginal Role Modelling Program, funded by Health Canada, has expanded to assist in identifying local heroes in Métis communities; their community development manual will be available and will identify and inspire other role models.

In this case, strong individuals made changes to their environment by celebrating and sharing cultural expression. The increased opportunity to learn about Métis culture has had an impact on both the participating individuals and the community at large. Participants have a renewed self-image and cultural esteem, making them psychologically stronger and able to deal with conflict. By stressing the importance of community involvement and connection, as well as giving children an opportunity to experience it, the Allards have also increased the children's beliefs in their personal abilities to participate as agents of change, thereby increasing their sense of industry and efficacy. At the community level, the response has been enthusiastic and racial tensions have eased as a result. Within the framework analysis, these individual and group dynamics feed upon each other and are mutually reinforcing. The policy implications of such community-based action argues strongly for movement toward personal balance by strengthening cultural pride and self-image. Celebration of Métis culture creates balance between the groups by offering everybody an opportunity to learn and understand. Even though the Allards may be solely responsible for providing that opportunity at present, it is possible that their actions will encourage local museums and schools to provide opportunities for guarding Métis culture. Institutionally guarded and supported cultural integrity in a multicultural context allows each group to be reflected in the formation of a Canadian identity. Finally, this case study illustrates the importance of proactive efforts in promoting healthy communities. Instead of a "last stand" reaction to school violence precipitated by racism, the Allards have built a bridge of understanding, acceptance and mutual exchange which has fostered respect.

Métis Addictions Council of Saskatchewan

The reciprocal influence of individuals and their environments is also being recognized at the institutional level, where substantial changes are taking place toward a more holistic approach. It is becoming increasingly clear to addiction counsellors that treating individuals in isolation of their families is not only frustrating but usually results in relapse. The Métis Addictions Council of Saskatchewan, Inc. (MACSI) is one of the oldest Métis health organizations in Canada, with the primary goal of assisting in lifelong mental, spiritual, physical and emotional recovery for all off-reserve Indigenous people in Saskatchewan. At MACSI, the keys to overcoming addiction are harmony and holism, which bring internal peace. Cultural reinforcement is central to these notions. Believing the individual needed to be treated as part of a family and community system, the centre ran a pilot program to educate families on the impact of addiction and how to assist with recovery. Family members were invited to attend lectures, video presentations and counselling sessions about addiction and recovery.

The Family Week initiative was funded by the province's Health and Social Services departments, although the bulk of MACSI's operating costs comes from the Alcohol and Drug Services section of the Saskatchewan Department of Health. The primary goals were to create a more supportive environment for recovery within the context of family; a safe place for families to relieve their guilt, shame and remorse and facilitate family healing. From MACSI's perspective, these goals were achieved. In a formal internal evaluation of Family Week activities, it was clear that families and clients were introduced to the dynamics of family wellness, enabling them to understand the mental, spiritual, physical and emotional effects of addiction. It shattered the "don't talk, don't feel, don't trust" code of silence in the dysfunctional family as well as providing an opportunity for healing goals to be set by the families. With improved communication and family functioning, it is anticipated that relapse will be reduced, although no long-term follow-up has been done.

Despite the lack of long-term follow-up, this pilot provides a model for other treatment centres wanting to incorporate family healing in addiction recovery and has been shared with referral agencies, neighbourhood schools and provincial correctional centres. It is also being adopted by Okimaw Ohci healing lodge for female offenders in Maple Creek, illustrating an important step by human service institutions in their efforts toward holism. The most important policy implications of this effort are that more holistic ways of healing individuals within their socioenvironmental contexts must be strengthened. Exceptional effort in this regard is required in the immediate future because of the overwhelming and relatively ineffective reductionist approach which has dominated curative efforts to date. Beyond family dynamics, learning the history which has led to the current climate of economic marginalization and cultural denigration also offers individuals the tools to understand that their addiction is a symptom of greater imbalance between groups. The balance that emanates from within when physical, mental, spiritual and emotional elements are nurtured can also influence the social environment.

Community Healing in Fishing Lake, Alberta

Fishing Lake, a small Métis settlement with roughly 460 residents, recently faced a turning point in its history when levels of violence became unacceptable and the community was prompted to act. Sparked by personal empowerment, a single community member participated in a self-esteem enhancement workshop, felt a complete turnaround in his life and made a commitment to share his experience at home. After recruiting twenty other community members, the group approached the settlement council for $20,000 in funding for a self-esteem enhancement retreat. Initially, the council was reluctant, so participants raised their own funds and adapted the program to be more appropriate to the Métis context by adding important historical information. A council member was among the first participants, offering a leadership role and, by example, encouraging other community politicians to participate. The initial group raised enough money to put another group through the session and by this time a paradigm shift had occurred. Further sessions were funded by the settlement council and the Brighter Futures initiative of Health Canada.

Rather than the usual issue-specific support group, *Healing the Spirit* created an understanding and supportive environment which encouraged individuals to embark on therapy, whatever their needs. Weekly healing circles were run by trained volunteers, and eventually a motion was passed stating that the entire leadership should go through the program. Over three years, 100 of the 460 active members of the settlement have participated in the self-esteem enhancement and personal empowerment training called Healing the Spirit. Both men and women, most of whom are adults, including virtually all of the political leadership, have participated.

Those who have participated are more emotionally expressive. There is a resurgence of spirituality and, for the first time, there are sweat lodges on the settlement. In fact, local bars in neighbouring towns have closed from lack of business. In addition, community ties have been renewed and, although help came from external sources, community members feel ownership of this healing journey, which comes with a new freedom and sense of possibility. Economic development is taking place and many individuals have removed barriers to the fulfilment of their potential.

Some families opposed spending money on the sessions. Like many other Indigenous communities, members silently carried the burden of having been physically and sexually abused and wanted to bury their pain. It is also possible that resistance was fed by those who had been abusive who were not prepared to be accountable for their actions. But, the need to heal overcame their fear and their initial anxiety turned to trust and acceptance. Community members recognize that political involvement was one of the keys to their success, particularly in assuring the involvement of the men. Enthusiasm and sheer numbers of participants have transformed the community. Although no formal evaluation was done, settlement members have shared their healing path at national conferences, with provincial social service agencies and even with American corporations. The settlement would very much like to document their experience formally and share it more broadly so that other communities could replicate their success. Ideally, community members could engage in training to offer self-esteem enhancement workshops. This would reduce dependence upon external consultants and could reduce some of the initial expense. Overall, the personal empowerment gained from learning history and restoring an internal balance between core elements of the self (physical, psychological, emotional and mental) removed the barriers to personal development. Many community members are pursuing education, small business endeavours and addiction-free lifestyles. Led by a small core, the possibility of internal healing spread throughout the community as other members watched their friends and neighbours embrace their newfound health. Vicariously, they learned that they too could tap the inner resources and resolve to change their lives. So powerful was the role-modelling effect that the community as a whole is much healthier, contributing to the demise of local bars.

These success stories illustrate the importance of cultural rejuvenation as a mechanism of improving personal balance as well as balance between groups. They also argue for the essential equilibrium which must be maintained in the treatment of individuals within their socioenvironmental contexts and the power of internal forces, including local leadership and individual healing, in reversing community destruction. Here, perhaps more than in any of the case studies offered, the influential strength of personal empowerment upon community dynamics and vice versa is best illustrated. Settlement members were inspired to heal after watching others endeavour and succeed. As more adults opted for a healing journey, the community began to change.

In each of the previous cases, however, healing partners had the advantage of being close to one another in a small town, service setting or contained community. But many Indigenous peoples now live in urban centres where the challenge of community development is great. The following case study provides an example of such a setting.

MOVEMENT IN WINNIPEG

In the last thirty years, the Indigenous population has become increasingly urbanized, with the most dramatic proportionate shift from rural- to urban-based populations in the last ten years. In fact, almost 70 percent of those claiming Indigenous origins live in cities or off-reserve (Statistics Canada 1991). Even though they live in blended communities, many retain their identity as Métis, First Nations or Inuit and find themselves in a tangled jurisdictional web as well as in a cultural and service void. Some argue that the health of Indigenous peoples is similar whether they reside in the city or in rural settlements, while others suggest that those who live in the city may be slightly better off than their rural counterparts (Secretary of State 1991). In any case, the city is not a place where Indigenous culture is strengthened or supported and access to human services not as universal as might be hoped. Although the provinces have not completely ignored Indigenous health concerns, many Indigenous Canadians do not enjoy the same guarantees to human services as other Canadians because of serious constitutional ambiguities which allow provinces to refuse services without federal cost-recuperating guarantees.

While both levels of government wrangle about who pays for what, many urban-based Indigenous peoples fall through the human service cracks. Winnipeg, however, seems to be at the forefront of urban Indigenous community development, and many interesting things are happening on the health horizon. Indigenous representation on the Winnipeg Social Planning Council as well as majority representation on the board of the Andrews Street Family Centre are evidence that municipal organizations can be responsive to the voice of urban-based Indigenous peoples. The Aboriginal Health and Wellness Board of Directors is striving toward an integrated system of human services where social and economic goals are intertwined. In fact, an Aboriginal Health and Wellness Centre is being planned which will be:

> fully culture-based, founded on traditional values and perspectives, where services and programs are parts of a continuum of resources made available to identify and support the aspirations, needs and goals of individuals, families and thus, the community (AHWCW 1995, 4).

Two of the central players in the development of integrated and holistic health systems in Winnipeg are the Aboriginal Centre and the Aboriginal Council of Winnipeg. The Aboriginal Centre is a central community gathering place with a wide range of services, organizations and businesses which have gathered through mutually cooperative efforts and with the support of both public and private sectors. The Aboriginal Council, formed roughly at the same time, is a status-blind entity which concerns itself with the full range of human services, such as employment, justice, education, sports and recreation, housing, health and social services (AHWCW 1995).

The underlying goals of this institutional development are as follows:
- strengthen opportunity for Indigenous culture to be institutionally guarded in the urban environment;
- integrate services so that the complexity of human well-being can be holistically addressed;
- form partnerships with allies who can facilitate these efforts, be they community-based, municipal or provincial officials.

Funding for most of these agencies comes from sources not traditionally involved in the provision of services to Indigenous Canadians, namely municipal and provincial governments.

The highly divisive categorization of Indigenous peoples thwarted the development of such status-blind organizations, and initially a hands-off provincial policy prevailed. Also, marginalization and dispersion, although relatively less severe in Winnipeg than in other Canadian cities, can inhibit the development of urban-based culturally sensitive institutions.

It is possible for other municipal and provincial partners to establish integrated urban-based services which are culturally appropriate to Indigenous peoples. Even federal partners have funded urban-based AIDS programs. What is unique about Winnipeg, which might make replication difficult, is that is has one of the largest proportions of Indigenous people of any Canadian city. When compared to Halifax, for example, the concentration and proportion of Indigenous peoples is significantly greater. Some of the most significant barriers to the development of collaborative urban-based efforts are the political/legal classifications and cultural diversity of Indigenous peoples. Many are resistant to the status-blind approach for a variety of reasons: they argue that it undermines treaty rights and melts Indigenous groups into a homogenous unit.

No formal evaluation of the urban movement in Winnipeg has occurred, but evidence of its impact is everywhere, from the Bear Clan Patrol, which is a community-run safeguard system supported by Mamawhichitata, to the advent of an Aboriginal Health and Wellness Centre. This kind of institutional development recognizes that health care and maintenance requires an integrated approach, functions to restore balance between groups by creating a more culturally hospitable context in the city and illustrates that municipal and provincial governments can establish partnership with Indigenous health authorities.

The policy implications of the Winnipeg movement suggest the importance of increased participation of municipal and provincial governments in the provision of human services to Indigenous peoples in urban centres, in strategic partnership with urban-based Indigenous health authorities. Funding arrangements should allow for the integration of the full range of services within the framework, and preventive and curative efforts should be prioritized within the group. Indigenous institutional development in Winnipeg works to create greater balance between groups by guarding cultural integrity in the urban context. It also facilitates greater balance in preventive and holistic approaches to health promotion.

But perhaps the greatest attention, institutional development and administrative transfer of control has occurred in the very narrowly defined human service of child welfare, both on-reserve and in the city. Many Indigenous health authorities administer child protection services, although subscription to provincial jurisdiction is imposed. The long history of this transferred control and its various manifestations illuminates why the development of internal moral authority and accountability is essential to the success of any health effort.

CHILDREN: OUR GREATEST RESOURCE

The Indigenous population is very young, with roughly 37 percent under 15 years of age, nearly twice the percentage of the Canadian population as a whole (Statistics Canada 1991). Stable fertility trends indicate that this will be an enduring population profile for decades to come. The social distress which will face this young cohort includes increases in nuclear family structures, divorce rate, births outside marriage, adoption and provincial wardship at alarming rates, and teen parenthood (Layne 1984; Ontario Native Women's Association 1989; Canada. Department of Indian Affairs and Northern Development 1989, 1992). There are substantially more single parents, most of whom are female: they raise an estimated 25–50 percent of all Indigenous children (Layne 1984). It is no secret that sexual abuse is a grave problem in this scenario. The good news is that solutions are within reach which involve immediate actions to safeguard and protect children in accordance with the way they were once guarded *collectively*—where all members felt a responsibility toward all children. These solutions are possible if internal and external agents, in strategic partnership, facilitate the resurrection of internal moral authorities.

Hollow Water Holistic Healing

Community-based services which are culturally and linguistically sensitive, where there is community ownership and opportunity for greater flexibility in program policy and delivery, can be superior to provincially run agencies. A substantial number of Indigenous communities successfully administer a wide range of affairs in which internal accountability is strong. Transferred services function to strengthen internal moral authorities but must never be confused as substitutes for these authorities. This is because, despite the flourishing healing movement, there is still an internalized colonialist social organization where political interference and government negligence renders the dependent at risk, allowing the most heinous crimes to occur without internal or external moral authority to check them. Within the group, inaction is excused by referring to the false notion of traditional behavioral codes such as noninterference (Brant 1990), without recognizing the effects of long-standing oppression on power structures within the community. Outside the group, inaction is explained away under the false notion that abdication of responsibility is somehow supportive of self-government, even though no political or legal structure supporting self-government exists.

The long-term goal is to address children's issues as a result of their devalued positions in families and communities by establishing balance between the genders and ages through the establishment and guidance of an internal moral authority. One of the important steps in the process is to strengthen and resurrect personal empowerment so that oppressive forces, be they internal or external, are understood and challenged. Both internal and external partners in balance must address the legacy of childhood suffering which manifests itself in a series of dysfunctional behaviours. Children who are abused and neglected are nine times more likely to take their own lives (Hibbard et al. 1990) and grow into dysfunctional adults, perpetuating what has become a vicious cycle of suicide and violence in Indigenous communities. First, Indigenous peoples must break the silence about current and historical violence, with support only when it is desired. Any resistance to disclosure, whether it be individual, institutional or governmental, is tacit approval of its continuation. Support should then come in the form of response to requests for help, guaranteed safety or partnership and, where appropriate (i.e., where a sufficiently strong moral authority exists which can guard victim safety), moral independence and egalitarian partnership should exist. In the balanced equation, exceptional leadership within families and communities which is recognized and supported by external allies is required.

This is exactly what happened at Hollow Water First Nation, out of which an especially creative story has emerged. Community members, motivated by several concerns, including family violence, and frustrated by adversarial justice systems and disruptive social services, initiated their own healing circles, which forced the issues out into the open. The movement was the result of early efforts by community-based human service workers and a member of the council who convened a meeting with the local leaders to discuss these concerns. A resource group was established, including community health service workers, provincial social services staff, church leaders, volunteers and community leaders who met weekly to determine how these issues could be resolved.

Their obvious strength was their willingness and initiative to tackle community problems with an integrated interdisciplinary approach where internal and external energies were pooled. Still, the team members felt they needed extensive training to help them on their community development journey. As their skills developed, they began their own sharing circle, where disclosures of sexual abuse emerged.

After the initial work of the resource group, an assessment team was established to address sexual abuse specifically, as it became clear that two-thirds of the community were survivors. Again, the assessment team consisted of community-based human service providers, volunteers, people specifically trained to tackle sexual abuse and external contributors, including the RCMP. While both genders were involved, it is the women who have been credited with the leadership role. Their team has developed the power of what has become known as *Community Holistic Circle Healing*, which views *"abuse as a problem of imbalance—individuals out of balance with themselves, nature and their community"* (New Economy Development Group 1993).

With respect to *community*, the people of Hollow Water believe that there is a significant interconnection among individuals in a group; therefore, individual abuse affects everybody. *Holistic* refers to personal and social balance: where individual physical, mental, emotional and spiritual elements are each nurtured with equal investment and harmony within the context of family and community. The *circle* symbolizes the recognition that the laws of nature, and even the dynamics of abuse, work in cycles. Finally, *healing* reflects the process of *"coming into balance from within."* This refers to the essential empowerment and personal peace which come from satisfying the holistic needs of the self as well as accepting the family and community responsibilities accorded to members of the group to ensure essential social and environmental harmony in the community (Hollow Water First Nation 1991).

Within this balanced form of personal place and social organization is the unwritten law that everyone is responsible for each other. This unwritten law is less about the privilege of having "rights" in the Western judicial sense than it is about having responsibilities toward family and community, where serving collective interests naturally takes care of individual interests. But perhaps the most attractive feature of *Community Holistic Circle Healing* is a culturally sensitive way of protecting the victim and making the perpetrator accountable to an *internal* moral authority consisting of mainly Ojibwa professional social workers and trained community members, while attempting to recreate collective harmony. This requires that the perpetrator restore balance through retribution as determined by internal authority and that the victim need not bear an unnecessary escape burden.

In its early phases more than a decade ago, the process operated exclusively upon community resources, with the support of leadership and community-based institutions. More recently, the process has received external recognition from federal and provincial justice systems who refer abuse cases to Hollow Water. This has led to collaboration with the courts whereby *Circle Healing* has become a presentencing and sentencing option with operational grants from the provincial Attorney General's office. *Circle*

Healing is also being supported with funds from Medical Services Branch of Health Canada. The impact and extent of the program has been expanded by federal and provincial funding sources who have supported the training of additional *Circle* healing facilitators.

Some community members resisted the healing movement and, albeit eventually supportive, the justice system was also initially resistant and sceptical. Eventually several gender-, age- and experience-specific healing circles were established. The Manitoba Department of Justice supports the Hollow Water approach, as it is clear that the recidivism rate of sexual offenders is much lower than it is following other rehabilitation programs:

> In nine years, 52 offenders have been enrolled in the healing program, along with 94 victims and more than 260 relatives of offenders and victims. In the same period, only five sexual offenders have gone to jail after their offenses were disclosed, mainly because they refused to acknowledge what they had done. Only two sex offenders have reoffended. Both were given penitentiary terms (Moon 1995).

An evaluation done by the Hollow Water First Nation revealed notable differences in community dynamics, including reduced substance abuse, a safer environment for children and a more open and communicative social climate for everyone (but most notably for children). In this first formal evaluation of circle healing, findings supported the continuation of this community-based, interdisciplinary approach where traditional and contemporary therapies are combined—not only because it proved to be a more effective means of soliciting disclosure and ending abuse, but also because offenders were held accountable internally, thereby eliminating the victim's escape burden. Other examples testify to the success experienced at Hollow Water, including the flood of visitors from across Canada and frequent callers requesting information about *Community Holistic Circle Healing*. It is not known how many of these visitors then apply this knowledge to their own situations, but it is clear that seeds of replication are being planted by such information exchanges. Furthermore, the community has been successfully able to engage healed offenders to help other offenders self-identify and plead guilty, especially those who are fighting it in the courts. Similarly, healed victims work with others to share their experience, ease the trauma and promote the healing path.

Some of the strongest sources of support include other Indigenous communities who have engaged in their own healing journeys— communities like Alkali Lake, British Columbia, which is noted for its incredible community turnaround to 95 percent sobriety. Other supporters, although initially opposed, include the RCMP and the courts. Last but certainly not least, the involvement and support of local churches and community leadership helped fuel the healing movement.

Part of the reason that child sexual abuse remains shrouded in secrecy is because the only alternatives which would alleviate the situation involve justice or child welfare systems. It is clear that incarceration is not a substitute for intervention specific to pedophilia, nor is it a substitute for the strong social sanctioning and group dynamics which are prohibiting and retarding this kind of behaviour in Hollow Water. Without such intervention, sexual offenders are very likely to reoffend, and neglectful communities, families and neighbours very likely to continue a pattern of silence. By themselves, punitive consequences or temporary child protection measures are woefully inadequate in addressing the root causes of family and group dysfunction. At Hollow Water, child sexual abuse is being disclosed in community settings and encouraged, even by those who have a history of offense! Usually, the identification of a sexual offender depends upon the assault survivor: the difficulty with this approach is that pedophiles generally have many more victims than records indicate (Abel et al. 1987; Hindman 1988; Marshall and Barbaree 1990). Treatment options should never replace accountability for a crime, but they must be provided along with accountability. Hollow Water provides an exceptionally balanced approach to dealing with family violence by attempting to restore individual well-being holistically by utilizing the power of social sanctioning to reestablish social harmony through the dictates of an internal moral authority. Accountability to the group has resulted in safer, more open environments. Where external accountability looms strong, children are not as lucky.

Why the System Failed Lester Desjarlais

In 1988, a 13-year-old boy named Lester Desjarlais hanged himself after a tormenting childhood of abuse, neglect and unstable foster placements. It might have otherwise been just another suicide in custody but when the coroner requested Lester's case files they were curiously missing from the Native child welfare agency responsible which prompted a lengthy and widely publicized inquiry. Over the course of many months, grave clinical errors, serious political interference and provincial negligence in the case were exposed.

There is a healthy fear that state intervention has not led to provisions that are in the best interest of Indigenous children, and this has bred a fierce territoriality when it comes to child protection. Still, Indigenous political interference with the process of ensuring a child's best interests can be a problem and has led, in some cases, to politically expendable children like Lester Desjarlais being left unprotected. Some claim that such political posturing in child welfare is a result of the fact that child welfare has come to be seen as a microcosm of self-government—one of the only places where authority can be flexed. But Lester's death is the direct result of service and governance systems designed to be externally accountable.

The characteristics of Hollow Water and the framework for its success are contrasted with the apparent failure to protect Lester Desjarlais in an environment where the intricacies of a community in denial and the influence of internal political forces were strong. They provide opportunity to analyze the contribution of within, and between group dynamics in breaking or maintaining the status quo. In the Hollow Water example, some important community dynamics existed, including:

- women at the forefront of the healing movement whose efforts were recognized and supported by involved local leadership;
- egalitarian and mutually respectful partnerships with external agents in the broader community, including important provincial players with the power to manoeuvre within the policy climate to allow the community moral independence;
- the development of an *internal accountability* mechanism which eliminated the victim escape burden and created an open climate for disclosure.

In contrast, Lester Desjarlais survived in a community where:

- efforts to break the silence, born mostly by women, were quashed by oppressive local governments;
- no internal accountability mechanism allowed for the application of social sanctions or victim protection;
- no support, involvement or responsible action on the part of external agents existed.

Looking closely at the factors which led to the unnecessary death of a young boy, community and institutional silence are the most salient. Sexual abuse thrives on secrecy. Community silence is often fed by the fact that services generally maintain and perpetuate the power imbalance which led to intervention in the first place. For example, the burden of escape is normally placed upon the child placed in temporary foster care or the battered woman sent to a crisis shelter. When accountability remains in the group and the goal is restoration of harmony, as in Hollow Water, then the victim need not escape but can be protected in his natural environment. Offenders pay restitution, yet also get the chance to heal in the context of their families and communities, creating an open environment where silence need not be maintained. Silence is also fed by the fear of violent repercussion, especially in a small community where anonymity may be impossible. In a community context where the issues are dealt with openly there is strong social sanctioning and subscription to internal moral authority. Anonymity is a nonissue because strict provisions exist to protect witnesses and their families within their communities.

In the unhealthy scenario, silence is enforced because perpetrators who occupy powerful positions in the community function to maintain an imbalance of power between victim and offender. Indigenous governments can operate without conflict of interest guidelines or improper interference protocol because their accountability is external and, in many cases, no internal check or balance exists. Where the influences of patriarchy are strong, women and children are not in empowered positions. While many people of both genders are in denial of their histories of abuse and violence, it was women who challenged this denial at Sandy Bay in an attempt to change Lester's life and those of other child victims (Giesbrecht n.d.) It is exactly this imbalance within the group coupled with external accountability which led to Lester's transiency, abuse and eventual death.

While the best and sometimes only way to break silence is from within, to limit collective responsibility strictly to Indigenous spheres would be a failure to recognize the *historical* responsibilities born by church and state for the current rates of sexual abuse. Furthermore, historical connections aside, no government or institution, Indigenous or otherwise, can claim impunity for the silence about violence in Indigenous communities. Such secrecy has been cultivated by dramatic changes within and between groups—changes which have denied Indigenous women their rightful place in their societies, created externally accountable systems of governance and diluted the potency of internal checks and balances.

Still, even if one supports the notion that years of cultural chauvinism have created conditions in which children are not safe, it is simplistic and unbalanced to assume that the withdrawal of cultural impositions will result in immediate healing. Poor parenting is individually willed and collectively endorsed. In the "out of sight, out of mind" existences of many remote Indigenous communities, only the communities can create or resurrect culturally appropriate challenges to check the plague of child suffering. Such an initiative must emanate from within. While it can and should be supported by external institutions, namely the federal government and historic mission churches, the most valuable and potent force will be internal healing forces, many of which have women at the forefront. No matter how benevolent the intent, paternalism is an insidious form of imbalance between groups which functions to maintain the stratification that limits any political, economic or internal clout which could guide communities toward health. Self-determination is about self-discipline through the means of a culturally appropriate central moral authority who can act immediately to balance the power within the group.

RAYS OF HOPE FROM THE NORTH

This case study has been drawn from Fletcher (1995), which describes an Inuit history of medical evacuation to distant, usually urban-based hospitals for treatment as a means of increasing service accessibility. Evacuation policy was conceived as an approach to widespread tuberculosis treatment, when many were transported from their communities to tuberculosis asylums in the south. So ingrained was the practice in the North that it was extended

to the very natural event of birth. For a time in northern Quebec virtually 100 percent of all births occurred in distant southern medical facilities (Fletcher 1995). This led to:
- decreased paternal and intergenerational involvement in birth;
- elimination of culturally appropriate birth practices;
- maternal fear and alienation; and eventually,
- concealment of pregnancy as a form of resistance to the evacuation policy.

Birthing was no longer a social event with extended family connection and cultural expression, but a medical event associated with earlier tuberculosis treatment (which, for some patients, had meant flying out and never returning). Although they were grateful for medical efforts in general, fly-out births seemed illogical to Inuit women, especially those who had had several community-based births prior to the evacuation policy. Fletcher (1995) also recounts a remarkable success story which began when the Kativik Regional Board of Health and Social Services, funded by the Province of Quebec under the James Bay Northern Quebec agreement, built the new regional hospital. It was an opportunity that Inuit women seized to reinstate their influence over the design and control of birthing practices by establishing the Povungnituk Maternity Centre.

Several key players were involved in the early phases of advocacy, including the Povungnituk Women's Association, southern academics, doctors with experience practicing in the North who had watched the development of other successful community health initiatives, and members of the health centre planning committee. However, staunch resistance was faced by the Corporation des médecins, and the overall political climate was less than hospitable to alternative birth practices or the endorsement of midwifery. Nonetheless, geographical isolation, together with solid, daring and committed local partnership between the Inuit and medical community facilitated the establishment of the centre without the endorsement of governments or professional associations. In fact, the Povungnituk Maternity Centre paved the way for the establishment of other midwifery pilot projects in Quebec.

While no formal evaluation has been done, it is clear that for the community the maternity centre serves several purposes. It:
- brings birthing back to the community and family;
- reduces maternal anxiety and loneliness at birth;
- allows for the father, children, and grandparents to participate in birth in a less intrusive environment;
- reduces the need to conceal pregnancy in order to increase autonomy.

The Inuit believe that paternal participation in birth is essential both to appreciating birth and understanding and accepting the responsibilities of parenthood. They link the high rate of single parenthood to the previous decades of fly-out births. Keeping childbirth in the community connects parents with culturally appropriate support services before and after birth, which can reduce the incidence of low-birthweight babies. In the maternity program, the power of community-based midwives is an argument for the greater involvement of Indigenous people in health care delivery, not only as professionals or paraprofessionals but also as peers. It is also clear recognition of the way services can work at cross-purposes with their goal when they isolate the individual from the context of family and community. Rather than costly evacuation, resources can be better applied to develop and expand community-based services which are holistic and preventive. Last but not least, the Povungnituk Maternity Centre is a contemporary example of committed partnership toward a shared goal where a comfortable blend of birthing support can be enjoyed.

In this case, balance between Inuit and southern groups led to a creative, cost-effective, family-friendly alternative to fly-out births which promoted greater balance within the group by allowing fathers, grandparents and other children to share the birthing process. The maternity centre is also an exceptional model of balance in human service delivery because it reinstates birth as a social event in the context of family and community, where opportunity for cultural expression—the greatest and most powerful preventive energy—is reinforced.

Personal balance as a means of achieving individual and community health was obvious in the celebration of Métis culture, personal empowerment efforts at Fishing Lake and healing circles of Hollow Water. Balance among groups functions to create opportunity for cultural exchange, including mutually supportive and respectful partnership which in turn leads to more culturally appropriate (holistic) and community-based human service delivery. Balance within the group restores internal harmony, eliminates the victim escape burden, and strengthens internal moral authority. Working towards balance in human service delivery, where efforts can be more holistic and preventive measures reduce the possibility of addiction relapse, increases service palatability, reduces bureaucracy, works better and feels right.

POLICY IMPLICATIONS

The health determinants framework is similar to Indigenous notions of holism in several fundamental ways. From both perspectives, health is a multidimensional construct reflecting the interaction of biological, social, environmental, cultural and political forces. However, framework solutions for Indigenous communities will not be simple or static. Nor, most importantly, will they be homogeneous: some important contextual modifications must be considered. *The broad goal is balance at various levels: on a personal level, between groups, within the group, and in human service energies.* The more practical and specific policy recommendations which follow are organized according to the various levels of balance that must be achieved and consider the actions that can be taken at the community, institutional and government levels. *Community* recommendations are those which are directed to Indigenous groups; *institutional* refers to influential, opinion-forming vehicles like corporations, media, professional associations, human services and educational facilities; and *governmental* refers to municipal, provincial and federal levels of government. Some recommen-dations are derived from the success stories analyzed, while others are taken from the framework, adapted for the Indigenous context.

Personal Balance

In many of the success stories, healing was initiated by individuals who tapped their unlimited inner capacity to survive and even thrive against seemingly insurmountable odds. They celebrated a rich cultural heritage without the endorsement of external groups, and, in partnership with committed, daring allies, reversed an intergenerational trend of child sexual abuse. They insisted, against the grain of powerful institutions, upon taking control of birthing practice. In each case, their culture featured prominently and their efforts fed their drive. These opportunities for efficacious action built self-esteem, courage and strength.

Community Action

The human potential in Indigenous communities is enormous. The endurance and resurrection of cultural strength despite the colonial legacy is a testimony to the Indigenous spirit. Community governments, com-mittees, boards, schools and families would be wise to invest in personal growth efforts which reinforce culture and make the world a more under-standable, manageable and meaningful place where opportunity for efficacious action is paramount. Feeding the spirit and mind with cultural teachings strengthens power from within and movement toward health. Effective interaction with the environment fuels self-esteem, confidence and the healing movement. To promote personal balance, *the following measures are recommended:*

- *Communities should establish or strengthen efforts to teach culture, language and colonial history: the world is a much more understandable place when historical colonial influences are understood.*
- *Local leadership should strengthen its support for community-based healing initiatives, because the ability to change the environment can only be exercised when there are opportunities to act.*
- *Local leadership and service agencies should increase their efforts to formally recognize and celebrate community heroes, because we learn not only by doing, but also by watching those who are most like us.*

- *Communities must claim and share ownership of a problem so that it will have meaning. When a problem belongs to us, we make the necessary investment required to develop solutions which work better and feel right.*

Institutional and Governmental Action

In the success stories presented here, cultural celebration and resurrection features prominently in the restoration and maintenance of personal balance. *Hence, it is recommended that:*

- *Major opinion-forming institutions and governments improve their efforts to guard the integrity of Indigenous cultures and languages with equitable resourcing.*

It is also clear that personal empowerment and balance are strengthened by the opportunity to act. In fact, nothing is more potent than action: therefore, barriers to individual and collective action must be dismantled. One of the most repressive barriers to individual action is directly related to income distribution policy which prohibits a workaday life. In order to quickly and easily eliminate this barrier, *it is recommended that:*

- *Social assistance policy be revised to be flexible enough to allow for workfare where it is desired.*

Similarly, when communities initiate healing efforts, coming to the negotiating table claiming full ownership of health problems and presenting culturally appropriate solutions, governments should be in a position to support their efforts. Practically and ethically, this community invitation to partnership is superior to the more traditional "top-down" approach where solutions are generated in distant bureaucratic venues and communities are invited (or expected) to participate. This barrier to collective action can be easily and quickly eliminated if:

- *Governments budget and plan to be* responsive *to local initiative and establish partnerships where they are invited and desired.*

People gain confidence in their own abilities when they see others like them succeed. Therefore, extraordinary efforts must be made to ensure that successful health models are shared with those who are still struggling. Local heroes are the best illustrations of the power from within. National campaigns, media, electronic information exchange or a World Wide Web vehicle should all be used to spread the good news. These can be funded by the state or privately. Specifically, *it is recommended that:*

- *All communications vehicles be enlisted to strengthen existing or establish new role-modelling programs and forms of information exchange among Indigenous communities.*

Balance between Groups

In addition to investment at a personal level, power gained through partnership moves institutions toward change. When ownership is shared, opportunity for efficacious action is created. Logically then, there must be greater balance between what is seen as possible from the outside and the possibilities which must be nurtured and fed from the inside. Because they are the most potent agents of change, the efforts of Indigenous peoples to achieve individual and community healing must be consistently recognized, supported and extended more broadly through responsive and responsible partnership. It has become clear that when Indigenous efforts are recognized and supported within their communities and by external agents, the impact on health status is most effective—because healing and renewal which originates from the inside is most palatable and enduring.

But balance between groups is about more than just shared ownership of problems. At the very core, balance between groups is about equity. Although human services may save a life, only access to an equitable level of opportunity will change that life. Indigenous Canadians are entitled to the same opportunities that other Canadians take for granted—like a workaday life, clean water, adequate housing and education for their children in the language of their choice. It is not unreasonable to expect to be as healthy as Canadians generally. In practical terms, this can be achieved by a more equitable distribution of economic opportunity, through resource co-management regimes and improved access to culturally and geographically appropriate housing. These measures should be accompanied by a recognition of and respect for Indigenous lifeways (including preservation of country foods) in the same institutionally guarded fashion as other founding peoples.

Community Action

It is true that many of the forces which have led to stratification among Canadians are directly related to colonization. But to identify power solely with external influence is to allow the opportunity for self-determination to slip away. In many cases, if the healing forces and agents of change in the Indigenous context would have waited for midwifery to be recognized, municipalities and provinces to get into the business of Indigenous human service delivery or Métis culture to be shared and celebrated, these things would never have happened. Canadian opinion polls regarding self-determination show that the time has never been better to take the initiative. The way to go about it is to seek out like-minded allies to advance and strengthen one's effort and then endeavour proactively to achieve one's goal in spite of inhospitable political or social climates. In the success stories presented, change happened because responsibility was reclaimed, control exercised and flexibility maximized—sometimes in partnership with external agents and other times independently. In other words, *it is recommended that:*

- *Communities take what they need and push forward without the endorsement of external agents, and find allies in the international, academic and broader Canadian context who can help change the politico-legal climate to support their healing efforts.*

Institutional and Governmental Action

There are really three levels at which action can take place, which can be called primary, secondary and tertiary. They differ in their degree of desirability as well as in their ability to effect enduring and substantive social change—with the primary level being the strongest in this regard. At the primary level, balance between groups is best achieved by movement toward more equitable Indigenous participation in resource management. Restoration of economic self-sufficiency and political equilibrium can only be achieved when Indigenous partners have an egalitarian hold on wealth extraction from natural resources. Dependency upon governmental transfer payments serves only to maintain the status quo. Rather, Indigenous groups should be active participants and powerful decision makers in managing and benefitting from the resource-rich land base to which they belong. At the primary level, *it is recommended that:*

- *Governments move toward more equitable distribution of economic opportunity by substituting the current system of support for Indigenous groups from a transfer payment system to one in which Indigenous peoples are egalitarian decision makers and beneficiaries in resource comanagement agreements.*

Until such resource management schemata are developed, secondary efforts must be undertaken to encourage balance among groups. These efforts should facilitate greater Indigenous participation in the economy, through equitable training and development investments. Such investments should sufficiently accommodate sustainable industries in which the focus allows for intimate relationships with the land to be maintained, goods and services are localized and there is a greater emphasis on collective gains. At the secondary level, *it is recommended that:*

- *institutions and governments increase training and development opportunities for Indigenous Canadians;*
- *economic development policy strengthen, encourage and support those businesses which meet local demand, feed collective gain and maintain traditional land relationships.*

Another very obvious disparity among Canadian groups is the strength with which institutions guard cultural integrity. With respect to improving, strengthening and guarding the image and integrity of Indigenous culture in the Canadian context, many participants can be involved. Of course, Indigenous groups are the source, and their ability to be self-directing and morally independent influences the extent to which they can express themselves culturally. Other powerful and important players include the media, schools and churches who, in partnership with Indigenous groups, can become very culturally hospitable institutions. To strengthen the degree to which Indigenous cultures are guarded by Canadian institutions, *it is recommended that:*

- *governments acknowledge and accept the right of Indigenous peoples to be morally independent;*
- *all opinion-forming institutions and communications media develop a formal policy statement which guards the integrity of Indigenous cultures;*
- *educational institutions in particular support the preservation of Indigenous languages and culture as well as eliminate colonizing language and history lessons from their curricula.*

Housing standards represent an area of great disparity among Canadians. In addition to being adequate, living space (housing and community layout) should also be culturally appropriate and "fit" with the geographic location and social mores of the group. Therefore, increased accessibility, creativity and flexibility in sewage and energy systems, as well as culturally sensitive design, are other secondary efforts which can yield significant impact. To achieve this end, *it is recommended that:*

- *governments and lending institutions allow for the expansion of adequate housing and encourage home ownership by immediately eliminating the policy barriers to mortgages on-reserve;*
- *all housing projects incorporate culturally appropriate structural changes and community planning;*
- *the development of alternative energy forms and sewage disposal systems be encouraged and strengthened by institutions and governments.*

Finally, balance among groups can be facilitated at the tertiary level through the promotion of greater institutional completeness in Indigenous communities. A community is institutionally complete when goods and services are primarily secured from, and produced by local sources (e.g., education, consumables, health, etc.). In other words, the development or transfer of administrative control of community-based services in education, justice and health can offer some equalization value, especially if moral independence is exercised. While moral independence is the ideal, in the immediate term, arrangements or protocols like that established between Hollow Water and the Manitoba Department of Justice offer greater flexibility than the scenario in which no community-based services exist. Some moral independence in administrative transfers could also eliminate the barriers to living a workaday life in social assistance–dependent scenarios. Consistently, those able to work are willing to do so and are prohibited from such efficacious action by welfare policy and inflexible contribution agreements. In short, at the tertiary level, *it is recommended that:*

- *Efforts to promote the development of institutional completeness at the Indigenous community level be strengthened through increased transfer of administrative control, with funding arrangements which are equitable and flexible, allowing for interdisciplinary structures to emerge where maximum moral independence can be exercised.*

Although popular at the federal level, the administrative transfer of human services at provincial and municipal levels has been thwarted by serious constitutional ambiguities which prohibit this development and allow for human service double standards to exist and flourish.[1] And while Indigenous community-based services are a great start, at the very least, provincial and municipal governments should ensure Indigenous representation in human service delivery structures. When invited and appropriate, provincial and municipal governments should also become more involved in supporting the health aspirations of Indigenous groups. Because the majority of Indigenous people now resides off-reserve, a new role is emerging for all levels of government. Therefore, *it is recommended that:*

- *The jurisdictional bifurcation of Indigenous human services be resolved so that all levels of government can freely accept responsibility for the provision of service; where provincial and municipal involvement is desired.*
- *Efforts be undertaken to ensure greater representation of Indigenous groups on human service boards.*

Balance within the Group

The erosion of the economic role of Indigenous women in their societies and the concomitant decrease in their power, coupled with culturally imperialistic notions of governance, have fed significant internal imbalances which in many cases are checked neither by culturally appropriate internal moral authorities, nor by outside means. Because much of the healing movement is led by women, the imbalance perpetuates the burden of illness. Creating balance within the group requires two things: the reinstatement of women in political life and the development of internal moral authority.

---

1. Elimination of the jurisdictional bifurcation plaguing Indigenous human services holds tremendous potential for advancing culturally appropriate health systems. For more information, the reader is referred to the works of James Frideres, Joyce Timpson and Alan Moskovich as well as the Report to the Ministers of Health and National Aboriginal Organizations by the Federal/Provincial/Territorial/National Aboriginal Organizations Working Group on Aboriginal Health, and Scott, K. 1993. Funding Policy for Indigenous Human Services. *The Path to Healing.* Royal Commission on Aboriginal Peoples.

Community Action

Communities must strive to integrate into economic and political life those marginalized by historical economic changes and patriarchal ideologies. More balanced gender representation in powerful decision-making positions would have a significant health impact in the Indigenous context. *It is recommended that:*

- *Indigenous governments move towards the reinstatement of women in political life and decision-making positions and increase their accountability to and support of healing initiatives led by women.*

Internal accountability must be strengthened through the development of moral authorities, conflict-of-interest guidelines, improper interference protocol and community-based dispute resolution mechanisms which have the power to check runaway individualism and corruption. For example, the establishment of a Council of Elders with veto power could serve as a check to the centralized power of community governments. Some Indigenous governments have an arm's-length tribal ethics office where members can report improper conduct for investigation: in these scenarios however, the ethics committee is supported by well-developed culturally appropriate systems of justice. Still, nothing prohibits the development of an internal moral authority under current politico-legal arrangements. *It is recommended that:*

- *communities develop culturally appropriate checks to current centralized power structures;*
- *conflict of interest guidelines and improper interference protocol be developed for all community authorities.*

Institutional and Governmental Action

The dilemma posed by external accountability can be resolved in a number of ways. A primary method of ensuring internal accountability is to ensure that Indigenous governments generate revenues from Indigenous peoples. This would be entirely possible in the primary scenario, in which Indigenous groups are egalitarian resource management partners with both levels of government as well as the private sector. This is because participation in a sustainable economy must be a parallel development to internal taxation. When governments secure revenues from their constituents, special interest groups have greater leverage. Currently revenues originate from *external* sources, which means that accountability remains external. For revenues to be obtained internally, Indigenous peoples must be able to participate fully in the wealth extracted from their territories. *It is recommended that:*

- *Egalitarian Indigenous partnership in resource management and benefits surfaces as a select recommendation to ensure group balance.*

Alternatively, community development toward institutional completeness could also serve as a system of checks and balances. For example, in contemporary democratic systems several entities function to balance central authority. They include, among others, the opposition, media, unions, professional associations, taxpayers, and even government-sponsored issue-driven councils like the Assembly of First Nations. Indigenous governments with administrative control of a variety of institutions (e.g., education, health, social services, justice and policing) could set up a similar system if greater powers and autonomy were afforded to local boards governing these institutions. While some Indigenous communities are strong, healthy places with well-developed mechanisms of internal accountability, there are others where the illness burden is great. The primary difference between those that are balanced and healthy and those still suffering appears to related to the degree of institutional completeness that they enjoy. Therefore, *it is recommended that:*

- *Movement toward institutional completeness be facilitated by providing increased opportunity for community-based services to develop.*

Balance in Human Service Delivery

The goal of Indigenous health efforts is not to replicate highly divisive, hierarchical, dependence-producing western approaches to wellness, but to provide a holistic approach with community-specific priorities. Rather than favouring models based on remedial, symptom-centred therapies, Indigenous communities could create healthy, balanced environments by integrating social and physical elements in the broadest sense, where health becomes the natural by-product of living a workaday life and growing in a functional family environment supported by institutionally guarded cultural integrity, and runaway individualism is checked by internal moral authority. But such balance between reactive and proactive energies can only be achieved when there is local control.

Community Action

Communities must seize opportunities for greater control even if political, legal and administrative structures are initially resistant: they need to develop strategic partnerships with like-minded allies who can advance their efforts. It is easier to get forgiveness than it is to get permission; and many policies which "govern" Indigenous affairs are antiquated and inappropriate; therefore, an old teaching with contemporary applications is "take only what you need." Translated into community action, this means establishing an adult care facility even if provincial accreditation cannot be obtained, selecting foster families based on culturally appropriate criteria despite institutional regulations, and the use and celebration of midwifery even though professional associations oppose it. Communities should do what feels right and works best. They should find those who can help make the policy climate more supportive. *Again, it is recommended that:*

- *Communities take what they need and push forward without the endorsement of external agents, finding allies in the international, academic and broader Canadian context who can advance their efforts.*

Institutional and Governmental Action

Consistently, Indigenous groups desire an approach to health which is holistic and integrated—one that makes sense in their world view. To achieve this kind of balance in human service delivery, however, greater opportunity for moral independence must be created—not only in funding arrangements but also in service approach. Indigenous partners are the experts, and they require the freedom to explore and map out health systems which are their own. Culturally relevant service systems are most powerful and preferred. Therefore the development or transferred control of human services at federal, provincial and municipal levels is required in combination with the movement of existing human service systems toward greater cultural sensitivity. To achieve these ends, *it is recommended that:*

- *all levels of government create opportunities for greater community integration of health goals through cross-departmental, alternative, flexible, umbrella funding arrangements;*
- *all levels of government recognize that moral independence may be required in human service delivery;*
- *indigenous representation on human service boards is ensured so that services can move toward greater cultural sensitivity.*

CONCLUSION

In a healthy future, Canadians in general would recognize that much work needs to be done to balance the relationship between themselves and Indigenous groups. Indigenous cultures and languages would be institutionally guarded both within the collective and in the broader Canadian context. Evidence of this institutionally guarded cultural integrity would be obvious in the history books, schools and other opinion-forming tools.

Autonomous Indigenous peoples could aspire to design healthy communities in a morally independent way where culturally cogent notions of responsibility to the group are strengthened and resurrected not as an 'intervention' but as a natural social order (i.e., where immediate individual interests would be balanced with long-term collective interests). In this vision, children thrive in safe, nurturing environments, everyone enjoys the personal benefits of living a workaday life, and Indigenous cultures are reinforced by broad social interactions, media representation and educational institutions.

Indigenous women would regain their stature in social, political and familial organizations. External control would be unnecessary because strong internal moral authorities would regulate unacceptable behaviours through culturally appropriate dispute resolution. Autonomous health care systems would not be "microcosms" of self-government or off-loading exercises, but would be supported by the recognition of an inherent right to be self-determining constitutionally, politically and socially.

Health is the consequence of strong, equitable social organization within and between groups as well as spiritual, emotional, mental and physical balance. Reconceptualizing health in these terms means integrating human development resources in the broadest sense to address all aspects of well-being in balance with reductive strategies where internal and external agents can partner freely. The promotion of integrated, holistic strategies which are informed by Indigenous values, respond to the burden of illness in the community, and balance this response with proactive effort will be the way to build healthy Indigenous communities.

Kimberly A. Scott*'s career spans a broad spectrum of activity including public health administration, program evaluation, historical research, policy analysis, teaching and training. She has written for organizations such as the Royal Commission on Aboriginal Peoples, the Canadian Medical Association and the Canadian Centre on Substance Abuse. She has offered courses with such organizations as the Health Promotion Directorate, Health Canada, and the Pauline Jewitt Institute at Carleton University. She is currently the director of Population Health, Medical Services Branch. She holds an M.Sc. from the University of Waterloo, a B.A. from Carleton University and, most dearly, the title Mom of a bright and beautiful daughter, Desirae.*

BIBLIOGRAPHY

ABEL, G. G., J. V. BECKER, M. MITTELMAN, J. CUNNINGHAM-RATHNER, J. L. ROULEAU, and W. D. MURPHY. 1987. Self-reported sex crime of nonincarcerated paraphiliacs. *Journal of Interpersonal Violence* 2(1): 3–25.

ABORIGINAL HEALTH AND WELLNESS CENTRE OF WINNIPEG, INC. March 1995. *Operational Plan.*

ANTONOVSKY, A. 1987. *Unravelling the Mystery of Health.* San Francisco (CA): Jossey-Bass.

ASSEMBLY OF FIRST NATIONS. March 1988. *Current First Nations Health Conditions: A Statistical Perspective.* Revised.

BANDURA, A. 1977. Self efficacy: Toward a unifying theory of change. *Psychological Review* 84(2): 191–215.

BRANT, C. 1990. Native codes of ethics and rules of behaviour. *Canadian Journal of Psychiatry* 35: 534–539.

CANADA. DEPARTMENT OF HEALTH AND WELFARE. DEMOGRAPHICS AND STATISTICS DIVISION. MEDICAL SERVICES BRANCH. 1986. *First Nations and Inuit of Canada, Health Status Indicators 1974–1983.*

_____. DEPARTMENT OF HEALTH AND WELFARE. 1991. *Health Status of Canadian First Nations and Inuit—1990.* Ottawa (ON): Medical Services Branch.

_____. DEPARTMENT OF INDIAN AFFAIRS AND NORTHERN DEVELOPMENT. 1981. *First Nations Conditions: A Survey.* Ottawa (ON): Published under the authority of the Minister. QS–5141–000–EE–A3.

_____. DEPARTMENT OF INDIAN AFFAIRS AND NORTHERN DEVELOPMENT. 1989. *Highlights of Indigenous Conditions 1981–2001, Part II, Social Conditions, 1989.*

_____. DEPARTMENT OF INDIAN AFFAIRS AND NORTHERN DEVELOPMENT. 1992. *Basic Departmental Data, 1992.*

_____. DEPARTMENT OF THE SECRETARY OF STATE. SOCIAL TRENDS ANALYSIS DIRECTORATE FOR THE NATIVE CITIZENS DIRECTORATE. 1991. *Canada's Off-Reserve Indigenous Population: A Statistical Overview.*

_____. STATISTICS CANADA. 1991. *Aboriginal Peoples Survey.*

DIEM, E. C., L. C. MCKAY, and J. L. JAMIESON. 1994. Female adolescent alcohol, cigarette and marijuana use: Similarities and differences in patterns of use. *International Journal of the Addictions* 29(8): 987–997.

FLETCHER, C. 1995. Inuit community-midwives in Povungnituk, Quebec: A case study of Aboriginal control of health care services. University of Montreal: Department of Anthropology, Faculty of Arts and Sciences. Unpublished M.Sc. thesis.

FRANK, J. W., and J. F. MUSTARD. 1994. The determinants of health from a historical perspective. *Health and Wealth, Proceedings of the American Academy of Arts and Sciences* 123(4): 1–19.

GECAS, V., and M. L. SCHWALBE. 1983. Beyond the looking-glass self: Social structure and efficacy-based self-esteem. *Social Psychology Quarterly* 4(2): 77–88.

GIESBRECHT, B. D., Associate Chief Judge. N.d. *The Fatality Inquiries Act Respecting the Death of Lester Norman Desjarlais.*

HIBBARD, R. A., G. M. INGERSOLL, and D. P. ORR. 1990. Behavioral risk, emotional risk, and child abuse among adolescents in a nonclinical setting. *Pediatrics* 86(6): 869–899.

HINDMAN, J. 1988. Research disputes assumptions about child molesters. *National District Attorney Association Bulletin* 7(4): 1–3.

HOLLOW WATER FIRST NATION. September 1991. *Community Holistic Circle Healing: Ni-pi-tai-osh (Sharing) "The Special Gathering".*

JIN, R. L., C. P. SHAH, and T. J. SVOBODA. 1995. The impact of unemployment on health: A review of the evidence. *Canadian Medical Association Journal* 153(5): 529–540.

KEATING, D. P., and J. F. MUSTARD. 1993. Social economic factors and human development. In *Family Security in Insecure Times.* Ottawa (ON): National Forum on Family Security.

KINNON, D. 1994. *The Health of the Métis People.* Royal Commission on Aboriginal Peoples: Research document.

LAYNE, N. 1984. Health promotion for First Nations/Inuit People: Discussion paper. Canada: Health Promotion Directorate, Department of Health and Welfare. Unpublished work.

_____. 1984. Potential years of life lost among registered First Nations in Canada, 1978–1983. Unpublished document prepared under the direction of the National Native Alcohol and Drug Abuse Program.

MARSHALL, W. L., and H. E. BARBAREE. 1990. The long-term evaluation of a behavioral treatment program for child molesters. *Behavioral Research and Therapy* 26(5): 383–389.

MOON, P. 1995. Native healing helps abusers. *Globe and Mail,* April 8, p. 1.

NEW ECONOMY DEVELOPMENT GROUP. 1993. *First Nations Children: Success Stories in Our Communities.* Health Canada Children's Bureau.

ONTARIO NATIVE WOMEN'S ASSOCIATION. 1989. *Breaking Free: A Proposal for Change to Indigenous Family Violence.* Thunder Bay (ON).

RENAUD, M. The future: Hygeia versus Panakeia. 1995. In *Why Are Some People Healthy and Others Not?*, eds. R. G. EVANS, M. L. BARER, and T. R. MARMOR. New York (NY): Aldine de Gruyter.

SCOTT, K. A. 1995. Indigenous Canadians: A substance use profile. *Canadian Centre on Substance Abuse: Annual Profile.*

SYME, S. L. 1994. The social environment and health. *Health and Wealth, Proceedings of the American Academy of Arts and Sciences* 123(4): 79–86.

WALLACE, J., and J. BACHMAN. 1991. Explaining racial/ethnic differences in adolescent use: The impact of background and lifestyle. *Social Problems.* 38(3): 333–357.

WHERETT, G. J. 1977. *The Miracle of the Empty Beds: A History of Tuberculosis in Canada.* Toronto (ON): University of Toronto Press.

WILKINSON, R. G. 1994. The epidemiological transition: From material scarcity to social disadvantage. *Health and Wealth, Proceedings of the American Academy of Arts and Sciences* 123(4): 61–77.

Community Solidarity and Local Development: A New Perspective for Building Sociopolitical Compromise

PIERRE HAMEL, PH.D.

Professor, Urban Planning Department
University of Montreal

SUMMARY

In assessing policies and programs designed to improve health, the broader context of health determinants is playing an increasingly important role, particularly with respect to factors having to do with living conditions, sociocultural considerations and socioeconomic integration. The problems of employment, social development and local economic development appear to be the key issues here.

Since the 1970s, in most large urban centres in industrialized countries, doubts about the Fordist accumulation model, the globalization of the economy and the use of advanced technologies in reorganizing production systems have had numerous adverse effects on local populations, particularly in former industrial neighbourhoods: the loss of vast numbers of jobs, rising unemployment, the emergence of new forms of poverty, growing violence and a general deterioration in living conditions. Public authorities seem to be overwhelmed by all of these closely correlated factors.

Because these transformations amount, politically and economically speaking, to a crisis in existing adjustment models, various initiatives have been put forward by members of the community to counteract the adverse impact of the rationalizations and restructurings forced upon social groups by decisions made elsewhere. This is what led to the establishment of community economic development corporations, which embarked on social restructuring efforts. The example under consideration in this study is the Regroupement pour la relance économique et sociale du sud-ouest de Montréal (RESO).

Ever since the 1980s, members of the community have been working to redefine citizenship as part of a review of the sharing of individual and collective responsibilities, and of a reassessment of accepted institutional rules. The process has led them to be critical of prevailing state and market logic, and to focus on the many different forms of social restructuring currently available, in the absence of a recognized adjustment model. What they have been doing therefore challenges the basic tenets of modernity.

How well are the community members who have become involved in recent years in local economic development strategies succeeding in improving living and employment conditions for workers in disadvantaged neighbourhoods? How have they been able to change government policies and programs? How do they view solidarity, justice, democracy and the sharing of responsibilities between the public and private sectors? To what extent have they achieved their objectives? Does the model of partnership with the state to which they subscribe inherently endanger their own objectives?

To answer these questions, and to report on recent work on local development and action by community members in job creation and support for entrepreneurship, we decided to examine the RESO example.

TABLE OF CONTENTS

INTRODUCTION

The transformations that Western societies have undergone, both socioeconomic and value related, raise many questions about the different forms of social integration and how to implement them. Economic globalization has led to one upheaval after another in work and management, and we still do not have a very good idea of what their impact will be (Drucker 1994); they will force many changes, including a redefinition of public administration models and policy priorities.

Health is not immune to uncertainty and challenges in such a context. Some research has emphasized the importance of considering social environment factors to explain the level of health of various social groups or health differences between them (Syme 1994; Marmot 1994). From this standpoint, the overall health of the population would appear to depend not only on access to care and quality of care, but also on the level of control that individuals and groups have over their working conditions and their living environment. Greater life expectancy also seems to be correlated with income equity (Frank and Mustard 1994).

In the postindustrial era, growth in the economies of industrialized countries no longer results simply from productive investment, but also from the drive and vitality of communities or socioeconomic environments, including health (Frank and Mustard 1994). In other words, in economies that are highly dependent on the tertiary sector, the overall components of the social, political, environmental and cultural context are the key to whether or not communities will be able to take advantage of opportunities that come about as a result of global change.

This study is based on three premises. Firstly, that poverty and economic and social underdevelopment have an adverse effect on health conditions for people who live in disadvantaged urban neighbourhoods. Second, social restructuring depends on the economic reintegration and the social integration of households, which are largely dependent on employment, in spite of the organizational and institutional difficulties involved in job creation in such neighbourhoods. Third, although we may be witnessing the withering away of the organic solidarity that has characterized industrial societies, it is gradually being replaced—as a result of a number of community initiatives—by new forms of solidarity that are based on a new division of individual and collective responsibilities.

That is why we decided on the Regroupement pour la relance économique et sociale du sud-ouest de Montréal (RESO) as an example of a success story. This community group, which is located in a former industrial zone in the Montreal area, took action on several fronts to improve living and working conditions for local residents. As a result, it was required to work in various types of partnerships with socioeconomic stakeholders, and to negotiate and reach a compromise with political authorities. In several respects, its experience has given us a better understanding of the strategies and types of action available to social players in disadvantaged urban neighbourhoods to create jobs and set in motion a social process to integrate the most seriously disadvantaged members of the community. It also sheds light on the nature of the contradictions of advanced modernity, which is being subjected to a serious crisis in terms of values and an adjustment model inherited from the Fordist model of industrial society.

The paper is divided into four sections and a conclusion. We begin by identifying the main components of the issues that will be used to focus on recent works on local development as well as the RESO example. Then, after addressing a number of semantic details, we place the main conclusions of recent works on local development into perspective. This step is useful in positioning the case being studied in its proper sociopolitical context, as well as in identifying what is currently at stake in local development in view of both the latitude available to community members on the one hand, and the overall determinants of health on the other. Third, we present a short case study, with due regard to the guidelines for success stories suggested by the Determinants of Health Working Group. Lastly, we describe the major policy implications that result from the RESO example and an analysis thereof. Conditions under which the example may be transposed to other settings depend on a combination of internal and external factors that are likely to appear together increasingly in the coming years because of the effects stemming from the transformation of our production system and the globalization of the economy.

THE ISSUES

In today's industrialized societies, which typically advocate a new type of relationship between personal life and all-encompassing systems (Giddens 1993), the challenges to economic and political players are not the same as those that were most conspicuous in the industrial era. The political class and governments have lost the legitimacy that not so long ago enabled them to make public choices without extensively consulting the people. At the time, they appeared to be the main proponents and advocates of a form of modernity designed to make up any ground lost from the economic or institutional standpoints. The march of history, wearing its progressive colours, appeared to everyone to be ineluctable. The state's mission caused little worry in terms of its purpose or its foundations.

As the year 2000 approaches, reality is very different. Governments have to face challenges that require a redefinition of the public administration model that was put in place after the Second World War, which was a compromise between the state and the marketplace. Indeed, the model went hand in hand with an increasingly restrictive vision of the economy (Laville 1993, 131), the limits of which we are only today beginning to grasp.

It is clearly from the institutional standpoint that it is easiest to see the problems faced by the state. Up until the mid-1970s, economic growth made it possible to both increase government regulation of the marketplace and at the same time significantly extend the social safety net. Of course, this was occurring at a time when the state was perceived as an engine of development rather than as an impediment to it.

Uncertainty is increasing as the consensus with respect to the redistribution role previously performed by the state is being challenged. Some believe that it is necessary to find a new foundation for government action to overcome the failure of legitimacy that has characterized it for several years in most Western countries.

This in essence is the debate between liberals and communitarians. Liberals believe that it is essential to defend universal values and to give precedence to the principle of law, which guarantees everyone access to public services; communitarians, on the other hand, hold that it is more important to recognize cultural identities and differences as rooted in social groups and to use them as a basis to settle conflicts between the general interest and individual interests. According to communitarians, freedom is not so much based on abstract principles as on community values rooted fundamentally in local forms of expression (Caney 1992).

The debate between liberals and communitarians has revolved around various issues such as the universality of public services, political rectitude and the integration of ethnic communities. It cannot be said that satisfactory compromises have been achieved yet. The debate has nevertheless focused on the difficulty, and indeed the inability, of institutions in their current form to meet new social demands. This is precisely what Bellah and his team (1992) have explored.

In examining the most common social problems, they ask themselves why American society is now unable to meet the expectations and demands of a growing portion of the population. Their analysis begins with the failure of public institutions. It also discusses the central principles and values of liberty, justice and democracy which have fuelled these institutions since their establishment.

Ethical issues and choices top their list of arguments. According to the authors, institutional dilemmas are above all moral dilemmas (Bellah et al. 1992, 16). If institutions are no longer able to solve social problems, it is because they have lost their moral foundation. Many explanatory factors are reviewed in connection with this subject. These include the world economic context, the existing legal system, the role of governments and attempts to reshape society. While the possible solutions require a renewal or redeployment of solidarity and social consensus, they also require a broadening of our methods of management and democratic representation.

Institutional models and options nevertheless remain limited by the recent transformations of the economic system. Thus the globalization of markets, the restructuring of employment, the greater role being played by information and new communications technologies, organizational changes in the workplace and their impact on urban development are also factors that have been raised in attempts to identify trends that will follow the Fordist model or the industrial development model (Dalton 1988). Moreover, according to Dahrendorf (1995), all of these upheavals have had significant impacts from at least three standpoints, namely job opportunities for all workers, social cohesiveness in civil society, and guarantees with respect to the exercise of political liberty.

In terms of economics, the world integration of markets has had direct repercussions on the living conditions of Canadians, as it has in the other industrialized countries (Reich 1991). The flexibility principle upon which the new "world economic order" will be based involves a series of structural adjustments as well as attempts by both business and governments to achieve increased competitiveness and productivity. Workers would also appear to have no alternative but to adapt to these new requirements. That at least is the claim of those who advocate an "economicist" vision of society.

The main problem stems from the fact that these adjustments lead to economic and social inequalities which unequivocally threaten the balances and solidarities established during the growth period of the 1950s and 1960s. As Dahrendorf (1995) notes, the recent economic changes that require social actors to show greater flexibility could not be introduced without challenging what was accomplished during the postwar growth years. The progress made during these years was as much economic, with numerous opportunities to individuals, as it was related to civil society in terms of solidarity and social protection, or again to freedom in political society. With globalization, new forms of exclusion appeared that created income inequalities. Here, rising unemployment and growing poverty threaten earlier forms of and opportunities for participation and even solidarity within civil society.

In such a context of insecurity and uncertainty, it is easy to see how civil and political liberties may be challenged. This is because the combined effects of increased world competitiveness and social disintegration causes fears and encourages the rise of a form of authoritarianism that is opposed to the expression of such freedoms (Dahrendorf 1995, 28).

Even with these difficulties, we can still yearn for prosperity, a civil society that can play a social integration role, and a politically dynamic society, namely one which can enforce the rule of law, protect political liberties and foster free expression. However, it would appear today to be increasingly difficult to pursue all three objectives at the same time.[1] Nor is

---

1. To remain competitive in growing world markets, First World countries will have to take measures that damage the cohesion of the civil society (adapted from Dahrendorf 1995, 13).

there a simple solution to these complex problems. Indeed, global solutions are likely to aggravate rather than improve the situation.

Seen from this standpoint, falling back on local development, namely giving local communities the resources they need to control their own development, may make it easier to redefine the framework for public action and hence give rise to a redefinition of government responsibility and forms of management. It may also make it possible to investigate concrete opportunities for action by all social actors together.

That is why the crisis in the welfare state adjustment model has led several social actors to turn towards new forms of community "solidarity," to compensate for the shortcoming of the redistribution mechanisms managed by the state. To be sure, these actors neither can nor wish to return to traditional forms of solidarity, which demanded strong and often direct reciprocity between the individual and the community. What they do advocate is extensive dialogue with the community in question, and transactions and relationships defined both as a complement to and in opposition to the bureaucratic management of social affairs. The issues involved in local development need to be stated with reference to these factors.

LOCAL DEVELOPMENT AND THE EMERGENCE OF COMMUNITY ECONOMIC DEVELOPMENT CORPORATIONS: LITERATURE SURVEY

Theoretical and Political Aspects of Local Development

The return to the local level that has been observed in all Western countries since the early 1980s is somewhat paradoxical. It has occurred at a time when the globalization of markets and culture have never been stronger. Ought we to see this as a result of government efforts to adapt to new post-Fordist adjustment mechanisms (Klein 1995) or is it simply pragmatic resistance or efforts by local actors to adjust to painful economic trends?

Local development is certainly inconceivable without the exercise of local power. The major problem nevertheless stems from the fact that it is very difficult to identify the main factors that shape the formulation of urban policies (Monkkonen 1988). In fact, even though we know that municipalities define their action on the basis of a variety of institutional logics— market logic, bureaucratic and democratic logic, corporate logic—we are still very poorly acquainted with the mechanisms that govern the development of consensuses that lead to local social and political transformations (Clarke 1995).

Theoretical studies carried out in recent years all emphasize the diversity and complexity of the processes in question. They also highlight the importance of giving close consideration to how the various categories of actors involved in formulating compromises and urban policies interact.

The indeterminacy of local power (Biarez 1989) is indisputably having an impact on opportunities for local development and on the practices that fuel it. However, the usual definitions of the local development concept do not often place an emphasis on this dimension, although researchers agree that this type of development is essentially a dynamic process (Blakely 1989, 59).[2]

Some authors, including Pecqueur (1989), argue that it is primarily a social component that can be expressed in the development of means to achieve solidarity for those who are excluded (Eme 1990, 30). This is a view that is not necessarily shared by all researchers—at least not in the same terms—nor by all local actors. Everything depends on the choices or on the nature of the commitment of the actors and researchers.

That is why some people make a clear distinction between the "liberal" and the "progressive" views of local development. The former emphasizes economic recovery and reconstruction to create jobs, whereas the second advocates economic investment based on social and democratic concerns (Fontan 1993). The progressive view also speaks of community economic development rather than local development.

Although this dichotomy is not unfounded, it does not remove all ambiguities. Thus, according to Boothroyd and Davis (1993), community economic development may opt for growth promotion, structural change or even community appropriation strategies. Others (Christenson, Fendley, and Robinson 1989) emphasize instead the fact that the concept of development already includes the ideas of improvement, growth and change.

Without taking this analysis of semantic details further, let us simply say that we base ourselves here on the representations, practices and strategies developed by community actors involved in transforming their environment. We assign a broad meaning to the concept of local development, including in it the distinctions made by these actors on the basis of local conditions and their ideologies. Although it is also possible to speak of "community economic development" to refer to the same reality, the latter expression does not always make it possible to remove the ambiguities and contradictions

---

2. Blakely's definition is as follows: "It is essentially a process by which local government and/or community-based groups manage their existing resources and enter into new partnership arrangements with the private sector, or with each other, to create new jobs and stimulate economic activity in a well-defined economic zone. The central feature in locally oriented or based economic development is in the emphasis on "endogenous development" policies using the potential of local, human, institutional, and physical resources. This orientation leads to a focus on taking local initiatives in the development process to create new employment and stimulating increased economic activity" (1989, 58).

with which the actors need to deal. The pragmatic approaches that they tend to prefer often cause further confusion.

This state of affairs stems largely from the fact that there is not, strictly speaking, any such thing as a theory of local development (Fasenfest 1991; Bingham and Mier 1993). Considered as a subject for both empirical and multidisciplinary study, however, local development has been addressed from various standpoints. According to Bingham and Mier (1993), such points of view emphasize a variety of areas, such as problem solving, the effectiveness of strategies, the responsibility of the various categories of actors involved, or equity. In short, a series of values associated with one specific analysis perspective.

The absence of a general theory of local development does not automatically mean that researchers do not share certain concerns, or even an heuristic corpus. Thus in spite of their divergent views, it can be said that researchers agree on three major principles: that local actors can change things if they engage in action; that there is a diversity of situations and problems, and hence a need for contextual variations in strategies (Hambleton 1991); and that an equitable view of development needs to be defended, even though justice does not mean the same thing for everyone (Mier 1993).

In addition, these three principles are more or less articulated around the major economic transformations of the past two decades. It should not be forgotten that the accelerated gross model introduced at the end of the Second World War in the form of "top-down development"—which is based more than anything else on the idea of continuing growth (Stöhr 1984)—entered a crisis period in the early 1970s. This required the Western countries to review their regional development policies, which had previous been defined in terms of modernizing industrial infrastructures and fostering labour mobility. After this, it began to appear desirable to introduce endogenous development policies oriented towards regional dynamism and local initiatives. This is what led the Organization for Economic Cooperation and Development (OECD), as early as 1974, to ask member countries to review their regional policies (Mormont 1989).

The changes observed regionally had their counterpart in the cities. However, the form and content of the changes were different. From the mid-1970s onward, the major urban centres, in particular former industrial centres, had to come to grips with phenomena like industrial redeployment, the tertiarization of their economies, urban sprawl and a redefinition of centrality. The result was a transformation of public intervention and urban policies.

Governments thus did not hesitate to decentralize in an effort to give greater responsibility to municipalities (Hamel and Jalbert 1991). Municipalities no longer hesitated to go beyond managing policies and programs developed by higher levels of government, and to take more initiatives in the form of entrepreneurship and partnerships between the public and private sectors.

In short, the introduction of such urban policies led to the replacement of the traditional administrative approach by a new "managerial" approach (Harvey 1989; Mayer 1989). These new trends, which appeared in the mid-1970s, strengthened during the 1990s. From this standpoint, the framework for public action at the local level can be said to have undergone a redefinition.

On the other hand, the emergence of local development, which goes hand in hand with greater local powers, did not necessarily result only from the crisis in the top-down development model. Even though this factor may have been an essential catalyst, the fact remains that local development depends more than anything else on the determination and initiatives of local actors.

From Issues to Practice

Several studies of local development have emphasized urban economic and social problems (Teisserenc 1994). As a multidisciplinary field of study, local development converges with a series of areas for intervention or issues which, barely 15 years ago, were not attached to it. Examples are architectural and urban heritage, public services and social policies. Researchers are also giving due regard to a number of political topics that cut across various fields such as citizenship, participation, democracy, and partnership. Each of these areas elicits questions not only about appropriate forms of action and strategies by local actors, but also about the values attached to them. Thus analysis of local development leads to a normative model of local public action (Heinz 1994).

It is not easy, however, to assess the scope of local development. Everything depends on what is being measured and on the evaluation methods chosen by the researchers (Wassmer 1994). A review of the main works published on local development since the early 1980s in four countries—Canada, the United States, France and the United Kingdom (Hamel 1995)—yields mixed results.

The example of Sheffield in England (Lawless and Ramsden 1990) is significant here. Indeed, even though the partnership between the public and private sectors—which is one of the preferred tools of local development—contributed in the Sheffield study to remaking the city's image and launching several projects, not all sectors and groups benefitted. There were winners and losers. The same is true in the United States, where a number of projects were primarily of benefit to private enterprise and the higher classes at the expense of people in disadvantaged neighbourhoods and most workers (Harvey 1989). Many researchers have pointed out that the concrete benefits from various forms of partnership between the public and private sectors in local development remain very limited for local residents (Levine 1989; Squires 1991; Stephenson 1991). The fact remains, however, that sometimes, as in Pittsburgh, the partnership made a direct contribution to the renewal of the urban core (Weaver and Dennert 1987).

It is nonetheless true that development factors vary considerably from one neighbourhood to another. Whether or not an experiment or project will be successful depends more than anything else on the extent to which the context is conducive to openness, dynamism and synergy. This may be explained by the historical factors that determine the possibilities for local institutional adjustment. In other respects, success depends on political factors that are the purview of the state and its relations with economic agents (Piven and Friedland 1984).

The role of actors and how they interact socially also merits consideration (LeGalès 1993) because some subjective factors can make a difference. These include quality of leadership in projects or organizations, or the extent to which the support of the locals has been obtained and mobilized. From this standpoint, the capacity of local communities to reach sociopolitical compromises is considered a strategic and even a key factor for the success of projects or local development policies (Jezierski 1990).

It is not easy to draw the boundaries of local development accurately. They are no longer restricted to ad hoc investment, such as the promotion of manufacturing (Pickvance 1990). What is important now is the creation of networks of actors in numerous areas: business services, research and development, promotion of the arts and culture, and development of new technologies and design (Quévit 1992). The ability of neighbourhoods to encourage innovation or to introduce the conditions needed to create a truly dynamic environment may depend on their ability to make use of technical and technological innovations by adapting them to their needs (Aydalot 1985).

In such a context, the formulation of public policy no longer comes about within an authoritarian technocratic framework but rather by means of more flexible managerial structures such as those that come from decentralization. Many institutional changes result from the shift. On the one hand, the state encourages competition between cities, which may lead to the emergence of a new form of local elitism (Peck and Tickell 1995), and on the other, a new "localism" is being affirmed which brings all endogenous forces into play (Quesnel 1995). This does not automatically mean a radical transformation in the power relationships between the state and local authorities. In many countries, it means not so much that the state has to submit to a subsidiarity principle as that it must redeploy its action with due regard to local features (Ascher 1992).

Despite the transformations underway, municipal administrations appear to be very reluctant to change their management structures. This is because the partnership between the public and private sectors often enables them to benefit from private expertise without changing their ways of doing things (Moore and Pierre 1988). Furthermore, by relying more and more on experts and thereby depoliticizing development decisions, the partnership limits the local democratic process (Ascher 1992).

In spite of the limitations on the public–private sector partnership, considered here to be an institutional model that makes it possible to fuel or promote a variety of local development strategies, many have noted that the approach fosters dynamic interaction between actors and sectors (Stephenson 1991). Furthermore, because of the flexibility which this partnership requires from public actors (Henry 1994), it tends to increase the autonomy of local public authorities and foster the intervention of community actors (Fainstein and Fainstein 1994). Indeed, it is through community participation that partnerships between the public and private sectors can break the circle that defends private interests and the primacy of marketplace logic (Jezierski 1990; Stephenson 1991).

That is why local development can create a new opportunity for social restructuring that can counter the dominant economic trends that engender various types of social polarization and exclusion (Dahrendorf 1995). Local development can thus become, from a political standpoint, "strategic" (Piore 1995), because local development offers concrete opportunities to many workers and excluded groups. It allows them to get involved in communications, exchanges and integration activities geared to production that they did not have access to before (Piore 1995).

From among all the works that consider the many components of local development, those that study the efforts of community actors and community economic development corporations may be considered separately. Like local development studies most, they are generally divided into those that examine the proliferation or fermentation of ideas and the research that reports on these projects.

In the United States in the early 1990s, the number of community economic development corporations was estimated at 2,000 (Wiewel, Teitz, and Giloth 1993). No systematic inventory has been prepared for Canada. It is highly likely that the relative number approaches that for the United States. In Quebec, in addition to the many local and regional coordination committees outside of Montreal, there are some 20 community development corporations that have turned their attention to giving life to their communities (Fontan 1993). Recently, in the city of Montreal, an inventory carried out by the Service du développement économique (1995) listed 68 agencies working with a variety of clienteles—women, youth, immigrants and cultural communities, adults—to encourage their entry into the labour market. The vast majority of these agencies grew out of the community or function in partnership with it.

For all these examples, one can speak of a genuine laboratory experimenting on both the social and institutional, and political levels. Within a given group, skills are being developed that make it possible to optimize results over the years. In addition, such skills are often transferred from one group to another.

These factors are repeatedly referred to in studies of these groups (e.g., Ross and Usher 1986), but other important aspects of their efforts are also mentioned. For example, although all these groups intervene directly or indirectly in employment and social integration, they are also highly diversified in terms of the resources they manage or generate, the activities or services they provide for their communities, and the nature of the links they maintain with their surroundings. Whether they use volunteers, some forms of patronage or "contractualization", like similar groups in Europe (Demoustier and Grange 1995), the relations they maintain with public institutions are in more than one respect ambivalent and contradictory. From this viewpoint, their actions converge with many social movements. Their action is also much more complex than most sociologists have thus far led us to believe, including those who from the outset have emphasized the importance of this dimension (Bartholomew and Mayer 1992).

On another front, several studies have highlighted the fact that these groups generally achieve the desired results (Mayer 1984) in spite of the many problems they have to overcome. Thus they generally succeed in obtaining the resources they need for their action. In addition, their success depends on a set of cumulative factors, including the training and skills of officials who can plan and administer budgets. A thorough understanding of the financial issues on which the completion of projects depends is also important. Finally, the agency's track record, its previous successes, can often be an indicator of successful performance. From this standpoint, it can be said that the skills and expertise of community agencies increase as they partake in concrete achievements (Mayer 1984).

These agencies play a unique role because of their familiarity with the community, their special skills in working in disadvantaged urban settings and their determination to take action to change things. Even though it is not infallible, and remains haunted by the spectre of social polarization, community action remains a worthwhile method of combatting the impoverishment of communities (Economic Council of Canada 1990). It is one area in which it is clear that economic efficiency and democracy go hand in hand (Fontan 1993).

Since the early 1980s, agencies involved in promoting the economics of their communities have refined their intervention tools and models. It is this that has led them to promote the idea of partnership with governments and business. It has made it possible for them to stop perceiving themselves as victims, a stance that often accompanied the confrontational ideology of the 1960s and 1970s, and to acquire the status of legitimate stakeholders (Hamel 1991).

Community action focused on managing social affairs or on development nevertheless continues to raise a good many questions. Many have noted that the institutionalization of community action involves some adverse effects that affect not only its ability to mobilize people, but also to change power relationships on the local political scene (Fainstein and Hirst 1995). Limited as they are by their localism, the actors must often agree to be co-opted or to negotiate compromises, hence an interpretation that downplays the extent of their action. On the one hand, there is disapproval of the increased risks associated with their use by the state, which means a definite threat for the independence considered essential if they are to be creative and innovative. On the other hand, it is admitted that they play a key role in the empowerment of civil society vis-à-vis the state (Wolch 1989).

Community economic development corporations grew out of several traditions. In Canada, there were farming, fishing and forestry cooperatives (Economic Council of Canada 1990). There was also the Desjardins movement in Quebec and the Antigonish cooperative movement in Nova Scotia—which meant experience dating back to the beginning of the century (Fontan 1993).

There is, however, another tradition, that of community action. As such, the tradition traces its roots to several influences. To begin with, political militancy by workers who, both in North America and Europe, established various forms of mutual assistance at the beginning of the worker movement (Julliard 1971); also worth noting is the associative movement in the form it took in Europe at the end of the nineteenth century (Salamon 1989). There is also community work and its renewal based on Alinski's confrontational concept, relying on mobilizing the have-nots of Chicago neighbourhoods in the 1950s (Boyte 1980). A final influence came from social movements to defend civil rights, which surfaced just about everywhere in the Western world, and in particular in the United States, most noticeably in the early 1960s.

All of these traditions centred on local communities, their initiatives and the various forms of solidarity that they developed. However, they did not evolve in isolation. From the mid-1960s onward in the United States, and at the same time in Canada with a program established by the Secretary of State known as the Company of Young Canadians, they received considerable institutional support, both from public agencies and private foundations like the Ford Foundation. These additional resources, and the administrative framework established, led community players in the area to review their internal organization and their intervention strategies, as well as their relationships with the state and political authorities.

Nevertheless, in the form they have today, which is what is of interest to us here, community economic development corporations go back to the 1970s. They focus both on the social component of development (Shragge 1993) and on the importance of its being rooted in a specific setting (Newman, Lyon, and Philp 1986). Seen from this standpoint, they promote a multidimensional view of development, in which economic factors are always related to social, political and cultural dimensions of communities (Douglas 1994). They are engaged in a battle again social exclusion, meaning that above all else, the economy needs to be democratized (Friedmann 1992).

As with local development, community economic development corporations are not a panacea. In many respects, they reflect the ambiguities and uncertainties of the crisis that public institutions are going through.

It must not be forgotten that their resources and their avenues for action are limited. What is more, the organizational and operational problems they have to overcome are both technical and practical, and involve socio-political aspects that relate to their vision of community affairs.

Their action remains circumscribed within a context of marketplace globalization, and is to a very large degree subordinate to the economic strategies of big business. In view of the trends towards economic polarization (Fontan 1995), their resistance often falls into the trap of the greater employment flexibility required by the dominant economic players. In other words, in spite of the vigilance of community actors, the risk remains great that a social integration objective may be diverted at the expense of flexible adaptation to an uncertain job.

One thing is certain, and that is that community actors alone cannot transform local communities. In addition to the direct contribution they make in terms of training, coordination, and the creation of businesses and jobs, these actors are engaged in an effort to change people's mindset (Mayer 1984). It is largely here that they can be seen to be innovative.

For leaders of community economic development corporations, the battle against exclusion has to begin with local development and the economic integration of the jobless through gainful employment. From here, they put forward a redefinition of citizenship and of the framework for public action which involves no longer recognizing or reiterating the rights inherent to the functioning of liberal democratic societies. What they advocate is a review of the sharing of collective and individual, public and private responsibilities in light of the new issues in society which, beyond class relationships, address the environment, the quality of development and living conditions, as well as racial and sexual discrimination. Within this set of issues, the question of health takes on a whole new meaning.

Local Development and Health

While the question of health is never broached directly in local development studies, it is certainly addressed indirectly, and from two standpoints: first of all, under the heading living conditions, which has become a major issue in the 1980s for neighbourhoods because of the need to remain or become competitive to attract businesses; it is also addressed in any discussions of employment. Since the 1980s, local administrations have been less concerned about controlling the urbanization process than about creating jobs. Local labour is considered a resource that plays a dynamic role in development, in relation to which qualitative considerations, including health, are important. That being the case, it is no longer acceptable to dissociate health from development (Paquet 1994).

This, moreover, is what the Canadian Institute for Advanced Research (CIAR) suggests when it says that collective health depends more on the ability of nations to "create" and "distribute" wealth than on the provision of medical services (CIAR 1991). The example of Japan is particulary revealing in this respect. Although the percentage of gross national product devoted to the health system is one of the lowest among the OECD countries, there has been a "remarkable increase in life expectancy" (CIAR 1991, 4). One interesting hypothesis to explain the phenomenon is the relatively small income gap between the poorest and richest groups in Japan compared to other countries.

Similarly, several studies have demonstrated that there is a strong correlation between the economic status or social class of a given population and its health (Townsend and Davidson 1982; Feinstein 1993; Marmot 1994). The Commission d'enquête sur les services de santé et les services sociaux noted that although the health of the population had improved over the past 15 years, there were still gaps between social groups and classes: [Translation] "A resident of Westmount can expect to live without any full or partial limitation on activities 11 years longer than a resident of St. Henri" (Government of Quebec 1988, 47). This was also corroborated by the most recent social survey carried out by the Montreal Centre Regional Health and Social Services Board (Chevalier and Tremblay 1995). In Greater Montreal between 1976 and 1991, the life expectancy differential between residents of disadvantaged neighbourhoods compared to "privileged" municipalities was not closed at all.

It is thus easy to understand why it is necessary to study more than the issue of access to medical care, both to explain inequalities with respect to health and to remedy the situation. Indeed, it is becoming increasingly clear that health results from the complex interaction of numerous factors operating at the socioeconomic, environmental and sociocultural levels. These determinants are also tied to individual biological, family and personal history factors. It is therefore clear that quality of care and access to care become additional factors that have an impact on improving health.

Even though several studies have highlighted the need to take the social determinants of health into consideration to improve the quality of life and health (Evans, Barer, and Marmor 1994), for example by reducing poverty and closing the income gap (Wilkinson 1986), the fact remains that in terms of public policy, health remains a societal choice. The arguments of those who defend special or corporate interests within the system can only be refuted if we can arrive at a better understanding of the relationships between health and development and broaden public debate.

Of the various aspects of the relationships between health and development, researchers in recent years have focused a good deal of attention on the link between health and employment. Generally speaking, we know that there is a positive correlation between employment and health (Graetz 1993; Wilson and Walker 1993; Ross and Mirowsky 1995; Turner 1995). In other words, having a job or finding a job improves health, even though a person's health may also help that person find a job. Several specific factors make it possible to have a better understanding of how employment or unemployment may affect health.

To begin with, the risk of being unemployed is not shared equitably throughout the population. People who have already been unemployed are much more likely than others to be unemployed again. All in all, it is a small percentage of the labour force that is chronically unemployed (Bartley 1994). Attitudes towards unemployment also vary from one setting to another. They are not as negative in settings where there is a greater likelihood of finding another job (Turner 1995), hence the importance of giving due regard to the dynamism of such settings and encouraging an active approach. Lastly, while having or finding a job can have a positive impact on health, the quality of the work and the level of satisfaction appear to be even more important. Thus people who leave school and take an unsatisfactory job do not really derive any benefit compared to those who do not find a job. Likewise, unemployed people who obtain an unsatisfactory job do not derive any significant health benefit from it (Graetz 1993).

These qualitative considerations are added to the residual effects that can persist once an unemployed person reenters the labour market (Turner 1995). Elsewhere, it has been found that it is not only employment itself that can benefit health. The support given to people looking for work—in the form of training, for example, to help them acquire new skills, or in the form of measures made available to them to provide them with a degree of financial security—may also help to reduce the negative impact of unemployment on health (Wilson and Walker 1993).

This was corroborated by the longitudinal study conducted between October 1986 and June 1990, which evaluated the rehabilitation and counselling program offered by La Relance inc. in Hull, a social integration firm that works with young people in trouble. The basic assumption in their work is that a person's self-esteem varies as a function of their own experience, which is directly influenced by the environments in which they live. The study monitored a group of 78 young representatives of the agency's clientele, namely young people with psychosocial problems looking for work (Bertrand et al. 1992, 46). The study used two experimental groups and one control group. Even though it is not possible here to summarize all the findings of the study, the main conclusions are very clear. The young people who participated in La Relance inc.'s program took the first steps towards improving their mental health. They also gradually improved their overall lifestyle and became more specific about the type of work they would like to do (Bertrand et al. 1992, 92). These, as it happens, are essential elements for successfully reentering the labour market. Thus the question of what connections there might be between employment and health leads us to give closer consideration to neighbourhoods and their ability to help people who are laid off or who find themselves without a job.

This was precisely the aspect considered by Gregory Pappas (1989) in the study that he carried out in Barberton, Ohio, an industrial town whose population peaked at 33,805 inhabitants in 1970, only to fall to 29,751 in 1980. Between 1979 and 1983, approximately 5,000 jobs were lost in this city because of the many plant closings caused by economic restructuring and industrial redeployment. The unemployment rate, which of course varied from one sector to another, hit 14.3 percent in 1982 for the county as a whole.

The scale of the layoffs over such a short time had a very harmful cumulative effect on the whole community. The training and employment opportunities available to workers in other cities were often unsatisfactory. Unemployment initially affected the personal identity of workers insofar as their previous beliefs in their skills and stability had been replaced by feelings of incompetence and instability (Pappas 1989, 82). Unemployment also reveals very clearly that for most people, work largely remains an element that provides a structure around which social life is organized as well as the preferred method of socialization. Thus beyond the sense of social usefulness which is often attached to work and which disappears when a job is lost, workers who are unemployed also experience withdrawal from many social activities, which makes them even more vulnerable.

When they lost their jobs, the Barberton workers had to ask themselves where they were going. Some had considered their job as a career which gave them a degree of stability and advancement based on their efforts and accomplishments. With the layoffs, they began to feel personal guilt, and this gradually transformed itself into collective guilt.

After taking jobs that did not pay as much or that had fewer opportunities for advancement, these workers had to redefine their work ethic because the new job did not necessarily give them as much satisfaction and was not necessarily suited to their personality.

To counter defeatism, to provide help to all the unemployed and to rebuild solidarity on a new foundation, some got involved in self-help groups and participation in a national movement. But the most significant project from the social and community standpoint was the establishment of a free health clinic for the unemployed. This made it possible to reestablish a social context in a disorganized environment and at the same time help to transform the whole community's social and political awareness.

The study also reports that during periods of unemployment, family networks can help by providing support. Family support, moreover, generally tends to attenuate the negative impact of losing a job.

In capitalist societies, work and consumer habits bring a degree of psychological security and a form of social integration. The collapse of such a world as a result of plant closings and massive losses of jobs in Barberton leads us to question the nature of the insecurity that characterizes modern societies—the moral crisis they are going through—and hence the possibilities for social restructuring available to them. The medical clinic experiment contributed to the emergence of new community values. Collective action and various forms of mutual assistance and solidarity convey a dual message. On the one hand, they reveal the limits of the marketplace and the state, as well as their inability to solve social problems, and on the other hand, possible avenues for reinventing society.

The Barberton example is not unique. Both in Europe and North America, we have since the mid-1970s observed the destructive effects of the globalization of production systems and markets on local communities, in particular in former industrial centres, both in terms of living conditions and opportunities for renewing industrial structures. At the same time, we note that local communities are not all adapting in the same way to the new economic context. Some appear to be succeeding better than others.

According to researchers, the most important factors in explaining this phenomenon are sociocultural and sociopolitical ones such as the level of cooperation from public authorities, the civic-mindedness of the community, citizenship, the closeness of the cooperation among the players, in a word, the deeply "patrimonial" nature of development (Barel, Arbaret-Schulz, and Butel 1982). As Putnam showed (1992) in a study of regions in Italy, the appearance and implementation of positive social integration measures depend on the existence of a tradition of cooperation and solidarity within civil society, and the reinstatement of such a tradition. It is also a condition which is indispensable to the overall development of society.

Here, the ability of regional authorities to play a concrete role is a function of institutional dynamism, which in turn is determined by the social context within which it exists. Thus in the regions and municipalities of northern Italy, where networks of associations are denser and where participation in public affairs occurs through horizontal structures rather than vertical and strongly hierarchical structures, such as those found in the south, various types of solidarity are created which strengthen civil responsibility vis-à-vis the common good. Indeed, the social contract is defined in moral terms rather than in legal terms.

Putnam (1992) is not alone in pointing to the importance of civic traditions in the drive and creativity of neighbourhoods or municipalities. In recalling the experience of Vienna at the turn of the century, Törnquist (1985) formulated a similar hypothesis. Sullivan (1995), who studied the economic transformations that the industrialized countries have undergone since the end of the Second World War, very largely shares Putnam's analysis. According to him, a community's power rests more than anything else on its ability to provide various forms of social integration. In the final analysis, it is what explains a community's success. "When it is present, as we have seen, all manner of things go well, while in its absence even the state and the market function poorly" (Sullivan 1995, 32).

It will be useful to study the RESO example to explore these aspects more concretely in the Canadian and Quebec context. RESO, which is considered by some researchers (Perry and Lewis 1994) to be the most dynamic community economic development corporation in Canada, is noted for its desire to encourage the social integration of those who are most disadvantaged. It is strongly rooted in its environment and has, since its establishment, shown a striking level of determination given the scale of the socioeconomic problems that the community to the southwest of Montreal has had to face. It may even be said that its action has had a direct impact on the redefinition of public strategies for economic renewal throughout the Greater Montreal area.

EXAMPLE OF A SUCCESS STORY: THE REGROUPEMENT POUR LA RELANCE ÉCONOMIQUE ET SOCIALE DU SUD-OUEST DE MONTRÉAL (RESO)

Actions on Nonmedical Determinants of Health

RESO is a community economic development corporation established in 1990 to foster renewal in southwest Montreal, one of the oldest industrial sectors of the city. In the past, it had been Canada's largest industrial centre, partly because the Lachine Canal gave access to the Port of Montreal and the St. Lawrence River. The area is currently suffering from several problems: aging industrial and urban infrastructures, loss of jobs and a general rise in poverty among the people who live there.

Chevalier and Tremblay (1995) analyzed the social and health survey conducted in Montreal Centre in 1992–1993. Their analysis clearly showed that people living in the disadvantaged or vulnerable area that includes southwest Montreal were in several respects more economically insecure and suffering from a higher level of psychological distress than families living in better-off neighbourhoods. Social support was also at a lower level than in the rest of the region (27 percent compared to 21 percent). In addition, health disparities by socioeconomic status, measured on the basis of factors like perceived financial status, accumulated assets and exclusion from the labour market, did not tend to decrease over time. Lastly, there was a very clear link between the social and health needs of people and their socioeconomic situation: [Translation] "Not only are the needs greater among the disadvantaged, but current intervention strategies are less effective with these groups" (Chevalier and Tremblay 1995, 247).

In view of the general decline in working and living conditions in the southwest, RESO officials did not hesitate to adopt a local development perspective that focused both on community solidarity and on the promotion of entrepreneurship. That is why they invited community agencies, business people, union and government representatives to work together with them in a concerted effort.

As RESO's view is that improving living conditions and urban development is an integral part of a renewal strategy, it did not hesitate to take action by contacting elected municipal officials, participating in public consultations and getting involved in urban disputes. For example, it worked to maintain the industrial zoning along the Lachine Canal to force the city of Montreal to speed up construction on the Wellington Bridge and to request public housing construction. All of these actions are based on the principle that quality of development plays a key role in countering the negative impacts of economic, social and urban deterioration, which often tend to mutually reinforce one another.

Since being set up, RESO has strived to prove [Translation] "that economic and social development are inseparable; that an industrial base can be maintained in Montreal; and that in the southwest, local solidarity provides a rationale for people from the community to control economic renewal" (Neamtan 1993). To achieve this, RESO relies on the participatory and community tradition that has existed for several decades in the Pointe-Saint-Charles, Petite-Bourgogne and Saint-Henri neighbourhoods.

To summarize, it can be said that in less than six years, RESO has succeeded in becoming a key player. It has even managed to alter government policies by forcing elected representatives to give proper regard to the needs of the neighbourhood. Most of all, it has been able to stop people from being defeatist and feeling that they are vulnerable to external economic forces. This does not necessarily mean that the negative economic trends have ceased to threaten the social integrity of this lifestyle, given the number of plant and business closings in recent years. However, people no longer allow themselves to be overwhelmed by a sense of powerlessness.

Reasons for the Initiative

To understand why RESO emerged, it is essential to examine not only the internal or subjective elements under which group action evolves, but also the contextual factors linked to the deterioration of the economic situation for the Greater Montreal area, particularly with respect to the city centre. From the viewpoint of internal elements, it is the growth of urban movements to address local democracy issues that explains why players in these movements decided to become involved in local development. The history of these movements, and the deeper motivations of those who orchestrated them, makes it possible to understand how their collective action has been redefined with a focus on partnership and pragmatism.

When established in the mid-1980s, community economic development corporations were rejuvenating the collective action of urban movements that had been started by citizens' committees in disadvantaged neighbourhoods in Montreal in the early 1960s (Hamel 1991). Three community economic development corporations were established on a pilot basis in three Montreal neighbourhoods with the financial assistance of the provincial government: Hochelaga-Maisonneuve, Centre-Sud and Pointe-Saint-Charles. The Programme économique de Pointe-Saint-Charles (PEP), the ancestor of today's RESO, had already focused its action on the objectives of employability, control over development by the local population and improving living and working conditions.

However, the institutional framework, the resources to which PEP had access and the area where it was acting were very different. Today, in addition to Pointe-Saint-Charles, RESO has extended its action to the following neighbourhoods: Saint-Henri, Petite-Bourgogne, Ville-Émard, Côte-Saint-Paul and Griffintown. It also has the support of the federal government and the City of Montreal.

When community actors and urban movements were mobilized in the mid-1980s around local development issues it was, even though there were a few signs of recovery, in the context of a steadily declining economic situation for residents of disadvantaged neighbourhoods. Not only was Greater Montreal encountering major restructuring problems, but the coordination of the main economic players and governments was ineffective or taking too long.

Like other run-down Montreal neighbourhoods, the southwest was hit hard by the changes to the core of the metropolitan region: industrial redeployment and the move of several businesses to the outskirts, a slowdown in and transformation of the manufacturing sector, the aging of the population and the exodus of the middle classes to the suburbs. All of these phenomena stemmed from the tertiarization of the economy, the relocation of economic activity to the west of the continent, Canada's poor competitiveness compared to other industrial countries, high levels of government indebtedness and the direct and indirect impacts of these elements on socio-economic dynamism.

Without going into RESO's history in detail, we note that PEP played an important role in setting up the Comité pour la relance de l'économie et de l'emploi du sud-ouest de Montréal (CREESOM). The committee, a federation of representatives of all socioeconomic players, including communities, unions, employers and municipal and government representatives, had a dual mandate to diagnose the situation in the southwest and to suggest possible ways to initiate a recovery.

The CREESOM recommendations released in April 1989 included assigning priority to raising the socioeconomic status of the population in terms of training and employability, consolidating the manufacturing sector, providing support for local entrepreneurship, adapting and coordinating government interventions, particularly to help those who were unemployed, and lastly, improving the living conditions and image of the southwest. The committee also recommended that RESO become the main coordinator of the proposed recovery measures.

In the spring of 1990, both levels of government and the city of Montreal showed their support for most of CREESOM's recommendations and agreed that RESO become the main authority responsible for local development in the southwest. They therefore agreed to invest more than $400 million over a three- to seven-year period (Secrétariat aux affaires régionales 1994).

The Actors

RESO is a nonprofit organization. For the municipal government and all its partners, its status is that of a community economic development corporation. Its board members are chosen by electoral colleges who meet before each general meeting to appoint their representatives. These colleges represent the whole area and the various partners at the same time. Out of 13 voting members on the board of directors, four come from community agencies, four from the business and financial institution sector, two from the unions, two selected from among the members of the corporation, and one personnel representative. The director general is an *ex officio* member of the board, but has no vote.

RESO ran a recruiting campaign in 1994–1995. The board of directors report dated October 24, 1995 stated that the agency had 823 individual members living or working in the southwest and 173 corporate members from both the public and private sectors, including the unions and community members. Among these were five large businesses, 55 small or medium-sized businesses, eight financial institutions, 48 community groups and 12 unions.

Increasing the number of members has become a RESO priority. It has therefore set up a committee of those who participate in its activities. In June

1995, it included [Translation] "entrepreneurial participants and was very active in fighting restrictions on recipients of income security" (RESO 1995).

At the moment, RESO has more than 40 employees, mostly women. This is an important characteristic insofar as many of its employable clients are female heads of households. RESO is increasingly giving consideration to the ethnic and cultural profile of local residents. For example, two women from the black community in Petite-Bourgogne were hired to work with the community on training and employability.

While several RESO staff members have university training, this is not a hiring criterion. RESO officials assign as much importance to sharing the corporation's objectives and orientation as to familiarity with the environment. Work experience also remains a major criterion.

There is very strong consensus on the board of directors concerning the agency's mission. Disagreements on fundamental orientations and choices are very rare, indeed virtually nonexistent.

RESO may be said to have acquired considerable legitimacy in its area, which does not necessarily mean that all businesses in the southwest share its vision and its social objectives. Many businesses do not recognize any immediate interest in RESO's actions or truly identify with the community. This is an indication of the limitations of local development as a way of addressing problems and as an intervention strategy. However, the fact that RESO has been able to broaden its membership base in recent years is clearly indicative of its drive.

Lastly, we note that the actors in question are also agencies with whom RESO has intervened or is currently intervening. In this study, we encountered four of these agencies.[3] Their social missions are varied: social reintegration, battling poverty, public education and occupational reintegration. The services provided to them by RESO are equally varied: help in starting up the agency or special projects, employee training and financing from an innovation fund to provide training and support for local initiatives. In all instances, even after interventions have come to an end, these agencies have continued to maintain links with RESO.

Analysis of the Results

According to Statistics Canada data, in 1991 the population in the southwest was 67,665. Average employment income was $21,181 compared to $22,308 for all of Montreal, $23,848 for all of Quebec and $24,716 for all of Canada. In addition, the percentage of low-income families was higher than for the

---

3. The agencies are the following: École Entreprise Formétal, Comité d'éducation aux adultes de la Petite-Bourgogne, the Garde-Manger pour tous inc. and the Auberge communautaire du sud-ouest.

city of Montreal as a whole (Côté et al. 1994, 29). But these overall indicators only give a rough idea of the serious problems faced by people living in the area. In 1992, out of a labour force estimated at 31,000 persons, there were 7,900 unemployment insurance beneficiaries and 9,000 social assistance recipients (Morin, Latendresse, and Parazelli 1994).

In view of the situation, it was urgent not only to implement a series of concrete measures for economic and social reintegration, but also to create conditions likely to have a medium-term impact on employability and on the dynamism of the community as a whole. This is what led RESO to exert pressure on public administrations to change the management criteria for their programs or to obtain additional resources to set new projects in motion.

RESO's interventions took many forms. Initially, it devoted itself to support for the jobless, in the form of mentorship or training programs— including programs in cooperation with the school commissions—to make it possible for some people to complete secondary school, to arrange business internships or to introduce a variety of measures to help people who wanted to create their own jobs and start their own businesses.[4]

The second step was to foster the creation and implementation of economic projects by supporting the introduction of new businesses or the development of new industrial projects, or again by contributing to the startup of community projects. Training was closely related to the creation of new services or businesses. RESO also participates in the Fonds de déve-loppement emploi-Montréal (FDEM) which to date has provided support to eight businesses in the southwest, representing the creation or maintenance of 40 jobs.

On the employability promotion front, in 1992–1993 RESO carried out a variety of activities with the following clienteles: information and referral, 928 persons; training orientation and follow-up, 242 persons; organizing workshops, 398 participants; local initiatives, seven projects with 109 participants; labour promotion, 87 placements and 45 business intern-ships, in addition to 17 permanent jobs and 164 part-time jobs at Price Club; training, 225 persons, in addition to participation in nine employ-ability projects financed by the Labour Adjustment Fund (Leduc et al. 1994).

During the same fiscal year, the data show the following accom-plishments with respect to business services: information and reference, 192 firms used the services of RESO; four small businesses received consult-ing services; 26 small and medium-size businesses received financial services; seven projects were financed under the Fonds de développement emploi-Montréal. For applicant training and finding workers, 20 firms made use of the service, in addition to placement activities, for a total of 104 regular

---

4. [Translation] "RESO's strategy has been to organize appropriate employability development services directly when these did not appear to be available within the neighbourhood" (Leduc et al. 1994, 15).

jobs and 164 part-time jobs. Twenty-eight entrepreneurs received assistance of various kinds, and 12 business plans were prepared (Leduc et al. 1994).

For a year now, RESO has been participating in an "experimental project" that gives it additional latitude and autonomy in managing public funds. The project is considered by its public partners to be a new form of partnership designed to close the gap between the requirements of bureaucratic management at the higher levels, and needs expressed by the community.

The "experimental project" has four parts: (1) a $500,000 economic development fund—for a three-year period—to finance various community activities to foster entrepreneurship, to create sectoral projects, to carry out studies, etc.; (2) the RESO Investissements inc. fund, which was established with the assistance of the Fonds de solidarité des travailleurs du Québec and the government, has $5 million in venture capital and can provide investment from $10,000 to $450,000 for the establishment or expansion of companies starting up or planning growth; it focuses on the manufacturing sector, as well as on service industries that could provide major benefits in terms of job creation; (3) the establishment of an innovation fund for training and for supporting community initiative for a period of three years, consisting of $3 million from the federal and provincial governments, administered by RESO under MOUs with community agencies—proposals are reviewed by a "facilitating committee" consisting of representatives from RESO and government agencies working in the area of employability, which must be part of a metropolitan framework and determine which areas of employment are already full; (4) an entrepreneurship program to provide assistance to self-employed workers.

Since being established in 1990, RESO has continued to expand and to take on new projects. From this standpoint alone, there can be no doubt that it is a success.

Replicability

There are currently seven community economic development corporations within the city of Montreal. RESO is, for the moment, the only one of these corporations to be managing an "experimental project."

This type of project could in all likelihood be extended to other parts of Montreal in the near future. Moreover, the investment tools managed by RESO exist elsewhere in other urban or regional communities. There are many advantages to decentralizing the administration of public funds in this way: community members are in a better position to determine the appropriateness of projects from a social standpoint, it strengthens networks and solidarity, and it increases the skills and expertise of community players.

The innovativeness of RESO's efforts lie less in its remarkable managerial effectiveness or its considerable ability to mobilize people, than in its analysis of individual and group responsibilities towards local development.

Works on local development emphasize that success is largely the result of the quality of leadership and the ability of local communities to reach compromises. In this, both RESO and the southwest have many strengths.

RESO's action depends on a tradition of continuity and on the conviction that communities possess knowledge and skills that other socioeconomic or institutional players do not have. It is largely this conviction, combined with a favourable political climate—a certain trend towards decentralization both federally and provincially—that made it possible to change the institutional framework with respect to the administration of government programs on manpower training and job creation. RESO was thus able to acquire latitude in training and in the establishment of firms that no community group had ever before been able to obtain.

For the experimental project, the federal and provincial governments agreed to give a community organization a great deal of leeway in the administration of public funds. Although it is not yet possible to determine all the implications of this innovation, it is clear that it significantly changes the framework for the administration of public funds.

As for the target groups, which here are the local residents as well as all the socioeconomic players, it may be said that RESO helped to set in motion profound changes in ways of reintegrating society's have-nots. By working towards mobilizing and coordinating the efforts of local actors, RESO changed the transaction and mediation process on both the socioeconomic and political levels. In a way, it has managed to counter the culture of inaction and defeatism.

Funding

As we mentioned earlier, funding is almost entirely public, namely from the federal government, the provincial government and the city of Montreal.[5] From 1990 to 1994, RESO's financing totalled almost $4 million. Its budget covered the agency's operations, as well as all of the services it delivered to the people and to business.

For the moment, RESO has no funding problems. Its activities are structured project by project, and new employees can be taken on as required.

In 1994, RESO obtained renewed funding for three years, once again under a tripartite agreement between the federal government, the provincial government and the City of Montreal. It was also granted additional funds for the "experimental project" that began in 1995.

---

5. In 1992–1993, RESO's budget was $2,169,248. The sources of funds for $1,111,248 may be identified as follows: OPDQ: $222,000; CIDEM: $165,000; CFP: $340,000; CEIC: $200,000; MICT (Quebec Department of Industry, Commerce and Technology): $55,000; ISTC: $50,000; other: $81,620 (Leduc et al. 1994).

Since being established, the organization's responsibilities, and the resources made available to it, have continued to grow. The September 1995 annual report mentioned the possibility of introducing a partial self-financing strategy. The organization certainly remains vulnerable in the sense that its survival depends entirely on public financing at this time. That is why the board of directors, which has been discussing the matter for two years, advocates the development of concrete tools to increase its financial autonomy. Thus some firms that succeeded in establishing themselves through RESO's support would be asked to pay fees on their profits once their profitability was established. Some business management services that require special expertise, such as the preparation of recovery plans, could involve charges. New chargeable services for small businesses could also be introduced in areas such as sales and promotion.

Indeed, can governments allow themselves to abandon RESO? It is always less expensive, except perhaps in the short term, to spend money on social integration than to allow urban neighbourhoods to become run down, because of the economic and social costs that result from such deterioration.

Nevertheless, the issue of financing under discussion here remains an important one, and one which largely goes beyond RESO's field of action. The issues involve not only the national manpower training policy, but also public strategies for social integration. In this area, Canada lags far behind countries like Austria and Germany. Unlike these countries, which spend as much on active measures like courses and internships as they do on passive measures like unemployment insurance and social assistance, Canada still spends only 20 percent on active measures compared to 80 percent on passive measures (Sansfaçon 1996).

We also know that manpower training alone is not enough to meet the new economic challenges. It is likewise necessary to foster entrepreneurship, create new companies, reduce deficits, improve management of our collective equipment, improve the local environment and strengthen commitment to civic responsibilities. RESO is affected by all of these aspects.

Evaluation

In 1994, like other CEDCs in Montreal, RESO was evaluated in the usual manner. The evaluation was carried out under the responsibility of the Comité d'harmonisation de Montréal, the authority responsible for the financing of CEDCs.[6] The evaluation was broken down into three parts:

---

6. The Comité d'harmonisation consists of representatives from the Government of Quebec, the Government of Canada and the City of Montreal. The evaluation was delegated to a subcommittee of representatives from the following partners: Société québécoise de développement de la main-d'œuvre, Human Resources Development Canada and the CEDCs (Comité d'harmonisation de Montréal 1994).

(1) a review of the accomplishments and the performance of CEDCs based on resources invested and objectives; (2) evaluation of the practices and foundations of local community development in an urban setting; (3) an economic overview of neighbourhoods and trends observed (Comité d'harmonisation de Montréal 1994).

In connection with part one, the evaluation raised several points, including the fact that the mobilization of CEDCs led to [Translation] "concrete actions in terms of direct services made available, the emergence of projects or the exploration of economic development opportunities" (Comité d'harmonisation de Montréal 1994, 12). The liaison function between private and public players was also noted. With respect to employability, the innovativeness of the CEDC has to do with their support on several levels: coordination and harmonization of several services, their ability to [Translation] "get the various players together to address the problems facing employment" (Comité d'harmonisation de Montréal 1994, 13). The CEDCs can also provide services to firms with 10 or fewer employees, and such firms had previously been neglected.

However, the committee also raised a number of problems. For example, it recommended a more detailed mission statement and a clearer description of a number of roles assumed by CEDCs. One such area was [Translation] "a clearer sharing of responsibilities" (Comité d'harmonisation de Montréal 1994, 14) between government and local partners.

With respect to part two, in addition to noting that the patterns varied from one CEDC to another, the committee highlighted a number of internal management problems as well as the fact that government standards were burdensome and inconsistent. For example, the partitioning of budgetary envelopes limits their flexibility in conducting activities. The committee further recommended that administrative requirements be harmonized among the various levels of government. This is precisely what the experimental project in which RESO is involved is designed to correct.

The Comité d'harmonisation's report made eight recommendations. One was that community economic development corporations improve their administrative continuity and that they obtain common management tools to better report on their activities and results. Likewise, the committee advocated the establishment of a framework for evaluation and the development of tools to measure results quantitatively.

This was the background to the committee's adoption in March 1995 of "a continuous evaluation framework for community economic development corporations." The framework consists of an evaluation that is participative, joint (qualitative and quantitative), progressive (ongoing), integrated (with consideration given to the interests of the partners and intervention levels) and, lastly, synthetic with regard to all community economic development corporation activities.

Indicators devised on the basis of this general framework are already being used to evaluate community economic development corporation activities. At the halfway point in October 1995, RESO had reached and even exceeded the vast majority of operational objectives for its range of services. The following are a few examples: in employability, the target for the year for reception and referral was 2,000 persons. By October, 1,000 persons had been referred. In employment counselling, the objective for the year was 600. In October, 716 persons had already been given guidance, with the breakdown as follows: reception (125), action plan (76) and employability development (515). For general training, an impressive success rate of 75 percent was achieved. The job integration level was also strong, with a success rate of 60 percent.

Performance was similar for business services. The objectives were met for reception and referral, and group training. For community management training, 15 agencies were to be contacted; at the halfway point, 28 had been contacted. For other programs to support entrepreneurship in small business, the objective for the year was to reach 80 persons. At the mid-point, 55 had been contacted. The objective for the year in business training in the manufacturing sector was eight firms and 160 workers. At the halfway point, five firms had been contacted and 232 workers were participating in training programs.

These few figures provide an overview of RESO performance, but they do not give the full flavour of the benefits to clients. The organization gives its clients the opportunity to undertake or pursue an economic integration process by making available to them the resources and the environment to which they would not otherwise have had access. It thus gives those who are initially motivated to find a job and who want to improve their position both personalized mentoring and the feeling that they are participating in a group project. These happen to be two elements that are indispensable to improving self-esteem, without which any integration efforts are doomed to failure.

The interviews we held with four organization that used RESO's services showed clearly that RESO is an essential factor in stimulating renewal and in giving hope once again to local residents. For these organizations, RESO is also a key source of information. It can disseminate or channel information both formally and informally. It also acts as a facilitator in groups' or businesses' action to develop or implement projects. Not least, thanks to the coordination processes and projects it sets in motion, RESO enables all of the socioeconomic players in the southwest to reinforce their identity, to enhance their mutual recognition of one another and to acquire greater legitimacy.

According to some, however, this partnership perspective engenders a transformation in community action and strategies which sometimes requires the community to put direct action or political pressures on the back burner.

Some also fear that RESO, because of its responsibilities and the size of the funds it manages, is beginning to function in a technocratic fashion that resembles the very methods it was attacking for several years. In fact, one stakeholder condemned the fact that RESO was not sufficiently critical of the companies it was supporting. This stakeholder felt that job creation was not an adequate objective and that it was also important to be concerned about the quality of the jobs created. For the moment, there does not appear to be any genuine debate about whether it is possible to create other forms of work and other ways of organizing work. The person in question nevertheless admitted that RESO had contributed a great deal to obtaining social and political recognition for communities.

Other Examples

There are several other community organizations in Canada whose work, like that of RESO's, is structured around local development. A well-known example is New Dawn Enterprises Ltd. of Cape Breton, Nova Scotia, which is considered the first community economic development corporation in Canada.

New Dawn, which was incorporated in 1976, emerged from an earlier experiment in cooperative development that in turn had grown out of community solidarity movements during the 1950s and 1960s in the area. The organizers of the project, who were concerned about the economic decline of the 1970s and who wanted to meet the needs of their community, began by buying an old building in downtown Sydney to accommodate a handicraft association that was looking for a facility where it could give courses. At the same time, they also had eight apartments built on the first floor.

Even though the people running the organization had no resources at the beginning, they were able to obtain funding for their project. They were thus able to contribute to the improvement of part of the deteriorating downtown area, to create jobs and to acquire experience that proved to be useful in launching other projects, according to one of the administrators.[7] The organization grew very quickly.

Today, New Dawn's significant property inventory enables it to make affordable housing available to low- or medium-income families, and at the same time to create jobs attached to nearby services, notably in the social and health areas. It currently owns over 230 housing units, and it

---

7. "Very soon, we bought other properties or borrowed money, made improvements, and provided much-needed housing for the community. To handle the day-to-day administration, we hired part-time staff, an approach made possible by the high level of voluntary committee involvement. Where possible, government "make-work" programs were tapped to make the project viable" (MacLeod 1986, 20).

helped to create two housing cooperatives and eight companies. The corporation administers assets worth over $14 million.

It plays an important role in the community, as it recruits its administrators and workers from several areas: unions, volunteers, community groups, business. Including members of the board of directors and volunteers who are active on its various committees, there were approximately 200 people working with New Dawn in 1993 (MacLeod 1995).

The organization's operating structure is decentralized. Its members can function either within or outside of its corporate legal framework. They can work on New Dawn committees or become affiliated in a way that gives them all the autonomy they need.

In 1990, when the Canadian Armed Forces' radar station in Sydney was closed down, the county of Cape Breton approached New Dawn to work in partnership with the municipality to convert the site and to transform the buildings there. The remarkable success of the redevelopment corroborated New Dawn's expertise. Also noteworthy is the fact that the corporation now has over 100 employees, with a total payroll of $1.7 million, less than 2 percent of which comes from government funds.

There are examples elsewhere in Canada too of the empowerment of economic and social local players. These include Colville Investments Corporation, a community economic development corporation established in Nanaimo, British Columbia in 1990 to help the community create jobs with a view to social development.

The organization provided financial support to start up local businesses, in particular those unable to obtain assistance from the usual sources of financing. It focuses specifically on marginalized people (Perry and Lewis 1994; Fontan 1993).

The corporation operates with funds from institutional sources like the municipality, as well as from noninstitutional sources. It has four permanent employees. Its annual budget is $150,000 and it created 161 jobs in 1990–1991.

Depending on the communities in which they are rooted, and their traditions, along with the nature of the socioeconomic problems they face, community economic development corporations use various forms of organization and group action. They formulate a variety of strategies and use many different tools to boost the economy and to effect social integration. They also share a common conviction, which is that it is necessary to democratize the economy.

POLICY IMPLICATIONS

As we have seen, local development is not a panacea, even when it leads to the participation of community actors. We have only to recall the key factors involved in the set of issues raised at the beginning of this study to understand the framework and possible avenues for group action to address the problems or crisis being faced by public institutions.

In short, in most industrial countries, the economic restructurings of recent years have generally worsened income inequalities between social classes and groups, leading to a variety of forms of social exclusion. This situation stems largely from the new needs for flexibility that have been engendered by the globalization of the economy and markets.

In such a context, people are being asked to assume more responsibilities with respect to their own futures. If governments have fewer resources than before to devote to the social safety net, they, like all social players, have doubts about what goals ought to be pursued and what forms of action ought to be used to implement them.

Although radical modernity may imply greater reflexivity, this does not mean that the actors involved have more control over their areas of endeavour. As Anthony Giddens (1990, 40) wrote, knowing no longer means being certain. Things have changed a great deal from the way they were only 35 years ago. Then, Quebec was in the throes of its "Quiet Revolution" and no one was in any doubt about the mission of the state. Its role was clearly to modernize society, beginning with public institutions. Innovations were expected both in planning and managing social matters. As for economic and urban development, there was broad consensus about the challenges.

Today, planning is in crisis. Planners no longer know what model to follow and they do not see very clearly what values they can base themselves on to reach the consensus needed to formulate public decisions and strategies.

Their framework, which is the same for everyone involved in social affairs, is one of uncertainty and risk (Beck 1992). And yet, the pluralism of identities, actors and lifestyles, whose expression should go hand in hand with an increase in civil and political liberties, is threatened by rigidities and worries that are attributable to the new economic imperatives (Dahrendorf 1995).

The community players involved in local social restructuring around the issues of employment and other aspects of local development are faced with a complex reality in which they are unable to control all the variables. Nevertheless, they unhesitatingly opted for partnership with public and private stakeholders to promote community renewal and dynamism.

The success of RESO and other local community development agencies like New Dawn has been impressive. Often against all odds, such agencies have been able to meet many of their objectives. They were thus able to acquire considerable legitimacy in their own communities, as well as political and institutional recognition. By focusing on local and community solidarity, and opting for a pragmatic approach, they were able to develop expertise and build solid support networks with both public and private stakeholders. Their action, as we saw with RESO, even succeeded in changing the way government employability, manpower training and business development assistance programs are managed.

In transforming the framework for public action, RESO had to change its own intervention strategies. We are no longer merely looking at ways to rethink government policy and program management strategies for local development. On the contrary, the task is now to transform them concretely with due regard to the demands of community players, which means that it is necessary to break out of the straightjacket of sectoral thinking—as well as top-down administrative standards—by taking the viewpoint of citizens and local environments into consideration.

In several respects, the socioeconomic position in which the southwest finds itself is similar to that of Montreal, an urban centre which is losing ground on all fronts. No one can predict when the situation will stop deteriorating, but one thing is certain, and that is that a wait-and-see attitude is not a solution.

RESO's convictions have led those who run the organization to gamble on concentrating on employment as a process and strategy for social restructuring, because this is the surest way of integrating most citizens in spite of the continued risk of social polarization. However, further deliberation about the quality of the jobs created and about what factors can make a given community dynamic in terms of job creation, is still required.

One of the first conclusions stemming from our analysis is that local development is continuing, and evolving, in a general framework that is at the same time regional, national and even increasingly international. In other words, even though local development, viewed from the social and community standpoints, contains many positive aspects, the fact remains that it is limited by the contradictions inherent in the economic system within which it functions.

Furthermore, neither local development nor solidarity, nor a tradition of civic commitment, can be imposed from above. While we may today be more aware of the links between health and socioeconomic status, we do not yet have any magic formula. What is certain is that we can provide communities with the resources they need to meet a growing number of social demands, which implies a number of things, including a redefinition of the framework for public action to reflect the sorts of changes set in motion by RESO.

Two comments are appropriate at the outset. First of all, it is important to recognize the specificity of the community setting, namely the high standard of its expertise. This means that one must also accept its characteristic ways of doing and learning. While the community may need more resources to meet social demands, what it needs above all is a political and institutional framework that is better suited to the requirements of local players. Moreover, by making additional resources available to community actors, governments must not give in to the temptation of imposing a generalized or standard bureaucratic framework. The energy of communities and their ability to play a key role in training, job creation, self-help or solidarity depend on the links they are able to maintain with all the players in civil society, based on its history and its integration in a given environment. For some years, the temptation has been great for governments to use local communities to manage social affairs sectorally at lower cost. This is a trap to be avoided.

Local development action is part of a complex process. Development does not result simply from investment; it depends more than anything else on the ability of local communities to renew themselves and to be vigorous on all fronts. This leads us to the importance of leadership among socio-economic players, as well as to the ability of local communities to reach compromises that result in the commitment of both public and private sector stakeholders . When it works, everyone appears to benefit. We have seen that community economic development corporations play an indispensable role in this.

For example, RESO's approach depends on quality leadership as well as on its familiarity with the community, links with the local setting and its roots in that community. Mentoring, training and business assistance projects are self-help practices in which citizens participate in the process alongside others, and this in turn generates personal commitment by participants and at the same time gives them a framework and a platform for solidarity, which is precisely what they need to acquire self-confidence and self-esteem, both of which are a prerequisite for action. It is a learning process for participants, as well as for RESO employees and managers, which is not of the same order as that which occurs in traditional employment settings. Under the current economic conditions, it is essential.

In connection with the program for action, it means that battling against inequality and efforts for social reintegration requires the commitment of individuals, even though they remain in an environment that conditions their behaviour. Individual and group action tend here to mutually strengthen one another.

Furthermore, RESO's example is an invitation to redefine the framework for public action to deal with current social issues and problems. Indeed, both the top-down model of development and the framework policies based on that model are from another age. While the welfare state crisis may well have sounded the death knell of a specific model of social protection, no satisfactory alternative models have been found to replace it. This does not mean that there are not a number of other social restructuring practices being worked on, but these are difficult to grasp because they have not yet been able to significantly change our collective understanding.

The fragmentation of society, combined with the crisis in public financing and the new imperatives of employment have given us the impression that incrementalism is the dominant trend. It is therefore important to quickly review the shape and mission of public services by asking ourselves how responsibilities ought to be shared between the public and private sectors, and what role the community setting has to play in economic and social integration.

From the health standpoint, we know that quality of life and working conditions, beginning with the opportunity to have a job, are becoming increasingly important. By focusing on community dynamism, RESO has defined its action in terms of that standpoint. At the same time, it advocates a transformation not only in government management, but in the whole framework for public action. Here, it recommends less top-down planning— as was common through the technocratic 1960s—and a greater emphasis on conditions that will make it possible for citizens to have better control over their living conditions.

The process raises questions in several areas, including how to manage social affairs, equity and social justice, state responsibilities and the control by politicians over decentralized ways of acting. In this, the RESO example encourages us to continue to think about how responsibilities ought to be shared between the public and private sectors. Moreover, while it may serve as a model for other communities or other regions, it must not be forgotten that it was successful precisely because it was closely based on the community tradition and context in which it was acting.

CONCLUSION

The policy implications of this study on community economic development corporations with respect to local development leave many questions about the redefinition of the framework for public action unanswered. In view of the new requirements for radical modernity, and the interests that are at stake, it is difficult to give a single answer that is likely to satisfy all of the stakeholders. However, two convictions remain. First of all, it is essential to make choices, and to realize that the problems that face us will not solve themselves. Second, the community is an essential partner in the debate on redefining the framework for public action. It possesses knowledge, expertise and a point of view that others do not have or cannot have because of the role they play on the political and institutional checkerboard.

Alone, community economic development corporations cannot solve all the problems that result from the economic and urban transformations that local communities have undergone as a result of globalization. Rising unemployment and new forms of poverty have caused communities to deteriorate, along with quality of life and the health of citizens. In such a context, it appears to be essential to focus on effective practices and strategies for economic and social integration and reintegration.

Even though the economic renewal of urban centres gives rise to forms of synergy that are difficult to anticipate, which in turn depend on external factors over which the local communities have no control, some conditions are necessary, and these are partly dependent on mobilizing these communities and on the compromises that they are able to reach. It was precisely to illustrate this possibility that we gave the example of community economic development corporations, and in particular the RESO example.

Pierre Hamel *is a professor at the University of Montreal. He is also a member of the Centre de recherche interuniversitaire sur les transformations et les régulations économiques et sociales. He is responsible for the Centre's series "Politique et Économie" at the University of Montreal Press. His research focuses on social movements and urban policy. His article "Urban Politics in the 1990s: Or, the Difficult Renewal of Local Democracy" will be published shortly in* International Political and Science Review.

BIBLIOGRAPHY

ASCHER, F. 1992. Projet public et réalisations privées, le renouveau de la planification des villes. *Annales de la recherche urbaine* 51: 4–15.

AYDALOT, P. 1985. L'aptitude des milieux locaux à promouvoir l'innovation technologique. Paper presented during the conference Technologies nouvelles: condition de renouveau des régions en crise. Brussels, April 1985.

BAREL, Y., C. ARBARET-SCHULTZ, and A.-M. BUTEL. 1982. *Territoires et cadres sociaux*. Paris: Centre de recherche sur l'urbanisme.

BARTHOLOMEW, A., and M. MAYER. 1992. Nomads of the present: Melucci's contribution to the "New Social Movement" theory. *Theory, Culture and Society* 4: 141–159.

BARTLEY, M. 1994. Unemployment and ill health: Understanding the relationship. *Journal of Epidemiology and Community Health* 48: 333–337.

BECK, U. 1992. *Risk Society: Towards a New Modernity*. London, Newbury Park: Sage.

BELLAH, R. N. et al. 1992. *The Good Society*. New York (NY): Vintage Books.

BERTRAND, J. et al. 1992. *Étude de l'impact d'un stage de réadaptation au travail sur la santé mentale et l'employabilité de jeunes adultes en difficulté*. Hull: La Relance Inc.

BIAREZ, S. 1989. *Le pouvoir local*. Paris: Economica.

BINGHAM, R. D., and R. MIER. 1993. *Theories of Local Economic Development: Perspective from across the Disciplines*. London, Newbury Park: Sage.

BLAKELY, E. J. 1989. *Planning Local Economic Development: Theory and Practice*. London, Newbury Park: Sage.

BOOTHROYD, P., and H. C. DAVIS. 1993. Community economic development: Three approaches. *Journal of Planning Education and Research* 12: 230–240.

BOYTE, H. C. 1980. *The Backyard Revolution: Understanding the New Citizen Movement*. Philadelphia (PA): Temple University Press.

CIAR. 1991. *The Determinants of Health*. Toronto (ON): Canadian Institute for Advanced Research.

CANEY, S. 1992. Liberalism and communitarianism: A misconceived debate. *Political Studies* 4(2): 273–289.

CHEVALIER, S., and M. TREMBLAY. Eds. 1995. *Portrait de santé des Montréalais : rapport de l'Enquête sociale et de santé 1992–1993 pour la région de Montréal-Centre*. Montreal (QC): Régie régionale de la santé et des services sociaux, Direction de la santé publique.

CHRISTENSON, J. A., K. FENDLEY, and J. W. ROBINSON. 1989. Community development. In *Community Development in Perspective*, eds. J. A. CHRISTENSON, and G. W. ROBINSON. Ames (IA): Iowa State University Press. pp. 3–25.

CLARKE, S. E. 1995. Institutional logics and local economic development: A comparative analysis of eight American cities. *International Journal of Urban and Regional Research* 19(4): 513–533.

COMITÉ D'HARMONISATION DE MONTRÉAL. 1994. *Recommandations du Comité d'harmonisation de Montréal concernant l'évaluation de l'expérience de développement local par les corporations de développement économique communautaire et rapport synthèse de l'évaluation*. Montreal (QC): Ville de Montréal.

CÔTÉ, F. et al. 1994. *L'évolution de la situation économique dans la ville et les arrondissements de Montréal: Évaluation des CDEC: volet 3*. Montreal(QC): CIDEM, Ville de Montréal.

DAHRENDORF, R. 1995. Can we combine economic opportunity with civil society and political liberty? *The Responsive Community* 5: 13–39.

DALTON, R. J. 1988. *Citizen Politics in Western Democracies: Public Opinion and Political Parties in the US, GB, West Germany and France*. Chatham (NJ): Chatham House Publishers, Inc.

DEMOUSTIER, D., and A. GRANGE. 1995. Dynamiques associatives dans quelques régions d'Europe: amorce d'une comparaison. *Coopératives et développement* 27(1–2): 25–36.

DOUGLAS, D. J. A. Ed. 1994. *Community Economic Development in Canada*. Two volumes. Toronto (ON) and Montreal (QC): McGraw-Hill Ryerson.

DRUCKER, P. F. 1994. The age of social transformation. *The Atlantic Monthly* 274: 53–80.

ECONOMIC COUNCIL OF CANADA. 1990. *From the Bottom Up: The Community Economic-Development Approach. A Statement by the Economic Council of Canada*. Ottawa (ON): Department of Supply and Services.

EME, B. 1994. Développement local et pratiques d'insertion. *Économie et Humanisme* 315: 29–37.

EVANS, R. G., M. L. BARER, and T. R. MARMOR. Eds. 1994. *Why Are Some People Healthy and Others Not*. New York (NY): Aldine de Gruyter.

FAINSTEIN, N., and S. FAINSTEIN. 1994. Le partenariat entre les secteurs public et privé dans le développement économique aux États-Unis. In *Partenariats entre les secteurs public et privé dans l'aménagement urbain*, ed. W. HEINZ. Paris: L'Harmattan. pp. 33–70.

FAINSTEIN, S. S., and C. HIRST. 1995. Urban social movements. In *Theories of Urban Politics*, eds. D. JUDGE, G. STOKER, and H. WOLMAN. London: Sage. pp. 181–204.

FEINSTEIN, J. S. 1993. The relationship between socioeconomic status and health: A review of the literature. *The Milbank Quarterly* 71: 279–322.

FASENFEST, D. 1991. Comparative economic development: A framework for further research. *Policy Studies Review* 10(2–3): 80–86.

FONTAN, J.-M. 1993. *Revue de la littérature en développement local et en développement économique communautaire*. Montreal (QC): Institut de formation en développement économique communautaire.

_____. 1995. Le développement économique communautaire québécois: éléments de synthèse et point de vue critique. *Revue internationale d'action communautaire* 32: 115–126.

FRANK, J. W., and J. F. MUSTARD. 1994. Perspective. *Daedalus* 123: 1–19.

FRIEDMANN, J. 1992. *Empowerment: the Politics of Alternative Development*. Cambridge (MA) and Oxford, U.K.: Blackwell.

GIDDENS, A. 1990. *The Consequences of Modernity*. Stanford: Stanford University Press.

_____. 1993. Modernity, history, democracy. *Theory and Society* 27: 289–292.

GOVERNMENT OF QUEBEC. 1988. *Rapport de la Commission d'enquête sur les services de santé et les services sociaux*. Quebec: Les Publications du Québec.

GRAETZ, B. 1993. Health consequences of employment and unemployment: Longitudinal evidence for young men and women. *Social Science and Medicine* 36: 715–724.

HAMBLETON, R. 1991. The regeneration of U.S. and British Cities. *Local Government Studies* 17: 53–69.

HAMEL, P. 1991. *Action collective et démocratie locale: les mouvements urbains montréalais*. Montreal (QC): Les Presses de l'Université de Montréal.

_____. 1995. Les hypothèses les plus probantes quant aux facteurs de réussite en matière de développement local. *Politique et management public* 13: 57–75.

HAMEL, P., and L. JALBERT. 1991. Local power in Canada: Stakes and challenges in the restructuring of the state. In *State Restructuring and Local Power*, eds. C.G. PICKVANCE, and E. PRÉTECEILLE. London: Pinter Publishers. pp. 170–196.

HARVEY, D. 1989. From managerialism to entrepreneurialism: The transformation of urban governance in late capitalism. *Geografiska Annaler* 71: 3–17.

HEINZ, W. 1994. Bilan: caractéristiques principales des partenariats du développement urbain. In *Partenariats entre les secteurs public et privé dans l'aménagement urbain*, ed. W. HEINZ. Paris: L'Harmattan. pp. 249–294.

HENRY, G. 1994. Conséquences du PPP pour la production des projets d'urbanisme. In *Le partenariat entre les secteurs public et privé: un atout pour l'aménagement du territoire et la protection de l'environnement?*, eds. J. RUEGG, S. DECOUTÈRE, and N. METTAN. Lausanne, Suisse: Presses Polytechniques et Universitaires Romandes. pp. 67–77.

JEZIERSKI, L. 1990. Neighborhoods and public-private partnerships in Pittsburgh. *Urban Affairs Quarterly* 26: 217–249.

JULLIARD, H. 1971. *Fernand Pelloutier et les origines du syndicalisme d'action directe.* Paris: Seuil.

KLEIN, J. L. 1995. Les mobilisations territorialisées et le développement local: vers un nouveau mouvement social? Paper presented at the session "L'avenir du Québec des régions" held during the 63rd ACFAS Conference, Regional Development Section, May 22–24, 1995.

LAVILLE, J.-L. et al. 1993. *Les services de proximité en Europe: pour une économie solidaire.* Paris: Syros.

LAWLESS, P., and P. RAMSDEN. 1990. Sheffield in the 1980s: From radical intervention to partnership. *Cities* August: 202–210.

LEDUC, M. et al. 1994. *Évaluation de l'impact des activités des corporations de développement économique communautaire — Rapport d'étape : portrait des activités des CDEC montréalaises.* Montreal: Ville de Montréal.

LEGALÈS, P. 1993. *Politique urbaine et développement local: une comparaison franco-britannique.* Paris: L'Harmattan.

LEVINE, M. V. 1989. The politics of partnership: Urban redevelopment since 1945. In *Unequal Partnerships: The Political Economy of Postwar America*, ed. G. D. SQUIRES. New Brunswick (NJ): Rutgers University Press. pp. 162–187.

MACLEOD, G. 1986. *New Age Business: Community Corporations that Work.* Ottawa (ON): Canadian Council on Social Development.

_____. 1995. Atlantic Canadian roots. In *Community Economic Development in Canada, Vol. 2*, ed. D. J. A. DOUGLAS. Toronto (ON) and Montreal (QC): McGraw-Hill Ryerson. pp. 23–52.

MARMOT, M. G. 1994. Social differentials in health within and between populations. *Daedalus* 123: 197–216.

MAYER, N. S. 1984. *Neighborhood Organizations and Community Development: Making Revitalization Work.* Washington (DC): The Urban Institute Press.

MAYER, M. 1989. Local politics: From administration to management. Cardiff Symposium on Regulation, Innovation and Spatial Development. University of Wales, September 13–15, 1989.

MIER, R. et al. 1993. *Social Justice and Local Development Policy.* London, Newbury Park: Sage.

MONKKONEN, E. H. 1988. *America Becomes Urban: The Development of U.S. Cities and Towns 1780–1980.* Berkeley (CA): University of California Press.

MOORE, C., and J. PIERRE. 1988. Partnership or privatisation? The political economy of local economic restructuring. *Policy and Politics* 16: 169–178.

MORIN, R., A. LATENDRESSE, and M. PARAZELLI. 1994. *Les corporations de développement économique communautaire en milieu urbain: l'expérience montréalaise.* Montreal (QC): UQAM, Département d'études urbaines et touristiques, Études, matériaux et documents 5.

MORMONT, M. 1989. Le local convié au développement. *Revue internationale d'action communautaire* 22: 151–166.

NEAMTAN, N. 1993. Plaidoyer pour la liberté d'inventer: le sud-ouest de Montréal défie les normes des bureaucrates. *Le Devoir*, interview with C. Leconte, June 21.

NEWMAN, L. H., D. M. LYON and W. B. PHILP. 1986. *Community Economic Development: An Approach for Urban-Based Economies.* Winnipeg (MB): University of Winnipeg, Institute of Urban Studies.

PAPPAS, G. 1989. *The Magic City: Unemployment in a Working-Class Community.* Ithaca and London: Cornell University Press.

PAQUET, G. 1994. Facteurs sociaux de la santé, de la maladie et de la mort. In *Traité des problèmes sociaux*, eds. F. DUMONT, S. LANGLOIS, and Y. MARTIN. Quebec (QC): Institut québécois de recherche sur la culture. pp. 223–244.

PECK, J., and A. TICKELL. 1995. Business goes local: Dissecting the business agenda in Manchester. *International Journal of Urban and Regional Research* (19)1: 55–78.

PECQUEUR, B. 1989. *Le développement local.* Paris: Syros.

PERRY, S. E., and M. LEWIS. 1994. *Reinventing the Local Economy: What 10 Canadian Initiatives Can Teach Us about Building Creative, Inclusive, and Sustainable Communities.* Vernon: Centre for Community Enterprise.

PICKVANCE, C. G. 1990. Introduction: The institutional context of local economic development: Central controls, spatial policies and local economic policies. In *Place, Policy and Politics: Do Localities Matter?*, eds. M. HARLOE, C. G. PICKVANCE, and J. URRY. London: Unwin Hyman. pp. 1–41.

PIORE, M. 1995. Local development on the progressive political agenda. In *Reinventing Collective Action: From the Global to the Local,* eds. C. CROUCH, and D. MARQUAND. London: Blackwell. pp. 79–87.

PIVEN, F. F., and R. FRIEDLAND. 1984. Public choice and private power: A theory of fiscal crisis. In *Public Service Provision and Urban Development,* eds. A. KIRBY, A. KNOX, and S. PINCH. London and New York: Croom Helm and St.Martin's Press. pp. 390–420.

PUTNAM, R. D. 1992. *Making Democracy Work: Civic Traditions in Modern Italy.* Princeton: Princeton University Press.

QUESNEL, L. 1995. La nouvelle politique: quand la citoyenneté cède la place au partenariat. In *Réflexions préliminaires.* Paper presented at the annual Learned Societies Conference, Montreal, June 1995.

QUÉVIT, M. 1992. Milieux innovateurs et couplage local-international dans les stratégies d'entreprise: un cadre pour l'analyse. *Canadian Journal of Regional Science/Revue canadienne des sciences régionales* 15: 219–238.

REICH, R. B. 1991. *The Work of Nations: Preparing Ourselves for 21st-Century Capitalism.* New York (NT): Alfred A. Knopf.

RESO. 1995. *Le sud-ouest innovateur pour un développement solidaire.* RESO Annual Report: Background and Future.

ROSS, C. E., and J. MIROWSKY. 1995. Does employment affect health? *Journal of Health and Social Behavior* 36: 230–243.

ROSS, D. P., and P. J. USHER. 1986. *From the Roots Up: Economic Development as if Community Mattered.* Toronto (ON): James Lorimer & Co.

SALAMON, L. M. 1989. The changing partnership between the voluntary sector and the welfare state. In *The Future of the Nonprofit Sector,* eds. V. A HODGKINSON, R. W. LYMAN, and ASSOCIATES. San Francisco and London: Jossey-Bass Publishers. pp. 41–60.

SANSFAÇON, J.-R. 1996. De l'emploi, mode d'emploi. *Le Devoir,* Saturday and Sunday, January 27 and 28.

SECRÉTARIAT AUX AFFAIRES RÉGIONALES. 1994. *Le sud-ouest de Montréal, suivi des mesures de relance.* Montreal, Région de Montréal.

SHRAGGE, E. 1993. *Community Economic Development: In Search of Empowerment.* Montreal (QC): Black Rose Books.

SQUIRES, G. D. 1991. Partnership and the pursuit of the private city. In *Urban Life in Transition,* eds. M. GOTTDIENER, and C. G. PICKVANCE. Newbury Park (CA): *Urban Affairs Annual Review* 39, Sage.

STEPHENSON, M. O. 1991. Whither the public-private partnership: A critical overview. *Urban Affairs Quarterly* 27: 109–127.

STÖHR, M. 1984. La crise économique demande-t-elle de nouvelles stratégies de développement régional. In *Crise & Espace,* ed. P. AYDALOT. Paris: Economica. pp. 183–206.

SULLIVAN, W. M. 1995. Reinventing community: Prospects for politics. In *Reinventing Collective Action: From the Global to the Local,* eds. C. CROUCH, and D. MARQUAND. Oxford: Blackwell. pp. 20–32.

SYME, S. L. 1994. The social environment and health. *Daedalus* 123: 79–86.

TEISSERENC, P. 1994. *Les politiques de développment local : approche sociologique.* Paris: Economica.

TÖRNQUIST, G. 1985. Créativité et développement régional. In *Redéploiement industriel et planification régionale,* eds. M. BOISVERT, and P. HAMEL. Montreal (QC): Université de Montréal, Faculté de l'aménagement. pp. 93–106.

TOWNSEND, P., and N. DAVIDSON. 1982. *Inequalities in Health: The Black Report.* Harmondsworth: Penguin Books.

TURNER, J. B. 1995. Economic context and the health effects of unemployment. *Journal of Health and Social Behavior* 36: 213–229.

VILLE DE MONTRÉAL. 1995. *Répertoire pour un parcours d'insertion au travail.* Montreal (QC): Ville de Montréal, Service du développement économique.

WASSMER, R. W. 1994. Can local incentives alter a metropolitan city's economic development? *Urban Studies* 31(8): 1251–1278.

WEAVER, C., and M. DENNERT. 1987. Economic development and the public-private partnership. *APA Journal* Autumn: 430–437.

WIEWEL, W., M. TEITZ, and R. GILOTH. 1993. The economic development of neighbourhoods and localities. In *Theories of Local Economic Development,* eds. D. BINGHA, and R. MIER. London: Sage. pp. 80–99.

WILKINSON, R. G. 1986. Socioeconomic differences in mortality: Interpreting the data on their size and trends. In *Class and Health: Research and Longitudinal Data,* ed. R. G. WILKINSON. London and New York: Tavistock. pp. 1–33.

WILSON, S. H. and G. M. WALKER. 1993. Unemployment and health: A review. *Public Health* 107: 153–162.

WOLCH, J. 1989. The shadow state: Transformations in the voluntary sector. In *The Power of Geography: How Territory Shapes Social Life,* eds. J. WOLCH, and M. DEAR. Boston: Unwin Hyman. pp. 197–221.

Environmental Health: From Concept to Reality

JOSEPH ZAYED, PH.D.

*Professor, Department of Occupational and Environmental Health
Faculty of Medicine
University of Montreal*

LUC LEFEBVRE, M.SC.

*Toxicologist
Public Health Directorate of Montreal-Centre*

SUMMARY

Health promotion and protection of the environment are closely linked. According to the Rio Declaration on Environment and Development, humans are at the core of sustainable development concerns. They deserve a healthy, productive life in harmony with nature.

However, beginning in the early 1970s, the rise in ecological disasters and environment problems has significantly increased the risks to public health. It was also during this period that a global concept of health first appeared based on four determinants: human biology, the environment, lifestyle and the organization of health care. More recently, a new conceptual framework has been proposed in which productivity and prosperity are among the key determinants of health. It is now appropriate to add to these elements the impact of the physical, chemical and biological environment on not only productivity and prosperity—notably by the direct contribution of natural resources to prosperity—but also on genetic makeup, since we know that some environmental pollutants have the potential to be genotoxic.

Today, it is often possible to establish a direct or indirect link between the health of the population and problems linked to air, water and soil pollution. In this context, promoting a healthier lifestyle is only one of the corollaries to improving environmental conditions, as shown by several success stories.

Success Stories

Children Contaminated by Lead

For several years, the Balmet company of Saint-Jean-sur-Richelieu, Quebec recovered the lead from used batteries: the company's facilities were located less than one kilometre from a residential community, home to approximately 600 children under the age of 10 years. The success story reports on the high level of contamination among the children and describes the intervention program introduced to alleviate the situation. This program made it possible to establish a link between two phenomena: the decontamination of the site and the reduction in blood lead concentrations in the children. In light of the findings, the company closed its doors and the government picked up the bill. This case illustrates how important it is to set up monetary funds to offset the fact that there is no policy on environmental pollution charges.

MMT in Gasoline

Lead was used in gasoline for many years. Because of this product's adverse effects on health, authorities worked together to introduce measures to reduce the population's exposure. Thus, in 1986, the Canadian government announced a plan to ban the use of lead in gasoline. In December 1990, it withdrew this product from the market and replaced it with MMT, although there had been insufficient research on the potential risks of this substance to public health. For socioeconomic reasons, the government is now looking to ban MMT from the Canadian market. However, such a move would create legal complications for the harmonization of the Canadian and U.S. markets. This case highlights the need to encourage preventive research on any health, environment or sustainable development issue, and to enhance communication between researchers, decision makers and the general public.

Rivière aux Pins

Rivière aux Pins runs through the heart of Boucherville, a suburb south of Montreal. Until about 15 years ago, the developed section of the river was considered a dump site and a symbol of urban pollution. The success story reports on the initiative of a local group of citizens that succeeded in reclaiming the river with the help of a grant from a federal agency, the assistance of municipal services and the support of the mayor at the time. The focus is on the alliances and mobilization of the people in the community which made it possible to clean up a polluted river.

The LaSalle Landfill Site

In the 1980s, LaSalle, Quebec was often in the headlines because of its landfill site, the first Canadian toxic waste disposal site to be located in a residential area. The success story recounts all of the restoration work carried out, including the demolition of houses. Concern, loss of trust by the public in government, the creation of citizen committees and the arrival of new actors set the scene for this story of exemplary intervention in the area of environmental health. This story inevitably concludes with an analysis of contaminated soil management policies and a review of the communication process between government authorities and the public.

Recommendations

The success stories lead to a number of recommendations: definition and consolidation of the mandates of joint environmental health committees; adoption of contaminated soil regulations; allocation of the necessary resources to and establishment of the structures for environmental protection organizations to enable them to control industrial emissions; creation of an environment fund; review of the standards and standardization of the regulations governing substances considered to be priority; establishment of a public consultation process for certain new toxic products.

TABLE OF CONTENTS

FIGURE

THE ISSUE

According to the first principle of the Rio Declaration on Environment and Development (WHO 1993), humans are at the core of sustainable development concerns. They deserve a healthy, productive life in harmony with nature.

Initially, the Industrial Revolution was viewed as a dream come true, one in which humanity triumphed over nature, ending hardship and eliminating disease. But there was a price to pay for this scientific and technical progress, both in terms of the new risks it placed on health and the new constraints it imposed on the environment (WHO 1990). Beginning in the early 1970s, the rise in environmental problems and ecological disasters significantly increased the risks to public health. The new field of environmental health sprang from the growing awareness of the interdependence of the health of the population and that of the ecosystem. It is based on a recognition of the potential impact of the environment on health, thereby highlighting the importance of the environment as a health determinant, especially if one subscribes to the theory that several factors contribute to the development of certain illnesses.

The Determinants of Health

The seventies also saw the emergence of a global concept of health as a result of the study of the causes of and factors inherent to morbidity and mortality and their impact on the health of Canadians (Lalonde 1974). This global concept of health went well beyond the narrow view of health as being linked exclusively to the health care system. It was based on four determinants: human biology, the environment, lifestyle and the organization of health care.

Recently, a new conceptual framework has been proposed which takes into consideration the dynamic interdependence of several factors (Evans and Stoddart 1990; Canadian Institute for Advanced Research 1991). The new element in this framework is the addition of the economy and prosperity as major determinants of health. According to the Canadian Institute for Advanced Research, health in today's society is closely linked to the ability of nations to create and distribute wealth.

Figure 1 reproduces the proposed concept and modifies it slightly to take into account the influence of the physical, chemical and biological environment on both productivity and prosperity—notably through the direct contribution of natural resources to prosperity—and on genetic makeup given that we know certain pollutants have a potential to be genotoxic.

Figure 1

The determinants of health

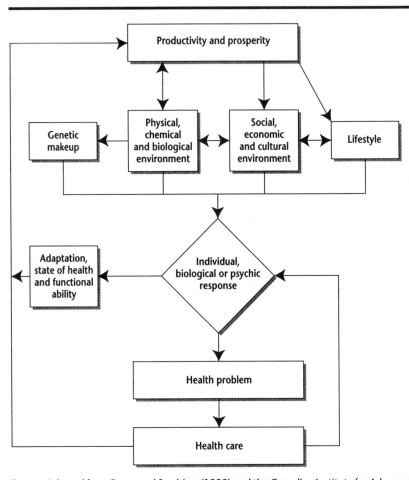

Source: Adapted from Evans and Stoddart (1990) and the Canadian Institute for Advanced Research (1991).

Environmental Health

Health is a complete state of physical, mental and social well-being and not just the absence of illness or infirmity (WHO 1946). Environmental health recognizes the role of the environment—and its physical, chemical and biological elements—in public health. It focuses primarily on the quality of the water, air, soil and foodstuffs. It can be defined as the study of the environmental factors likely to influence the health and well-being of humans (Chandrakant 1995)

The environment has always had a significant impact on public health. Droughts, hurricanes and earthquakes are phenomena often linked, directly or indirectly, with the state of the health of the populations affected by them. Even today, such natural disasters—sometimes amplified by poor land management—seriously threaten certain populations. Nevertheless, the twentieth century has seen spectacular progress in the improvement of overall health, as evidenced by the rise in the average life expectancy rate, especially in industrialized countries (Canadian Institute for Advanced Research 1991). Vaccination programs, healthier eating, a higher standard of living, better working conditions, greater accessibility to health care and a better social climate are the main reasons for this progress.

Today, chemical substances represent the main concern of environmental health. In 1984, a study by the U.S. National Research Council revealed that no toxicological information was available for approximately 80 percent of commercial chemical products. While their known effects on public health are less immediate and less spectacular than those linked to natural disasters, they do exist. Most often, they have adverse systemic (affecting the respiratory, cardiovascular, gastrointestinal, haematologic, hepatic and renal systems) and immune effects, not to mention the neurological, genotoxic, teratogenic and carcinogenic effects.

These insidious effects, for which there is increasing documentation, clearly show the extent of the link between the environment and health. While air, water and soil pollution are part of an interdependent system in the biosphere, we will examine each type of pollution separately.

Air Pollution

Numerous accidents and their impacts on mortality and morbidity have sharpened interest in the deleterious effects of air pollution. Among the most significant incidents were those which occurred in London in 1880 and 1952 and which killed nearly 1,000 and 4,000 people respectively (Gosselin et al. 1986). These two events were caused by a temperature inversion which prevented toxic gases from escaping into the air and trapped them at low altitudes.

In Canada, interest in this type of pollution was heightened by the increase in atmospheric emissions primarily from the use of fossil fuels. Transportation (responsible for more than 50 percent of air pollution in Canada), industry (approximately 25 percent) and heating (slightly more than 10 percent) have led to a significant increase in air pollutants (Pampalon 1980). These emissions are linked mainly to six major pollutants found in the urban environment: sulphur, carbon and nitrous oxides, volatile organic compounds (such as hydrocarbons), suspended particulates and ozone (Tolba et al. 1992). It is estimated that, within a few years, the number of automobiles in the world will climb from 540 million to almost one billion

(MacKenzie and Walsh 1991). Significant improvements will be needed in the performance and efficiency of antipollution devices if emission and air quality standards are to be respected.

Numerous links have been established between exposure to these pollutants and the development of illnesses (Whittemore 1981), especially respiratory tract illnesses (asthma, chronic bronchitis and pulmonary emphysema). It should be noted, however, that research to date has been unable to identify with any precision a single causative substance. The effects appear to be caused more by the synergy of air pollutants and may have other contributing factors, such as tobacco consumption and exposure in the workplace.

At present, researchers and the population are focusing on three types of pollution: destruction of the ozone layer (by CFCs) which could lead to increased skin cancer; pollution of the ambient air by tropospheric ozone (caused primarily by pollution from vehicular traffic) which may lead to increased respiratory problems (Lippman 1989); and contamination by suspended particulates (< 5 μm) which can be inhaled and can travel to the alveolar level.

Water Pollution

There are three primary sources of water pollution: industrial waste, agricultural waste and sewage. The famous cholera epidemic in London in 1854 was the catalyst for recognition of the potential risk to public health posed by contaminated water.

Most of the harmful effects of water pollution are caused by biological agents from animal and human excrement. Cholera, diarrhea, typhoid and paratyphoid fevers are examples of the main water-borne infections: each year millions of people around the world are affected by these diseases (WHO 1992).

The risks from physicochemical sources are just as real although less apparent. There are several reasons for this: the incidence of illness is lower than with biological agents, the dormant period of the illness is often very long, the appearance of a health problem cannot be attributed to a single contaminant and may have multiple causes, and lastly, we do not know the fundamental mechanisms which lead to chronic pathologies. Nevertheless, more than 700 chemical compounds have been detected in drinking water (Shy 1985). Nitrates (incidence on haemoglobin), mercury, lead (neurological problems) and cadmium (hypertension) are products that are frequently linked to health problems.

Diagnosis of Minamata disease was probably the key element in establishing a cause and effect relationship between a chemical agent and public health. This illness is a chronic neurological disorder which was first reported in the area around Minamata Bay in Japan. In 1968, it was determined that the disease was caused by mercury which the Chisso company was discharging in its effluents. The population was exposed to the mercury through the consumption of contaminated fish and shellfish. The mercury concentrations in these species were 10 to 10,000 times higher than the concentration in the ambient environment. It should be noted that, between 1974 and 1990, the Chisso company was required to assume 60 percent of the costs of dredging and cleaning up some 1,510,000 m^2 of the bottom of the bay.

Other contaminants pose problems which are beginning to impact on public health. These include organic products with a very high persistence, such as PCBs (polychlorinated biphenyls), dioxins and furans, as well as several pesticides for which we do not yet have sufficient information on their long-term effects. One example is the immunotoxic effects of several pesticides and organophosphorous insecticides which can inhibit acetylcholine, a neurotransmitter found almost everywhere in the body (Repetto and Baliga 1996).

Soil Pollution

Soil pollution is caused by the use of chemical products—pesticides and fertilizers—in farming and forestry practices, as well as from the dumping or burial of industrial (mainly mining wastes) and domestic waste (household garbage).

The direct relationship between soil pollution and health problems is relatively weak and relates mainly to children who, because of their habit of putting everything in their mouths, have a higher incidence of exposure. In general, exposure of the population to soil contaminants occurs indirectly through the food chain, that is, by ingesting contaminated food or water (for example, pesticide residue on edible plants and in livestock).

A relatively new source of contamination can be added to the already long list of soil contaminants. This newest contaminant is radioactive waste for which burying appears to be the most realistic solution. However, the stability of radioactive matter will make it a potential source of public health problems for generations to come.

Lastly, the consumer mentality of Canadians makes them the largest producers of garbage in the world (Government of Canada 1991). As a result, the number of landfill sites continues to grow just as the population is displaying increasing concern about them, primarily because of the dangers from the toxic substances buried in these sites.

Added to these concerns is the problem of decommissioned or closed dump sites in which dangerous wastes have been improperly disposed of (Government of Quebec 1993), and for which the Government of Quebec has had to establish decontamination and restoration programs.

Scientific Uncertainty

The present state of the environment stems in part from the inability to predict the potential risk of new developments and technologies (WHO 1990). Indeed, although modern societies generally bring about considerable and varied change, their collective projects fluctuate and the long-term effects of these changes are seldom predictable. As for the short-term effects, they are often fraught with uncertainty. The dormant period poses one of the major difficulties to being able to link the disease to the cause (Hertzman 1994).

Furthermore, the inability to isolate one substance from among the many substances to which populations are exposed makes any potential etiological link uncertain. Added to this are the doubts inherent to extrapolating to humans the results obtained with laboratory animals and, *a fortiori*, to a highly diverse population with interindividual variations. Indeed, the toxic effect of a pollutant can be altered by any number of determinants and factors—genetic makeup, diet, age, gender, weight, immune system and the consumption of drugs, cigarettes and alcohol. The uncertainty is even greater because the scientific community finds itself undergoing profound change while, at the same time, being confronted with ethical and economic issues (Renaud 1993).

The so-called exact sciences are no longer the authority in the field (Evans and Stoddart 1990). They no longer have the desire nor do they claim to be striving to achieve a coherent design for the world, one in which everything can be explained or solved. Anything that changes can be challenged since it can only be defined with difficulty. There is uncertainty about the extent of the direct and indirect risks to human health attributable to certain agents in the environment. For many substances, we do not know if there are thresholds to the adverse effects. We are far from having explored fully the potential toxicity of all of the chemical substances to which populations are being exposed (U.S. NRC 1984). Widely used substances that were long considered to be innocuous have been found to have harmful effects.

For this reason, the World Health Organization has tested some 1,000 substances over the past 20 years and has identified the environment as a key sector in the new health paradigm (WHO 1992). Far greater effort has to be made in this area: a moratorium should be placed on the manufacture of new substances. One thousand substances represent a mere drop in the ocean of those found in today's environment (Tolba et al. 1992).

Health Promotion

The link between the environment and public health has come to the fore in the past decade. As a result, protection of the environment has become one of the key determinants in improving public health. Indeed, protection of the environment is the main strategy of health promotion (Chandrakant

1995). Both public policy and the initiatives introduced to date are aimed at mobilizing the population and organizations to prevent or reduce the effects on health of exposure to pollutants.

In general, public policy encourages intersectoral action in terms of legislation, regulations and standards. Moreover, community organizations, by educating the public and taking social action, represent the mainstay of health promotion (Rose 1987). Lastly, promotion of a healthier life style is a corollary to improving environmental conditions (WHO 1990).

As the Ottawa Charter states (WHO 1986):

> Health promotion is the process of enabling people to increase control over, and to improve, their health. To reach a state of complete physical, mental and social well-being, an individual or group must be able to identify and realize aspirations, to satisfy needs, and to change or cope with the environment. Health is, therefore, seen as a resource for everyday life, not the objective of living...

The emergence of this new paradigm of health promotion requires innovative approaches which combine environmental protection with the public taking charge of its health; this apporach will have to be facilitated by the application of appropriate normative measures (Epp 1986).

There is a downside to environmental health that must be avoided: there is a growing tendency to disregard environmental problems which do not present immediate risks to public health. In the long term, such disinterest may have negative repercussions both for the environment and for health.

A number of recent cases of intervention at the local, provincial and national levels show that it is sometimes possible to act and to change things. This report discusses four cases which involve different issues and have different scopes; the purpose is to encourage the adoption of more effective means for enhancement of the environment and health in general.

SUCCESS STORIES

Children Contaminated by Lead

Actions on Nonmedical Determinants of Health

In the late 1980s, the history of environmental health in Quebec was marked by the case of children in Saint-Jean-sur-Richelieu being contaminated with lead. The contamination was caused by the industrial activities of the Balmet company involving the recovery of lead from used batteries. The company was located less than one kilometre from a residential community of

6,000 inhabitants, 600 of whom were children under the age of 10 years. The community was affected by the contamination.

In terms of public health, the population at risk was the children and pregnant women. The nervous system of children is more sensitive to lead than that of adults. Further, because children play outside and may have the habit of putting things in their mouths, they run a significantly higher risk of contamination. It is generally acknowledged that children ingest an average of 200 mg of soil per day compared to 10 mg for adults. In the case of pregnant women, the fetus is more vulnerable to lead because of its rapid development.

In Saint-Jean-sur-Richelieu, a clear link between the source and the target was established instantly: monitoring of blood lead concentrations in children in the community established a correlation between the various environmental interventions—cleaning the streets and houses, decontaminating the soil and pavement at the company's site—and the drop in blood lead concentrations among the children.

While it was relatively easy to verify the link between exposure to lead and the effects on physical health, there are other incidences which are much more difficult to assess. For example, the psychological and physiological effects of the stress experienced by the families involved remain undetermined.

Reasons for the Initiative

The population was aware that environmental contamination existed in 1987, almost a year before the issue reached the media. The community had complained about the stockpiling of the batteries at the Balmet site on several occasions.

In 1988, after several warnings from the ministère de l'Environnement du Québec concerning the noncompliance of its facilities and its operations, the Balmet company was forced to carry out a soil study and to propose viable options for restoration.

The study conducted during the summer of 1988 revealed significant lead contamination throughout the company's property, and the Département de santé communautaire (DSC) du Haut-Richelieu immediately took over the case. Because of the number of children living near the company and the risk of exposure to dust from the property, the DSC asked Environnement Québec to evaluate the level of soil and surface contamination outside of the company's property.

The results of this study revealed soil contamination within a 500 metre radius of the industrial site that was several times higher than the C criteria of the Contaminated Sites Rehabilitation Policy and which required immediate attention. Lead dust from the contaminated soil was found in vegetable gardens, raising the concern of the population.

A variety of measures were proposed given that there were about 600 children under the age of 10 years living within a kilometre of the site: an epidemiological study on the children's exposure to the lead, a moratorium on the consumption of home-grown fruits and vegetables, an analysis of the lead content in these foods, the closing down of the company's activities as soon as possible and, lastly, the implementation of a remedial plan (DSC Haut-Richelieu 1990).

Environnement Québec informed the DSC of the situation on Thursday, August 24, 1989. The following Monday, the DSC organized an information meeting with pediatricians, gynaecologists and general practitioners-obstetricians working at the Haut-Richelieu hospital. The purpose of the meeting was to provide medical information, especially as regards the health risk, and to identify the groups at risk. A press conference and public meeting were held the same evening and the next day.

One week later, interventions with the population began. Nurses from the Centre local des services communautaires (CLSC) visited homes to give families the information directly and to schedule visits to collect blood samples from children under the age of 10 years and from pregnant women living less than 150 metres from the company.

Blood samples were taken from a total of 186 children and 22 pregnant women. Since the results clearly indicated the need for further testing, a second and third phase were initiated with residents living between 150 and 400 metres from the company and 400 to 600 metres away respectively. In total, blood samples were taken from 662 children, 62 pregnant women and 21 adults.

According to health organizations, the normal blood lead concentration in children between the ages of six months and five years is between 50 and 80 µg/l; less than 5 percent of children should have a lead level higher than 150 µg/l and none normally should have a concentration higher than 200 µg/l (CDC 1991).

In Saint-Jean-sur-Richelieu, 21 children were found to have blood lead concentrations higher than 200 µg/l, including two with concentrations higher than 400 µg/l and six between 300 and 400 µg/l, and 27 had blood lead concentrations between 150 and 200 µg/l. These values illustrated the seriousness of the problem. It should be noted that only one child showed obvious signs of toxicity (CTQ 1989).

All of the families with children with high lead concentrations were offered psychosocial support to prevent anxiety attacks, after-attacks and traumatic reactions as a result of the situation. In addition, because of the large quantities of lead dust inside homes, the DSC recommended that 96 homes be cleaned, that is, in all instances in which the potential for exposure was high.

Stronger action was taken in the case of the two children whose blood lead concentrations exceeded 400 µg/l. One of the two and his family had to move, while the other changed daycare locations.

Actors

Although there are always a large number and variety of intervenors in situations such as this, the key actors are essentially in the environmental (ministère de l'Environnement du Québec) and public health (DSC, CLSC, Centre de toxicologie du Québec) sectors. While a joint environment-health committee already exists to deal with emergencies, there appears to be a need to endow it with the means to ensure more effective emergency response operations. All of the other public agencies involved in the case played much smaller roles.

The Info-Santé service set up by the CLSC, and which was used extensively to keep the public informed, made it possible to maintain an ongoing and close link with the whole of the population affected.

Analysis of the Results

While responsibility for the contamination rests in first step to the company, it would appear that the seriousness of the problem is the responsibility of the ministère de l'Environnement du Québec since its pollution control measures were clearly inadequate. Moreover, given the risks to public health, it is unacceptable that the Department waited more than a year before acting.

As for the interventions themselves, given the seriousness of the problem, it was important that action be taken quickly and that it be coordinated. We can report that intervention was quick and that coordination among the many intervenors was satisfactory.

The only negative aspect of the story was the behaviour of the Balmet company. When confronted with the extent of the restoration work required and the related cost, the company walked away from its obligations by simply declaring bankruptcy.

In the circumstances, this type of disappearing act is unacceptable. The government must acquire the means to make corporations accept their responsibility with respect to the environment. One possible solution would be to set up an environment fund. Every corporation would pay into the fund an amount proportional to the risk to the environment presented by its activities. The greater the evidence of effective environmental management, the lower the amount paid into the fund, and vice versa.

Such a fund would provide environmental and public health agencies with the means to deal adequately and consistently with all situations.

Replicability

To the extent that a population is exposed to pollutants arising from industrial activity and these substances represent a risk of toxicity to public health, it is possible to generalize the actions taken at Saint-Jean-sur-Richelieu. However, it is important to understand that, without a compensation policy for environmental pollution, the success of the intervention depends solely on the seriousness of the risk identified.

Consequently, in a similar situation in which the results might have revealed a lower risk, one might wonder whether public funds would have been allocated to remedy the situation.

Moreover, as long as the focus is on remedial action, it will be difficult to propose and implement a prevention program. The identification of health risks before the effects become evident and the establishment of monitoring and prevention mechanisms are the most effective ways of managing environmental health. The story of the children of Saint-Jean-sur-Richelieu is on the limit of prevention and treatment.

Funding

While the costs of the operation should have been assumed by the company, it declared bankruptcy. Consequently, the bill was picked up by the various government agencies responsible for the case, and the costs incurred by the health agencies (DSC, CLSC, physicians, health professionals) were charged to their operating budgets. The CLSC estimated the costs associated with the use of the Info-Santé service at $15,000. The cost of cleaning the 96 homes, estimated at $320,000, was covered by the ministère de la Santé et des Services sociaux. For its part, the Conseil régional de la santé et des services sociaux de la Montérégie area covered the costs of evaluating the results of the public health program ($15,000).

Environnement Québec assumed all of the costs associated with the soil decontamination work, as well as those for the soil analyses of private property ($62,000), the development of a restoration plan ($22,000), the preparation of the plans and designs ($70,000) and the removal of the contaminated soil (official cost unknown).

Evaluation

As with a number of other cases in the environmental health field, the social impact is a whole other element when public health is at stake, especially when the population at risk is children. This is an element that must be taken into consideration when analyzing the speed of the interventions and the large number of intervenors.

While Environnement Québec oversaw all of the operations, the participation of the health sector was crucial. It was this sector, through the DSC, which evaluated the situation and ensured the effectiveness of the on-site interventions. Two types of evaluation were used: ongoing individual medical and biological monitoring and an epidemiological study to monitor changes in the blood lead concentrations in the children and the return to normal conditions.

The quality of the interventions in this case was certainly satisfactory. But one question remains. The long-term effects, both physical and mental, not only of the contaminant but also of the stress caused by this type of situation, will probably never be known.

MMT in Gasoline

Actions on Nonmedical Determinants of Health

Lead is probably one of the pollutants most commonly known to the Canadians. Its physicochemical characteristics explain its multiple uses, including in batteries, munitions, paints, solders (pipes, cans) and gasoline (Royal Society of Canada 1986).

Lead was used in gasoline primarily because of its antiknock properties; the automobile has been one of the largest sources of emissions for a long time. Only a few years ago, environmental pollution from lead was a worldwide problem and several studies had clearly demonstrated its toxicity, especially for children (U.S. Department of Health and Human Services 1990).

Faced with this reality, the Canadian government decided to ban the use of lead from its market. Unfortunately, at the time of its decision to use MMT, research on the potential risk to public health associated with MMT and with exposure to its combustion products in emission gases (notably manganese particulates) were insufficient. Health and Welfare Canada nevertheless gave its approval for the use of MMT; at the time, it described the potential risks as being very low.

Recently, automobile manufacturers have revealed that MMT reduces the useful life of some engine components (especially the catalytic converter) which might interfere with the antipollution device in automobiles. They believe that this situation might lead to an increase in nitrous oxide and carbon monoxide emissions with the related environmental pollution and risks to public health. This type of pollution would essentially be harmful to the respiratory system. Curiously, this concern has not been raised in nor supported by any study published in scientific journals, although the economic and environmental impacts are considerable.

Reasons for the Initiative

It was because of the potential toxicity of lead that public pressure mounted to find ways to reduce lead pollution and its effects on humans.

This is why the Canadian government directed a great deal of energy to this problem and various national committees and commissions were established (Royal Society of Canada 1986) in an effort to reduce or eliminate lead in the Canadian market.

A series of legislative and regulatory measures were introduced in the 1970s and 1980s by the Canadian government to achieve this goal. One of the first measures dates back to 1975. It involved the regulatory control of the lead content in paint (Hazardous Products Act)—more specifically, in the paint used on toys, on children's furniture and in other domestic uses. During the 1980s, new regulations were introduced requiring the gradual elimination of tin cans using lead solders. The first products targeted were cans used for foods consumed by children: baby formula, fruit juices and tomato-based products. In 1985, the Government of Canada announced that, beginning in 1988, all new light transport vehicles had to have a catalytic converter. This was a major decision that was based on evidence of a definite link between lead from automobile emissions and environmental pollution. In 1986, just one year later, the Minister of the Environment for Canada launched a plan to eliminate lead in automobile gasoline by 1992. This goal was achieved in December 1990 (Environment Canada 1991).

However, gasoline must be mixed with a substance with antiknock properties. Consequently, Canada had to replace lead with MMT. In actual fact, this substance had been in use since 1976 and it gradually replaced lead until the latter's complete elimination in 1990.

MMT is manufactured in the United States and is used as an antiknock agent in gasoline sold to Canada. However, because of its potential risks to public health and to the environment, Canada announced in 1995 that it would be withdrawing it from the market (bill on manganese-based additives). Paradoxically, Bulgaria, Argentina and New Zealand were planning to introduce its use. In the United States, recent court decisions would indicate that MMT will be in use soon, probably in 1997. Although this product is manufactured by our neighbours to the south, its use was prohibited until October 1995 because of concerns of the Environmental Protection Agency (EPA) about its harmful effects on health.

The recent decisions of the American courts have prompted the Canadian government to do an about-face on its plan to ban MMT: the bill tabled in the House of Commons died on the order paper in January 1996 after having received second reading. Curiously, a new bill addressing the same issue was tabled in March 1996.

As much as the government's action with respect to lead was rational and supported by scientific evidence of the toxicity of this product, its action with respect to MMT appears to be somewhat ad hoc. It is difficult to see how a balance will be struck between the environmental, economic and political issues.

Actors

A review of the chronology of MMT identifies four initial actors: Ethyl Corp., which manufactures and markets the product; Health Canada, which gave the green light for its use; the Government of Canada, which developed the necessary legislation; and the Canadian Petroleum Products Institute, which was a key player in the decision for the use of MMT.

In the United States, Ethyl Corp. has had a great deal of difficulty convincing the EPA to grant it a permit to use MMT in the United States. It was only very recently (in 1995), after rejecting several applications from Ethyl Corp. over several years, that the EPA was forced by a court decision to award a use permit. It should be noted that the EPA was lobbied hard by both automobile manufacturers and environmental groups, including the Environmental Protection Fund, which fought against MMT because of the potential risk to public health linked to its combustion products.

Aware that there was inadequate scientific data on the potential risks of MMT, several public agencies and corporations decided to fund a research program to investigate this issue. Health Canada, Environment Canada, the ministère de l'Environnement et de la Faune du Québec, the Natural Sciences and Engineering Research Council of Canada, the Canadian Petroleum Products Institute and Ethyl Corp. itself funded research conducted over several years in Canada, the only country in the world using MMT. Cities such as Montreal and Toronto, with their high density vehicle traffic, thus became open-air laboratories.

In the meantime, automobile manufacturers exerted increasing pressure on the Government of Canada to ban MMT, arguing that it reduced the useful life of some vehicle components, thereby interfering with the operation of the antipollution device.

Analysis of the Results

The elimination of lead from gasoline was widely accepted by Canadians. Indeed, all of the government's efforts to reduce lead exposure and pollution levels were well received. Just over 10 years ago, the average blood lead concentration in Canadian children was around 120 µg/l, while today, it is around 60 µg/l. There has been a rapid and substantial reduction.

The decision to ban lead from the market was based on unequivocal scientific evidence. However, this does not appear to be the case with MMT.

Although it is readily agreed that the original studies used by Health Canada to justify its recommendation were insufficient, today there is new data which alleviates one of the two concerns about MMT.

According to recent research (Loranger and Zayed 1994, 1995; Loranger et al. 1994, 1995; Brault et al. 1994; Zayed et al. 1994), it appears that the manganese pollution from MMT is relatively low and has no major environmental repercussions. The potential public health risk is also minimal. A recent Health Canada report (Wood and Egyed 1994) comes to the same conclusion.

As for the second concern about increased oxides of nitrogen and carbon monoxide emissions, very few scientific studies have as yet been carried out or published on this matter.

Consequently, it appears that Canada's decision to ban MMT cannot logically be based on scientific evidence of any substantial risk to the environment or to public health. This decision could be strictly political.

Replicability

The experience with the elimination of lead shows that an informed decision may be received favourably. In spite of advances in science, it cannot predict everything nor offer ironclad prognoses. Some things can only be learned and discovered through experience. Consequently, since the impact on the environment and potential effects on public health of lead were not known and established at the time the decision was made to allow its use, we can understand the error.

The same is not true of MMT. Just as the initial decision to use this substance in Canadian gasoline was made prematurely, so the decision to ban its use is without basis. The tabling of the bill on MMT and its subsequent abandonment clearly show that the government is not basing its decision on scientific evidence.

Funding

The market for lead or MMT in gasoline represents billions of dollars worldwide. Even for the American economy, the stakes are not negligible. That is why it is not unreasonable to spend a few million dollars to ensure that a new product has no harmful effects. However, when we know that almost all of the studies have been conducted by the corporation interested in marketing the product, there is reason to question whether the data is totally reliable and has been properly interpreted, and whether all possibility of bias can be ruled out.

Evaluation

The outcome of this case is still unknown. We will have to be patient and take a step back in order to be able to evaluate it properly. However, the preliminary assessment clearly shows that the Government of Canada must develop a mechanism by which it can ensure the rational development and marketing, from an environmental standpoint, of any new product. This mechanism must encourage preventive research on any issue relating to health, the environment and sustainable development, ensure the participation of citizens in the decision-making process relating to environmental health projects and, to a lesser degree, encourage and improve communication between researchers, decision makers and the general public.

Rivière aux Pins

Actions on Nonmedical Determinants of Health

Uncontrolled urban growth has had serious repercussions on the quality of life of individuals. Clearly, noise, air pollution and lack of green spaces are factors which can affect public health to varying degrees.

The exodus to the suburbs is not surprising and is based, in part, on a desire to overcome the many shortcomings of urban communities. A significant proportion of people living in the suburbs are very concerned about their quality of life and do not hesitate to become involved politically or to act directly to preserve and enhance that quality of life.

That is what happened in the case of Rivière aux Pins. Located in the heart of Boucherville, a suburb south of Montreal, this river has one of the most sensitive and richest aquatic ecosystems in the metropolitan area. However, until about 15 years ago, the one kilometre developed section of this river was a veritable garbage dump. Citizens used it to dispose of objects they wanted to get rid of quickly; this behaviour was so prevalent that the river rightly became a symbol of urban pollution. The challenge was to restore this natural environment and ensure its protection in the long term.

Reasons for the Initiative

As it is always alarming to be a powerless witness to the destruction of a natural setting and to its transformation into an open dumping ground, the residents had expressed their concern to elected officials on numerous occasions. Although they acknowledged the badly deteriorated state of the river, officials had always bluntly refused to intervene.

This attitude is not surprising. Often, improvement of environmental conditions depends less on political power and legislative authorities, although their support is essential, than on direct action by citizens.

As a result, the community itself came together and found the technical and financial means to restore the natural habitat that had been polluted by mismanaged urban development and a lack of interest by politicians in environmental problems. This action was particularly important because the local population was growing quickly, as was residential development and its corollary, urban pollution. Concerted action was also needed by the residents and their municipal representatives to ensure that the municipality made rational decisions concerning the environment.

In order to promote this initiative and to ensure that their goals were achieved, the residents adopted an intersectoral approach supported by the determination of various units of the municipal government, in particular those dealing with urban development and communications.

Actors

It was in this context that the Comité d'aménagement naturel de Boucherville was established. The committee's activities clearly reflected the approach preferred by the World Commission on the Environment and Development, which identified the need to ensure optimal utilization of natural resources in the interest of sustainable development (World Commission on the Environment and Development 1988). Accordingly, local action taken as part of a general move to protect the environment constitutes a health determinant.

The Comité d'aménagement naturel de Boucherville consisted of 13 people, including two university professors, a lawyer, an industrial hygienist, a landscape architect, a botanist and an accountant. The nature and variety of the professions represented enhanced the credibility of the committee at the meetings called throughout its project to restore Rivière aux Pins.

The project received support from the lakes and rivers branch of the ministère de l'Environnement et de la Faune du Québec and the city's urban development department. Sympathetic to the project, local newspapers increased the number of articles on the state of the river and its potential uses after the cleanup.

The first step was to remove from the river all solid objects which were showing above the surface of the water. Five people were hired for three weeks to accomplish this task. After promoting the cleanup work and obtaining the support of the urban development department, the city of Boucherville offered its assistance and that of the public works department. Several city workers were assigned to collect all of the waste. By becoming an active participant in the project, the city positioned itself to reap any future political benefits.

Over and above the obvious political interest of municipal authorities, the committee realized that, as time went by, the city was showing greater and greater interest in the project itself and demonstrating a real willingness to contribute to enhancing the quality of the environment. For example, it was involved in the planting of trees and shrubs and provided tables for a picnic area.

In order to spark the interest of the residents of Boucherville, the Comité d'aménagement naturel decided to organize a special community day in the spirit of an old-time barn raising and invite everyone to plant a tree along the riverbank. More than 200 people showed up and were given a tree to plant in the places indicated on the development plan. People gave many reasons for joining in the event: "We believe in helping others", "We want to teach our children the importance of protecting the environment," "We want to help create an environment where it is good to live."

Analysis of the Results

Ten tons of waste were removed from the river, over a distance of only one kilometre—bicycle frames, oil tanks, bathtubs, toilets, wheelbarrows, bottles (in industrial quantities) and many other objects.

Several hundred trees and shrubs were planted along both riverbanks. This stabilized the banks and beautified the site, thereby restoring an unclean river to its natural appearance. Of course, this was only a physical restoration, there still needed to be a cleanup of the river itself, an intervention that had been called for for a number of years mainly because of pollution from waste oils.

As has been the case with similar interventions initiated by community groups, it was the involvement of several municipal departments that was the key factor in the political decision to support the project. Indeed, this involvement was vital to the promotion and success of the project.

Lastly, this local action clearly shows that partnerships between the community and municipal government are a way to maximize community involvement. It is a way for everyone to benefit.

Replicability

Several other similar projects carried out in Quebec have had equally positive results. Whether it is associations of fishermen or public health committees, the protection of lakes or the protection of the environment, all of the goals involve enhancement of the quality of life.

The time has come to acknowledge the unique and vital role which community groups play in protecting the environment and monitoring ecosystems. This recognition has to be more than mere talk. It must be accompanied by strong financial support, that is uncomplicated and accessible. Such support is legitimate and justified given the major environmental and socioeconomic benefits.

Funding

In order to carry out its project, the Comité d'aménagement naturel applied for a grant of about $35,000 from Employment and Immigration Canada. The grant was approved and the committee then asked municipal authorities to contribute a matching amount in services. The city agreed, bringing the total amount for the project to $70,000—not to mention the innumerable hours of volunteer time put in by the members of the committee.

There is no doubt that the work of the committee would have been made significantly easier had restoration programs been in place at any of the levels of government. Such programs would have made it possible to focus local energies and would have made access to financial resources easier. In the absence of such programs, the success of similar projects will continue to be uncertain and will depend on the goodwill of citizens.

Evaluation

Today, Rivière aux Pins is an enjoyable and accessible recreational area. Its banks are adorned by hundreds of trees and thousands of shrubs. Since the completion of the cleanup project, the city has built a bicycle path along the river. It is planning to continue developing the area by building several small facilities for water sports.

Although no statistics are available, the large number of people visiting the river is a good indication of the project's benefits. The city has given the committee approval to increase and to enhance the services linked to this urban park.

LaSalle Landfill Site

Actions on Nonmedical Determinants of Health

In the 1980s, LaSalle was a name that was always in the media because, like the Love Canal in the United States, it had the first toxic landfill site in Canada located in a residential area (Bonnier 1987).

LaSalle is located southwest of Montreal Island, Quebec between the St. Lawrence River to the south and the Lachine Canal to the north, less than nine kilometres from the Port of Montreal. Because of its easy access, this municipality experienced rapid and significant demographic, commercial and industrial growth. Like several other cities, it had a landfill site for local waste disposal. It seems, however, that a number of industries used the site to dispose of toxic waste.

A few years later, homes were built on the site which had been redeveloped for residential purposes, although significant quantities of toxic products still remained in the soil. These substances included volatile organic compounds (benzene, toluene, xylene, trichloroethylene and tetrachloro-ethylene), oils and greases, polycyclic aromatic hydrocarbons (benzopyrene, pyrene and chrysene) and polychloride biphenyls (PCBs) (Foratek International Inc. 1985).

Not only were these substances contaminating the soil but they also posed a threat to the water table because of the permeability of the soil and the migration of the substances toward the canal of the Montreal's water supply system, the main source of drinking water for the residents of Montreal Island. They therefore posed a risk to public health.

Reasons for the Initiative

In 1983, as part of its hazardous waste management policy, Environnement Québec set up a task force to study and restore hazardous waste disposal sites. The group's mandate was to establish an exhaustive list of all sites in Quebec likely to have received hazardous waste. The initiative was similar to that already conducted in other countries, including the United States and the Netherlands.

One year after it was formed the task force presented a list of the various disposal sites in Quebec. Of the 345 hazardous waste disposal sites on the list, 41 were located on Montreal Island. However, because of the complexity of certain cases, the status of 19 sites could not be completely documented. The former LaSalle landfill site was one of these. After being used as a landfill site from 1940 to 1959, it had been covered with about three metres of clean soil and then closed.

However, from the task force's inquiries and several accounts, there was reason to believe that during its final years of operation, industries in LaSalle had apparently used this site to dispose of barrels containing toxic waste. However, no one was able to determine the exact location of the dump site, nor the exact nature of the products disposed of.

The problem was compounded by the fact that thirty residential homes and five commercial buildings had been built on this contaminated site between 1965 and 1984.

For these reasons, a comprehensive study was conducted to determine the exact nature of the contaminants and evaluate the risk to the environment and public health. A highly contaminated area was identified. Eight homes were standing on this site.

No further announcements about the situation were made after the task force's report was published in 1984; only representatives of Environnement Québec were fully aware of the situation. It was not until early in 1985 that other senior officials, including the director of the Département de la santé communautaire in Verdun and the municipal authorities of LaSalle, were informed. In June 1985, Environnement Québec decided that the findings of the supplementary studies warranted declaring a state of emergency in the area concerned. A coordinating committee and a health committee were then set up.

It was not until a public meeting was held with the Minister of the Environment for Quebec and the mayor of LaSalle in July 1985 that the full extent of the situation was made known to everyone. At the meeting, the findings were presented and opinions offered as to the public health risk. The creation of the coordinating committee, a medical clinic and a special information and assistance office for residents was also announced.

A number of measures were then initiated: a toxicological study, medical examinations, monitoring of the air quality in the homes and comprehensive soil analyses.

Surprisingly, the situation did not create much concern among the residents affected. Only nine people visited the medical clinic between July and September 1985. Fortunately, none of the examinations turned up any health problems that could be linked to the contaminants in the soil. Given the lack of demand, the medical clinic was closed at the end of September 1985.

The air quality analyses in the homes did not reveal any significant pollution. While these results indicated that the pollutants had not migrated into homes, the level of soil contamination and the risk to health from long-term exposure was sufficiently high to warrant taking remedial action within a relatively short time period.

In late September, a second public meeting was held. The main results were presented and it was clear that soil decontamination was necessary. This process would require the demolition of eight houses and the relocation of dozens of families for the six months or so that the work would take, that is, from April to September 1986. The Quebec government offered the residents affected financial assistance or compensation.

It was after this second meeting that communication between provincial authorities (the ministère de l'Environnement du Québec) and municipal authorities broke down and all of the planned interventions came to a standstill. This period of silence, waiting and procrastination can be attributed in part to the provincial elections and to the change in government. It appears that the new political entities were questioning some of the commitments made by the previous government, leaving municipal authorities and health officials to assume full responsibility for the situation. Nor did the government follow through on the financial commitments that it had made earlier.

Faced with the inaction of the political powers, the citizens of LaSalle banded together to set up a committee called ARRET (Association des résidants refusant toute émanation toxique). The environmental group, Société pour vaincre la pollution, sounded the alarm, claiming that Montreal's drinking water was in danger because of the migration of the pollutants in the soil.

In an effort to solicit a reaction from Environnement Québec, the health committee issued statements that the nature and toxicity of the substances identified posed a very serious danger and that the failure to clean up the contaminated soil constituted a threat to the residents and was placing unacceptable stress on them.

Finally, after five months of silence, the government approved an order providing financial assistance. The announcement was made on April 30, 1986 by the Minister of the Environment for Quebec and the mayor of LaSalle.

The government order was the signal for the start of a soil restoration program. This was a two-stage program that would take two years. In the first phase, the contaminated areas were completely cleaned and restored during the summer of 1986. The toxic waste from the excavation of the site was stored on the former site of LaSalle Coke. In early August 1986, all of the cleanup work had been completed. Unfortunately, the work required the evacuation and temporary or permanent relocation of the residents of 84 homes. The second phase began in the summer of 1987 and mainly involved the burial of the contaminated soil in sealed containers.

Actors

This was clearly a complex case: the interventions spanned a three-year period during which a number of actors became involved. The ministère de l'Environnement du Québec was the leading agency in the intervention.

Initially, this was an environmental matter spearheaded by Environnement Québec's task force. However, the results concerning the nature of the contamination were unexpected and surprising. The presence of a population that could be exposed to this contamination and the risk to public health made this a potentially explosive situation.

Several public agencies, lobby groups, committees of experts and individuals had to deal with a population which grew increasingly cynical as the evaluation work progressed.

The diversity of the agencies involved in the case became evident with the release of the initial data on the nature of the contamination: municipal officials, the Direction de la protection civile du Québec, the ministère des Affaires sociales, the ministère des Affaires municipales, the ministère de la Santé et des Services sociaux and the Département de santé communautaire—they all received the information.

In addition, the Communauté urbaine de Montréal (CUM), Environment Canada, the Commission de santé et sécurité du travail (CSST) and several consultants were involved in carrying out the additional soil analyses, the monitoring of the air quality, the necessary analyses and the decontamination work.

People from the area affected were also called on for help, but the most important role fell to the health committee and to the Centre de toxicologie du Québec, which had to determine the toxicity of the substances uncovered at the site and interpret the results in terms of the risk to health. The health committee included experts in toxicology from the University of Montreal, Laval University, McGill University and the Armand-Frappier Institute.

Lastly, the action taken by the residents and by the SVP environmental group (Société pour vaincre la pollution) was the catalyst that ensured the interventions continued at a time when political interest appeared to wane.

Analysis of the Results

One need only look at the data on the quantity of contaminated soil— 125,000 m³ buried about three metres under the surface of the ground—to realize the seriousness of the problem.

In spite of the extent of the soil contamination, air quality in the houses was not significantly affected and did not apparently pose any risk to public health. Nevertheless, uncertainty about the effects of long-term exposure, even at very low concentrations, was sufficient to justify major intervention in this case.

Indeed, it was the potential impact on public health which weighed heavily in decisions. Initially, the intervention launched by the task force was essentially environmental. If not for the recommendations made by the health organizations (Département de santé communautaire and the Centre de toxicologie du Québec), the outcome might have been quite different, especially given the change in government which had an impact on all of the decisions and interventions.

One shadow remains: why was communication cut off after the second public meeting? This is an important question in that it added to the inherent difficulties of the situation, as well as to the fear and the stress caused by the uncertainty. This breakdown in communication and the hesitation to begin taking action by implementing the planned restoration program can be attributed to the fact that there were no contaminated soil management regulations and standards which set forth the levels of intervention. Operating on a case-by-case basis, the government undoubtedly feared that major intervention might establish a precedent creating a legal and moral obligation to intervene in other similar cases.

Replicability

Inadequate information on soil quality in areas redeveloped for housing means that we have seen only the tip of the iceberg in terms of problems with contaminated soil in developed areas. These problems will multiply in the years ahead.

Since there are still no regulations governing the restoration of contaminated soil, financial institutions have adopted guidelines which partially make up for this inadequacy. Loans for new residential, commercial or industrial developments are not approved unless developers can assure the lending institution of the soil quality. This practice should at least avoid the possibility of similar situations in the future.

Funding

Public and parapublic agencies involved in this case did not have special budget envelopes for this type of intervention. Consequently, they were forced to tap the resources of their regular operating budgets.

The Government of Quebec picked up most of the bill. It provided initial funding of $500,000 to LaSalle so that it could ensure the health and safety of the population affected (technical studies, temporary accommodation for some residents, etc.). Further funding of $8.3 million was given to the city by the Government of Quebec to cover the costs of restoring the soil quality of the site.

Evaluation

The LaSalle case is the first of its kind in Canada. It is the first toxic landfill site in a residential community.

Eight houses were demolished—contaminated buildings for which no other solution was available. The next step is to gain a better understanding of the determinants of health relating to interior climate and ambient air quality in homes and buildings in order to set standards to be incorporated in building design and construction codes, as well as in product safety.

There are also questions about the conduct of the parties involved. Why did residents not react after the first public meeting when Environnement Québec had declared a state of emergency? What prompted the residents to mobilize later on?

Lastly, the need for regulations governing contaminated soil management must be acknowledged. The roles and responsibilities of the various departments, branches and agencies must be clearly defined and appropriate intersectoral links established. The levels of intervention must also be defined in order to speed up decision making about the action to be taken.

The government itself acknowledged that such regulations were needed when, in 1988, it proposed a contaminated site rehabilitation policy. Its intent was to establish the need to restrict the use of former industrial land and the importance of undertaking restoration work following the closure of industrial facilities. This policy was to have served as the basis for developing contaminated soil management regulations; unfortunately, a directive was the only outcome and it certainly does not have regulatory force. More than ten years after the LaSalle incident, there are still no regulations. As a result, problems with contaminated soil are managed on a case-by-case basis; such an approach opens the door to conflicting solutions and the methods used to achieve them. The time is both appropriate and opportune for the government to act in this area.

RECOMMENDATIONS

The purpose of the success stories highlighted is to enhance the management of environmental health. They recommend ways to create an environment which protects and promotes health. It should be noted, however, that these recommendations do not take into consideration the jurisdictions of the various levels of government and would have to be reworked to respect the respective areas of responsibility.

1. for emergency situations, define and strengthen the mandate of joint committees on environmental health;
2. for all other situations, establish a mechanism to encourage information sharing among the various government bodies—including departments and branches—and the stakeholders;
3. enact long-promised regulations on contaminated soil management;
4. review the structures and resources of environmental protection agencies to control industrial emissions while supporting recent environmental assessments by corporations (self-assessment);
5. set up an environment fund financed by corporations, with contribution rates based on the potential for contamination and the risks to the environment;
6. continue evaluating certain priority substances in order to amend the environmental standards and to standardize relevant regulations within a reasonable time frame;
7. establish a consultation process which will enhance communication of information to individuals and communities and their involvement in the decision-making process with respect to the use of new chemical products. Consideration must be given to the quantities involved and their toxicity.

These recommendations must be part of a general framework in which:

- the government would recognize the principle that any damage to the environment can affect health;
- Canada, like European countries, would adopt a charter on environmental health and would enumerate the directions likely to promote the enhancement of physical environments in order to provide a rational foundation for a healthy lifestyle. The supporting framework for this charter would be a description of the priority action to be taken to reduce pollution and to restore the environment and the internal policies to promote the judicious use of resources

and products. Such action would give meaning and form to the principle of sustainable development which Canada already supports;

- the government would recognize the vital role of the population in the protection of the environment and the monitoring of ecosystems;
- the government would encourage the participation of non-government organizations and the industrial and scientific communities in national activities to support efforts and initiatives for sustainable development to the benefit of health and the environment.

Joseph Zayed *obtained his Ph.D. in community health, specializing in environmental toxicology. He is an associate professor in the Department of Occupational and Environmental Health at the University of Montreal. His research focuses on the evaluation of environmental contamination and population exposure. He is also director of postgraduate studies in environment and prevention. He is an ad hoc member of the Bureau d'audience publique sur l'environnement and has been involved in three commissions.*

Luc Lefebvre *has a master's degree in occupational and environmental health. He works as a toxicologist at the Montreal-Centre Department of Public Health. He is responsible for writing and evaluating public health notices in regard to environmental problems involving dangerous materials. He is also a member of the regional intervention team for technological emergencies that may endanger public health. Mr. Lefebvre is also a guest professor at various courses on environment and on toxicological risk assessment at the University of Montreal and at the University of Quebec in Montreal.*

BIBLIOGRAPHY

BARBEAU, A. 1984. Manganese and extrapyramidal disorders (a critical review and tribute to Dr. George C. Cotzias). *Neurotoxicology* 5: 13–36.

BONNIER, J. G. 1987. *Exposé historique de l'ancien dépotoir municipal de ville LaSalle 1984–1987.* Département de santé communautaire, Centre Hospitalier de Verdun.

BRAULT, N., S. LORANGER, F. COURCHESNE, G. KENNEDY, and J. ZAYED. 1994. Bioaccumulation of manganese in plants: Influence of MMT as gasoline additive. *The Science of the Total Environment* 1553: 77–84.

CANADIAN INSTITUTE FOR ADVANCED RESEARCH. 1991. *The Determinants of Health.* Publication no. 5, Toronto (ON): Canadian Institute for Advanced Research.

CENTRE DE TOXICOLOGIE DU QUÉBEC. 1989. *L'exposition au plomb des enfants du quartier N.D.A. de Saint-Jean-sur-Richelieu.* Report.

CHANDRAKANT, P. S. 1995. *Public Health and Preventive Medicine in Canada.* Ste-Foy (QC): Les presses de l'Université Laval.

COMMISSION MONDIALE DE L'ENVIRONNEMENT ET DU DÉVELOPPEMENT. 1988. *Notre avenir à tous.* Éditions du FLEUVE, Les publications du Québec.

DSC HAUT-RICHELIEU. 1990. *La contamination environnementale par le plomb d'un quartier résidentiel à Saint-Jean-sur-Richelieu. Volume I.*

ENERGY AND ENVIRONMENTAL ANALYSIS. 1995. *Clearing the Air: Urban Smog Emission Trends in Selected Canadian Metropolitan Areas. Final Report.* Ottawa (ON): CAA.

ENVIRONMENT CANADA. 1991. *Canada's Green Plan.* Ottawa (ON).

EPP, J. 1986. *Achieving Health for All: A Framework for Health Promotion,* Ottawa (ON): Health and Welfare Canada.

EVANS, R. G., and G. L. STODDART. 1990. Producing health, consuming health care. *Social Science and Medicine* 31(12): 1347–1363.

FORATEK INTERNATIONAL INC. 1985. *Étude de caractérisation partielle de l'ancien dépotoir de ville de LaSalle à LaSalle.* Report 671.

GOSSELIN, P., D. BOLDUC, E. DEWAILLY, J. GOSSELIN, P. LAJOIE, D. LALIBERTÉ, and M. SERGERIE. 1986. *Salubrité de l'environnement au Québec. Bases théoriques et pratiques.* Québec (QC): Les publications du Québec.

GOVERNMENT OF CANADA. 1991. *The State of Canada's Environment.* Ottawa (ON): Department of Supply and Services Canada.

HERTZMAN, C. 1994. The lifelong impact of childhood experiences: A population health perspective. *Health and Wealth, Journal of the American Academy of Arts and Sciences* 123(4): 167–180.

LALONDE, M. 1974. *A New Perspective on the Health of Canadians: A Working Document.* Ottawa (ON): Department of National Health and Welfare.

LIPPMAN, M. 1989. Health effects of ozone: A critical review. *J Air Pollut Control Assoc.* 39(5): 675–695.

LORANGER, S., and J. ZAYED. 1994. Manganese and lead concentration in ambient air and emission rates from unleaded and leaded gasoline between 1981 and 1992 in Canada: A comparative study. *Atmospheric Environment* 28: 1645–1651.

———. 1995. Environmental exposure to manganese from mobile sources: A multimedia assessment. *Int. Arch. Occ. Environ. Health* 67: 101–110.

LORANGER, S., J. ZAYED, and G. KENNEDY. 1995. Contribution of methylcyclo-pentadienyl manganese tricarbonyl (MMT) to atmospheric Mn concentration near expressway: Dispersion modeling estimation. *Atmospheric Environment* 29(5): 591–599.

LORANGER, S., G. DEMERS, G. KENNEDY, E. FORGET, and J. ZAYED. 1994. The pigeon (*Columba livia*) as a monitor of atmospheric manganese contamination from mobile sources. *Archives of Environmental Contamination and Toxicology* 27: 311–317.

MACKENZIE, J., and M. WALSH. 1991. *Driving Forces: Motor Vehicle Trends and Their Implications for Global Warming Strategies and Transportation Planning*. Washington (DC): World Resources Institute.

MINISTÈRE DE L'ENVIRONNEMENT DU QUÉBEC. 1985. *Ancien dépotoir de LaSalle : bilan de la situation et stratégie d'intervention*. Report, July 1985.

_____. 1993. *État de l'environnement au Québec, 1992*. Montreal (QC): Guérin.

PAMPALON, R. 1980. *Environnement et santé. Éléments d'une problématique québécoise*. Québec (QC): Gouvernement du Québec, Ministère des Affaires sociales.

RABINOWITZ, M. et al. 1985. Environmental correlate of infant blood lead levels in Boston. *Environmental Research* 38: 96–107.

RENAUD, M. 1993. The future: Hygeia versus Panakeia? *Health and Canadian Society* 1(1): 229–249.

REPETTO, R., and S. A.BALIGA. 1996. *Pesticides and Immune System: The Public Health Risks*. Washington (DC):World Resources Institute.

ROSE, G. 1987. Environmental factors and disease: The man-made environment. *Br Med J* 294(6577): 963–965.

ROYAL SOCIETY OF CANADA. 1986. *Lead in Canadian Environment: Science and Regulations, Final Report*. The Commission on Lead in the Environment.

SHY, C. M. 1985. Chemical contamination of water supplies. *Environmental Health Pespectives* 62: 399–406.

TOLBA, M. K., O. A. EL-KHOLY, E. EL-HINNAWI, M. W. HOLDGATE, D. F. MCMICHAEL, and R. E. MUNN. 1992. *The World Environment 1972–1992. Two Decades of Challenge*. London: United Nations Environment Programme, Chapman & Hall.

U.S. DEPARTMENT OF HEALTH AND HUMAN SERVICES. 1990. *Toxicological Profile for Lead*. Agency for Toxic Substances and Disease Registry.

_____. 1991. *Strategic Plan for Elimination of Childhood Lead Poisoning*. Centers for Disease Control.

U.S. NATIONAL RESEARCH COUNCIL. 1984. *Toxicity Testing*. Washington (DC): National Research Council.

WHITTEMORE, A. S. 1981. Air pollution and respiratory disease. *Annu. Public Health* 2: 397–429.

WHO COMMISSION ON HEALTH AND ENVIRONMENT. 1992. *Our Planet, Our Health*, Geneva, Switzerland: World Health Organization.

WOOD, G., and M. EGYED.1994. *Risk Assessment for the Combustion Products of Methylcyclopenta-dienyl Manganese Tricarbonyl (MMT) in Gasoline*. Ottawa (ON): Environmental Health Branch, Health Canada.

WORLD HEALTH ORGANIZATION. 1946. *Basic Documents*. 26th ed. Geneva, Switzerland: WHO, 1976.

_____. 1986. *Ottawa Charter for Health Promotion*. Copenhagen, Denmark.

_____.1990. *Environnement et santé: la Charte européenne et son commentaire*. First European Conference on the Environment and Health, WHO Regional Publications, European Series No. 35, European Regional Office, Copenhagen, Denmark.

_____. 1993. *WHO World Staregy for Health and the Environment*. Geneva, Switzerland: WHO/ EHE/93.2, World Health Organization.

ZAYED, J., M. GÉRIN, S. LORANGER, P. SIERRA, D. BÉGIN, and G. KENNEDY. 1994. Occupational and environmental exposure of garage workers and taxi drivers to airborne manganese arising from the use of MMT (methylcyclopentadienyl manganese tricarbonyl) in unleaded gasoline. *American Industrial Hygiene Association* 55: 53–58.

Issues

Preventing Violence: School- and Community- Based Strategies

MARLIES SUDERMANN, PH.D., C.PSYCH.
PETER G. JAFFE, PH.D., C.PSYCH.

London Family Court Clinic and the University of Western Ontario

SUMMARY

Violence is a significant concern for the majority of Canadians. Vulnerable groups, such as women, children and visible minorities, have special concerns. Violence against women is a major health issue in our society. For example, women are more than four times more likely to be injured by their own male partner than in a motor vehicle accident. Research in Canada points to the fact that 29 percent of women have experienced violence in a current or former marital relationship (Statistics Canada 1993). Women are more likely to be killed by their partner or ex-partner than by anyone else in the community (Statistics Canada 1993). Their children who witness violence are at risk of a host of short- and long-term emotional and behavioral adjustment problems. Aside from the immediate risk to physical and psychological well-being, violence against women costs the Canadian economy at least $4 billion per annum in the justice, health, social service and employment sectors.

Violence is also a concern for both female and male children and youth at school. Research in Canada, as well as in other countries, such as Norway, indicates that bullying and peer-to-peer violence are pervasive, serious concerns in schools and neighbourhoods. Influences such as the increasingly violent media to which children are exposed may heighten the level of physical and psychological violence in schools and communities, although reliable statistics on school violence are only now becoming available.

Primary prevention, if proven effective, would be the most preferable intervention to stem this tide of violence. School-based violence prevention is a promising primary prevention strategy for addressing violence in general, as well as violence against women and girls. The present paper reviews several school-based violence prevention programs with positive evaluation results. Common features of the successful programs are identified, as well as gaps in our knowledge about the effects of such programs. Directions for future evaluation and development of such violence prevention initiatives are suggested.

Secondary prevention efforts that target high-risk populations, such as children raised in violent families, are also discussed. Recent innovations that include a specialized group counselling program offer some hope for longer-term reductions in violence.

This paper also explores policy implications with respect to methods governments, communities, individuals and legal bodies can use to support violence prevention efforts, with special reference to violence against women. Issues of government, legal and community responses to violence against women are also addressed.

TABLE OF CONTENTS

INTRODUCTION

As a major cause of concern for the majority of Canadians, violence is second only to the economy. This concern has been increased by a number of well-publicized murders and the development of articulate victims' groups that demand a more accountable and effective justice system. At the same time, several school boards, parents' groups and teachers' associations have expressed concerns about increasing violence in schools and among young people in general. There has been a move toward zero tolerance of violence, as well as toward policies and programs geared to reducing violence and creating safer schools.

Violence is a social issue that attracts discussion from divergent viewpoints and considerable public debate. Some analysts have suggested that we are living through a "paradox" in this field because our level of awareness has been heightened beyond the actual statistical increase in violent crime (Howard 1996). This suggestion is based in part on increased media reporting and sensationalization of violence, although the homicide rate has been declining since 1975 in Canada. On the other hand, there is some debate about the accuracy of violent crime statistics and some indication that youth crime has increased over the past 10 years.

No matter what conclusion Canadians reach about violence, some agree (in part because of economic restraint) that building more prisons and hiring more police will not solve the problem in the long term. Canada is second only to the United States among industrialized nations in the use of incarceration. (If prisons worked, the United States would be the safest country in the world.) The United States locks up four times as many citizens per capita as Canada and has four times the homicide rate (Horner 1993). Canadian provinces spend 90 percent of federal funding allocated to them for correctional services on custody of young offenders. The number of police officers in Canada has declined gradually over the past 5 years. With limited resources, police services have had to focus on the most serious crime. Energy is increasingly directed toward improving use of resources and seeking more proactive approaches to reducing violence (e.g., prevention programs).

Several federal government committees have offered broad directions for prevention programs, with some unifying themes. The 1993 Parliamentary Standing Committee on Justice and the Solicitor General emphasized the importance of primary and secondary prevention efforts. Primary prevention would focus on broad-based community and school strategies to ensure better beginnings for young children and a reduction of violence as a form of entertainment. Secondary prevention would focus on high-risk populations, such as disadvantaged youth raised in abusive families.

In the words of Drs. S. Hart and D. Dutton of the committee (Horner 1993, 10):

> Childhood abuse breeds abusers… abused children are three times more likely than the rest of the population to become violent adults. Physically abused children are five times as likely to be violent as adults towards a family member…

The Canadian Panel on Violence Against Women came to very similar conclusions on the basis of visits to 139 communities and submissions from 4,000 citizens and groups (Canadian Panel on Violence Against Women and Children 1993). The final panel report stressed the importance of recognizing different levels of vulnerabilities and encouraging a climate of zero tolerance toward violence. The panel made links between violence and inequality similar to those made by the Ad Hoc Advisory Committee for a National Strategy on Community Safety and Crime Prevention (1993), which found that "crime and victimization are directly linked to inequality and injustice" (Ad Hoc Advisory Committee for a National Strategy on Community Safety and Crime Prevention 1993, 1). The panel stressed the importance of every government agency, institution and community member taking action to address these issues. It placed special emphasis on the school as a forum for prevention efforts, as well as on high-risk youth (such as children witnessing or experiencing violence in families) as a target for secondary prevention programs.

One major conclusion drawn from an overview of the literature on violence is that it is important to integrate government and community efforts to reduce violence in general and violence against women in particular. Although these fields of study developed through the efforts of separate groups of academics, practitioners and social activists, they converge in identifying the need for better, more extensive prevention efforts. The vast majority of violence happens at the hands of family members, not strangers. When strangers do perpetrate violence, they have clear histories of abusive family backgrounds.

The Impact of Violence on Health and Safety

Violence is a concern related directly to health and safety. Both injuries and deaths from actual violent acts, as well as the psychological *sequelae* of violent acts, such as post-traumatic stress disorder, have a serious health impact on our society. In addition, the fear or threat of violence and lack of a safe, secure environment can result in severe psychological stress, resulting in negative mental health and behavioral outcomes. For example, Osofsky and colleagues (1993), in their review of the effects on children of living in chronically violent family and community environments, concluded that such environments contribute to a wide range of mental health and behavioral impairments, including: difficulty concentrating at school, memory impairment resulting from intrusive thoughts, anxious attachments to mothers, restricted emotions and "acting tough" to deal with emotions, lack of social and emotional responsiveness, and severe constriction in activities and thoughts for fear of reexperiencing traumatic events. Children growing up in violent homes and communities also learn to use violent behaviour in situations of conflict. Steinhauer (1995) identified children's observing family violence as an important factor in the development of juvenile delinquency. A tendency toward conduct disorder and use of interpersonal violence in children who witness wife assault has repeatedly been identified by researchers (Jaffe et al. 1990).

Violence against women, specifically wife assault, has been identified as a major physical and mental health problem in our society (Canadian Panel on Violence Against Women 1993; Statistics Canada 1993). Violence committed by wives against their husbands also occurs with some frequency (Straus and Gelles 1995), although it is not as fearful or injurious to men because of the strength and power differentials between men and women. Some forms of violence committed by parents against their children are still viewed as justifiable discipline in our society, although tolerance of disciplinary violence is declining (Straus and Gelles 1995). As a result of vastly increased reporting rates over the last 10 years, some people fear that our society is experiencing an epidemic of wife assault and child abuse. However, the real reason for the increased reporting rate is a shift toward greater awareness and less tolerance of these forms of violence. Recently, our society also became concerned about violence in schools, and media violence and its effect on children, youth and vulnerable adults.

The health impacts of different forms of violence should be studied more widely. Estimates of the physical and psychological trauma and impairment resulting from different forms of violence, as well as estimates of the costs of treating the immediate and long-term aftermath of violence in the health, social service, criminal justice and education systems, are only beginning to emerge and require further study.

To our knowledge, the broad-based negative effects of all forms of violence on community levels of stress, well-being and self-efficacy have not been extensively studied. The ways these psychological factors, in turn, affect various indices of health also need further study. However, the current public concern with, and mobilization around, violence issues supports the contention of the widespread nature of such effects.

The first section of this paper, "Key Conclusions from the Literature," focuses on the health effects of violence, with a special focus on violence against women, children who witness wife assault, and school-based violence. Primary prevention of these forms of violence through successful, evaluated, school-based violence prevention programs is reviewed in the section

"Success Stories in the Prevention of Violence against Women and Other Forms of Violence." The section "Interests at Stake in Promoting or Impeding Change" lists the interests at stake in promoting or impeding change in violence. The final section, "Policy Implications," indicates policy directions to assist in primary prevention of violence in relationships and of school-based violence, as well as more effective community responses to violence in relationships.

KEY CONCLUSIONS FROM THE LITERATURE

Wife Assault

Wife assault has only recently received acknowledgment and study as a health issue. In a well-conducted random telephone survey, Statistics Canada (1993) found that 29 percent of women have experienced violence at the hands of a marital partner. This groundbreaking study also found that, of women who reported violence in a current marriage, 34 percent feared for their lives at least once during the relationship (Canada. Statistics Canada 1993). The American Medical Association recently published data indicating that U.S. women were four times more likely to suffer physical injury at the hands of their own male partner than from a motor vehicle accident (American Medical Association 1992). Straus and Gelles (1986), on the basis of the second of their large-scale U.S. surveys, estimated that the incidence of severe husband-to-wife violence is 11.3 percent of U.S. women each year. Severe, repeated violence takes place in an estimated 1 out of 14 families (Dutton 1988).

The health costs of violence against women are undoubtedly very great. Violence against women produces many physical injuries, as indicated in the American Medical Association (1992) study, and a significant number of deaths are also associated with violence against women. For example, Statistics Canada (1994) reported that, from 1974 to 1992, a married woman in Canada was nine times more likely to be killed by her spouse than by a stranger and that, in this same period, 1435 women were killed by their husbands, whereas only 451 husbands were killed by their wives.

The physical, verbal and emotional abuse and lack of control over their lives experienced by abused women significantly affect the broad determinants of health. The women's fear, anxiety and lack of control over their own lives, characteristic of the abusive situation, are, for many women, more harmful than the actual physical injuries.

To gain compliance and avert separation, many abusers threaten their wives with serious violence and consequences against their children. Stalking and harassment after separation are commonplace. Child visitation after separation, and the postseparation period as a whole, are times of elevated risk to battered women. Under such circumstances, health, problem solving, and parenting are all under serious risk and pressure. Wolfe and colleagues (1986) found that mothers residing in a shelter for battered women scored significantly higher on the General Health Questionnaire than women from nonviolent families. In addition, current residents of the women's shelter scored significantly higher on the General Health Questionnaire than former residents. Symptoms measured by the General Health Questionnaire include somatic problems, anxiety, insomnia, social dysfunction and depression. Scores for family disadvantage and negative life events were higher among women with either current or past shelter residence than among women with nonviolent marriages. In this study, family disadvantage scores covered family income, number of residence changes, reliance on social assistance and several other factors. This study suggested that, although it is very stressful in the short term, separating from an abusive partner results in improved maternal health after separation, even if family disadvantage continues after the separation and the end of shelter residence. However, as the authors pointed out, longitudinal studies are needed to confirm the findings of this cross-sectional study.

The traditional practices of the medical system in Canada and other Western countries have failed until recently to identify or respond to wife assault in an overall effective manner. For example, in one study (Tearmann Society for Battered Women 1988, cited in the report of the Canadian Panel on Violence Against Women 1993, 205, 275), 60 percent of abused women who sought medical assistance received a drug prescription, usually a tranquillizer. The prescription of psychoactive medication may worsen the coping abilities, parenting capacities and safety of a battered woman, rather than improving them. Numerous studies document the under-identification of wife assault in medical settings and the high rate of women presenting themselves in medical settings with issues related to wife assault (Ontario Medical Association Committee on Wife Assault 1986). For example, Hilberman and Munson (1978) found, in a study of 120 women referred for psychiatric treatment in North Carolina, that 60 (50 percent) of the women revealed that they were abused by their male partners but that only 4 (3 percent) had been identified as abuse victims before being referred for psychiatric attention. A rate of diagnosis of 1 in 25 cases of wife assault was found in a study at a Yale surgical emergency department (Stark et al. 1981). Although many physicians are becoming more attuned to the issue of wife assault and associated health care needs, a recent study of both rural and urban Ontario doctors indicated that, by their own estimate, these doctors believed that they identified fewer than 50 percent of such patients in their own practices (Ferris and Tudiver 1992). When consistent screening of women in medical settings is implemented, the increase in identification of woman abuse is often startling. For example, a three-question abuse screen instituted in public prenatal clinics at two U.S. sites yielded a 17 percent (1/6) prevalence rate of physical or sexual abuse during pregnancy, with 60 percent of abused women experiencing recurrent abuse (McFarlane et al. 1992, 3178). The conclusion of these authors was that "Straightforward, routine clinical assessment is recommended as essential in preventing potential trauma, interrupting existing abuse, and protecting health."

Children Who Witness Violence: Wife Assault

Another way violence affects health is through its effects on the children who witness violence. Research has recently begun to address the health and behavioral outcomes for children who live in violent homes and witness their mother being abused, as well as for children who witness or experience violence in their communities.

Children who witness wife assault at home are affected in a serious and broad-ranging manner. Harmful effects may occur in the areas of emotions, behaviour and school competence. These children tend to experience depression, anxiety, somatic complaints with no identifiable physical cause, peer conflicts, social isolation and preoccupation, noncompliance with adults, conduct disorder, conflict with the law, and a host of other behavioral problems (Fantuzzo et al. 1989; Jaffe et al. 1990). Many children experience full-blown post-traumatic stress disorder (Lehmann 1995), including symptoms of severe anxiety, chronic fear, hypervigilance, avoidance of thoughts or settings that remind them of the traumatic event, irritability and, in some cases, explosive anger. The effects on a particular child or youth will be mediated by the age of the child or youth, the child's strengths and coping style, gender, severity and frequency of violence witnessed, whether the violence has stopped, whether there is danger of its resuming, and the severity of attendant stressors, especially the effects on the mother's parenting availability as a result of her own trauma, among other factors (Fantuzzo et al. 1989; Sternberg et al. 1993; Sudermann and Jaffe 1997). Children who witness violence at home live in a war zone, and the aggressor is frequently their own father or father figure. These children often have no safe place where they can escape the violence and most often experience strong familial and social pressure to tell no one about the violence.

Until very recently, most police interventions, family physicians' and emergency physicians' mental health services, and school programs could not meet the needs of women or child witnesses of violence. Child protection legislation in many jurisdictions still makes little reference to children who witness violence as a group in need of protection (Echlin and Marshall 1995).

Children Who Witness and Experience Community Violence

Studies in large urban centres of the United States have recently begun to address the mental health and behavioral effects on children of severe, chronic community violence (Reiss et al. 1993). In the 1980s, many centres in the

United States had a marked increase in the rates of homicide, drug-related offenses and other violent crimes, greatly exceeding those of most Canadian neighbourhoods. Among children living in such settings, researchers are identifying many serious mental health and behavioral problems, including poor attachments to caregivers, aggressive behaviour, memory and concentration impairments resulting from avoidance or intrusive thoughts, and constriction in emotional responsiveness. These children's school competence and social relationships with peers are severely compromised. For many of these children, some of the most serious effects are associated with the combination of witnessing family violence in their homes and experiencing the risks of living in a violent neighbourhood (Osofsky et al. 1993).

Adult Male Victims of Violence

Men are also victims of violence. Although the murder rate for men in Canada is consistently higher than that for women, men and women suffer equally high rates of victimization overall from other criminal offenses involving violence (Canada. Statistics Canada 1992). However, the patterns of offenses, perpetrators and location of offenses are very different for men and women. Men perpetrate more than 90 percent of violent crimes. Women tend to be victimized in their own homes and by men they know or are acquainted with (husband, common-law partner, boyfriend, date or other family members and acquaintances), while men are much more likely to be victims of violence in public places. While 43 percent of female assault victims are attacked by a current or estranged male partner, only 3 percent of male assault victims are attacked by current or estranged female partners. Eighty-four percent of those accused of killing men in 1992 were men, and 96 percent of those accused of killing women were men.

Dating Violence

Studies of dating and early relationship violence repeatedly show that young women are overwhelmingly the victims in these forms of violence. For example, a study of high school students in grades 9–13 found that of students who were dating, 21.4 percent of females experienced physical violence and 23.3 percent experienced sexual violence in a dating relationship. The corresponding figures for male students were much lower, at 7.2 and 3.3 percent (Sudermann and Jaffe 1993). Studies at the university and college levels have consistently found high rates of violence against women in dating and acquaintance situations (Koss et al. 1987; DeKeseredy and Kelly 1993). Other studies have found that violence during courtship and marriage frightens women much more than it does men, and that the greater potential for men to injure women, as a result of men's greater strength, size, and social power and control, must be taken into account in addressing gender differences in the effects of violence (Mahlstedt et al. 1993; O'Leary et al. 1994).

Violence in Schools

Many people in Canada, as well as in the United States and Europe, are now concerned about violence in schools as well as in communities. Numerous strategies for addressing school-based violence are being developed across Canada (McDougall 1993). Research on the nature and prevalence of school-based violence is still in the early stages, and few reliable statistics are available in Canada, as many incidents are never reported or recorded. A study by Ryan and colleagues (1993) in two Ontario schools showed that students are concerned about violence at school. However, no comparable data from past years are available to compare with the current concerns and experiences of students.

Large-scale studies in Norway by Olweus (1992, 1993) indicated that about 15 percent of students in that country are involved in school violence, either as bullies or as victims of bullying. Olweus found that boys at every age studied were more likely to become bullies than girls (Olweus 1993). Olweus refers to data from Sweden and Britain that indicate similar or greater rates of bully-victim problems. Pepler and Craig (1995) found similar rates of bully-victim problems in a sample of Toronto elementary schools. Using video and audiotaped observation of elementary school playgrounds during recess, Pepler and colleagues (1993) found a disturbing rate of peer-to-peer violence among both boys and girls. Also interesting and disturbing was her finding that even students who appeared well adjusted and non-violent in class frequently behaved aggressively in the school playground. Like Olweus, Pepler found that, while both boys and girls engaged in both physical and verbal bullying, boys were more likely to engage in physical bullying and girls were more likely to use subtle verbal and emotional (indirect) bullying.

Primary Prevention

Given the high prevalence of violence and the negative health effects of both violence and witnessing violence, prevention often receives a high priority for dealing with this issue. As our knowledge about the causes of violence grows, more effective primary prevention and early intervention against violence are becoming possible. Violence prevention efforts can encompass a great variety of primary, secondary and tertiary prevention activities, but the present paper will survey school-based primary prevention strategies delivered on a whole school level, and secondary prevention for children and adolescents who have witnessed violence at home. Primary prevention strategies delivered in a very broad-based manner have several advantages. These strategies reach a maximum number of students and teachers, with the result that new attitudes and skills can be widely disseminated. They are nonstigmatizing, that is, no children need be singled out or labelled as "problem" children to deliver the service. Also, by targeting the whole school, the strategy affects school climate and the attitudes and behaviour of those who tend to be bystanders or passive supporters of violence, as well as students who are already violent or are at risk of becoming violent. Broad school-based strategies for prevention of violence also tend to be cost effective because they are often delivered in the context of routine school programs with regular staff and routine educational opportunities. Students do not need to withdraw from regular school activities if violence prevention is incorporated into regular school activities.

Price and colleagues (1989) surveyed primary prevention programs in an effort to identify model programs for the American Psychological Association Task Force on Promotion, Prevention, and Intervention. They identified several characteristics associated with successful programs. First, these programs tended to rely on a good understanding of the problems and risks encountered by the participants. Second, these programs were designed to have a long-term impact, changing the life trajectories of the participants at a transition point in their lives. Third, the successful programs were focused in their objectives and employed evaluation strategies. Finally, these programs used and strengthened natural supports in the participants' environments and taught new coping skills.

One important issue with broad-based violence prevention strategies, as with other kinds of broad-based health promotion and illness prevention strategies, has been that of proving the effectiveness of outcomes, especially since the ultimate goals of primary prevention programs often pertain to long-term objectives ranging over the life span of the participants. The violence prevention programs discussed in the following section have achieved success in implementation and have achieved positive outcomes in short-term evaluation studies. Comprehensive, long-term evaluation of outcomes of primary prevention programs such as these is difficult to achieve because of the large number of subjects, the hidden nature of much interpersonal violence, and the presence of many other factors in the social environment that affect violence and victimization rates. Nevertheless, because of the relatively low cost and broad-scale impact of these programs, those with positive short-term evaluation results are well worth considering while we wait for long-term evaluations.

SUCCESS STORIES IN THE PREVENTION OF VIOLENCE AGAINST WOMEN AND OTHER FORMS OF VIOLENCE

Primary Prevention Programs

ASAP: A School-Based Antiviolence Program

Description of the program – The approach taken in A School-Based Anti-violence Program (ASAP) was developed by the London Family Court Clinic, together with London, Ontario, educators and community members as a school-based violence prevention program with a special focus on gender issues in violence and violence in intimate relationships. An extensive implementation manual is available (Sudermann et al. 1993, 1996). The three main characteristics of ASAP are (1) educator and staff development and awareness; (2) community involvement; and (3) student programs. Special violence awareness events, curriculum integration of violence awareness, prosocial skills development, and promotion of attitudes favouring nonviolence are emphasized. Central to the approach is the in-volvement of school-based committees of educators, parents, students and community members in planning the implementation of the program.

Values underlying the project – ASAP is based on recognition of gender issues in violence and on inclusion of the issues of family violence, woman abuse, dating violence and sexual harassment as important elements in fundamental violence prevention. Naming violence against women and girls is advocated in the program, as opposed to silence and omission of gender issues in understanding violence. Violence is seen as connected to issues of power sharing, equity of all kinds, and a commitment to respect for diversity in the community and school. The central viewpoint of ASAP is that most violent acts arise from inappropriate attempts to gain power and control. ASAP promotes power sharing, respect for others, and teaching of prosocial skills in conflict resolution and social relations as an alternative to violence.

Another important value of ASAP is the need to place the responsibility for and the decision making around violence prevention with the commu-nity, parents and students, as well as with educators. Violence is seen as a community and societal issue, and the program is designed to involve community members, parents, students and educators in the school-based prevention of violence.

Reasons for the initiative – ASAP began as part of a community-based model for addressing violence against women. As policing initiatives and services for women in abusive relationships moved toward community coordination, a need for primary prevention of violence against women became apparent. As the project developed, it also became apparent that many strategies and values related to prevention of wife assault and dating violence resembled those of general violence prevention. Initiatives such as peer mediation, social skills training and conflict resolution training, problems such as bullying, and equity issues such as gender equity and cultural equity were incorporated into the program.

Actors-participants – ASAP was developed with the help of the London Family Court Clinic, together with three area school boards and supportive community agencies, which took part especially as the local front-line women's services in cases of wife assault. ASAP used a model that includes empowering teachers, school administrators, students, parents and community agencies to take ownership of the programs and develop new variations and adaptations suited to their schools. In this way, the programs continue after the initial sponsors are no longer involved. Planning the interventions is the responsibility of school committees, supported by community agencies. School committees may include students and parents as well as teachers and administrators. Community agencies provide volunteer speakers and discussion leaders.

Parent-teacher organizations, such as the Home and School Association, have been most supportive. Teachers' associations, particularly the Ontario Women Teachers' Federation, have also been involved. Initial support for evaluation of ASAP initiatives came from the Ontario Ministry of Community and Social Services and the Ontario Ministry of Education (now Education and Training).

ASAP has been supported by local media, particularly the *London Free Press*, with publicity for positive initiatives for violence prevention developed over the years and issues of violence against women. The Ontario Ministry of Education and Training has sponsored several conferences for educators and community members in southwestern Ontario, and these conferences promoted networking and implementation of violence prevention strategies. The federal government, through Health Canada (then Health and Welfare Canada), supported a crucial stage in the development of ASAP when it suggested disseminating ASAP ideas and practical procedures by producing a manual and a video, and organizing 10 national conferences. Dissemination conferences were hosted by various national, provincial and local organizations at national sites, and community organizations, teachers and parents were invited to the conferences.

The development of the intervention: secondary level –The goals of the ASAP violence prevention program were to provide knowledge about the incidence and causes of family and dating violence, to shape more prosocial attitudes in these areas, to offer knowledge of community agency resources for those currently affected by the problem, and to generate ideas from students about how they could mitigate the effects of such problems. Physical, sexual and verbal abuse were all targeted issues, and the roles of violence in the media and in sports in perpetuating acceptance of violence were also addressed.

The initial phases of ASAP saw the development of an administration-based planning committee (including representatives from the London Board of Education, the London Family Court Clinic, and elementary and secondary school officials) and school-based planning committees (comprising keen teachers, students and administrators), as well as several information presentations and workshops for people interested in or affected by the high school intervention program. Participants in presentations or workshops in the initial implementation included: all principals in London, staff delegates from every elementary and secondary school in London, all staff at each of the high schools receiving the program, the London Home and School Association, parents of students at the five target high schools and, finally, community resource personnel, who participated in the workshops as speakers and discussion group facilitators.

Special violence awareness events were held at each area high school, usually including a theatrical production related to violence in relationships, followed by in-class discussions, with the help of volunteer discussion leaders, many from community agencies. During discussions, students developed school-based action plans for the prevention of violence. School-based counselling and referral services were made available on site at the time of the program for students who made personal disclosures or appeared distressed.

Development of elementary school programs – In the last 3 or 4 years, ASAP has grown most in the elementary schools. Following some conferences held as part of advanced professional development sessions at the Board of Education for the city of London, existing, but isolated, initiatives related to violence prevention in elementary schools became more coordinated and activated. The programs that focused on violence in relationships, wife assault and sexual harassment became more coordinated and integrated with general violence prevention and equity initiatives such as peer mediation, peer counselling and support, antibullying programs, and gender and cultural equity programs. Today, the model in many London-area elementary schools, both those of the Board of Education of the city of London and those of the London and Middlesex separate school board, is to hold an annual violence prevention week or month, accompanied by a yearlong integration of related antiviolence, social skills and curriculum initiatives.

Evaluation of the effectiveness of the ASAP violence prevention program – Two large-scale evaluations of ASAP violence prevention initiatives conducted in schools in London, Ontario, have been undertaken and are described here. Both of these evaluations focused on the effects of special violence awareness events on student knowledge, beliefs and behavioral intentions with regard to violence, particularly violence in relationships.

The first study (Jaffe et al. 1992) evaluated the impact of violence prevention events at four high schools, which focused on wife assault and dating violence. Two schools employed a full-day intervention, and two schools employed a half-day intervention, both of which followed the pattern described previously.

A random sample of students, stratified by grade and academic level, was selected from each of four high schools. A total of 737 students completed the evaluation surveys. A 48-item questionnaire, the London Family Court Clinic Questionnaire on Violence in Intimate Relationships, was constructed for the evaluation, as no suitable instruments could be identified in the literature. This questionnaire was designed to tap knowledge about wife assault, beliefs and attitudes about violence in marital and dating relationships, and behavioral intentions to intervene in dating violence. Questionnaires were administered 1 week before the intervention, about 1 week after the intervention and, at two schools, also at 6 weeks after the intervention.

Results indicated significant changes in the desired direction for female students on 11 of the 48 items and no changes in the undesired direction, with stability of these positive changes found at delayed follow-up. Knowledge, attitudes and behavioral intentions all showed areas of positive change for females. Eight of 48 items showed significant change among males in the positive direction, including changes in knowledge, attitudes and behavioral intentions. However, seven of the attitude items and one behavioral intention item showed change in the undesired direction among males, with the majority of these negative changes relating to attitudes about dating violence.

Students showed significant and consistent differences in attitudes toward violence in intimate relationships, with females having more positive attitudes than males, both at pre- and postintervention. Also, more females than males were aware of violence in their own or a peer's dating relationships (60.5 percent of females versus 47.5 percent of males). These findings indicated that females may be more sensitive to issues of violence in relationships and more supportive of women's equality in intimate relationships. The results also indicated that females benefitted more than males from the intervention and that, in particular, females showed more positive attitude changes following the intervention. This study, together with reports from the classroom, suggested that future directions for intervention might include adaptations to reduce male defensiveness and backlash. The study also showed that both the knowledge and attitudes of students can be positively affected by a relatively brief intervention.

A second evaluation of an intervention program for violence in intimate relationships was completed in two high schools from different Ontario school boards (Sudermann and Jaffe 1993). These two schools, one from the public school board and one from the separate school board in London, Ontario, cooperated in planning a half-day program on preventing dating violence with a high level of student input in planning and organizing the events. The student planning committees decided to make dating violence prevention the focus of the intervention. Peer support groups from each school, together with school administrators, presented separate programs for the junior grades (grades 9 and 10) and senior grades (grades 11 to OAC [Grade 13]). The junior group viewed a video on dating violence prevention and saw a play by a student drama group. Classroom discussion followed. Senior students attended their choice of two workshops from those offered by 22 community presenters on topics related to preventing violence in relationships.

All students at each school completed a revised 32-item version of the London Family Court Clinic Questionnaire on Violence in Intimate Relationships before and after the intervention. In the postintervention test, students also wrote comments and suggestions about the program. The total sample comprised 1,547 students: 672 in grades 9 and 10 and 875 in grades 11–13. Of these, 1,112 were present at the pretest, intervention and posttest stages, and this smaller sample was retained for analysis, yielding 488 in grades 9 and 10 and 624 in grades 11–13.

For students in grades 9 and 10, significant positive changes in knowledge, attitude and behavioral intentions occurred for both females and males. Results for females showed positive changes on 8 of 29 items, and results for males showed positive changes on 7 of 29 items. Among males, only one item showed significant change in the undesired direction ("poverty causes family violence"). This question was not a specific target of the intervention, which was focused on dating violence, rather than family violence.

For students in grades 11–13, positive changes occurred on 7 of 29 items among females and on 2 of 29 items among males. Changes in the undesired direction occurred on one attitude item among males and on a different attitude item among females in grades 11–13. These were again family violence items, which were not emphasized in the dating violence intervention. For both junior and senior students, marked gender differences in attitudes were found, with females having more positive attitudes at pre- and postintervention.

Also of considerable interest were the results of three questions addressing the experience of violence in dating relationships. Females reported experiencing considerable verbal, physical and sexual abuse in dating relationships. Of 44.3 percent females who indicated that they were currently dating, 57.3 percent reported experiencing verbal abuse in a dating relationship; 23.3 percent, sexual abuse; and 21.4 percent, physical abuse. The comparable percentages for boys were 32.6 percent for verbal abuse, 3.3 percent for sexual abuse and 7.2 percent for physical abuse. Student comments about the intervention were overwhelmingly positive and supported the relevance of the topic for adolescents.

Overall, the results from this study showed positive results for the intervention for the male and female junior students and positive results for the female senior students. Senior male students did not respond as positively. This may be because some older male students may already be entrenched in dating violence patterns, so that the program caused them to feel defensive and resistant. Another explanation may be that the videoplay format was more effective for males than the elective workshop format employed with the older students.

A future direction suggested by this study would be to disentangle the confounding of age and type of intervention in research designs. It also seems well worth studying the benefit of intervention with younger, pre-dating males, possibly in grades 7 and 8.

ASAP has been evaluated less at the elementary level. Some preliminary evaluations with students in grades 4–6 indicate that significant gains in attitudes, knowledge and beliefs occur after an elementary violence prevention week (Sudermann and Watson 1993).

Many aspects of the ASAP violence prevention program still require evaluation. Areas requiring attention are: the effect of the intervention on actual student behaviour—perpetrating different forms of dating violence, avoiding or ending violent relationships, using verbal, physical and sexual violence in dating relationships, using violence in peer relationships, and engaging in sexual harassment and verbal abuse at school and in peer relationships—and the effect on students' families of the interventions that concern witnessing family violence. With regard to the effect of the interventions on students' families, the local women's shelter gave feedback indicating that referrals and admissions to the shelter increased during the weeks immediately following violence prevention events at schools. Long-term follow-up of the effects of the violence awareness events, as well as evaluation of subsequent curriculum integration of violence prevention material, is also needed. Many schools in the London, Ontario, area now have annual or ongoing violence prevention initiatives, and the cumulative effect of these initiatives should be evaluated.

Analysis of what made the program successful – An important aspect of ASAP is that it directly addresses issues of violence against women as well as the societal influences, such as media violence and sexism, that support violence. The program directly links to issues of equity, diversity, and power and control. In contrast, many other violence prevention approaches and materials we have encountered seem to focus more narrowly on social skills or anger management at the individual level, without addressing the broader social issues that are the substrate of violence. Also, ASAP has implementation guidelines that give strategies for involving and transferring control over the program to schools, parents and communities. The program is flexible and multifaceted, and uses a manual that contains extensive information on integrating resources such as videos, books and curricula on a wide range of topics that contribute to violence prevention. Violence prevention probably requires such a flexible, comprehensive promotion program, since violence is a complex, multidetermined phenomenon.

Funding–The ASAP intervention is essentially low cost because it builds on existing educational services and community organizations. To develop the ASAP manual and video and make the evaluations described previously, support was provided by the federal government (Health Canada), as well as the Ontario ministries of Education and Training, and Community and Social Services. Additional support in developing and disseminating the program has come from foundations (the Richard and Jean Ivey Foundation and the Donner Canadian Foundation) and corporations (the Ontario Hydro Corporate Citizenship Fund and the *London Free Press*).

To implement ASAP in an area without such a program, the cash outlay for start-up would be very small—that is, for the purchase of an ASAP manual. The costs associated with the commitment and time of teachers, administrators, community agency personnel, other community members and parents could be redirected from existing programs or offered as volunteer service.

Replicability of the initiative: cross-Canada indicators – ASAP is being implemented in many sites across Canada. For example, Calgary, Alberta is currently engaged in a citywide school-based implementation aided by municipal support. Two sites have conducted evaluations of their implementations.

To conduct a partial replication of ASAP in several Ontario high schools, Hilton and colleagues (1994) organized several special violence awareness events resembling ASAP events for high school students. However, it is unclear how much preparatory work, such as teachers' professional development and community-support development, was done before the awareness events were implemented. The content of the awareness events for students focused less on issues of violence against women than on general violence issues. This apparently fitted better with the comfort level of teachers, which may reflect a need for professional development of teachers before students' events take place. Z. Hilton (personal communication) reported that the evaluation, a pre-post design employing questionnaires, indicated a disappointingly small positive change in student attitudes after the intervention. However, this evaluation also indicated no backlash effect.

Both the initial ASAP evaluation studies with high school students (Jaffe et al. 1992; Sudermann and Jaffe 1993) found that, when the intervention specifically targets violence against women, some males, usually a small group, resent the message and respond negatively on the questionnaire. Their responses seem to move in a direction opposite to that intended in the intervention. Although ASAP specifically implies that most males do not support violence, a backlash with regard to attitudes about violence against women is likely to accompany the initial stages of successful ASAP interventions. If the issues of gender equity and male roles in violence are not presented, no backlash will arise.

A replication and evaluation done in a Saskatchewan elementary school yielded good implementation and positive results (Tenold-Phillips 1995). This implementation at the elementary level included the use of all of the elements recommended in ASAP, including extensive in-service training for teachers, community input and evaluation. Prosocial skills training, peer mediation and conflict resolution were implemented with students. A pull-out program for high-risk students was added. Specific results of the questionnaire evaluation were not available at the time of writing, but recommendations of the summary report indicated that the implementation was considered to have had positive effects on both student behaviour and the schoolwide teaching and learning climate. Important potential initial barriers overcome included the issues of insufficient teacher and class time, and teachers' commitment. The extensive in-service training for teachers and community meetings were seen as central to the success of the program in the face of these obstacles.

The Olweus Norwegian Antibullying Program

Description of the program –The Norwegian Antibullying Program, led by Dr. Dan Olweus, is becoming widely recognized as a model for nation-wide implementation of school-based violence prevention. This program, which focuses on peer-to-peer bullying that occurs at school, is associated with a long-term research program on the dynamics of bullying and the characteristics of bullies and victims. The program institutes measures in schools to inform teachers and parents about bullying, and encourages actions at the school, classroom and individual levels to reduce bullying and help victims. These actions include: using teachers' professional development, holding meetings with parents' groups, improving playground supervision, ensuring more consistent (but nonaggressive, noncorporal) consequences for bullying behaviour, talking individually with bullies and victims, involving the parents of bullies and of victims immediately after incidents, involving students in formulating classroom rules against bullying, and teaching students not to tolerate bullying and to support and include victims in social groups. The program has achieved national implementation in Norway and has been shown, in well-conducted research studies, to reduce bullying by about 50 percent. Dr. Olweus' work spans a considerable period and has enjoyed comprehensive support from governments and education systems in Norway.

Reasons for the initiative –The Norwegian Antibullying Program was prompted by a cluster of three teen suicides related to bullying at school. These tragic events galvanized public opinion to support a national anti-bullying initiative in schools. A 1983 large-scale survey of students, at the start of the initiative, revealed a 15 percent prevalence rate for bully-victim problems among students in Norwegian comprehensive schools, or

84,000 cases of students who were either victims or bullies. These findings and related research about the impact of bullying on victims and on the long-term outcomes for bullies further mobilized support for the project.

Values underlying the project – Olweus (1992, 3) indicated that one of the primary values underlying the project is that "bully-victim problems... concern some of our fundamental democratic rights. Every individual should have the right to be spared oppression and repeated, intentional humiliation, in school as in society at large." In addition, the program views bullying as intentionally antisocial behaviour in which the bully chooses to break social norms of behaviour to gain pleasure or other rewards. Olweus rejected a treatment or skills deficit model for understanding antisocial behaviour. Rather, he emphasized that the antibullying program comprehensively strengthens sanctions against bullying behaviour and strengthens social norms in favour of inclusive, prosocial behaviour.

Actors-participants – The antibullying program is designed to involve and affect the school as a system, including not only students but also teachers and parents. The program is also intended to affect the school's climate and social norms. As mentioned previously, the antibullying program was implemented on a national scale right from the beginning, through all primary and junior high schools in the country. This was a result of leadership from national education authorities. Dr. Olweus and colleagues have also played a key role in providing research information and evaluation that has shaped the program, highlighted the issue of bullying for the public, and measured and demonstrated the program's effectiveness.

The development of the intervention – The initial development of the program was based on an analysis of bully and victim characteristics. Olweus had shown in his previous research that bullies were generally confident and, if they were boys, they tended to be physically stronger than others their age. No evidence of underlying self-esteem or anxiety problems was found for bullies. They tend to come from family settings where violence was condoned or modelled and there were low levels of parental supervision and involvement. Victims were found to be anxious and socially isolated, to lack confidence in their abilities, and to have a tendency not to respond assertively to aggression.

Based on these findings, the intervention was designed to mobilize firmer, more consistent responses to bullying behaviour while supporting victims and encouraging a school climate in which "neutral" students, who are involved only as bystanders or witnesses, do not tolerate bullying.

After considerable observation and evaluation of the program, Olweus considered the following measures crucial to the effectiveness of the antibullying program (Olweus 1993):

1. awareness and involvement of adults with regard to bully-victim problems;

2. a survey of bully-victim problems at the start of the implementation;
3. a school conference day devoted to bully-victim problems;
4. closer adult supervision during recess and lunch hour;
5. consistent, immediate consequences for aggressive behaviour of students;
6. generous praise for prosocial, helpful behaviour of students;
7. specific class rules against bullying;
8. class meetings to discuss bullying;
9. serious individual talks with bullies and victims;
10. serious talks with parents of bullies and victims; and
11. a meeting of the school parent-teacher (home and school) organization on bullying.

The measures implemented first in the national program included provision of written material for all teachers and parents on bullying and what could be done about it through the program. Low-cost videos were also made available for rent or purchase to promote the awareness component of the program.

Evaluation – Extensive, large-scale evaluation is a noteworthy feature of this program. In addition to a nationwide survey on bullying problems conducted in 700 schools at the start of the intervention in 1983 to establish the preintervention incidence of the problem, intensive evaluation has been conducted with students from 42 schools in Bergen, Norway. The Bergen schools received feedback on their preintervention rates of bullying as part of a bullying awareness intervention. Thereafter, evaluation through the same student self-report questionnaire was repeated annually for 3 years. The study included no untreated control group, as the intervention began simultaneously in all schools across the country. Cohorts were used for comparison with baseline data as they advanced through the grade levels annually. Thus, for example, grade five students' scores after 1 year of intervention were compared with the previous year's grade five students, who had no intervention at that time. To guard against differential attrition by individuals who were at high risk for bullying, only students for whom data were available for each of the three evaluation times were employed in the analyses. However, as it turned out, this did not affect the outcome data.

The results showed large decreases in reports of bullying, both of the students themselves and of others they observed. Self-reported victimization was reduced by 50 percent over the 3-year period, and similar reductions occurred in reports of observed bullying of others. Self-reports of engaging in bullying behaviour declined similarly. Olweus also reported a reduction in antisocial behaviour, such as vandalism, and a marked improvement in social climate at schools. Teachers reported more positive social relationships among students, improved order and discipline, and better attitudes on the part of students toward schoolwork. Acceptance and support of the program by teachers was very good, even though it involved more work for them in some ways. For example, the program introduced higher expectations of teachers for supervision of the schoolyard and hallways, and more contacts between teachers and parents regarding individual bullying incidents. Nevertheless, teachers viewed the program as realistic and beneficial.

Another interesting finding from this research was that classes with better implementation of the program (classes where more components of the program were in place) showed more reduction in bullying. Olweus reported a correlation of $r = 0.51$ between implementation level and reduction in bullying. He also pointed out that a nationwide preintervention incidence rate of 84,000 cases of bullying per annum means that a 50 percent reduction indicates at least 40,000 fewer bullying incidents.

Funding – The detailed costs for this program are not known. Some of the initial direct costs included the provision of the written material to teachers and parents. Schools covered much of the personnel and administration costs. Evaluation costs were also incurred in the large-scale initial survey and in the subsequent Bergen study.

Replicability – Considerable international interest has been shown in the Norwegian Antibullying Program, and implementation is being tried in several other countries, including the United Kingdom, Sweden and Canada. Evaluation results from these replications are also being prepared. An implementation study in several schools in the Toronto Board of Education was conducted by Pepler, Craig, Ziegler and Charach (1994). This study found less dramatic results than Olweus's evaluation of the Norwegian program. A major difference in the two programs was that the Norwegian program began on a national scale immediately, whereas the Toronto study involved only a few schools in one board of education.

Other Evaluated Prevention Programs

Another violence prevention program that has been evaluated was the Minnesota Coalition for Battered Women School Curriculum Project (Jones 1987). This program consisted of 5 to 6 days intervention for students in grades 7–12 targeting both attitudes and knowledge about wife assault and dating violence. Results showed positive changes in knowledge but no attitude changes. This result may reflect the relatively brief, five-item assessment measure employed. The documentation for this program evaluation is not readily available, as even the original authors are now having difficulty locating their paper on the evaluation.

Another study of a school-based violence prevention program was recently done in Florida, and the results will soon be published (M. MacGowan, personal communication). In this study, middle school students (like junior high school students) in four schools participated in a brief violence prevention initiative. In one school, a formal evaluation was conducted. In this school, an experiment was conducted with treatment and control groups. Attitudes and knowledge of students were assessed before the intervention, immediately after the intervention and 3 weeks after the intervention. Students at the school that participated in the formal evaluation received one full week of violence prevention programming. The main focus of the intervention was bullying, with some focus on dating violence issues. We are awaiting a more detailed description of this intervention, which should be available soon. The results indicated a significant effect of the intervention, some of which was seen at a 3-week follow-up (M. MacGowan, personal communication). The results showed a significant gender x time interaction, with the attitudes of boys improving less than those of girls, and with boys maintaining their gains less well than girls at the 3-week follow-up.

Another formal evaluation of a brief violence prevention effort was done by Mahlstedt and colleagues (1993). These investigators conducted a dating violence intervention with 331 college students from introductory psychology classes. The design included a treatment condition that focused on dating violence prevention from a feminist perspective and a control condition that focused on education about stages in a relationship. Participants received 2 hours of intervention, including presentation of information and small group discussion. Attitudes and knowledge were assessed immediately after the intervention and 3 weeks after the intervention. The results showed a significant gender effect, with females having more positive attitudes and beliefs in the absence of any intervention, as assessed from comparison group data. In this study, males improved more than females in the period following the intervention, but they also lost more of their gains at the 3-week follow-up.

Another program related to violence prevention being widely implemented is the Second Step Social Skills Curriculum (Committee for Children 1992). Second Step consists of materials and procedures to teach social skills such as perspective taking and empathy, understanding feelings, communicating effectively in social situations with peers, problem solving and impulse control. Teaching is done through direct classroom instruction, using specific materials and lesson plans provided with the curriculum. Programs are now available for three age levels—preschool, junior elementary and senior elementary—and a program for parents has recently been introduced. The program is designed to decrease aggressive behaviour through improving social skills. Second Step contains ideas for evaluation by program users, but the techniques suggested are rather complicated and difficult to implement. Some small-scale initial evaluation studies yielded mixed results with regard to behaviour changes among children, but indicated very high teacher regard for the potential of the curriculum (Larson 1994).

One program that integrates prevention of several types of abuse is the Response by Schools to Violence Prevention (R.S.V.P.) Program (1993), developed in Hamilton-Wentworth, Ontario by the Community Child Abuse Council of Hamilton-Wentworth. This set of manuals and resource books for educators addresses child, woman and elder abuse, and other related topics. It is designed to be used in schools. As far as we know, no formal evaluation of this program is available.

Conclusions from This Review of Violence Prevention Programs

It is interesting to note that Olweus' antibullying program has many aspects in common with the ASAP violence prevention program. Similar measures have been found to be effective in implementing both programs, including a coordinated, systemwide approach and the use of teachers' professional development, involvement of parents, evaluation, and school planning committees. One difference between ASAP and the Olweus program is that the latter does not address violence against women, sexual harassment or gender differences in bullying. Olweus' own research on incidence and prevalence of bullying indicates large gender differences in this behaviour, with boys being more likely to be bullies of both male and female victims. In his research he finds that girls also bully, but they do so less often than boys and use less physical bullying. Girls are more likely than boys to use exclusion from the social group as a form of bullying.

As can be seen from the above review of the literature, very few researchers have systematically studied preventive interventions in wife assault, dating violence or general violence. Where evaluations have been done, the one constant is a significant role of gender in the reactions and needs of the participants. Future research should address the reasons for this effect. Also, evaluations should extend beyond brief, one-time interventions to the study of large-scale, long-duration interventions such as ASAP.

Secondary Prevention Programs

In addition to primary prevention, secondary prevention programs are required to address the needs of children and youth who have witnessed violence in their family. As outlined in the literature review, children who witness wife assault are recognized as a high-risk group in terms of emotional and behavioral adjustment. Boys are at particularly high risk of repeating violent behaviour toward women learned by observing their fathers (Jaffe et al. 1990). Among both boys and girls, subtle messages about the acceptability of violence as a solution to interpersonal conflict are absorbed when children witness wife assault and other forms of domestic violence. Specific interventions for this group of high-risk children and adolescents can be viewed as an effective secondary prevention initiative because of the potential to prevent violence in these children's relationships.

Secondary prevention or early interventions for this group are only now emerging, and few have been evaluated in any depth. One of the more detailed programs is outlined in Peled and Edleson (1995). In analyzing the important ingredients of this program, Peled and Edleson (1995) suggested interrelated goals, such as the following:

- breaking the secret of the violence in the family by learning how to share the experience, defining the violence, and understanding the range of feelings evoked;
- learning to protect oneself by developing safety-planning skills and assertive conflict resolution skills;
- ensuring a positive experience in the group by creating a safe, structured, enriching program; and
- strengthening self-esteem by developing support from other group members and validating children's thoughts and feelings.

Peled and Edleson (1995) assessed the impact of these groups with a qualitative evaluation and reported that the four main goals of the groups can be achieved in 10 sessions, according to assessments by participants and group leaders. However, Peled and Edleson emphasize that these children are not "fixed" in the 10 sessions. The children will continue to work through and experience the aftereffects of witnessing violence at home.

Another group program, which addresses the needs of children and adolescents who witness violence in London, Ontario, was recently evaluated with positive results (Marshall et al. 1995). The groups in this program also ran for 10 sessions and included an experienced group coordinator-leader, together with volunteers from community agencies. The groups were sponsored by a child protection agency and a children's mental health centre, and clients either referred themselves or were referred through these agencies. Children participated in mixed-gender groups for younger children, older children and teens. The goals of the groups included the following:

- increasing the participants' adaptive functioning and mitigating the effects of social-behavioral problems resulting from witnessing violence;
- creating change sufficient to prevent violence in the children's future relationships; and
- ensuring that the children learn skills to keep themselves safe during recurrences of violence in their family environment.

The groups were evaluated through a questionnaire especially con-structed to reflect the goals of the groups, which was administered to the children and adolescents before and immediately after they participated in the groups. As well, parent and child participants completed questionnaires to assess their satisfaction with and perceptions of the groups. Thirty-one children aged 7–15 years participated in this initial study, with a mean age of 11.6 years. About half of the participants were girls, and the other half were boys. Results indicated that children improved in their ability to identify abusive actions and that, at posttest, children had learned safer strategies for dealing with abusive episodes at home. For example, far fewer children indicated that they would try to intervene directly if they witnessed violence between their parents again, and children had a greater repertoire of help-seeking skills, such as calling police, calling the emergency number or seeking help from neighbours, friends or other adults. At posttest, fewer children condoned any kind of violence, including peer-to-peer violence. Children also improved in their knowledge of nonviolent conflict resolution skills. At posttest, fewer children believed that they were the cause of their parents' fights. Client satisfaction with the groups was high in both children and mothers.

The long-term impact of groups such as these in preventing violence and improving the emotional adjustment of the children should be assessed. As Peled and Edleson have pointed out, children need more than a 10-week program to deal with the experience of witnessing violence. Nevertheless, these groups showed positive results in the initial evaluations and represent some of the first systematic community efforts to address secondary prevention of violence in relationships. These groups clearly represent an important secondary prevention technique for targeting a high-risk population.

INTERESTS AT STAKE IN PROMOTING OR IMPEDING CHANGE

Many groups and interests support violence prevention efforts. These groups include:
- feminist women's advocacy organizations, women's shelters and related community organizations;
- some provincial and national teachers' professional associations;
- some health care providers;
- individuals and organizations concerned with gender equity and violence against women;
- children's mental health agencies that are aware of the effects on children of witnessing violence;
- victims' rights organizations; and
- men's organizations dedicated to eliminating violence against women.

Many individuals and organizations, once they are aware of the scope of violence against women and the effects on children of witnessing violence, support school-based violence prevention. Other groups and individuals also support the general concept of reducing violence through prevention at schools, but need to be convinced that violence against women and related issues of gender equity and racial or cultural equity are topics that require emphasis.

Some groups resist initiatives promoting violence prevention, and these may include:
- educators and policymakers who resist values-based education in schools;
- educators and health care providers opposed to working toward gender equity and cultural or racial equity and tolerance;
- those who believe that education should focus narrowly on specific skills, without education for citizenship and broader life success;

- those who benefit from the status quo and from denying that violence against women is a problem society should correct;
- those who generally resist change in education and social values; and
- those who profit from portraying violence on television and in videos, video games, music and other media.

The major challenge faced by governments and communities in ending violence is to find ways for groups to collaborate better in their efforts. All involved parties need to recognize common interests, such as:

1. Violence is violence, whether it happens at the hands of family members or strangers. Homes must take priority for safety, as must the streets.
2. Certain community members are more vulnerable and likely to be victimized than others.
3. Certain victims are less likely to seek help from the police or any outside intervention than others.
4. Violence is a major health issue with significant economic consequences.
5. Proactive responses (e.g., police and correctional services) are more expensive than primary prevention.
6. Violence is learned behaviour that is condoned and glorified by many exponents of societal attitudes and behaviour, such as the entertainment industry.
7. Prevention efforts must involve children and adolescents, as they are future perpetrators and victims (e.g., the initiatives of the National Crime Prevention Council).
8. No single agency (e.g., police or shelter) can end violence by itself. Only a collaborative approach involving the whole community has any potential for success.

POLICY IMPLICATIONS

The overall conclusions from our review of the literature and success stories stress the importance of linking efforts to reduce violence in general with efforts to reduce violence against women. The vast majority of violence happens within families and intimate relationships. The childhood history of violent offenders indicates that the violence perpetrated by strangers is clearly linked to violence in the home.

The major policy implications of this study relate to governments and communities and their efforts to develop environments conducive to primary and secondary prevention. The implications for these two types of prevention will be addressed in turn.

Policy Implications for Primary Prevention

Governments and communities need to create a strong belief in zero tolerance of violence and strong public support for nonviolence. Zero tolerance has to include all aspects of society, including schools, parenting, inter-personal conflict resolution, and the media and entertainment industries. As public awareness, knowledge and attitudes about the causes of violence develop, specific primary prevention programs and interventions against violence in all its forms will be much more successful. Ultimately, the positive effects of such broad-based changes in public attitudes and practices regarding violence would be dramatic. Alternatively, if we fail to encourage zero tolerance of violence and establish policies to prevent violence, we may face seriously deteriorating social conditions and health, which are now evident in many communities and neighbourhoods in the United States.

One area in need of immediate attention is that of the media and entertainment industries. We live in a culture that expresses serious concern about violence but is prepared to accept violence as a form of entertainment. This entertainment surrounds us in sport, television, video games, movies and advertising. Although the Canadian Radio Television and Tele-communications Commission took some small steps in the right direction by approving the V-chip technology to help parents control the extent of the violence their children are exposed to on television, a more active and comprehensive campaign is needed. We need to address media violence used to entertain all members of our society (and to make profits), not just offer alternatives only a minority of informed and concerned parents will use. We need broad-based cultural change and public education about the negative effects of media violence, together with incentives for the production of high-quality, nonviolent entertainment that promotes prosocial values and skills. The ever-increasing, broad-based social and cultural impact of the media is difficult to overestimate. Consideration should be given the question of whether the community should have an input into the content of the media, rather than having the media controlled by a few corporations and powerful individuals.

We suggest that all levels of government engage in an active media campaign against violence as a form of entertainment. Although we spend millions of dollars advertising the dangers of smoking, labelling cigarette packages and highlighting the links between smoking and cancer, we do little to point out that the strength of the relationship between television violence and aggressive behaviour is comparable with that of the link between smoking and cancer (Ebon et al. 1994). Violence must be understood as a major health issue that requires a health promotion campaign analogous to that given to tobacco use. We need to help Canadians understand the impact of entertainment violence on our youth (as well as on high-risk adults) as a significant desensitizing and modelling influence for very inappropriate and dangerous behaviour.

Governments cannot do it alone. Primary prevention will require that consumer groups and parent committees recognize the power of their financial decisions and the support these give to advertisers, products and programs.

Extensive community action across Canada is needed to bring about social change in this area.

Another major forum for community change has to be Canadian schools. All provincial governments should recognize violence prevention as a high priority in schools and collaborate with partners such as parents and community agencies. The provincial governments should identify violence prevention as a high priority and assign financial resources to prevention programs. Without such a policy change, these initiatives will fall to the budgetary cutting room floor in these times of severe restraint; violence prevention programs will be seen as nonessential in contrast to basic classroom functions and mandatory subjects. However, the long-term cost of school violence and the expense of reactive responses, such as the security guards and metal detectors that are now prevalent in U.S. schools, will be overlooked. The school-based violence prevention programs reviewed in this study require no major funding initiatives. However, they do require leadership from provincial ministries of Education and teachers' federations, as well as broad public support. The Norwegian nationwide implementation of the antibullying program serves as a model for what can be done with public support and government leadership.

This policy change—emphasizing and supporting violence prevention at schools—can be addressed in a positive, proactive manner by suggesting that schools cover the "4 Rs": reading, writing, 'rithmetic and relationships. School-based violence prevention programs must specifically address violence against women, including wife assault, children witnessing violence, dating violence and sexual harassment. Just dealing with bullying in general or general violence at schools is not enough. School-based violence prevention programs need to make connections with equity issues and respect for all cultural groups. The message has to be that teaching respect, tolerance and conflict resolution is part of the school's responsibility, as it is the parents' duty. Building more young offender custody centres and changing the Young Offenders Act will not be effective by themselves.

A more radical policy approach to demonstrating governments' commitment to primary prevention in the education system would be to make a portion of the grants of individual school boards depend on each school's filing a violence prevention plan. Given the widespread concern of teachers and parents, grassroots support could be found for this policy, conditional on a philosophy of collaboration rather than of dumping the issue of violence solely on the backs of teachers.

Obviously, provincial government policies in this area would be followed by similar policies at each school board. These changes would be supported by directives to public officers of health to include violence as a public health issue, as did the U.S. Centre for Disease Control in Atlanta and recent publications from the American Medical Association that define the issue of violence as a major health problem. Public health units across Canada work closely with school boards and could reinforce these policy changes.

Secondary Prevention

The major policy implications related to secondary prevention concern the recognition of high-risk children and adolescents who are growing up in violent families. Policy development must ensure that these youth receive special programs to reduce, in the long run, the incidence of violence in the community.

The first of these policy implications concerns the training of front-line professionals such as teachers, police officers and family physicians about family violence and its effects on children. Although most professionals have some understanding of physical and sexual abuse and mandatory reporting requirements, they have limited awareness of the impact of witnessing violence. Education programs in medical schools, police colleges and continuing education programs should emphasize this current literature (e.g., Peled et al. 1995) to create better early identification and prevention programs.

Looking at the policy implications for schools in greater detail, we suggest that teachers be made aware of the prevalence of children who are witnessing violence at home. It is important that the school system adopt policies and protocols to guide and support teachers and administrators who deal with disclosures. Teachers and administrators may fear making family situations worse by doing the wrong thing, and they may not be familiar with the appropriate community agencies to assist children and their parents in this situation.

School policies and protocols are important and should be widely disseminated in easy-to-access, quick-reference formats. Sample protocols are provided by ASAP (Sudermann et al. 1993, 1996), and these can be adapted to local needs, in consultation with both schools and community agencies.

When a child discloses having witnessed violence at home to a teacher, the teacher must be prepared to respond appropriately. Appropriate responses include: attentive, nonjudgmental listening; asking the child whether he is safe and helping the child to develop a personal safety plan in the event of renewed violence; refraining from promising a "quick fix" to the problem; reporting abuse as mandated by local child welfare legislation; reassuring the child that he did right to tell someone about the problem; consulting appropriate resource people and agencies; depending on the situation, possibly contacting a parent of the child in a safe manner (e.g., individual interview at the school) if this role is not adopted by a school social worker or community child protection worker; and seeking personal support from colleagues and supervisors, as needed, to help handle the situation.

Police services need to implement more detailed training on wife assault and domestic violence. The topic of children who witness violence and woman abuse is rarely included. Since police are often the only mobile, around-the-clock crisis intervention service, officers who receive domestic violence calls must be aware of the impact on the children who are present. As with teachers, networking between police and community service providers for abused children and women's services is important.

Identifying children who witness violence has many implications for social services and mental health facilities. The ways service providers conceptualize the importance and urgency of the problem, and the significance of the trauma, of witnessing violence are important. To consider such policy issues, one may think through vital questions such as:

1. Do children who witness violence need protection?
2. If children need protection, what interventions should the state consider?
3. Do children who witness violence need specialized assessment and treatment services?

In Canada and the United States, child protection services are highly inconsistent about responding to reports of children witnessing violence. In some jurisdictions, legislation explicitly indicates that child witnesses to violence should be deemed children in need of protection but, in most cases, there is no legislation or explicit policy to make these children a priority. Legislative and policy initiatives are needed to ensure enough resources to make child witnesses a priority. If these children are deemed in need of protection, then appropriate services and community collaboration adequate to ensure meaningful intervention must be provided.

A related question is: What happens between separated parents when there are disputes over child custody or visitation, and allegations of domestic violence? In such circumstances, courts try to set up a custody or visitation plan that best serves the children's interests, rather than having the state intervene to decide whether the children need protection. Typically, the woman is the abused partner and is trying to limit visitation by a former husband to minimize contact with and effects of his violence. In such cases, women may find themselves before judges who see no link between a man's roles as husband and father, and may consider the mother an "unfriendly parent" for mentioning the violence.

Child custody and domestic violence are increasingly important topics for debate and judicial education. For example, by 1995, the majority of U.S. states had enacted custody statutes to require courts to consider domestic violence when developing custody and visitation orders. The many controversies and perspectives in this area range from concern about false allegations used to help women gain advantage in custody disputes to consistent disregard for the reality of violence in making custody orders.

A major concern is that women and children are most at risk while parents are separated but not divorced, and that, in many cases, the violence does not end but escalates during this time. At the extreme, women's advocates are concerned that some custody and visitation orders further endanger women by promoting contact with abusive ex-partners and creating opportunities for ongoing threats and harassment. In custody disputes without violence, judges are trying to reduce hostilities and encourage parents to work together for the sake of the children. However, when there are allegations of violence, judges are challenged to make safety a priority and find a way to balance the rights of fathers with the needs of children for safety and security. In these circumstances, specialized resources are essential, such as custody assessment services and supervised visitation centres with staff trained in domestic violence.

Many parents turn to children's mental health centres and counselling services to "fix" their children, as if they were dropping off the car at the garage for the day. It is often difficult to convince parents that the children's adjustment problems may be caused by their own behaviour and attitudes. A prime example of this problem is the limited awareness and understanding among adults of the impact on children and adolescents of witnessing violence.

At the London Family Court Clinic, most of the youngsters charged with assault grew up in homes where violence and abuse of power and control in relationships were normal. If secondary, prevention programs received as much attention as the Young Offenders Act, there would be less youth violence.

Policy development should include making mental health professionals aware enough of these issues to ask the basic questions about conflict resolution and violence. When centres put this perspective into their intake forms and raise the question in initial interviews, it signals parents that this topic is important and relevant. It is also vital to gather the same information directly from children and adolescents, since parents tend to underestimate both the extent of the violence their children have been exposed to and the actual impact of this experience.

To help them understand that they are not alone and develop skills to survive traumatic experiences, policy development should encourage group counselling programs for children exposed to violence.

CONCLUSIONS

This paper reviews the extensive concerns and debate about violence in society and the search for effective strategies to reduce violence. We propose that efforts to reduce violence in general and efforts to reduce violence against women should be brought together by examining the strong links in this field. Most violence happens within families and intimate relationships. Most strangers who are violent have childhood histories of witnessing violence.

We propose that the most effective strategies to reduce violence include primary and secondary prevention programs. Primary prevention programs stress reaching out to people of all ages to help them recognize violence as a major health problem and identify links between violence and entertainment that encourages violence. Canadians need to recognize that the link between violence on television and youngsters' aggression resembles the link between smoking and cancer. Primary prevention efforts should focus on schools as a forum for innovative programs. Several broad-based school programs offer hope for effective interventions.

Since we live in a time of limited resources, we conclude that it is also important to have secondary prevention programs, which target high-risk youth such as children and adolescents who witness violence in their families. Innovative group programs that focus on this population have demonstrated positive outcomes.

We urge all levels of government and community organizations to develop policies and programs to foster primary and secondary violence prevention programs. We conclude that effective policy and legislative changes must recognize:
- the extent of violence in society and the extent to which we socialize boys to condone and celebrate violence;
- students' right to speak freely about all kinds of violence, including sexism, racism and emotional and psychological abuse;
- it is cheaper and more effective to use proactive approaches to violence, such as prevention, an examination of school climates policies, and leadership to promote equality and safety, than to take a reactive approach;
- that safe homes are as important as safe streets, and that a great deal of violence that students experience occurs in their family environment;
- that violence in relationships often begins in early courtship and dating relationships, which are adolescents' opportunity to practice what they have learned in their family of origin about the nature of conflict resolution, and power and control issues between men and women;
- that violence and inequality are linked, and that, in our society, some individuals are more vulnerable and likely to be abused than others; and
- that ending violence requires commitment and collaboration among all community members and cannot be left to the justice, social service or education systems.

Marlies Sudermann, *Ph.D., C.Psych., is an adjunct clinical professor in the Department of Psychology at the University of Western Ontario. She is the director of Violence Prevention Services at the London Family Court Clinic in London, Ontario and consultant clinical psychologist at Harmony House, a senior young offender facility for young women, as well as at Madame Vanier Children's Services, a children's mental health centre. Dr. Sudermann also serves as director of the London Custody and Access Project. She serves on the Board of Changing Ways, a men's abuse treatment agency, and on the London Co-ordinating Committee to End Woman Abuse. Dr. Sudermann is the first author of* A.S.A.P.: A School-Based Anti-Violence Program *(1993, 1996). She has published numerous scholarly articles, chapters, and evaluation reports. Her current research interests include evaluation of groups for children who have witnessed violence, and prevention of dating violence, child welfare, woman abuse, and bullying. She frequently speaks to community and professional groups.*

BIBLIOGRAPHY

AD HOC ADVISORY COMMITTEE FOR A NATIONAL STRATEGY ON COMMUNITY SAFETY AND CRIME PREVENTION. 1993. *Community Safety through Crime Prevention.* Ottawa (ON): Supply and Services Canada.

AMERICAN MEDICAL ASSOCIATION. 1992. Violence against women. *Journal of the American Medical Association* 267: 107–112.

CANADA. STATISTICS CANADA. 1992. Gender differences among violent crime victims. *Juristat Service Bulletin.* Cat. no. 85–002. Ottawa (ON): Minister of Supply and Services.

———. 1993. The violence against women survey. *The Daily.* Ottawa (ON): Minister of Supply and Services.

CANADIAN PANEL ON VIOLENCE AGAINST WOMEN. 1993. *Changing the Landscape: Ending Violence—Achieving Equality (Final Report).* Ottawa (ON): Minister of Supply and Services.

COMMITTEE FOR CHILDREN. 1992. *Second Step: A Violence Prevention Curriculum.* Seattle (WA): Committee for Children.

COMMUNITY CHILD ABUSE COUNCIL OF HAMILTON-WENTWORTH (published by author). 1993. *R.S.V.P.: Response by Schools to Violence Prevention.* Hamilton (ON).

DEKESEREDY, W. S., and K. KELLY. 1993. The incidence and prevalence of woman abuse in Canadian university and college dating relationships. *Canadian Journal of Sociology* 18: 137–159.

DUTTON, D. G. 1988. *The Domestic Assault of Women: Psychological and Criminal Justice Perspectives.* Boston (MA): Allyn & Bacon.

EBON, L. D., J. H. GENTRY, and P. SCHLEGEL. 1994. *Reason to Hope: A Psychosocial Perspective on Violence and Youth.* Washington (DC): American Psychological Association.

ECHLIN, C., and L. MARSHALL. 1995. Child protection services for children of battered women: Practice and controversy. In *Ending the Cycle of Violence: Community Responses to Children of Battered Women,* eds. E. PELED, P. G. JAFFE, and J. EDLESON. Thousand Oaks (CA): Sage Publications. pp. 170–185.

FANTUZZO, J. W., L. M. DE PAOLA, L. LAMBERT, T. MARTINO, G. ANDERSON, and S. SUTTON. 1989. Effects of interparental violence on the psychological adjustment and competencies of young children. *Journal of Consulting and Clinical Psychology* 59: 258–265.

FERRIS, L. E., and F. TUDIVER. 1992. Family physicians' approach to wife abuse: A study of Ontario, Canada practices. *Family Medicine* 24: 276–82.

HILBERMAN, E., and J. MUNSON. 1978. Sixty battered women. *Victimology* 2: 460–470.

HILTON, Z., G. T. HARRIS, and M. RICE. 1994. Evaluation of an educational intervention on aggression in high school students' relationships: Change without backlash. Penetanguishene (ON): Mental Health Centre. *Research Reports* 11(6).

HORNER, B. 1993. *Crime Prevention in Canada: Towards a National Strategy—12th Report of the Standing Committee on Justice and the Solicitor General.* Ottawa (ON): Supply and Services Canada.

HOWARD, R. 1996. The paradox of violence. *The Globe and Mail,* 2 Mar.

JAFFE, P. G., D. WOLFE, and S. WILSON. 1990. *Children of Battered Women.* Thousand Oaks (CA): Sage Publications.

JAFFE, P., M. SUDERMANN, D. REITZEL, and S. M. KILLIP. 1992. An evaluation of a secondary school primary prevention program on violence in relationships. *Violence and Victims* 7: 129–146.

JONES, L. E. 1987. *Dating Violence among Minnesota Teenagers: A Summary of Survey Results.* St. Paul (MN): Minnesota Coalition for Battered Women.

KOSS, M. P., C. A. GIDYCZ, and N. WISNIEWSKI. 1987. The scope of rape: Incidence and prevalence of sexual aggression and victimization in a national sample of higher education students. *Journal of Consulting and Clinical Psychology* 55: 162–170.

LARSON, J. 1994. Violence prevention in the schools: A review of selected programs and procedures. *School Psychology Review* 23: 151–164.

LEHMANN, P. 1995. Post-traumatic stress disorder in children who have witnessed their mothers being assaulted. Paper presented at the Children's Aid Society of London and Middlesex, London (ON).

MACDOUGALL, J. 1993. *Violence in Schools: Programs and Policies for Prevention.* Toronto (ON): Canadian Education Association.

MAHLSTEDT, D., D. J. FALCONE, and L. RICE-SPRING. 1993. Dating violence education: What do students learn? *The Journal of Human Justice* 4: 101–117.

MARSHALL, L., N. MILLER, S. MILLER-HEWITT, M. SUDERMANN, and L. WATSON. 1995. *Evaluation of Groups for Children Who Have Witnessed Violence.* London (ON): Centre for Research on Violence Against Women and Children.

MCFARLANE, J., B. PARKER, K. SOEKEN, and L. BULLOCK. 1992. Assessing for abuse during pregnancy: Severity and frequency of injuries and associated entry into prenatal care. *Journal of the American Medical Association* 267: 3176–3178.

O'LEARY, K. D., J. MALONE, and A. TYREE. 1994. Physical aggression in early marriage: Prerelationship and relationship effects. *Journal of Consulting and Clinical Psychology* 62: 594–602.

OLWEUS, D. 1992. Bullying among school children: Intervention and prevention. In *Aggression and Violence throughout the Lifespan*, eds. R. DeV. PETERS, R. J. MCMAHON, and V. L. QUINSEY. Thousand Oaks (CA): Sage Publications. pp. 100–125.

———. 1993. *Bullying at School: What We Know and What We Can Do.* Oxford, U.K.: Blackwell Publishers.

ONTARIO MEDICAL ASSOCIATION COMMITTEE ON WIFE ASSAULT. 1986. Wife assault: A medical perspective. *Ontario Medical Review* 53(12): 771–791.

OSOFSKY, J. D., S. WEWERS, D. M. HANN, and A. C. FICK. 1993. Chronic community violence: What is happening to our children? In *Children and Violence*, eds. D. REISS, J. E. RICHTERS, M. RADKE-YARROW, and D. SCHARFF. New York (NY): The Guilford Press. pp. 36–45.

PELED, D. 1996. *A Peak behind the Fence: What We Have Learned about Bullying.* Paper presented at York University Conference, Putting the Brakes on Violence. August 1996.

PELED, E., and J. L. EDLESON.1995. Process and outcome in small groups for children of battered women. In *Ending the Cycle of Family Violence: Community Responses to Children of Battered Women*, eds. E. PELED, P. G. JAFFE, and J. L. EDLESON. Thousand Oaks (CA): Sage Publications. pp. 77–96.

PELED, E., P. G. JAFFE, and J. L. EDLESON. Eds. 1995. *Ending the Cycle of Family Violence: Community Responses to Children of Battered Women.* Thousand Oaks (CA): Sage Publications.

PEPLER, D. J., and W. M. CRAIG. 1995. A peek behind the fence: Naturalistic observations of aggressive children with remote audiovisual recording. *Child Development* 31: 548–553.

PEPLER, D.J., W. M. CRAIG, and W. R. ROBERTS. 1993. Aggression on the playground: A normative behaviour? Paper presented at the biennial meetings of the Society for Research in Child Development, Mar. 1993, New Orleans (LA).

PEPLER, D. J., W. M. CRAIG, S. ZIEGLER, and A. CHARACH. 1994. An evaluation of an antibullying intervention in Toronto schools. *Canadian Journal of Community Mental Health* 13: 95–110.

PRICE, R. H., E. L. COWEN, R. P. LOZON, and J. RAMOS-MCKAY. 1989. The search for effective prevention programs: What we learned along the way. *American Journal of Orthopsychiatry* 59: 49–58.

REISS, D., J. E. RICHTERS, M. RADKE-YARROW, and D. SCHARFF. 1993. *Children and Violence.* New York (NY): The Guilford Press.

RYAN, C., F. MATTHEWS, and J. BANNER. 1993. *Students' Perceptions of Violence: Summary of Preliminary Findings.* Toronto (ON): Central Toronto Youth Services,

SMITH, M. D. 1990. Patriarchal ideology and wife beating: A test of a feminist hypothesis. *Violence and Victims* 5: 257–273.

STARK, E., A. FLITCRAFT, and D. ZUCKERMAN. 1981. Wife abuse in the medical setting: An introduction for health personnel. *Domestic Violence Monograph.* Series no. 7. Washington (DC): National Clearinghouse on Domestic Violence. pp 1–54.

STEINHAUER, P. 1995. Model for the prevention of delinquency. Paper presented to the National Crime Prevention Council, Ottawa (ON), December 1995.

STERNBERG, K. L., M. E. LAMB, C. GREENBAUM, D. CICCHETTI, S. DAWUD, R. M. CORTES, O. KRISPIN, and F. LOREY. 1993. Effects of domestic violence on children's behaviour problems and depression. *Developmental Psychology* 29: 44–52.

STRAUS, M. A., and R. J. GELLES. 1986. Societal change and change in family violence from 1975 to 1985 as revealed by two national surveys. *Journal of Marriage and the Family* 48: 465–479.

_____. 1995. Societal change and change in family violence from 1975 to 1985 as revealed by two national surveys. In *Understanding Partner Violence: Prevalence, Causes, Consequences, and Solutions,* eds. S. M. SMITH and M. A. STRAUS. Minneapolis (MN): National Council on Family Relations. pp. 15–29.

SUDERMANN, M., and P. G. JAFFE. 1993. Violence in teen dating relationships: Evaluation of a large-scale primary prevention program. Paper presented at the Annual Meeting of the American Psychological Association, Aug. 1993, Toronto (ON).

_____. 1997. Children and adolescents who witness violence: New directions in intervention and prevention. In *Child Abuse: New Direction in Prevention and Treatment across a Life Span,* eds. R. De V. PETERS, R. J. MCMAHON, and D. WOLFE. Thousand Oaks (CA): Sage Publications.

SUDERMANN, M., and L. WATSON. 1993. *An Evolution of an Elementary Violence Prevention Initiative.* London (ON): London Family Court Clinic. Unpublished document.

SUDERMANN, M., P. G. JAFFE, and E. HASTINGS. 1995. Prevention programs in secondary schools. In *Ending the Cycle of Violence: Community Responses to Children of Battered Women,* eds. E. PELED, P. G. JAFFE, and J. EDLESON. Thousand Oaks (CA): Sage Publications. pp 232–254.

SUDERMANN, M., P. G. JAFFE, and E. SCHIECK. 1993, 1996. *A.S.A.P.: A School-Based Anti-Violence Program.* London(ON): London Family Court Clinic.

TEARMANN SOCIETY FOR BATTERED WOMEN. 1988. *Medical Services or Disservice? An Exploratory Study of Wife Assault Victims' Experience in Health Delivery Settings.* New Glasgow (NS): Tearmann Society for Battered Women,

TENOLD-PHILLIPS, B. 1995. Implementation of "A School-Based Anti-Violence Program". Prince Albert (SK).

WOLFE, D. A., L. ZAK, S. WILSON, and P. G. JAFFE. 1986. Child witnesses to violence between parents: Critical issues in behaviourial and social adjustment. *Journal of Abnormal Child Psychology* 14: 95–104.

Suicide in Children, Adolescents and Seniors: Key Findings and Policy Implications

RONALD J. DYCK, PH.D.

Alberta Health
Government of Alberta

BRIAN L. MISHARA, PH.D.

Department of Psychology
University of Quebec at Montreal

JENNIFER WHITE, M.A.

Cooperative University–Provincial Psychiatric Liaison
University of British Columbia

SUMMARY

Suicide in Canada is a significant social concern and major public health problem that requires attention. Suicide results in one of the highest rates of potential years of life lost. The rates of suicide and suicidal behaviour have been steadily increasing over the years, and only recently have they plateaued. For every completed suicide, there are an estimated 10–100 suicide attempts. In an extensive study on parasuicide in a major Canadian city, the rate of parasuicide for a one-year period was higher than in any of the 17 major cities in Europe where similar data were collected. Moreover, the impact of these events extends far beyond the suicidal person: family members, friends, neighbourhoods, workplaces, schools, health care providers and systems, and communities are all affected.

To determine future directions in addressing this significant issue, the National Forum on Health, established by the Government of Canada, commissioned this paper to examine suicidal behaviour among three populations: those of children, adolescents and the elderly. The literature is reviewed with a view to identifying key conclusions from a population health framework, and examples of successful and not-so-successful interventions are described. Finally, recommendations for policy directions are provided.

Suicidal Behaviour among Children and Adolescents

Suicidal behaviour among children and youth is clearly complex and must be understood within a multidimensional framework that takes into account the individual, familial, social, economic and cultural contexts. In reviewing the literature, several key findings can be highlighted that provide insights into suicidal behaviour among these populations. The following conditions in interaction with one another appear to pose the greatest risks for the emergence of vulnerabilities that can set the stage for suicidal behaviour among both children and adolescents:

- *negative early family experiences characterized by loss, difficulties in attachment, parental psychopathology, and family history of suicide and abuse;*
- *school problems, including academic failure;*
- *environmental disruptions during critical transition periods;*
- *peer difficulties, including loss of friendships;*
- *cultural attitudes that are accepting of suicide as a coping mechanism, including sensationalized media reporting of suicide;*
- *effects of low income and poverty;*
- *ease of access to means of self-destruction, such as firearms;*
- *the presence of a psychiatric disorder, previous suicidal behaviour, learning disability, and cognitive deficits; and*
- *the lack of trained gatekeepers in the community.*

Several additional conditions specifically related to adolescent suicidal behaviour include the breakup of relationships, suicidal behaviour among peers and significant others, substance abuse, and reticence to seek help for oneself or one's peers.

Suicidal Behaviour among the Elderly

Suicide among the elderly must also be understood within a multidimensional framework in which a risk for suicide results from the complex interaction of risk conditions, personal vulnerabilities, and precipitating conditions that can trigger suicidal behaviour. Key findings from the literature suggest that the following conditions in interaction with one another can serve not only to set the stage for, but also to precipitate, suicidal behaviour:

- *loss of economic viability that can result from such events as retirement or loss of a job;*
- *an accumulation of losses such as loss of spouse or social network, including friends, confidants, relationships, social roles, self-esteem and efficacy, meaningful work, one's own residence (home), and structure in one's life;*
- *availability of firearms and other means for self-destruction;*
- *the presence of an affective disorder, especially depression;*
- *reluctance or inability to seek help;*
- *cultural attitudes that are accepting of suicide, especially among the elderly who are ill;*
- *presence of chronic illness or physical disability;*
- *lack of appropriate services employing care providers trained in suicide intervention and prevention and recognition of depression in older persons;*
- *lack of community gatekeepers adequately trained in suicide intervention;*
- *anticipation of nursing home placement; and*
- *presence of factors in institutions for long-term care, such as size of the population of residents, rate of staff turnover and per diem rates.*

The findings from the research literature inform our understanding of the complexity of suicidal behaviour among children, adolescents and the elderly, and the identification and description of initiatives designed to address the various risk and precipitating conditions from a nonmedical perspective are given consideration. Six programs are reviewed that have relevance to the specified groups. The first is a school-based program, the School Transition Environment Project (STEP), which is a structural intervention targeting youth at a critical transition point in their lives. Results from this program suggest that environmental manipulation can reduce academic failure, behavioral problems, dropout rates, delinquency, poor health practices, violence, psychosocial difficulties, suicide and depression, and substance abuse among students, and levels of stress and absenteeism among teachers. Improvements can be found in prosocial behaviour, safety and order in the schools, attitudes opposed to substance abuse, academic outcomes, achievement scores, and successful transitions across school levels and to work.

The second of these programs, the Alaska Community-Based Suicide Prevention (CBSP) project, is an example of how suicide prevention can be facilitated in small, northern communities with 1,000 people or fewer. Results from this program reveal that changes can be realized in small communities by funding community-based projects that encourage community involvement and participation. In five case study communities, suicide rates are declining; community members have become more knowledgeable about suicide and self-destructive behaviour; community-based responses for dealing with self-destructive behaviour have been initiated; healthier behaviour has been adopted; and the changes in communities are being institutionalized. Other changes include more community members being able to identify and appropriately refer a suicidal person; more members of the community reporting assisting a child experiencing difficulty;

increased abstinence and a decrease in abusive drinking; and an increased perception among residents that they have control over local problems.

The third is a multidisciplinary approach to identifying and locating the isolated and at-risk elderly: The Gatekeeper Model for the Isolated, At-Risk Elderly. This approach uses people (nontraditional gatekeepers) who come into contact with these high-risk elderly people through their work and are appropriately trained to make referrals. While the results of this program are more difficult to measure, several findings point to success. Increases have occurred in the community health centre's caseload of these underserved and hard-to-reach elderly people; nursing home bed shortages are no longer experienced in the county; 40 percent of the referrals to a related in-home case management program are the result of the gatekeeper system.

The fourth is a bereavement support group for older widowers: the Suicide-Action Montreal Program for Widowers. Using well-trained volunteers, the program targets men over age 55 who have experienced the death of a spouse less than two years before their participation. At the time of writing, the results of this program are not available. Suffice it to say that participants were asked to complete several questionnaires designed to measure their level of bereavement, well-being, situational anxiety, and depression before their entry into the program, after six months of participation, and one year later.

The fifth, the High/Scope Perry Preschool Program, has as its primary goal the development of at-risk children's skills and dispositions that can serve as a foundation for adaptive functioning in school and result in school success. From immediate and long-term (at age 15, 19 and 27) follow-up studies, the results include improved academic performance, more social and emotional maturity, greater commitment to school, better jobs obtained, fewer unemployed, less public assistance received, and fewer arrests.

Lastly, the Postvention Effort[1] in New South Wales (Australia) was an attempt to reduce levels of risk for suicidal behaviour following the deaths by suicide of two students. Specified postvention activities were undertaken in the schools within seven days of the suicides. Evaluation results of these efforts revealed that eight months after these suicides, no differences were found between students who received the intervention and those who did not. Several explanations for these lack of differences are offered.

A number of critical policy directions emerge from the review of the key findings from the literature and the identification of several success stories that have the potential for influencing suicidal behaviour in the target populations. First, it is clear that to continue to reduce rates of suicide among the elderly and to influence child and adolescent suicide rates, we must address the issue of social and economic environments. Attention must be given to the issues of low income, so that the cycle of poverty can be broken; the manner in which suicide

---

1. Postvention activities are typically initiated after a suicide attempt or completion.

is depicted in the electronic and print media; the creation of environments and living conditions that increase social support, promote healthy coping, and reduce the negative effects of loss; the development of guidelines, regulations and legislation that ensure the safe storage or reduce access to firearms and dangerous medications; and the ongoing commitment to community participation and involvement in improving the quality of life of its citizens.

Second, to enhance the potential for health and well-being and to improve early identification, crisis intervention, and treatment for those who are suicidal (or potentially suicidal), it is necessary to implement appropriate and effective strategies for teaching cognitive and social-emotional skills to all people; increase the awareness among adults of the potential for children to take their own lives; provide suicide prevention training for all gatekeepers; include suicide awareness education for students, using a comprehensive school health approach; and ensure that professional faculties (health related) at universities and community colleges provide training in suicide intervention skills and in suicide prevention.

Third, service delivery issues need attention. Specifically, mental health professionals must be given specialized training in the assessment and treatment of those at risk for suicide, interventions in first-episode affective illness, and assessment for comorbidity of affective illness and substance abuse; a thorough assessment of possible drug interactions, especially among the elderly, must be undertaken; the elderly must be made aware of resources that they can access; and services must be made available, appropriate and accessible to the youth population.

Fourth, there is a need to emphasize not only the evaluation of prevention and health promotion programs proposed to reduce vulnerabilities to suicide, but also multidisciplinary research approaches to examine this multidetermined behaviour.

TABLE OF CONTENTS

APPENDIX

FIGURE

INTRODUCTION

Approximately 3,500 people kill themselves in Canada each year, and many more attempt suicide. Since the 1970s, Canadian suicide rates have been consistently higher than U.S. rates. Moreover, like the United States and most European countries, suicide in Canada has consistently ranked among the top 5–10 leading causes of death for the last several years. It accounts for more than 15,000 potential years of life lost among youth aged 15–19, and represents the second leading cause of death among young people aged 15–24. What these statistics often fail to reveal, however, is the additional cost to society in lost economic productivity, lost potential, and the human suffering and emotional burdens associated with having a loved one attempt, or die by, suicide (Health Canada 1994).

In response to deep concern about the high rates of suicidal behaviour, task forces and royal commissions have been established, national conferences and consultations have been held, centres for the prevention of suicide have been established, community, regional and provincial suicide prevention strategies have been developed and implemented, and research on the epidemiology and treatment of suicide has been conducted (Health Canada 1994). Recommendations from these efforts tend to centre around several key intervention strategies: early identification and crisis intervention, treatment, postvention and survivor support. To support these efforts, recommendations also focus on the need for solid research and evaluation, as well as public education and gatekeeper training.

It is becoming apparent that we must provide services to intervene in a suicidal crisis and provide treatment and support in the event of a suicide attempt or a suicide death, and approaches must also be developed to reduce the conditions that create vulnerability to suicide. With the number of children and families in need of intensive mental health services (an estimated 35–50 million people in the United States), the increasing number of births among teens, the current levels of substance abuse, children living in poverty, and family violence, there will never be enough resources to address such needs (Silverman and Felner 1995). If we are to significantly reduce these problems, it is necessary to consider suicidal behaviour through a wide lens. Such a perspective moves beyond an exclusive emphasis on individual risk factors, psychopathology, crisis intervention and treatment, to take the key socializing factors and broad determinants of health into account.

While no particular factor can be considered singularly responsible for causing suicidal behaviour, it is important to understand that an array of individual, social and environmental factors interact with one another in a complex and nonlinear fashion to create a vulnerability to suicide. These predisposing factors, or "risk conditions," serve to set the stage for the possible emergence of a range of emotional and behavioral disturbances that includes suicide. More acute stressors or precipitating factors interact with these predisposing conditions, serving to exacerbate the risk for suicidal behaviour. Sudden in their onset, these precipitating conditions can often trigger a crisis.

Unlike the prevention of some diseases, such as coronary heart disease, where the risk factors are specifiable and for the most part modifiable (e.g., diet, smoking, exercise), suicide prevention does not have the benefits of such specificity and precision. The prevention of suicide must be approached from the perspective of a comprehensive, multicausal, nonspecific, developmental pathway (Silverman and Felner 1995). Consequently, the purpose of this paper is to identify from the research literature those risk conditions that could lead to vulnerabilities to dysfunction and to specify some of the primary precipitating factors that in interaction can result in suicidal behaviour among children, adolescents and the elderly. Furthermore, it is our intent not only to describe several success stories in relation to the prevention of suicide from a perspective of broad-based determinants, but also to point out policy directions that emerged from the review.

CHILDREN AND SUICIDAL BEHAVIOUR—RISK CONDITIONS

Social and Economic Environments

Role of the family – There are several studies of the family characteristics associated with suicidal children; however, the extent of the influence of family variables is subject to debate. Morrison and Collier (1969) felt that childhood suicidal behaviour is invariably a symptom related to "underlying family disruption" (140). Pfeffer (1986) cautioned that it is often difficult to obtain objective information about the families of suicidal children because of secretiveness and distortions about the cause of death, feelings of personal blame and guilt, and anger at the deceased child. For example, Calhoun, Selby and Faulstick (1980) asked 119 adults to read one of two newspaper articles describing the deaths of a 10-year-old: in one instance, the child died by hanging; in the other, by a viral disease. They found that parents of the child who died by suicide were less liked by the adult participants, and the parents were also blamed more for the child's death.

Despite these research limitations, several studies have reported on family characteristics associated with the risk of childhood suicide. A number of studies have suggested that the families of suicidal children are more likely to be characterized by parental separations, divorces or one-parent family situations (Shaffer 1974; Tishler, McKenry, and Morgan 1981; Cohen-Sandler, Berman, and King 1982; Garfinkel, Froese, and Hood 1982; Murphy and Wetzel 1982). For example, Morrison, and Collier (1969) reported that 76 percent of 34 children seen in an outpatient clinic following a suicide attempt had experienced a significant loss, separation or anniversary of loss within 2–3 weeks before the suicide attempt. In a study comparing suicidal children aged 5–14 years with nonsuicidal, depressed children and children with other psychiatric diagnoses in an inpatient setting, Cohen-Sandler and colleagues (1982) found that suicidal children had experienced more stressful life events, such as parental divorce and hospitalizations of a parent, than the other groups.

Several authors have suggested that there is a link between suicidal behaviour in children and parental violence and sexual abuse. For example, in a study comparing physically abused, neglected and "normal" children, Green (1978) found that 40 percent of the physically abused children had engaged in self-destructive or suicidal behaviour, compared with 17 percent of neglected children and 7 percent of the control group. The self-destructive and suicidal behaviour usually followed an incident of being beaten by a parent. Adams-Tucker (1982) suggested that suicidal behaviour is more common among children who are victims of sexual abuse.

Another research area concerns the possible relationship between suicidal behaviour and psychopathology in parents. For example, Garfinkel, Froese and Hood (1982) reported that preadolescents with suicidal behaviour more frequently had family histories of alcohol and drug abuse, depression, and suicidal behaviour. There are numerous anecdotal reports of children engaging in suicidal behaviour among families where a parent either committed or attempted suicide. For example, Pfeffer (1986) presents several case histories that she interprets as children imitating parental suicidal behaviour by attempting suicide themselves.

Mishara (1996) reported that 5 out of 65 children aged 6–12 years knew of someone who died by suicide, although these children were not told by a parent or other adult about the suicide. These were all instances of a death by suicide in the family reported as troubling to the child but not overtly discussed with an adult. More than 20 years ago, Furman (1974) described how parents are generally secretive when a spouse dies by suicide and almost invariably lie to the child about the nature of the death, usually by saying that the death was due to illness or an accident. Although children are rarely told about the true nature of the suicidal death, children often know and yet are unable to discuss it because of a reluctance or inability on the part of the surviving parent to discuss the situation openly and honestly.

Role of the media – In a study by Mishara (1996), children learned about suicide primarily from discussion with other children and through experiences with suicide depicted on television. Three-quarters of the 7-and 8-year-olds had seen or learned about suicide on television. All of the 9-, 10-, 11- and 12-year-olds said that they had seen or learned about suicide from television. In this study, more than 80 percent of children often reported talking about suicide. However, their discussions were usually with other children. It was rare that a parent or teacher would explain suicide to them.

In television programs that children watch, suicides are often depicted as heroic acts that must be carried out when a fictional character is cornered or without a means of escape. There are also cartoon examples of mock suicides, where a character uses a suicide threat to obtain an unreasonable request. For example, a Bugs Bunny cartoon showed the rabbit threatening to shoot himself if another cartoon character did not hand him a carrot he desired. This suicide threat was successful in obtaining the carrot, although the rabbit showed afterward that it was only a toy gun, with which he could not have killed himself.

Role of economic factors – Economic environmental risk factors for childhood psychiatric disorders may also be considered as possible risk factors for childhood suicidal behaviour. Offord (1990) and Offord, Boyle and Racine (1989) identified economic disadvantage as a major risk factor for childhood psychiatric disorders, including low family income and welfare status; urban residence, including overcrowding; and residence in public or subsidized housing. Offord reported that male children are at higher risk than female children and that children of particular minority or immigrant groups are at increased risk because of their economic and social circumstances. We can understand that the effect of poverty is to increase the susceptibility of a child to future suicidal behaviour by increasing the likelihood that the child will develop a wide range of vulnerabilities associated with increased risk of suicide.

Individual Capacity and Coping

Cognitive development – To better understand suicide among children, it is useful to understand how children develop an understanding of death. The low numbers of reported suicide among children may arise in part from a reluctance on the part of coroners to classify children's deaths as suicides because they believe that children do not understand enough about death to truly commit suicide. However, there is extensive research literature on the development of children's conceptions of death. In the 1940s, probably as a result of the war, Sylvia Anthony (1940) and Maria Nagy (1948) interviewed children concerning their concepts of death and reported a series of stages in the acquisition of a "mature" understanding of death. For the youngest children, death was akin to a sleep-like state, from which one can be awakened, as in the fairy tale "Sleeping Beauty." For the youngest children it was possible to avoid death by being adept or careful, and dead people were sometimes considered to have thoughts, feelings and behaviour that more mature children ascribed only to the living.

Since this early research, there has been much debate about the exact nature of the stages in the acquisition of a mature concept of death. For example, Melear (1973) found that some younger children had a more "mature" understanding than several of the older children. Raimbault (1975) reported that children who suffer from a terminal illness develop a sophisticated understanding of death, even at a young age. Koocher (1973) found that the concept of death was related to levels of cognitive development, classified according to a Piagetian schema, rather than chronological age. Despite the debates concerning the possibility of defining clear-cut stages, researchers generally agree that an understanding of death develops gradually. More recent research has evaluated the concept of death according to five subconcepts: aging, irreversibility, universality, finality and causality (e.g., Orbach et al. 1985). Aging, the idea that people die eventually when they grow old, tends to be understood before any other concept. Irreversibility, the idea that once a person is dead they cannot come back to life, is usually understood next, followed by universality, the fact that everyone dies. Finality, the idea that death is an end state, and causality, the concept that death is an inevitable part of living and is not just because of some external accident, develop later. Grenier (1986) refined these subconcepts and developed criteria for a mature concept of death: finality (which includes irreversibility), state of death (which concerns how complete is the cessation of biological functions), universality, unpredictability and causality.

Grenier (1986) found that the more experiences children had related to death (e.g., prolonged separations, death of an animal or pet, death education at school), the more mature their concept of death in general. In her study of 52 6- to 9-year-olds, Kane (1975) found that death concepts tended to be more mature when children experienced a death in the immediate family, and younger children (age 3–6) tended to change their concept of death the most as a result of the loss of a family member. Our review of the literature suggests that the concept of death develops gradually and is related to experiences with death. One can ask whether the concept of suicide develops in a similar manner. More particularly, when do children begin to understand suicide and how does their understanding relate to their comprehension of death, as well as their experiences of death and suicide?

Normand and Mishara (1992) conducted an interview study of 60 French-speaking children in public elementary schools in Montreal in grades 1, 3 and 5. They evaluated the children's understanding of death, experiences related to death, and the word *suicide*, their experiences related to suicide, and their attitudes toward suicide. In this study, school personnel were concerned that if a child did not know the meaning of the word *suicide*, then the interview with these children should be stopped immediately, rather than pursuing the investigation of the child's understanding by replacing the word *suicide* with expressions such as *ending one's life* or *killing oneself*. In this particular study, the researchers complied with the teachers' wishes and agreed to end the interview without further investigation if the child did not know the meaning of the word *suicide*. Only one of the 60 children chose to terminate the interview before its completion because he felt "too sad to talk about death" (his mother had died a few months earlier). Otherwise, children generally discussed death and suicide easily, with no negative emotional reactions.

Normand and Mishara (1992) found that 87 percent of the children understood the concept of the universality of death, that is, that everyone will die some day, even without having had an accident or having contracted an illness. Almost 90 percent of the children understood that death is final, that it is impossible to come back to life. Slightly more than half of the grade school children (53 percent) recognized that death is unpredictable. Ninety percent of the children reported causes of death that were external, such as accidents or smoking cigarettes. Only 10 percent cited internal processes as being the cause of death. Forty percent of the children felt that people who were dead could feel emotions such as "good" or "sad," even though they could not see or move, and one-third felt that people who died continued to live in some manner in another setting, such as Heaven. In this study, children had a mature concept of death by the age of 9 or 10. In the study by Normand and Mishara, only two of the 20 first graders knew the meaning of the word *suicide* and only 50 percent of the third graders knew what *suicide* meant. However, 19 of the 20 fifth graders knew the meaning of the word. Because of the possibility that children may understand killing oneself but not know the word *suicide*, Mishara (1995) conducted a follow-up study that differed from the study by Normand and Mishara (1992): children who did not understand the meaning of *suicide* or *to commit suicide* (in French, *se suicider*) were asked if they knew about *killing oneself.* Children who knew about *killing oneself* but who did not recognize the word *suicide* were then interviewed in detail about suicide, replacing *killing oneself* for *suicide* throughout the interview. Mishara (1996) conducted a more detailed investigation that involved 65 children in grades 1 through 5. Although none of the 6-year-olds in this sample knew about suicide, one-third of 7-year-olds knew about suicide or killing oneself and 87 percent of 8-year-olds, 81 percent of 9-year-olds, and all (100 percent)of the children aged 10 and older knew about suicide. Five of the 65 children (7.7 percent) reported that they knew someone who had committed suicide, and 9 of the children (13.8 percent) had considered killing themselves.

Although virtually all children know about death, their understanding of death differs from what adults generally believe to occur when someone dies. For younger children, death is not necessarily final. Death is seen as similar to events that children see in television cartoons: the characters may be crushed to the thickness of a piece of paper but then they can jump up and come back to life. Death is not inevitable: if we have a good doctor or are careful (e.g., crossing the street carefully or avoiding bad guys), we can avoid dying. Not everyone dies—death is not universal; and death is seen as being caused only by exterior events. Many of the attributes we reserve for the living, such as feeling sad, are ascribed to the dead by younger children. But more important is the fact that children can often accept the coexistence of different, seemingly contradictory concepts of death without any trouble. A child can understand that everyone dies some day and at the same time believe that, if you are careful, you may live forever. A young child may believe that people who die can never come back to life, that death is final, but if you want to come back *very much* and your friends shake you *very hard*, you can wake up from death. All this suggests that suicide may have a very different meaning for a child who may not see death as a complete cessation of life from which one can never return.

A child's understanding of suicide may also have a significant influence on the child's own potential for suicidal behaviour. An immature understanding of death may put children at risk of engaging in suicidal behaviour if death is not seen as irreversible. Also, a child's understanding of suicide may influence the child's overall adjustment and development throughout childhood and adolescence. An illustration of this is the case of an 8-year-old boy whose presenting problem was an eating disorder. The child was much below the average weight for his height and age. He was reported as giving away the contents of his lunch box every day, and his parents said he hid food from meals, rather than eating, and gave this food to other children in the neighbourhood or at school. Although the child lived in a poor neighbourhood where nutrition was not generally good, he came from a "better-off" family, proud that they were able to provide quality food for their child. In discussions, he said that he gave food to the other children because they "wanted" his food. Further investigation revealed that when he was 4 years old his older half-brother (then 16 years old) committed suicide by hanging himself. It was this young boy who had discovered the body. The parents had told the child that this was an accident. However, the child remembered clearly that his older brother had asked his father to borrow the car that day and was refused shortly before killing himself. Four years later, the boy was afraid that if he did not give his friends his food, which they had asked for, something as disastrous might happen to them, in the same way that his half-brother had killed himself because his father did not give him something he had wanted. The child even went so far as to generalize this behaviour and did not wait for the others to ask but insisted on giving them his food as often as possible, whether they asked or not.

In this instance, a young child reached his own understanding of why a tragic loss had occurred in his family in a situation where no one explained what had really happened. Four years later, this understanding was expressed by what was erroneously diagnosed as an eating disorder. The child responded well to therapy, whose goal was to help the child develop a more mature (and perhaps more sophisticated) understanding of his brother's death and why people may kill themselves.

It is naive to think that children do not know about suicide. They not only know about suicide but also develop an understanding of why and how people kill themselves. This understanding is a function of their level of development and their experiences with death and suicide. In our society, and probably in all societies, we rarely teach children about suicide and tend not to discuss suicide openly. Even when there is a death by suicide in the family, the child is usually told nothing or given an inaccurate explanation, such as that an accident has occurred. However, even though explanations of suicidal death are not given, children often know what happened and find their own ways of understanding why the person committed suicide. Their explanations may be based on personal hypotheses, discussions with others (generally other children) or from experiences with suicide in television or movies.

Problem-solving skills – Asarnow, Carlson and Guthri (1987) and Orbach, Rosenheim and Hary (1987) suggested that young people who engage in suicidal behaviour use poor problem-solving methods or lack problem-solving skills. Orbach, Rosenheim and Hary (1987) and Levenson and Neuringer (1971) further contended that suicidal young people have a more rigid cognitive style and are less capable of seeing alternative solutions when faced with difficult life experience.

Health Services

It is evident that children acquire an understanding of suicide at an early age, despite the fact that the topic is rarely discussed. There are indications that about 3 percent of children may threaten suicide in talking with their parents. However, few deaths among children are classified as suicides. It may be that children rarely commit or attempt suicide. However, there are suggestions that a significant number of the accidental deaths and injuries in childhood may have involved suicidal intent that was ignored because of the erroneous belief that children do not understand enough about suicide and death to intentionally attempt to kill themselves. People who provide health and counselling services to children, as well as educators, may profit from training to understand the reality of children's understanding of suicide and to recognize the potential for children to engage in suicidal behaviour. In addition, it is important to provide age-relevant support for children who have suffered a loss by suicide.

Summary of Key Findings

Children learn about suicide at an early age, usually from media depictions of suicides and suicidal behaviour and through discussions with other children. However, children may often have an understanding of death that differs from adult conceptions. Such childhood conceptions of suicide and death may influence childhood behaviour, as well as these children's adolescent and adult suicidality.

Suicides are infrequent among children according to official statistics; however, these data may underestimate actual child suicide rates.

Children's problem-solving skills and family characteristics, including low family income, family psychopathology, abuse, loss, violence and other family disruptions, are related to childhood suicidal behaviour.

ADOLESCENTS AND SUICIDAL BEHAVIOUR—RISK CONDITIONS

Social and Economic Environments

Role of the family – One of the earliest and most significant social influences on a young person's development is the family. Studies have revealed an association between the following family-level characteristics and youth suicidal behaviour: early parental loss (Adam, Lohrenz, and Harper 1982; Spirito et al. 1989b; Pfeffer 1990), attachment pathology (Adam 1986; Richman 1986; van der Kolk, Perry, and Herman 1991), parental mental illness (Brent et al. 1988; Pfeffer 1990; Spirito et al. 1989), parental abuse and neglect (Bayatpour, Wells, and Holford 1992; Riggs, Alario, and McHorney 1990), and a family history of suicide (Garfinkel, Froese, and Hood 1982; Spirito et al. 1989b). Family-related precipitants to suicidal behaviour among youth include serious conflict with family members, death or divorce of parents, or perceived rejection by one's family (Brent et al. 1988; Hoberman and Garfinkel 1988b; Graham and Burvill 1992). Furthermore, when family members fail to take adolescents' talk about suicide seriously when they are ill equipped to intervene appropriately because they lack knowledge and skills, adolescents are at further risk.

Role of the school – A key environmental influence on youth development is school. A history of school problems and the stress of disruptive transitions in school have both been cited as potential risk conditions for youth suicidal behaviour (Hoberman and Garfinkel 1988b; Felner and Adan 1988). Other school-related factors that have been associated with suicidal behaviour among youth include failure, expulsion and overwhelming pressure to succeed (Brent et al. 1988; Hoberman and Garfinkel 1988b).

Role of peers – Peers are very influential in shaping youth behaviour, and there is a significant body of research that highlights the risk for imitative suicidal behaviour among adolescents who have been exposed to a peer's suicide (Gould et al. 1990; Brent et al. 1993; Hazell 1993). Furthermore, this "contagion effect" appears most likely to affect youths who are already vulnerable or who tend to identify strongly with the one who committed suicide. Long-term problems with peer relationships and a history of anti-social behaviour and isolation have also been associated with youth suicidal behaviour (Shafii et al. 1985; Marttunen, Aro, and Lonnqvist 1992). Rejection from peers, the breakup of a significant relationship, or the loss of a confidant have each been identified as precipitants to youth suicidal behaviour (Brent et al. 1988; Hoberman and Garfinkel 1988b; Davidson et al. 1989). Adolescents who fail to act when confronted with a suicidal peer, dismissing it as insignificant or failing to inform an adult, can exacerbate the risk of suicide.

Role of the media – Sensational media reports and fictionalized accounts of suicide have been shown to have a facilitating effect on the rates of suicide, particularly among teenagers (Gould and Shaffer 1986; Phillips and Carstenson 1986). However, not all media reports increase suicidal risk (Berman 1988). Clearly, the processes and mechanisms through which imitative suicidal behaviour among youth takes place are complex, and depend on a variety of interactive variables, such as the characteristics of exposed persons, including their preexisting vulnerabilities, the nature of the stimulus itself and environmental conditions.

Cultural attitudes – Cultural attitudes about suicide and suicidal behaviour have also been investigated to determine their effects on youth suicidal behaviour (Kienhorst et al. 1992). In a comparison of Canadian and U.S. youth, Domino and Leenaars (1989) reported that young Canadians more frequently saw suicide as an acceptable and normal response to problems, compared with their U.S. peers. Apparently, Canadian youths also feel less optimistic about the value of intervention, perceiving suicide as a private matter, a finding that has serious and obvious implications for whether youth in Canada will seek help for themselves or for a friend during a suicide crisis.

Social integration – The social conditions found to be associated with youth suicidal behaviour include social isolation, instability, religious detachment, and loss of social integration (Sakinofsky and Roberts 1987; Trovato 1992). Canadian research has revealed some important findings in this area. Trovato (1992) reviewed suicide mortality rates among young Canadians aged 15–29 for the 1971 and 1981 census periods. He found a positive association between "religious detachment"—measured by the number of respondents who indicated "no religious affiliation" in the census—and suicide rates among young males for the two time periods. The apparent protective function served by religious affiliation may have more to do with having enduring social ties to the religious community, which would serve to increase social integration and reduce overall isolation, rather than any specific effect of being religious.

Economic factors – The influence of the economy on suicide rates has been studied by examining the effects of unemployment (Platt 1984) on suicidal behaviour. Leenaars and Lester (1995) reported that in the years when unemployment was high, divorce more common, and birth rates lower, suicide rates were higher among young Canadian males.

Suicidal behaviour among youths has also been linked to low-income status. In one study, a significant correlation was found between white male adolescent suicide and family dissolution, as well as between the white adolescent male suicide rate and the percentage of white children living in poverty (McCall 1991). Furthermore, the effects of poverty on children and youth are often linked to a series of other risk conditions, such as low birthweight, low levels of preschool stimulation, poor school readiness, school problems and failure, psychiatric disorders, low self-esteem and substance abuse (Canadian Institute of Child Health 1994), all of which can create a vulnerability to suicide and suicidal behaviour among adolescents.

Physical Environment

Availability of lethal means – Having immediate and easy access to the lethal means to kill oneself obviously creates a potentially lethal environment for suicidal and vulnerable youth. Among males, the most common method to commit suicide is to use a firearm. In Canada, firearms are used by 45 percent of male suicides under the age of 20, while 18 percent of young women use a gun to kill themselves (Health Canada 1994). The choice of such an instantly lethal method is of particular concern for young people who may be especially vulnerable to acting impulsively in a crisis.

Two studies in particular have highlighted the association between the access of youth to firearms and higher rates of completed suicide in this age group (Brent et al. 1988; Sloan et al. 1990). In comparing two groups of suicidal adolescents with similar levels of affective disorders, Brent and his colleagues (1988) found that the availability of firearms in the home was significantly more prevalent among adolescents who eventually killed themselves. Another study (Sloan et al. 1990) revealed that the rate of suicide by handguns among 15- to 24-year-olds living in Seattle was shown to be 10 times greater than that of their Canadian peers, who live in a country where handgun regulations are more restrictive.

Environmental and structural factors – The structural and environmental organization of a school setting can also affect student performance, quality of life, and, indirectly, the emergence of mental health problems and suicidal behaviour (Felner and Felner 1989). For example, school conditions, such as overall climate, classroom sizes, disciplinary policies, size of the school population, and structural organization, have been shown to have an effect on academic achievement, behavioral and emotional problems, and other associated dysfunctions, such as drug abuse and crime (Moos 1979).

Personal Health Practices

Substance abuse – The abuse of alcohol and drugs by young people is a fairly well-established risk factor for suicide and suicidal behaviour (Berman and Schwartz 1990; Adcock, Nagy, and Simpson 1991; Pfeffer et al. 1991). Motto (1980) suggested that the increased use of alcohol and drugs among youths may be a significant contributing factor to the rising rate of youth suicide since the 1970s. Brent and his colleagues (1988) suggested that at least one-third of adolescents who kill themselves are intoxicated at the time of their suicide, and many more are likely to be under the influence of drugs. In a study of adolescent suicide attempters, Berman and Schwartz (1990) found that substance abusers were three times as likely to make a suicide attempt as a normative population of youths who were not substance abusers with whom they were matched for age and sex.

Risk-taking behaviour – Risk-taking behaviour, such as impaired or reckless driving, has also been associated with suicidal behaviour among youths (Adcock, Nagy, and Simpson 1991; Martunnen, Aro, and Lonnqvist 1992). Such high-risk behaviour tends to be more common in males, and in some cases, may represent actual suicide attempts.

Help-seeking behaviour – Reluctance to seek help for oneself during times of stress and crisis may also contribute to suicide risk. This has been identified as a particular concern with young males who seem less willing than females to communicate their pain and emotional distress to potential helpers (Shaffer et al. 1990).

Related to this is the apparent reluctance of adolescents to solicit support from an adult when the adolescents are concerned about a potentially suicidal peer. In a survey exploring adolescents' experiences with suicidal peers, it was revealed that only 25 percent told an adult when a fellow student was feeling suicidal (Kalafat and Elias 1992).

Individual Capacity and Coping

Psychiatric disorders – A history of previous suicide attempts and the presence of a psychiatric disorder are well-established risk conditions for youth suicidal behaviour (Brent et al. 1988; Shaffer et al. 1988; Spirito et al. 1989b; Pfeffer et al. 1991). In a follow-up study of adolescent suicide attempters, 10 percent went on to make a subsequent attempt within the first three months of the original attempt (Spirito et al. 1992). Other studies suggest that anywhere between 10 and 14 percent of suicide attempters may go on to complete suicide (Diekstra 1989; Spirito et al. 1989b).

The most common psychiatric disorders among adolescents who have committed suicide are affective disorders, conduct disorders or antisocial personality disorders, and substance abuse (Brent et al. 1988; Shaffer 1988). The cooccurrence of disorders—in particular, affective disorders, substance abuse, and conduct disorders—is common among adolescents, and this type of comorbidity is often associated with an elevated risk for adolescent suicide (Shafii et al. 1985; Brent et al. 1988).

Cognitive deficits and coping strategies – Learning-disabled youngsters, and those who have deficits in interpersonal problem-solving skills, maladaptive coping styles and poor impulse control, have all been found to be at higher risk for suicidal behaviour (Hoberman and Garfinkel 1988b; Rourke, Young, and Leenaars 1989; Kienhorst et al. 1992). Although several studies have found that suicidal adolescents report having experienced more stressful life events, several recent investigations have shown that there are no significant differences between stressful life events experienced by suicidal and non-suicidal young people (Khan 1987; Spirito, Overholser, and Stark 1989). Given these findings, several authors have suggested that the coping mechanisms that adolescents use to deal with stressful life events may be the determining factor in suicidal behaviour (Curran 1987).

Clum, Patsiokas and Luscomb (1979) proposed that suicidal risk increases in individuals who have poor problem-solving abilities and are unable to think of alternative methods for dealing with stressful events. Investigating these potential cognitive influences on suicidal behaviour, researchers have concluded that suicidal adolescents use fewer cognitive coping skills (Asarnow, Carlson, and Guthri 1987), more frequently use social withdrawal as a means of coping with their problems (Spirito et al. 1989b), and demonstrate poorer problem-solving abilities (Curry, Miller, and Anderson 1992; Fremouw, Callahan, and Kashden 1993; Orbach et al. 1985; Levenson and Neuringer 1971).

Health Services

Comprehensive approach – A comprehensive service delivery strategy for preventing youth suicide highlights the range of services that should exist in, or be accessible to, a community, including mental health promotion, prevention and early intervention, crisis intervention, treatment, and bereavement and postvention services (White et al. 1991). The community services should be well known to adolescents, and key gatekeepers should be well prepared and trained to deal with potentially suicidal youth.

Use of services – If developmentally appropriate services do not exist or if adolescents are unaware of existing community services, the adolescents will be less likely to reach out for help in a crisis. One study found that adolescent suicide attempters were less likely to be aware of crisis services than adults who had attempted suicide (Greer and Anderson 1979).

Crisis response services need to meet the needs of both males and females in a suicidal crisis. Studies reveal that young men use the services of crisis hotlines much less frequently than young women (Shaffer et al. 1988), and furthermore, they tend to be less satisfied than women with the help that they receive (King 1977).

Skilled gatekeepers – Another critical consideration in a comprehensive service delivery strategy for preventing youth suicide is ensuring that those individuals who are most likely to come into contact with potentially suicidal youth have the skills and training to recognize suicide risk, assess the seriousness of the situation, and make an appropriate referral. Key gatekeepers that should have training in this area include school staff, parents, child welfare workers, community volunteers, coaches, police and clergy.

Other key service-level components that can contribute to the overall effort to prevent youth suicide in a community are supporting policies such as interagency protocols between schools and mental health centres for dealing with high-risk youth or postvention policies within the school system for managing the aftermath of a student suicide (Tierney et al. 1991; White 1994).

Summary of Key Findings

Youth suicidal behaviour is clearly complex, and like other human behaviours, it must be understood within a multidimensional framework that takes the individual, familial, social, economic, and cultural contexts intoaccount. Key findings from the literature suggest that the following con-ditions, in interaction with one another, pose the greatest risks for vulnerabilities leading to youth suicidal behaviour:
- negative early family experiences, characterized by loss, attachment problems, parental psychopathology, and family history of suicide and abuse;
- school problems, including academic failure and stressful environmental disruptions during key transition periods;
- peer difficulties, including the breakup of relationships, loss of friendships, and suicidal behaviour among peers;
- sensationalized media reports of suicide;
- cultural attitudes accepting of suicide as an option for dealing with problems;
- religious and social alienation;
- low income and poverty;
- easy access to firearms;
- substance abuse;
- reluctance to seek help for oneself or a peer;
- a history of previous suicidal behaviour;
- psychiatric disorders;
- learning disabilities and cognitive deficits; and
- lack of appropriate services for youth and trained gatekeepers in a community.

THE ELDERLY AND SUICIDAL BEHAVIOUR—RISK CONDITIONS

Social and Economic Environments

Age composition of the population – Canada is undergoing a dramatic shift in the makeup of the population. The proportion of persons over 65 years of age increased from 7.6 percent in 1961 to 11.6 percent in 1991, a 53 percent increase. The proportion of elderly people (65 years of age and over) to youths (10–24 years of age) climbed by 78 percent from 1961 (31.1 percent) to 1991 (55.5 percent), again reflecting an aging population. The old age–dependency ratio, defined as the ratio of the population 65 or more years of age to the working-age population (15–64 years of age), indicates that in 1961 there were 13.1 older adults for every 100 working-age persons, whereas, in 1991 there were 17.2 older adults for every 100 working-age persons, a 31 percent increase.

With such a shift in the age composition, the dynamics and experiences of specific populations such as that of the elderly may be rather different. For example, in a population that is increasing numerically, older persons may come to see themselves as superfluous and disadvantaged if society cannot incorporate them into the life and activity of the community (Osgood 1985). Easterlin (1980) proposed that as a cohort increases in size, competition for available resources becomes more intense. Thus, as the cohort of elderly persons increases in size, greater competition for resources would be expected, resulting in increased hardship for older persons and a concomitant increase in potential for suicide.

Preston (1984) suggested that in the United States the opposite may be true. He found that the growth in the elderly population is associated with improving conditions, as reflected in increases in social security and health care resources. Examining Preston's ideas further, McCall (1991) used time series regression models to assess the relationships between various social factors and suicide rates. In support of Preston's analysis, McCall's findings demonstrate the need to ensure the economic security and the availability of health care for the elderly to maintain decreasing suicide rates.

In Canada, where the proportion of elderly people in the population is increasing, conditions appear to be improving for the elderly. The Canada Pension Plan and other pension plans, old age security, universal health care, and social housing programs across the country, are but a few examples of the potential improvement of the economic circumstances of the elderly. Based on an analysis of the proportion of elderly living below the poverty line, it is clear that the economic circumstances of the elderly are indeed improving. Between 1980 and 1990, the percentage of elderly people living below the poverty line decreased from 33.6 percent to 19.3 percent, a 43 percent drop (Poverty profile 1980–1990: report by the National Council on Welfare, 1992). During this same period, suicide rates among elderly persons decreased from 17.6 to 13.2 per 100,000 population, a 25 percent decrease. A correlational analysis revealed that the rate of suicide and the level of poverty among older Canadians were significantly related ($r = .78$, $P < .05$), suggesting that the economic viability of the elderly is important to reducing the suicide rate.

Although an increasing number of the elderly are living above the poverty line, reduced income as a result of retirement continues to be a significant factor in increasing the vulnerability to suicide for a segment of older persons in the population (Lepine 1982). Limited income may require a downward adjustment in the standard of living that may negatively affect the quality of life, housing, friendships and social support systems. Financial difficulties may also lead to anxiety, depression and a sense of hopelessness about the future, and a sense of helplessness regarding one's capacity to do anything about it. These feelings have consistently been identified in the literature as precursors to suicidal behaviour.

Retirement – Retirement appears to have a widespread effect on older persons who later go on to commit suicide (Miller 1978). By its very nature, retirement causes a major loss of the occupational role that can result in an identity crisis and in a loss of status, meaning in life, self-respect, friendships and feelings of connectedness to society and to organizational and community life (Blau 1973).

Although retirement is often identified as a major contributor to suicidal behaviour among older persons (Lepine 1982), there appears to be little evidence to support a direct connection. According to Miller (1978), it is unclear whether elderly persons commit suicide because they are unhappy with retirement or suicidal elderly choose to retire early. Bagley and Ramsay (1993), in a community mental health survey, found that older persons were not particularly distressed by retirement or the loss of income associated with retirement. Similarly, Abrahams and Patterson (1978–79) found in a survey of elderly people that just over half of respondents were enjoying their retirement, even though most had been forced into it. However, approximately one-third "had got used to it" (13), and 14 percent were distressed. It is this latter group that may be at greatest risk for suicide.

Widowhood – Such role changes can have an even greater negative impact on those already distressed over retirement if this is accompanied by other losses. For example, if in addition to retirement, older men experience the death of a spouse, they may experience greater distress. They have not only lost an identity provided by their occupational role, but they have also lost a family or spousal role that provided a sense of personal significance, friendship and social support. Indeed, researchers have found that widowhood in older men is related to suicidal risk, particularly during the first two years after the loss (MacMahon and Pugh 1965; Berardo 1968; Bock and Webber 1972b; Benson and Brodie 1975; Miller 1978; Stroeber and Stroeber 1983).

Widowhood may have different effects on women and men (Parkes 1972). While a woman's life expectancy increases after the death of her husband, Parkes (1972) demonstrated that in the first year after a wife's death, the risk of death increased among men by 40 percent. This may be because husbands tend to be older than their wives and to have a shorter life expectancy and poorer health than older women. Moreover, in the present generation of the elderly, it is still women who deal with daily activities such as shopping and meals after men retire. Lopata (1973) explained the difference in reactions of men and women to widowhood by the fact that men tend to have fewer intimate relationships and supports and may rely more heavily on their spouse as a confidant. Consequently, the death of one's wife can result in a substantially reduced social world (Rosow 1967; Osgood 1985) and involvement in community life. Women, on the other hand, tend to have more family ties and other friendships, and are more likely to have a confidant to help them through stressful situations.

Social support – Lack of social support may be an important risk factor for suicide in the elderly, particularly when combined with other loss-related risk factors such as widowhood and retirement. The data from the Quebec Health Survey of 1992–93 showed that people who indicated having a confidant had significantly less suicidal ideation (3.6 percent) than those who indicated having no confidant (6.3 percent). Similarly, those who evaluated their social supports as poor were more likely to have considered suicide in the 12 months preceding the study (9.6 percent) than those who evaluated their level of social support as high (2.6 percent). Having someone to confide in and having family, friends and acquaintances to assist in dealing with crises, can buffer or reduce health problems, including suicidal behaviour. Research shows that living alone, being single, being widowed, being unable to build relationships outside the family, not having a confidant with whom to share experiences, and being without visitors are associated with suicide among the elderly (Barraclough 1971; Bock and Webber 1972a; Lonnqvist 1977; Abrahams and Patterson 1978–79; Miller 1978; Jarvis and Boldt 1980; Cattell and Jolley 1995; Draper 1995; Haight 1995).

Cultural and societal factors – A predominant attitude in Canada and the United States appears to place a good deal of value on youth and things that prolong a sense of being young and frown on growing old and being an elderly person. The elderly are often perceived as useless, dependent, frail and nonproductive; they are considered "over the hill" and should be "put out to pasture" (Osgood 1985; Evans, Fogle, and McDonald 1987). As Osgood suggests, the elderly cannot keep up with technological advancement and so are unable to make more than a little contribution, and their wisdom gained from years of experience is no longer valued by the young who live in a very different world than their grandparents. Consequently, self-esteem and sense of self-efficacy of some older persons are affected negatively and they become increasingly vulnerable to suicidal behaviour.

The attitudes of the public and care providers toward suicide, assisted suicide and euthanasia can also be important factors in suicide among the elderly. Evans, Fogle and McDonald (1987) found that attitudes toward elderly suicide were permissive, especially when there is perceived terminal illness.

Because of these seemingly prevailing attitudes, older people may worry that they could be coerced into suicidal behaviour by family members, society in general, or care providers. Research has indicated that while more than 90 percent of nursing home inhabitants were opposed to euthanasia or its legalization, 50–60 percent of these same inhabitants were fearful of being euthanized (Bostrom 1989; Fenigsen 1989). It is apparent that the elderly are concerned about how prevailing attitudes will be put into practice.

Although elder abuse and neglect of the elderly have been cited as factors possibly related to suicidal behaviour (e.g., Osgood 1985), there is little direct empirical evidence to conclusively link elder abuse or neglect to suicide. Podnieks and Pillemer (1990) found that approximately 4 percent of all Canadians age 65 years or over reported that they were victims of some form of mistreatment or abuse by members of their family. The review by Hudson and Johnson (1986) of 31 empirical studies on elder abuse concluded that women are more often victims of abuse than men and that victims tend to be over 75 years old. Elderly persons who live with others are more often at risk of abuse (Pillemer and Finkelhor 1988). Studies by O'Malley and colleagues (1979) and Lau and Kosberg (1979) found that 75 percent of victims of abuse have some form of physical or mental disability and that 75 percent of these individuals have also experienced stressful life events.

The noteworthy low levels of elderly suicide among Aboriginal persons are related to issues of culture, attitudes and elderly suicide. Harris and McCullough (1988) found that suicide across the life span of Aboriginal people in Canada was highest in the 15–19-year-olds and below the Canadian rates after the age of 60. Could it be that the suicide rate is found to be so low for Aboriginal elderly persons because of the respect given to the elders in First Nations communities and the overall level of support from families, friends and the community? Clearly, from the perspective taken in this paper, the answer would have to be a tentative yes, with the proviso that further investigation is needed.

Role of the media – Assessing the impact of television news stories about suicide on suicide rates, Stack (1991) found that news stories of elderly suicides had a significant impact on the suicide rate of those aged 65 years and over. The mechanisms that facilitate imitative behaviour of the elderly are unclear but could include such factors as the characteristics of the suicide, the specific vulnerabilities of the viewer, and specific features of the environment such as the availability of the means.

Physical Environment

Environmental and structural factors – In addition to specifically enriched environments (Mishara and Kastenbaum 1973), there are other environmental factors that could be expected to have an effect on suicide and suicidal behaviour. Since feelings of isolation and loneliness can contribute to suicidal behaviour in the elderly, any factors that affect interaction between staff and residents and among the residents may influence well-being and suicidal behaviour. Greenwald and Linn (1971) argued that levels of communication, satisfaction and activity declined as the size of the facility increased.

Osgood (1992) examined several environmental factors that could contribute to suicidal behaviour among residents of long-term care facilities. She surveyed a random sample of administrators of 1,080 facilities for information about the characteristics of their facility and suicidal and intentionally life-threatening behaviour. Higher staff turnover rates (50 percent or greater per year), higher numbers of residents (e.g., more than 100 residents), lower per diem costs, and religious or other facilities (as opposed to private or public), were associated with higher number of deaths by suicide.

Nursing home placement – In Canada, a relatively small proportion of the elderly (less than 5 percent of those aged 65 years and over) reside in institutions such as nursing homes and long-term care facilities. Nonetheless, the anticipation of nursing home placement can precipitate suicidal behaviour among the elderly. Loebel and colleagues (1991) found that in addition to other contributing factors to suicide among the elderly—such as depression and chronic or painful illness—nursing home placement was the most consistently identified precipitant.

On the other hand, nursing home placement can also serve as a protective factor for some vulnerable older persons (cf. Conwell 1994). Examining suicide rates among elderly residents of long-term care facilities, Osgood and Brant (1990) found lower rates in this population than among elderly persons living in noninstitutional settings. Any conclusions drawn from these preliminary findings should be treated with caution.

Availability of lethal means – In several death file review studies (Miller 1978; Jarvis and Boldt 1980; Cattell and Jolley 1995), researchers have found that the elderly prefer to use more violent means, such as firearms and hanging, in committing suicide. Men tend to use firearms and hanging more, whereas women use hanging and drug overdose. Some have argued that strict control of firearms could significantly reduce violent deaths in general and deaths by suicide in particular. Lester (1983, 1984, 1988a), in examining the relationship between handgun control laws and suicide deaths, found that states with stricter firearm controls had lower suicide rates across age groups, including among older persons.

The elderly also tend to have other means of ending their life, including such indirect self-destructive behaviours as self-starvation, misusing medications and not following physician orders, voluntarily withdrawing and isolating themselves, and mismanaging their diets, particularly if they are diabetic (Miller 1978; Nelson and Farberow 1980).

Personal Health Practices

Substance abuse and misuse – A history of alcoholism and current alcohol use may be implicated less often in suicidal behaviour among older persons, but it remains a factor to be considered. Investigators have found that older attempters are more likely to abuse alcohol (Lester and Beck 1974). Conwell, Rotenberg and Caine (1990), in a death file review study of persons who completed suicide, found that up to 10 percent of persons aged 65 and over had alcohol in their blood at the time of death. Of these, approximately 71 percent had blood levels of 0.10 percent or higher.

Mishara and Kastenbaum (1980) and Mishara and McKim (1989), in their reviews on alcohol use and abuse among the elderly, indicated that it is much less likely for an alcohol problem of an older person to be identified by either family or professionals. One reason for this is that the usual symptoms or indications of a drinking problem do not apply as easily to older persons. For example, trouble at work, an important indication of alcohol problems among younger people, is not an issue for an older person who is retired. The aggressive behaviour associated with alcohol-related troubles among those who drink in public is less of an issue, since elderly people more frequently drink alone. Very often the health and mental health problems associated with alcohol are viewed as "normal" physical problems, forgetfulness associated with aging, rather than being correctly identified as symptoms of alcohol consumption.

Both over-the-counter and prescription drugs have been implicated in suicidal behaviour among the elderly. Because of age-related changes in the absorption, distribution and elimination of drugs, older persons are generally more vulnerable to drug interactions and adverse reactions to medicines and drugs (Mishara and McKim 1989). Several national surveys (e.g., Health and Welfare Canada, Statistics Canada 1981; Québec, Santé Québec 1995) indicate that more than two-thirds of Canadians over age 65 are using prescription and over-the-counter medicines weekly. On average, these older persons use five different drugs, including over-the-counter medicines and those prescribed by physicians. Although research results indicate that psychological distress is least prevalent in persons over age 65 (Québec, Santé Québec 1995), as a group the elderly use the most psychotropic medications. Tranquillizers and medicines to help with sleep are prescribed more often for the elderly than any other medication. The most common adverse reactions to medication and its side effects mimic senile psychosis, such as Alzheimer's disease; the most common symptoms include problems with memory and cognition.

Most older persons in Canada have at their disposal medications that can be used to end their lives. The symptoms of the inappropriate use of medication may be interpreted by older persons as irreversible problems associated with aging, rather than reversible symptoms resulting from inappropriate drug use. Sometimes it is difficult to determine whether a death from a minor drug overdose is an accident or a suicide. Similarly, lack of compliance with a prescription routine is also difficult to interpret; one may not know whether the individual failed to take a necessary medicine because of a desire to die prematurely or if it was unintentional. Numerous authors (e.g., Cooper, Love, and Raffoul 1984) found that a substantial number of older persons (in this study 43 percent) failed to comply with prescribed medication routines and that most of the errors were of omission, not taking the drugs (in this study 90 percent). Noncompliance may be related to the cost of the drugs, as well as a number of other factors, including misunderstanding of instructions from the physician and an inability to open childproof containers. However, some individuals who fail to comply indicate clearly that they wish to die and for this reason refuse to take necessary medication (Mishara and McKim 1984).

Help-seeking behaviour – Reaching out for help and assistance may be particularly difficult for the elderly. Such difficulty in reaching out may be the result of a lack of confidence in obtaining help from a telephone call to a seniors' crisis line, lack of knowledge about where to find help or how and whom to contact for help, or an inability to express the need for help to available care providers, such as physicians. For example, crisis centres and helplines generally report that relatively few older persons in Canada call to obtain help during a suicidal crisis. This may be due to habits and beliefs in the current cohort of older persons, who grew up at a time when telephones were not readily available and it was not generally regarded as acceptable to tell one's troubles to a stranger on the telephone or to seek mental health services unless a person was quite "crazy."

Nonetheless, the majority of older persons who commit suicide see their physician within several months of their death (Lepine 1982), usually for a physical problem. In an early study of suicide among the elderly, Barraclough (1971) found that approximately 90 percent of older persons who committed suicide had visited a physician within three months of death; 70 percent within a month; and almost half, during their last week. Although the proportions vary, visiting physicians within a short period of time before their suicide is a common finding (Miller 1978; Cattell and Jolley 1995).

Individual Capacity and Coping

Coping resources – Although aging is related to physical decline and an increased risk of chronic illnesses, most of the changes associated with aging are quite gradual and only affect maximum capacities, while impairing none of the usual activities in daily living. Although the maximum speed a person can run may diminish and the maximum number of words a person can memorize all at once may decline, it is rare for elderly people to run as fast as they can or memorize as many words as possible in the course of their daily lives. Furthermore, most elderly people compensate for any perceived declines by adjusting their behaviour. People who begin to forget certain things may begin to keep a list, or individuals experiencing a loss of energy may enroll in an exercise program or change their diet and reduce their weight. It has been suggested (Mishara and Riedel 1994) that older people have a much greater capacity for coping and adaptation to life stresses because of their greater experience in dealing with problems. A loss for an adolescent may seem like the end of the world and result in suicidal ideation or behaviour. A similar loss for an older person may be viewed with the wisdom that comes from having experienced and survived many life crises. Contrary to current stereotypes, results from various surveys across Canada indicate that older persons give more instrumental support to their family members than they receive. They are more likely to give money to their children than receive money from them; they are more likely to help their children with home repairs than to receive help. The stereotype of the dependent older person incapable of coping with life stresses is not unsupported in research studies on the elderly in Canada.

However, as in any other age group, some elderly individuals exhaust their coping resources and are extremely troubled by losses they have experienced. Biological changes, such as a loss of sensory acuity across the senses, decreasing motor abilities, loss of hair and teeth, and chronic diseases that are often accompanied by pain and incapacitation, make life difficult to bear. Social changes, such as the loss or death of a spouse or friend, loss of associations with work, organizations or community activities, and giving up one's home to enter an institution, can often lead to frustration, anxiety, anger, grief, loss of self-esteem and self-efficacy, isolation, loneliness, depression, and despair. As these accumulate, the elderly's ability to cope may well be exhausted, and suicide becomes an option.

Mental illness – Depression is often associated with older persons who are experiencing the numerous personal, social and physical losses discussed above (Wasylenki 1980). Indeed, research indicates that between 60 and 80 percent of older persons who commit suicide suffered from depression (Jarvis and Boldt 1980; Gurland and Cross 1983; Dyck and White 1990; Cattell and Jolley 1995).

But not all research supports the conclusion that the elderly are more vulnerable to mental ill health. Studies report a decline in depressive symptoms with age (Frerichs, Aneshensel, and Clark 1980; Lieberman 1983), with rates lower than those of young or middle-aged adults, and lower lifetime prevalence rates of psychiatric disorders in general and affective disorders in particular (Bland, Newman, and Orn 1988). Conwell, Rotenberg and Caine (1990), in a death file study of 246 completed suicides of persons over the age of 50, found that psychiatric histories were less common with increasing age.

Taken together, these studies do not describe a consistent pattern of the relationship between mental ill health and aging or between mental ill health and suicide in an aging population. Such inconsistency in findings can be explained in part by methodological differences, use of different populations, and differences in types of measuring instruments (D'Arcy 1986).

Other forms of mental illness that relate to cognitive functioning may bear some relation to suicidal behaviour. Organic mental diseases are more common among older persons and are characterized by disturbances or deterioration in memory, problems in intellectual functioning and judgment, difficulties in orientation, and superficial or labile emotions. The most common organic mental disorders are Alzheimer's disease and cardiovascular-related diseases, which result in gradual irreversible deterioration in functioning. Fear of developing an irreversible dementia, such as in Alzheimer's disease, has been cited as a possible factor in suicide. For example, one of the individuals whom Dr. Kevorkian "helped" to end her life feared that she was suffering from Alzheimer's and indicated that this was her reason for wanting to end her life. In some instances, the fear is unfounded because an acute reversible brain syndrome is mistaken for an irreversible syndrome, such as Alzheimer's. Many people fearing they have Alzheimer's disease have committed suicide. There are also undocumented reports that suffering from more advanced mental deterioration reduces the risk of suicide, since it is more difficult to carry out the task.

Chronic disease and physical illness – Several investigators (Jarvis and Boldt 1980; Draper 1995) have documented the contribution of physical illness and chronic disease to suicidal behaviour among the elderly. Terminal illness, chronic illness (e.g., cardiovascular disease, diabetes, respiratory diseases) and physical disability that result in increased dependence on care providers, chronic pain, and increased likelihood of institutionalization have been linked to depression and suicide (Shulman 1978; McCartney 1978; Conwell, Rotenberg, and Caine 1990; Frierson 1991; Draper 1995). With increasing age, the proportion of suicides among the elderly known to be terminally ill also increases (Jarvis and Boldt 1980).

Health Services

Use of existing services – Based on death file reviews, elderly suicide completers used a variety of services, including hospitals and physicians (Cattell and Jolley 1995). However, they appear to have underused mental health services, even though depressive disorders are the most common psychopathologies of later life (Barraclough 1971; National Institute on Aging 1987; Conwell, Rotenberg, and Caine 1990).

Skilled gatekeepers – As already discussed, most elderly people who commit suicide visited their physician within weeks or months of their death. Yet physicians appeared not to recognize the potential for suicide. It is not known at this time whether they failed to recognize the potential because of failure on the part of their patients to indicate their suicidal intentions or because the psychopathology presented was less clear as a result of its atypical nature (Conwell, Rotenberg, and Caine 1990) or because physicians did not know what the appropriate intervention should be or where to find it. Some evidence suggests that physicians and other gate-keepers receive little formal training in suicide prevention or intervention. The original Task Force on Suicide in Canada (Health Canada 1994) conducted surveys of the faculties of medicine, nursing, social work and psychology at Canadian universities to assess the level of education provided on suicide and its prevention. The task force found suicide education limited in all the specified faculties at the undergraduate level but that there seemed to be a somewhat stronger focus at the graduate level. It was also found that suicide was treated less as a separate issue and more as a general topic related to depression.

Summary of Key Findings

Some of the key findings from the literature are as follows:
1. Suicide rates among the elderly in Canada have been declining over the last decade, which also happens to coincide with the decrease in the number of elderly living below the poverty line ($r = .79$). In other words, economic viability of the elderly is a protective factor against suicide.
2. Social support, especially that of having a confidant, is influential in reducing suicidal behaviour among older persons. Retirement, loss of spouse and friends through death, and loss of home can have tremendous negative effects on the elderly and increase their vulnerability to suicide.
3. While institutional placements can be protective of vulnerable and suicidal elderly people, conditions within these settings can also induce greater risk for suicide. Institutions with larger populations, high staff turnover, higher per diem costs, and religious and "other" facilities have been associated with higher rates of suicide among the elderly.
4. Permissive attitudes toward suicide in the elderly have been demonstrated both within the general public and among care providers. These attitudes have the potential to influence both the type of intervention provided to a potentially suicidal older person and the speed with which it will be provided.
5. Availability of firearms and medications enhances the risk of suicide among the elderly.
6. Mental illness, especially depression, and chronic illness may place some elderly persons at risk for suicide.
7. Although many elderly people visit a physician within weeks of their suicide, their intentions at those times are not identified, and appropriate interventions are not undertaken.
8. Both alcohol and drug use have been implicated in suicide and suicidal behaviour among the elderly.
9. That suicide in the First Nations elderly population is so low can serve as a model for the rest of Canada concerning the ways to view, respect and support older persons.

NOTEWORTHY PROGRAMS

Judging the Success of Suicide Prevention Efforts

Programs that have as their ultimate goal the prevention of suicide and suicidal behaviour are difficult to evaluate for many reasons. First, completed suicide is a phenomenon with a low base rate when considered at local or community levels, which makes it difficult to detect changes attributable to the efforts of specific programs. Second, the events we have prevented from occurring are very difficult to measure in any reliable way; in this case suicidal behaviour. Third, many efforts to prevent suicide are designed to target younger children and their key socializing environments by building their social competencies, strengthening their families and improving conditions in their schools and communities. The effects of such programs on later suicidal behaviour will not be known for several years after the intervention. Fourth, suicide and suicidal behaviour outcomes do not follow a linear or simple causal pathway, with specific markers leading predictably to the point of disorder or death. This makes it challenging to identify the appropriate intermediate targets for change and the corresponding outcome measures that would be most suitable for purposes of evaluation.

As highlighted in the previous section, suicidal behaviour is multiply determined, and a wide range of antecedent risk conditions can interact to create a potential for suicidal behaviour. Evaluating the effectiveness of efforts to prevent suicide means having an appreciation of the complexity of that behaviour, understanding the multiple developmental and dynamic pathways that lead to conditions of risk or vulnerability in a population, and developing appropriate intermediate and long-term outcome measures.

Silverman and Felner (1995, 103) suggested that by approaching program development and evaluation from a "developmental pathway-antecedent risk condition perspective," planners of suicide prevention programs are in a better position to monitor the effects of their efforts on the "key conditions that are earlier in the developmental pathway." In this way, the challenges of low rates of occurrence and the delay between the intervention and expected onset of the problematic behaviour can be circumvented because one can determine whether the program is effective without having to place exclusive reliance on rates of completed suicide as the only outcome measure.

The School Transition Environment Program

Actions on nonmedical determinants of health – The School Transition Environment Program (STEP) was initiated in Illinois and has two main goals: (1) to reorganize the school routines to reduce the degree of flux and complexity encountered by the student; and (2) to restructure the roles of homeroom teachers and guidance personnel (Felner and Adan 1988). Specific strategies include assigning STEP students to the same classes so that there is a high degree of constancy and overlap among the STEP students; keeping the STEP classrooms in proximity to one another; and broadening the homeroom teacher's role to include administrative duties and guidance counselling. The aim is to cultivate a climate in which students feel a strong sense of belonging and perceive their school as a stable, supportive, orderly and understandable environment.

Reasons for the initiative – The normative transition from one school to another, such as from junior high to senior high, has been associated with significant shifts in psychological and academic adjustment among adolescents, including increased absenteeism, decreased academic performance, decreased emotional well-being, and increased potential for substance abuse, delinquency and other behavioral and social problems (Felner, Ginter, and Primavera 1982; Felner and Adan 1988). STEP is intended to facilitate students' transition from one school environment to another by modifying particular elements of the school setting.

Actors – STEP was originally undertaken in a large urban high school, and students entering it were primarily from low socioeconomic and minority backgrounds. Criteria for selecting teachers for STEP include those who regularly teach the incoming students' academic subjects; those who volunteer to participate; and those whose classrooms are situated in proximity to one another. Teacher preparation before the school term includes one full day of skills development training which is devoted to enhancing teachers' academic and social-emotional counselling skills. This training can be provided by guidance counselling staff or outside professionals. A second day of teacher preparation is devoted to team building activities.

Results – After one full year of the program, matched control students showed significant decreases in academic performance and increases in rates of absenteeism, compared with STEP students. Control students showed declines in their self-concept scores, while STEP students' scores remained stable. STEP students perceived the school environment as more stable, understandable, well organized, involving and supportive (Felner and Adan 1988). A welcome but unexpected finding from STEP was the participating teachers' overall satisfaction with the program. The teachers reported feeling better about the school environment, and they showed improvements in their attitudes toward teaching in general, as well as toward their students.

Replicability – In an effort to replicate these findings, other STEP initiatives were undertaken in a variety of other school settings (Felner, Adan, and Evans 1987). A broader range of outcome measures were used in these subsequent studies to include such factors as depression and other emotional problems, anxiety, and conduct disorders; school behaviour problems; delinquency and substance abuse; suicidal ideation; and grades, absences and self-concepts. The findings from these studies confirmed those of the initial STEP initiative: STEP students showed fewer declines in academic performance, fewer decreases on indicators of positive mental health, and fewer increases in emotional and behavioral difficulties, compared with control students.

STEP programs are intended for large schools that serve students who come from a number of different feeder schools, where the risk of confusion, stress and social disorganization is much greater than it would be in smaller schools. As well school populations characterized by lower academic and socioeconomic levels appear to benefit the most from the STEP model.

Funding – Another critical consideration in understanding STEP's success is its ability to be implemented with minimal cost and to place few demands on a school's resources. The implementation of the STEP program requires a reorganization of the school environment, as well as some initial preparatory training time for participating teachers. It does not demand the development or implementation of new curricula and is minimally disruptive to teaching schedules. These characteristics make it particularly attractive to school administrators and teaching staff.

Evaluation – A key strength of STEP is that it has been in place for several years and has been well evaluated. Furthermore, the project has provided substantial longitudinal data for a broad range of outcome measures, and several studies have been published (Felner, Ginter, and Primavera 1982; Felner and Adan 1988).

Alaska's Community-Based Suicide Prevention Project

Actions on nonmedical determinants of health – Between 1989 and 1993, the Alaska Department of Health and Social Services, Division of Mental Health, provided funding for the development and implementation of community-based suicide prevention programs in small Alaskan communities. Each funded project was unique and reflected the diverse culture and needs of the community within which it was developed:

> The Community-Based Suicide Prevention Projects do not look like mental health programs nor do they provide an array of mental health "services." Rather than have a name, these projects have a mission. Rather than provide services to individuals, these projects direct interventions to the community at large. Rather than being run by professionals who are not from the community, these projects are coordinated by local people who work to improve the community where they live and will probably always live. Rather than provide help to individuals or groups, these projects work to show individuals and groups how to help themselves (Bernier 1994, 6).

Reasons for the initiative – Following the completion of the "Interim Report of the Senate Special Committee on Suicide Prevention" (Hensley

1988), the U. S. Department of Health and Social Services undertook the development of a rural human services program based on the concept of using community development to tackle the well-documented problems of suicide and drinking in small Alaskan communities. According to Bernier (1994, 1), the report highlighted the limitations of the existing methods for dealing with suicide and self-destructive behaviour, noting that "the current model of human services delivery to Alaskan villages is not working" and that the current model relies heavily on "itinerant, non-Native professionals based in regional hub communities."

Small rural communities, defined as communities with fewer than 1,000 people, have rarely received state funding for local initiatives. There are approximately 171 communities throughout Alaska that fit this criterion. The Community-Based Suicide Prevention (CBSP) project has been particularly successful in supporting initiatives in these rural communities.

Actors – Senator Hensley's 1988 report compiled information on suicide and other forms of self-destructive behaviour, highlighted the results from public hearings held across the state, and documented the state's capacity to respond to the issue of suicide. One of the major themes of the report was the notion that suicide in the villages could be understood only within the social context of these small rural communities. Furthermore, to address the complex social factors and stresses, the report recommended that policies should support initiatives generated by the communities themselves.

While the report provided no clearly articulated regulation, the legislative intent was honoured through the conceptualization, implementation and ongoing operation of the CBSP project. This was achieved because "the individuals within state government who are responsible for program implementation internalized the goals of the program, have the professional skills and experience to effectively monitor program implementation, and have first-hand experience in communities where project activities are funded" (Bernier 1994, 1). In many ways, it has been the willingness and commitment of the state government to support local control and community ownership that has led to the success of the CBSP project.

The project manager, through the Division of Mental Health, established a series of operational goals for funding, which reflected the spirit and intent of Senator Hensley's report and the needs of communities most affected by suicide. For example, the emphasis was placed on community involvement and community-based initiatives, rather than demonstrating adherence to particular service goals or achieving specific targets.

Recommendations for funding individual projects, including funding levels and policies, were provided to the Division of Mental Health by an interdepartmental team, which served to strengthen a "non-categorical approach to funding" (Bernier 1994, iv). Small communities were actively encouraged to apply for funding, and technical assistance was provided in completing grant applications.

Results – After four years, the CBSP project in Alaska has generated some very promising results, including the following:

1. Suicide rates in communities with CBSP projects in place have apparently declined at a faster rate than the statewide suicide rates for Alaskan Natives.
2. Through the CBSP projects, local people have become more knowledgeable about the problems of suicide and self-destructive behaviour, and ongoing community programs of activities not involving alcohol have been developed.
3. Several important community-based responses for dealing with self-destructive behaviour have been initiated including increased referrals for at-risk persons, development of support groups, and organization of local action groups and task forces to respond to suicide and self-destructive behaviour.
4. CBSP projects have positively influenced the behaviour of individuals who live in their communities, including increasing the number of proactive responses toward people perceived as being at risk and increasing the adoption of healthier behaviour.
5. Continuously funded projects that have been functioning for almost five years are institutionalizing change in their communities, which is apparent in the development of local support groups and youth or adult advisory boards, the involvement of local governments in addressing suicidal behaviour, and the existence of broad-level community support.
6. Specific changes noted among the five case study communities include more local residents being able to identify and appropriately refer a suicidal person, more community members reporting having provided assistance to a child experiencing personal problems, increased abstinence and a decrease in abusive drinking, and an increased perception among community residents that they have control over local problems.

Permanence of the changes – Thirty-five percent of the projects have been continuously funded since 1989. Even though many of these small rural communities lack the formal infrastructure to support community-based initiatives, they have maintained programs of sufficient quality and scope to warrant continued state funding. It is clear that these communities are strongly committed to the CBSP projects, and reliance on state support was kept to a minimum. For example, it is estimated that communities will leverage U.S.$0.76 for every U.S.$1.00 of state funding, despite the fact that there is no required match for these projects.

Funding – Over the past five fiscal years, up to U.S.$860,000 has been allocated each year to directly support community-based suicide prevention projects through the Division of Mental Health. Average funding awards were approximately U.S.$15,000, with between 47 and 60 projects being funded each year. Seventy percent of project funding went to communities with fewer than 500 people, and nearly 100 percent of all funds were spent in communities with populations of fewer than 1,000 people.

Increased community involvement and support was indirectly facilitated through the fairly low levels of funding. Communities were encouraged to seek out contributions in kind, as well as other sources of support in the community, to augment state funding.

Evaluation – The evaluation had three levels: case study, community assessment, and community self-assessment. Five communities served as case studies, and baseline data were collected along a number of dimensions, through the following: site visits, community profiles, baseline statistics, key informant interviews, project coordinator interviews, household survey on knowledge, attitudes and behaviour, and adolescent focus groups. Eight communities participated in the community assessment. Baseline data were also collected in these communities but along fewer dimensions than those included for the pilot communities. Forty-one communities were administered the self-assessment survey at the project's inception and at five-year follow-up. Suicide deaths and suicide attempts were recorded for all participating communities. A summary of the evaluation design, overall findings and copies of the instruments are included in the final report (Bernier 1994).

The Gatekeeper Model for the Isolated, At-Risk Elderly

Actions on nonmedical determinants of health – The Gatekeeper Model was developed in Spokane, Washington, to identify and refer elderly people who were underserved or unserved altogether by community-based agencies (Raschko 1990). The elderly targeted for this program were those living in their own homes, and suffering from physical illnesses, significant memory impairment, emotional problems, including depression, and environmental and social stress. Furthermore, these elderly people demonstrated difficulty with personal care and activities of daily living, and were socially isolated and generally lacked a personal support system. The major strategy employed was to use the people who, through their daily work activities, come into contact with these high-risk elderly people and provide these workers with training so that they could identify and appropriately refer those in need to community-based services.

Reasons for the initiative – According to Raschko (1990), there were three major reasons for the program. These include the following:

1. it is difficult to identify and locate isolated, resistant, high-risk elderly people who have no support system to act on their behalf;
2. the majority of community-based agencies are organized to have persons from the target population access services by coming to the agency, rather than the agency going out to locate at-risk elderly people and providing the services in their own home; and

3. the high-risk elderly feel shame, suffer depression, fear that they will lose control over their lives, and are anxious about being removed from their homes and placed into a nursing home. Consequently, the at-risk elderly tend to be unserved or underserved.

Actors – Because the people in the program's target group are isolated and have few social supports, nontraditional gatekeepers need to be used to identify these at-risk elderly and make appropriate referrals. These gatekeepers work for corporations, businesses and social agencies that have contact with the target population. Included as gatekeepers are meter readers, repair personnel working for major utility companies, residential property appraisers, telephone company personnel, apartment and mobile home managers, postal workers, police, firefighters and pharmacists. It was important that gatekeepers received ongoing training and feedback on referrals to maintain a high level of service.

Once an at-risk older person is identified, the people working in the In-Home Multidisciplinary Assessment/Evaluation program are notified and a comprehensive in-home evaluation is conducted. The case manager and team leader conduct the initial visit and evaluation and bring a psychiatrist and internist, when required. A service and treatment plan is developed and initiated, which may include medical, psychiatric, socio-economic, environmental manipulation, and medication interventions. The success of this integrated approach is the result of the collaboration of these various agencies, organizations and preventive, supportive and rehabilitative services in providing services (Raschko 1990).

Analysis of results – While program outcomes have not been particularly well documented, there is some evidence that it is fulfilling the original intent, that is, to reach the isolated, at-risk elderly. First, while it was estimated that approximately 4 percent of the national population in the United States consisted of underserved persons 60 years of age and over, 21 percent of Spokane Community Health Center's caseload consisted of these under-served elderly people. Second, no shortage of nursing home beds was experienced after 1984 in Spokane county, partly a result of this program and the collaborative efforts of the network of services that support it. Third, the relationship between the Eastern Washington Area Agency on Aging and the Spokane Mental Health Center is unique among mental health centers. Fourth, it has been shown that 4 out of every 10 admissions to the in-home case management program are the result of the gatekeeper system.

Identifying at-risk elderly through nontraditional gatekeepers appears to have achieved some beneficial results. This may be due to the following:
- recruiting, training and supporting a wide variety of gatekeepers not only expands the sphere of contact with the target population but also increases the likelihood that these gatekeepers will remain motivated to identify and make referrals;

- having a network of organizations and agencies provides the opportunity to share the work and the satisfaction of being helpful, as well as being able to learn from each other; and
- having a place to which the gatekeepers can refer the elderly and have every confidence that the person will be seen and given assistance.

Replicability of the initiative – This particular approach is relatively easy to replicate, given three very important elements: 1) cooperation from businesses and agencies or organizations within a community to encourage staff who come into contact with the isolated elderly to participate in such a gatekeeper program; 2) an available and coordinated network of services that can manage the health and social service issues of the identified at-risk elderly; and 3) the training of, and ongoing support for, staff who volunteer to serve as gatekeepers.

Funding – Two integrated components of the Spokane Mental Health Center's Elderly Services Program are Telephone Information and Referral and the Multidisciplinary In-Home Evaluation, Treatment and Case Management. Since the Gatekeeper Model is an important part of the Multidisciplinary In-Home Evaluation, Treatment and Case Management component, it derives its funding from those organizations that fund the integrated components, namely, the Eastern Washington Area Agency on Aging, the Washington State Mental Health Grant-in-Aid, and the National Institute on Drug Abuse. While budgets are not available, the Gatekeeper Model requires very little funding to operate, since it is largely volunteer based, rather than staff intensive.

Evaluation – There is little information at this time about intensive evaluation. However, the results discussed above indicate that this approach is increasing the number of those isolated, at-risk elderly who are being identified, referred, and provided with the necessary services. Nonetheless, more information is required regarding the longer-term benefits for these older persons who receive services.

Suicide-Action Montreal Program for Widowers

Reasons for the initiative – Men over 65 constitute one of the highest risk groups for completed suicide in Canada. For men, one of the periods in which the risk for suicide is greatest is in the two years after the death of a spouse. Despite the high risk of suicide in this group, few older men call the hotline at Suicide-Action Montreal for help with crises. Therefore, Suicide-Action Montreal developed an initiative to reach this group through a bereavement support group for elderly widowers.

Actors – The widowers' program was developed by Suicide-Action Montreal, the volunteer-based regional suicide prevention centre serving the metropolitan Montreal area. The program was funded by a special grant from the United Way to create a pilot suicide prevention program for the elderly.

Objectives – The objectives of the widowers' program were to "accompany" widowers to help them with the grieving process and to attempt to transform the process of grief into an experience of personal growth, primarily by teaching the individual to be better acquainted with resources and supports available in his environment. The program was based on the goals proposed by Worden (1982). According to Worden's model, each of the following tasks needs to be accomplished to resolve the loss: (1) acceptance of the reality of the loss; (2) expression of the pain related to this loss; (3) adaptation to the environment where the partner is absent; and (4) withdrawal of emotional energy from the relationship and reinvestment of this energy in other relationships.

This program used volunteers with at least 100 hours of experience in intervention with suicidal persons at Suicide-Action Montreal. Volunteers received training to prepare them to accompany widowers based on a program developed by Suzanne Le Poidevin in her research on bereavement at the London Hospital Medical College in the United Kingdom. Volunteers received training on the nature of the bereavement process, as well as on methods of counselling the bereaved, cognitive techniques in problem solving, and techniques for use in face-to-face communication that were adapted to the program for accompanying widowers.

Participants in the program were men over age 55 who had experienced the death of a spouse less than two years before they entered the program. The program lasted eight months, during which there were 12 meetings (every two weeks), followed by two other meetings one month apart. Meetings lasted 1.5 hours at the home of the widower or at the suicide prevention centre. Widowers were recruited from those who called Suicide-Action Montreal, and a brochure describing the program, which was distributed throughout the Montreal area through various health and mental health services, as well as through social organizations that had contact with older persons.

Analysis of results – At the time of this writing, analyses of the results of this program are currently being conducted. Participants are evaluated before their first meeting with the volunteers, after six months of participation in the program, and one year after the beginning of the program. Evaluation is conducted by four instruments: Parkes' Bereavement Scale, Perceived Well-Being Scale, Situational Anxiety Scale (from Spielberger) and the Geriatric Depression Scale.

Replicability of the initiative – This is a program that is fairly easy to conduct in a number of different settings, using volunteers from different organizations.

Funding – This is a relatively cost-effective program, since it involves volunteers and the only expenses are those related to printing a brochure and training and supervising of volunteers.

Evaluation – The evaluation is described in the analyses of the results. The primary problem with the evaluation is that there were no direct or indirect measures of suicidality and no long-term evaluation of outcomes to provide an indication of the effectiveness of the program in preventing suicide. Furthermore, there was no control group for comparison.

The High/Scope Perry Preschool Program

Actions on nonmedical determinants of health – The High/Scope Perry Preschool Program was initiated in Michigan and has as its primary goal the development of children's skills and dispositions to serve as a foundation for adaptive functioning in the school setting (Schweinhart and Weikart 1988). Children targeted for this program were those at risk for school failure because of the lack of education and income of parents and children whose home environments were considered stressful. Thus, the major strategies employed included using a developmentally appropriate curriculum based on child-centred activities, ensuring a small student-teacher ratio, using staff trained in early childhood development, involving parents as partners with the staff, and attending to the noneducational needs of the child and family. Overall, the aim of the program was to increase the potential for school success of children at risk for school failure.

Reasons for the initiative – According to Schweinhart and Weikart (1988), early childhood education can serve to break the poverty cycle that places children at risk. Developing adaptive functioning skills and abilities that improve school performance can interrupt the path from child poverty, to school failure, to juvenile delinquency and crime and, eventually, to adult poverty and its associated social problems. Indeed, school failure has been associated with not only childhood poverty but also later adult poverty (Schweinhart and Weikart 1988).

Schweinhart and Weikart (1988) suggested that intervention during early childhood may provide the greatest benefit. During early childhood, children are sufficiently mature in the physical, social and mental domains for providing appropriate and relevant opportunities to learn thinking and social skills and to develop a sense of curiosity and persistence at tasks. These opportunities will give them the foundation for school success.

Actors – The High/Scope Perry Preschool Program was undertaken in an urban setting where 3- and 4-year-olds from families of low socioeconomic status were assigned randomly to the program or a control. Most children attended the program five mornings per week for seven months for each of two years. In addition, home visits were conducted by a staff person every week of the program. The classroom group consisted of approximately 25 children with a staff-child ratio of between 1:5 and 1:6. It should be emphasized that staff were well trained in childhood develop-ment and education.

Moreover, they were active in developing opportunities for parent involvement in their child's experience.

Because the High/Scope curriculum was judged developmentally appropriate and based on Piaget's perspective on children as active and self-initiating learners, this curriculum was selected as the basis for instruction. No workbooks as such are used; rather, at the beginning of each class, each child, together with his teacher, develops a plan, carries out that plan, and then develops another plan to be carried out, and so on. After carrying out several plans, the child meets with the teacher to review what the child has done. In this process, the children are enabled to initiate and carry out their own learning activities, as well as to make their own learning decisions.

Analysis of the results – The Perry Preschool Program has been carefully examined in both short- and long-term outcomes. The High/Scope Educational Research Foundation's long-term Preschool Curriculum Comparison study included a comparison of three preschool curriculum models (direct instruction model, High/Scope model, and a typical nursery school model), and investigators found that all three programs produced increases in mean intelligence quotient scores (Schweinhart, Weikart, and Larner 1986). Moreover, they found that by age 15, participants in both the High/Scope and the nursery-school groups engaged in significantly fewer acts of delinquency than the direct instruction group.

Following up participants in the Perry Preschool Program, investigators found that in comparison with those with no preschool, participants in the program achieved better academically and were rated by teachers as being more socially and emotionally mature (Weikart, Bond, and McNeil 1978). Furthermore, participants demonstrated greater commitment to schooling and valued schooling more by the age of 15 (Schweinhart and Weikart 1988).

By age 19, participants were found to score higher on measures of literacy and life skills. In addition, they had better jobs and less unemployment, received less public assistance, saved money routinely, were arrested less often, and reported fewer pregnancies and births.

In a recent report, researchers followed up the Perry Preschool Program sample of children to age 27 (Schweinhart et al. 1993). Compared with nonparticipants, program participants were arrested less often and were more likely to earn $2,000 or more per month, own their own home, have a second car, and graduate from regular or adult high school or receive a General Education Development certification. Moreover, fewer participants received welfare assistance or other social services.

The approach used in the High/Scope Perry Preschool Program clearly prepared children from low-income families to succeed not only in school but also in society as a whole. Schweinhart and colleagues (1993) suggested several reasons for the significant and lasting results of the program. First, children were given the opportunity and responsibility to determine their own learning activities and to make decisions about their own learning.

Second, emphasis on parental involvement in the child's learning and development was considered critical in the support of the child's development of skills and abilities. Finally, Schweinhart and colleagues suggested that curriculum training for teachers, provision of the necessary tools for monitoring children's developmental progress, and overall support from senior staff provided a positive environment for children to maximize their learning potential.

Replicability – On the basis of the long-term results of this program, it is apparent that the High/Scope Perry Preschool Program has had a positive impact. Other preschool programs that have been examined and have used similar child-initiated learning frameworks have also met with success. Schweinhart and Weikart (1988) reviewed early childhood programs and concluded that the effective programs have several components in common. These include

- a curriculum that is developmentally appropriate and based on child-initiated learning;
- a small teacher-student ratio (e.g., less than 1:10);
- staff well trained in both early childhood development and the child-initiated learning curriculum;
- parent involvement;
- attention to other needs of the child that are not educational; and
- an appropriate evaluation process.

It is not difficult to see that these criteria are easily applicable, transferable and operational in most settings, given the necessary political will to establish priorities in this area.

Funding – While specific information about funding is not available at this time, Schweinhart and colleagues (1993) stated that the cost per participant in 1992 U.S. dollars was U.S.$12,356, based on five children for each staff member. If the number of children per adult were increased to eight, the cost per child per year would be reduced to approximately U.S.$5,500, with little, if any, loss in the quality of the program. Recommendations from the National Head Start Association's Silver Ribbon Panel indicated that a similar cost per child per year was an appropriate expenditure.

Schweinhart and colleagues also conducted a cost-benefit analysis of the program and its long-term effects. Using constant 1992 U.S. dollars, discounted annually at 3 percent, the investigators found that for every dollar invested in the High/Scope Perry Preschool Program, U.S.$7.16 was returned to taxpayers.

Evaluation – The High/Scope Perry Preschool Program has undergone extensive study and evaluation. Research and evaluation documents can be obtained through the research literature or by writing directly to the High/Scope Educational Research Foundation, 600 North River Street, Ypsilanti, MI, 48198-2898, United States. In total, the Foundation has produced six monographs, a colour videotape illustrating the age-27 findings, and a paper describing the cost-benefit analysis.

A Postvention Effort in New South Wales, Australia

Actions on nonmedical determinants of health – Postvention activities are typically initiated after a suicide attempt or completion and generally are implemented in populations of youths who tend to be at greatest risk for imitative suicidal behaviour. Postvention efforts are designed to reduce levels of immediate distress in populations that have been exposed to a death by suicide and are often delivered in the school setting. Postvention plans usually include the following elements: support and factual information presented to school staff; coordinated delivery of information to the student body regarding the suicide; provision of support and counselling to students; monitoring, assessment and identification of high-risk students; coordinated management of information to parents and media; and linkages to mental health resources in the community.

Reasons for the initiative – Findings from the literature suggest that there is valid reason to believe that certain students may be at heightened risk for a range of disorders, including suicidal ideation, following their exposure to a peer suicide. Brent and colleagues (1993) found that students exposed to a student suicide had higher rates than those of matched controls of the onset of the following disorders: major depression, post-traumatic stress disorder, and suicidal ideation, with a plan or an attempt.

In this particular case, postvention activities were initiated in two schools in New South Wales, following the deaths of two students by suicide (Hazell and Lewin 1993). The first suicide occurred in February 1990, and the second in March of the same year.

Actors – The postvention effort was conducted at two high schools in New South Wales within seven days of the suicides. Students were selected for participation by school staff and were chosen primarily on the basis of their relationship to the deceased. A total of 63 students received the postvention intervention. A child psychiatrist or trainee psychiatrist conducted the 90-minute sessions to groups of 20–30 students. Sessions focused on students' understanding of the events leading up to the suicide; managing rumours; exploring personal reactions to the death; and acknowledging that some students may feel suicidal. Specific information was given regarding ways to get help. School staff participated in debriefing sessions following the sessions with students, and plans were made to closely monitor those students identified as potentially high risk.

Results – Eight months after the suicides, students at the schools were asked to complete questionnaires to assess the following: proximity to attempted and completed suicide; suicidal ideation and behaviour before and after the peer deaths; recent emotional and behavioral symptoms; risk-taking behaviour; drug use; and attendance at postvention counselling sessions or other related services. Students who received the intervention were matched with students who did not participate in the postvention sessions and compared on a range of outcome measures. No differences were found between the two groups on the outcome measures listed above.

One of the reasons that no differences were found between the two groups might be the recruitment strategy. The authors noted that "A key problem appears to have been the appropriateness of criteria for selection for postvention counselling, since proximity to completed suicide alone was a relatively weak predictor of subsequent suicidal ideation and behaviour" (Hazell and Lewin 1993, 108). Other possible reasons for the failure to find a difference between the two groups include the following: the intervention itself was very brief in duration (90 minutes) and had no follow-up; the outcome measures did not examine the specific content of the session which was primarily focused on coping with the immediate crisis; and finally, the long interval between the intervention and the administration of the questionnaire (eight months) may have contributed to the lack of noted effects.

Replicability – These results cannot be generalized to other postvention efforts. The intervention that was implemented in this particular case represented a pilot project and was rather limited in its scope (Hazell and Lewin 1993).

Funding – No specific information is available for this particular initiative; nonetheless, it is reasonable to assume that the costs of the intervention itself are minimal. There may, however, be costs associated with administering questionnaires and follow-up surveys.

Evaluation – Despite the finding that there were no differences between counselled and noncounselled students in this study, the value of this effort is in the fact that it was evaluated. Very few postvention activities have been formally evaluated (Shaffer et al. 1988).

IMPLICATIONS FOR POLICY

It is evident from our analysis of the research on risk factors that since suicide is a complex multidetermined phenomenon, effective suicide prevention must involve multiple complementary strategies. This section includes only those priority strategies that, if enacted, are most likely to result in a significant reduction in suicide, suicidal behaviour and the impact of suicide on individuals and society. Some of the recommendations are specific to suicide, while others are more general and are likely to also affect a wide spectrum of social and health problems. No single strategy is likely to be effective for all individuals or groups at risk. However, when considered together, these policy recommendations constitute a comprehensive action plan for the reduction of suicide in Canada. The recommendations fall into four categories: social issues–environments; training; service delivery; and research and evaluation.

Social Issues/Environments

1. Several social and environmental interventions have significant potential to reduce the risk conditions that set the stage for the development of vulnerabilities to suicidal behaviour. These include decreasing poverty, strengthening families, decreasing all types of abuse in families, and creating healthy school and community environments. It is necessary, therefore, to address issues of low income, so that the cycle of poverty and all its consequences can be broken.

2. Children learn about suicide at an early age, primarily from depictions of suicidal behaviour on television. They generally discuss suicide but usually with other children and rarely with parents or educators. What children learn about suicide at this young age develops and becomes transformed into their teenage and adult conceptions of suicide. Therefore, the manner in which suicide is depicted in television, particularly the "how to" for children, needs to be guided by a thoughtful consideration of the research findings.

3. Media reports have been shown to have a potentially facilitative effect on suicidal behaviour. Therefore, print and broadcast media should be governed by policies outlining how to present information pertaining to suicide and suicidal behaviour (Canadian Association for Suicide Prevention 1994).

4. The environments within which people live can have a significant impact on personal levels of stress. Persons faced with poverty, abuse, instability, failure and losses (including death, suicide by a family member, peer, neighbour or teacher), require considerable skills, abilities and support to cope effectively. The surrounding environment can influence how well people experiencing such stress are able to deal with these situations. Therefore, it is important to create environments and living conditions that increase social support, promote healthy coping and reduce the negative effects of loss. It is also important to ensure that appropriate postvention policies are in place in the community, schools and other institutions, as well as access protocols to the mental health agencies and professionals.

5. The availability of the lethal means for suicide is an important consideration in suicide prevention.
   a) Males tend to use firearms in their attempts to take their lives. Therefore, any public policy or legislation that reduces access to firearms and reduces the number of homes in which firearms are available is likely to reduce suicides.
   b) Teens, especially females, tend to take their lives by consuming medications available in their homes and many homes contain enough unused medications to kill oneself. Any attempt to eliminate or to safely store dangerous medications at home will reduce suicide. Because some of these medications are acquired through prescription,

increasing physicians' knowledge and awareness about suicide, prescribing practices and suicide assessment may also reduce self-destructive behaviours through drug use.

6. Just as suicide may reflect the relative health of an individual, the level of suicide in a community may be an indicator of the relative health of that community. Given that a sense of control over the events of one's life is important for good health, then a sense of contribution, participation and involvement in the life of a community is important in developing and maintaining a healthy community. Therefore, it is necessary to ensure community involvement and participation should be ensured at all levels of suicide prevention program development and implementation. As the Royal Commission on Aboriginal Suicide has suggested, it is important that the community be given the opportunity to take control over its affairs to heal itself.

Training

1. Conflict resolution, problem solving and communication skills and abilities are important elements for achieving health and well-being. Because there is evidence that these skills are more deficient among suicidal individuals, appropriate and effective strategies should be engaged for teaching cognitive and social-emotional skills to people of all ages. Preschool programs, especially for at-risk children, that emphasize self-initiated learning approaches is one cost-effective approach.

2. It is often difficult to understand and accept the fact that children commit suicide. This is reflected in the underreporting of suicide in official statistics. Therefore, adults, including coroners and medical examiners, need to increase their awareness of the potential for children to take their own lives.

3. Suicide should be reduced by increasing awareness and knowledge of suicidal behaviour and the contributing factors, and developing the skills needed to identify and assess the risk and intervene effectively during a suicidal crisis. Therefore, it is necessary to (1) provide suicide prevention training for all gatekeepers (e.g., teachers, community workers, nursing home staff, police, paramedics, clergy); (2) include suicide awareness education for students in a comprehensive school health approach (such a program should follow recommendations suggested by the Centers for Disease Control and Prevention [1992] and be evaluated carefully); and (3) ensure that professional faculties at universities and community colleges (e.g., medicine, nursing, psychology, social work, gerontology) provide training in suicide intervention skills, in particular, and suicide prevention in general.

Service Delivery

1. Given the high rate of psychopathology among suicide completers, standards of professional practice in mental health should emphasize the following: conducting a thorough diagnostic interview to improve assessment and treatment of those at risk for suicide; taking all suicidal threats and behaviour seriously; aggressively intervening in first-episode affective illness; and assessing for the existence of comorbidity of affective illness and substance abuse (Brent and Perper 1995).
2. Drug interactions should be assessed, especially for elderly patients, who often take multiple medications.
3. Because older Canadians do not tend to avail themselves to the fullest of the crisis services that are available, the elderly should be informed of the services available, and other appropriate crisis services should be developed for the elderly.
4. Since adolescents who kill themselves typically have not received mental health treatment and the majority of attempters do not receive any formal intervention after their attempt, there is a need to reconsider the current service delivery system to ensure that services are available, appropriate and accessible to those in the youth population.

Research and Evaluation

1. Despite the proliferation of suicide prevention programs, little evaluative research has been done to help determine the most effective programs for different populations. In particular, long-term outcome studies should be undertaken of prevention and health promotion programs proposed to reduce vulnerabilities to suicide.
2. Much research in suicidology has a very narrow focus and concerns only a small segment of this complex, multidetermined problem. Perhaps, the limited view of this complex behaviour contributes to the inability of current research to inform effective intervention policies. Therefore, it is necessary to encourage multidisciplinary research strategies to investigate this multidetermined behaviour.
3. Finally, according to Hertzman (1995, 12), "It turns out that many of the most promising social interventions are rather modest in character: the redefinition of community development as a strategy for population health; the value of positive mentors and good recreation programs for the young; a few decent opportunities at a 'second chance' to make a successful transition from childhood to adulthood; and a strong social support network to buffer the stresses of middle and later life."

Ronald J. Dyck, *Ph.D., is the executive director, Corporate Services Division, Alberta Health, Government of Alberta, and is an associate clinical professor in the Department of Psychiatry, University of Alberta. As the former provincial suicidologist for the Province of Alberta, he was instrumental in facilitating the ongoing development and implementation of the province-wide, comprehensive suicide prevention program. In addition to these responsibilities, Dr. Dyck continues his involvement in various suicide-related research projects as well as serving as the coprincipal investigator for the Alberta Heart Health Project.*

Brian Mishara, *Ph.D., is a professor in the Psychology Department and a researcher in the Laboratory for Research on Human and Social Ecology (LAREHS) at the University of Quebec in Montreal. His numerous publications include research on the effectiveness of suicide prevention hot lines, theories of the development of suicidality, and the recent books,* Le Vieillissement *(Aging) (with R. Riedel) and* Drugs and Aging *(with W. A. McKim). Professor Mishara was a founder of both Suicide Action Montreal, the Montreal regional suicide prevention center, and the Quebec Association of Suicidology. He is past president of the Canadian Association for Suicide Prevention, was coorganizer of the 1993 Congress of the International Association for Suicide Prevention, and is the recipient for 1994–1995 of the Bora Laskin Canadian National Fellowship on Human Rights Research for his work on human rights issues regarding the involvement of physicians and family members in assisted suicide and euthanasia.*

Jennifer White, *M.A., is the director of the British Columbia Suicide Prevention Program, Cooperative University–Provincial Psychiatric Liaison (CUPPL), Department of Psychiatry, University of British Columbia. Previously, she held the position of youth suicide prevention coordinator with Alberta Health from 1991 to 1994, where she was responsible for program development, planning, consultation, and monitoring in the area of youth suicide prevention. She also worked in a clinical capacity as a suicide intervention counsellor at SAFER, a counselling agency in Vancouver, from 1988 to 1991. From 1984 to 1988, she worked as a child and youth care counsellor in a large residential facility in Calgary.*

BIBLIOGRAPHY

ABRAHAMS, R. B., and R. D. PATTERSON. 1978–79. Psychological distress among the community elderly: Prevalence, characteristics and implications for service. *International Journal of Aging and Human Development* 9(1): 1–17.

ADAM, K. 1986. Early family influences on suicidal behaviour. *Annals of the New York Academy of Sciences* 487: 63–76.

ADAM, K., J. LOHRENZ, and D. HARPER. 1982. Early parental loss and suicide ideation in university students. *Canadian Journal of Psychiatry* 27: 275–281.

ADAMS-TUCKER, C. 1982. Proximate effect of sexual abuse in childhood: A report in 28 children. *American Journal of Psychiatry* 139: 1252–1256.

ADCOCK, A. G., S. NAGY, and J. A. SIMPSON. 1991. Selected risk factors in adolescent suicide attempts. *Adolescence* 26(104): 817–828.

ANTHONY, S. 1940. *The Child's Discovery of Death: A Study in Child Psychology.* London, U.K.: Kegan, Paul, Trench, Trubner & Co.

ASARNOW, J. R., G. A. CARLSON, and D. GUTHRI. 1987. Coping strategies, self-perceptions, hopelessness, and perceived family environments in depressed suicidal children. *Journal of Consulting and Clinical Psychology* 56: 361–366.

BAGLEY, C., and R. RAMSAY. 1993. Suicidal behaviour in contrasted generations: Evidence from a community mental health survey. *Journal of Community Psychology* 21(1): 26–35.

BARRACLOUGH, B. M. 1971. Suicide in the elderly. In *Recent Developments in Psychogeriatrics*, eds. D. W. KAY and A. WALK. Ashford, Kent, U.K.: Headly Brothers.

BAYATPOUR, M., R.WELLS, and S. HOLFORD. 1992. Physical and sexual abuse as predictors of substance use and suicide among pregnant teenagers. *Journal of Adolescent Health* 13: 128–132.

BENSON, R. A., and D. C. BRODIE. 1975. Suicide by overdose of medicines among the aged. *Journal of the American Geriatrics Society* 23: 304–308.

BERARDO, F. M. 1968. Widowhood status in the United States: Perspective on a neglected aspect of the family life-cycle. *The Family Coordinator* 17: 191–203.

BERMAN, A. L. 1988. Fictional depiction of suicide in television films and imitation effects. *American Journal of Psychiatry* 145: 982–986.

BERMAN, A., and R. H. SCHWARTZ. 1990. Suicide attempts among adolescent drug-users. *American Journal of Diseases of Children* 144: 310–314.

BERNIER, J. 1994. *Community-Based Suicide Prevention Program: An Innovative Strategy to Reduce Suicide and Drinking in Small Alaskan Communities. Final Evaluation Report.* Juneau (AK): Department of Health and Social Services.

BILLE-BRAHE, U., B. JENSEN, and G. JESSEN. 1994. Suicide among the Danish elderly. *Crisis* 15(1): 37–43.

BLAND, R. C., S. C. NEWMAN, and H. ORN. 1988. Prevalence of psychiatric disorders in the elderly in Edmonton. *Acta Psychiatrica Scandinavica* 77(suppl. 338): 57–63.

BLAU, Z. S. 1956. Changes in status and age identification. *American Sociological Review* 21: 198–203.

_____. 1973. Aging, widowhood, and retirement: A sociological perspective. In *Old Age in a Changing Society*, ed. Z. BLAU. New York (NY): Franklin Watts. pp. 21–36.

BLAZER, D. G., J. R. BACHAR, and K. G. MANTON. 1986. Suicide in late life: Review and commentary. *Journal of the American Geriatric Society* 34(7): 519–525.

BLAZER, D. G., L. K. GEORGE, R. LANDERMAN, M. PENNYBACKER, M. L. MELVILLE, M. WOODBURY, K. G. MANTON, K. JORDAN, and B. LOCKE. 1985. Psychiatric disorders: A rural/urban comparison. *Archives of General Psychiatry* 42: 651–656.

BOCK, E. W., and WEBBER, I. L. 1972a. Suicide among the elderly: Isolation, widowhood and mitigating alternatives. *Journal of Marriage and the Family* 34.

_____. 1972b. Social status and relational system of elderly suicides: A re-examination of the Henry-Short thesis. *Life Threatening Behaviour* 2(3): 145–159.

BOSTROM, B. A. 1989. Euthanasia in the Netherlands: A model for the United States? *Issues in Law and Medicine* 4: 467–486.

BRENT, D., and J. PERPER. 1995. Research in adolescent suicide: Implications for training, service delivery, and public policy. *Suicide and Life-Threatening Behaviour* 25(2): 222–230.

BRENT, D., J. PERPER, C. GOLDSTEIN, D. KOLKO, M. ALLAN, C. ALLMAN, and J. ZELENAK. 1988. Risk factors for adolescent suicide. *Archives of General Psychiatry* 45: 581–588.

BRENT D., J. PERPER, G. MORITZ, C. ALLMAN, J. SCHWEERS, C. ROTH, L. BALACH, R. CANOBBIO, and L. LIOTUS. 1993. Psychiatric sequelae to the loss of an adolescent peer to suicide. *Journal of the American Academy of Child and Adolescent Psychiatry* 32(3): 509–517.

CALHOUN, L. G., J. W. SELBY, and M. E. FAULSTICH. 1980. Reactions to the parents of a child: A study of social impressions. *Journal of Consulting and Clinical Psychology* 48: 535–536.

CANADA. STATISTICS CANADA. 1982. *Population: Age, Sex and Marital Status.* Catalogue no. 92–901. Ottawa (ON): Minister of Supply and Services Canada.

CANADIAN ASSOCIATION FOR SUICIDE PREVENTION (CASP). 1994. *Recommendations for Suicide Prevention in Schools.* Calgary (AB): CASP.

CANADIAN INSTITUTE OF CHILD HEALTH. 1994. *The Health of Canada's Children: A CICH Profile.* Ottawa (ON): Canadian Institute of Child Health.

CARLSON, G. A., J. R. ASARNOW, and I. ORBACH. 1987. Developmental aspects of suicidal behaviour in children. *Journal of the American Academy of Child and Adolescent Psychiatry* 26:186–192.

CATTELL, H., and D. J. JOLLEY. 1995. One hundred cases of suicide in elderly people. *British Journal of Psychiatry* 166: 451–457.

CENTERS FOR DISEASE CONTROL AND PREVENTION. 1992. *Youth Suicide Prevention Programs: A Resource Guide.* Atlanta (GA): U.S. Department of Health and Human Services.

CHOINIÈRE, R., W. PICKETT, and B. L. MISHARA. Forthcoming. Les suicides et les tentatives de suicide. In *Pour la sécurité des jeunes canadiens: des données statistiques aux mesures préventives*, ed. G. BEAULNE. Ottawa (ON): Santé Canada.

CLUM, G. A., A. T. PATSIOKAS, and R. L. LUSCOMB. 1979. Empirically based comprehensive treatment program for parasuicide. *Journal of Consulting and Clinical Psychology* 47(5): 937–945.

COHEN-SANDLER, R., A. L. BERMAN, and R. KING. 1982. Life stress and symptomatology: Determinants of suicidal behaviour in children. *Journal of the American Academy of Child Psychiatry* 21: 178–186.

CONWELL, Y. 1994. Suicide and aging: Lessons from the nursing home. *Crisis* 15(4): 153–154, 158.

CONWELL, Y., M. ROTENBERG, and E. D. CAINE. 1990. Completed suicide at age 50 and over. *Journal of the American Geriatric Society* 38: 640–644.

COOPER, J. K., D. W. LOVE, and P. R. RAFFOUL. 1984. Intentional prescription nonadherence (noncompliance) by the elderly. *Journal of the American Geriatrics Society* 30(5): 329–333.

CURRAN, D. K. 1987. *Adolescent Suicidal Behaviour.* New York (NY): Hemisphere Publishing Corporation.

CURRY, J. F., Y. MILLER, and W. B. ANDERSON. 1992. Coping responses in depressed, socially maladjusted, and suicidal adolescents. *Psychological Reports* 71: 80–82.

D'ARCY, C. 1986. Aging and mental health. In *Aging in Canada: Sociological Perspectives*, ed. V. MARSHALL. Toronto (ON): Fitzhenry and Whiteside. pp. 424–450.

DAVIDSON, L., M. ROSENBERG, J. MERCY, V. FRANKLIN, and S. V. SIMMON. 1989. An epidemiologic study of risk factors in two teenage suicide clusters. *Journal of the American Medical Association* 262(19): 2687–2692.

DIEKSTRA, R. 1989. Suicidal behaviour among adolescents and young adults: The international picture. *Crisis* 10: 16–35.

DOMINO, G., and A. LEENAARS. 1989. Attitudes towards suicide: A comparison of Canadian and United States college students. *Suicide and Life-Threatening Behaviour* 19: 160–172.

DRAPER, B. M. 1995. Prevention in suicide in old age. *The Medical Journal of Australia* 162: 533–534.

DYCK, R. J., and J. WHITE. 1990. A ten-year case file review of elderly. Unpublished manuscript.

EASTERLIN, R. A. 1980. *Birth and Fortune: The Impact of Numbers on Personal Welfare.* New York (NY): Basic Books.

EVANS, A. L., D. O. FOGLE, and C. V. McDONALD. 1987. Cultural attitude towards suicide of the aged. Annual meeting of the American Association of Suicidology. San Francisco (CA).

FELNER, R., and A. ADAN. 1988. The school transitional environment project: An ecological intervention and evaluation. In *Fourteen Ounces of Prevention: A Casebook for Practitioners*, eds. R. PRICE, E. COWEN, R. LORION, and J. RAMOS-MCKAY. Washington (DC): American Psychological Association. pp. 111–122.

FELNER, R., and T. FELNER. 1989. Prevention programs in the educational contexts: A transactional-ecological framework for program models. In *Primary Prevention and Promotion in the Schools*, eds. L. BOND, and B. COMPAS. Newbury Park (CA): Sage Publications. pp. 13–49

FELNER, R., A. ADAN, and E. EVANS. 1987. Evaluation of school-based primary prevention programs. Unpublished manuscript.

FELNER, R., M. GINTER, and J. PRIMAVERA. 1982. Primary prevention during school transitions: Social support and environmental structure. *American Journal of Community Psychology* 10: 277–290.

FENIGSEN, R. 1989. A case against Dutch euthanasia. *Hastings Centre Report*, 22–30. Special Supplement 19(1): suppl. 22–30, Jan.–Feb.

FREMOUW, W., T. CALLAHAN, and J. KASHDEN. 1993. Adolescent suicidal risk: Psychological, problem-solving, and environmental factors. *Suicide and Life-Threatening Behaviour* 23: 46–54.

FRERICHS, R. R., C. S. ANESHENSEL, and V. A. CLARK. 1980. Prevalence of depression in Los Angeles County. Paper presented at the Society of Epidemiological Research, Minneapolis (MN), June 1980.

FRIERSON, R. L. 1991. Suicide attempts by the old and the very old. *Archives of Internal Medicine* 151: 141–144.

FURMAN, E. 1974. *A Child's Parent Dies.* New Haven (CA): Yale University Press.

GARFINKEL, B. D., A. FROESE, and J. HOOD. 1982. Suicide attempts in children and adolescents. *American Journal of Psychiatry* 139: 1257–1261.

GOULD, M., and D. SHAFFER. 1986. The impact of suicide in television movies: Evidence of imitation. *New England Journal of Medicine* 315: 690–694.

GOULD, M., S. WALLENSTEIN, M. KLEINMAN, P. O'CARROLL, and V. MERCY. 1990. Suicide clusters: An examination of age-specific effects. *American Journal of Public Health* 80(2): 211–212.

GRAHAM, C., and P. BURVILL. 1992. A study of coroner's records of suicide in young people, 1986–1988 in Western Australia. *Australian and New Zealand Journal of Psychiatry* 26: 30–39.

GREEN, A. H. 1978. Self-destructive behaviour in battered children. *American Journal of Psychiatry* 135: 579–582.

GREENWALD, S. R., and M. W. LINN. 1971. Intercorrelations of data on nursing homes. *The Gerontologist* 11: 337–340.

GREER, S., and M. ANDERSON. 1979. Samaritan contact among 325 parasuicide patients. *British Journal of Psychiatry* 135: 263–268.

GRENIER, G. 1986. L'acquisition d'un concept de mort évolué chez l'enfant en fonction des expériences vécues d'une part et du développement des concepts de vie, d'inclusion et d'âge d'autre part. Unpublished M.Sc. thesis. Montreal (QC): Université du Québec à Montréal,

GURLAND, B. J., and P. S. CROSS. 1983. Suicide among the elderly. In *The Acting Out Elderly*, eds. M. K. ARONSON, R. BENNETT, and B. J. GURLAND. New York (NY): Haworth Press. pp. 456–465.

HAIGHT, B. K. 1995. Suicide risk in frail elderly people relocated to nursing homes. *Geriatric Nursing* 16(3): 104–107.

HARRIS, J., and R. S. MCCULLOUGH. 1988. *Health Indicators Derived from Vital Statistics: Status Indian and Canadian Populations 1978–1986.* Ottawa (ON): Health and Welfare Canada, Medical Services Branch.

HAZELL, P. 1993. Adolescent suicide clusters: Evidence, mechanisms and prevention. *Australian and New Zealand Journal of Psychiatry* 27: 653–665.

HAZELL, P., and T. LEWIN. 1993. An evaluation of postvention following adolescent suicide. *Suicide and Life-Threatening Behaviour* 23(2): 101–109.

HEALTH CANADA. 1994. *Suicide In Canada: Update of the Report of the Task Force on Suicide in Canada.* Ottawa (ON): Minister of Health.

HEALTH AND WELFARE CANADA, STATISTICS CANADA. 1981. *The Health of Canadians: Report of the Canada Health Survey.* Ottawa (ON): Ministry of Supply and Services, catalogue 82-538E.

HENDIN, H. 1982. *Suicide in America.* New York (NY): W. W. Norton and Co.

HENSLEY, W. 1988. *Interim Report of the Senate Special Committee on Suicide Prevention.* State of Alaska (AL): Senate Special Committee.

HERTZMAN, C. 1995. Child development and long-term outcomes: A population health perspective and summary of successful interventions. Working paper no. 4. Toronto (ON): The Canadian Institute for Advanced Research.

HOBERMAN, H. M., and B. D. GARFINKEL, B. D. 1988a. Completed suicide in children and adolescents. *Journal of the American Academy of Child and Adolescent Psychiatry* 27: 689–695.

_____. 1988b. Completed suicide in youth. *Canadian Journal of Psychiatry* 33: 494–502.

HUDSON, M. F., and T. F. JOHNSON. 1986. Elder neglect and abuse: A review of the literature. *Annual Review of Gerontology and Geriatrics* 6: 81–134.

JARVIS, G. K., and M. BOLDT. 1980. Suicide in the later years. *Essence* 4(3): 145–158.

KALAFAT, J., and M. ELIAS. 1992. Adolescents' experience with and response to suicidal peers. *Suicide and Life-Threatening Behaviour* 22: 315–321.

KANE, R. 1975. Children's concept of death. Ph.D. thesis. Cincinnati (OH): University of Cincinnati,

KHAN, A. U. 1987. Heterogeneity of suicidal adolescents. *Journal of American Academy of Child and Adolescent Psychiatry* 26(1): 92–96.

KIENHORST, C., E. de WILDE, R. DIEKSTRA, and W. WOLTERS. 1992. Differences between adolescent suicide attempters and depressed adolescents. *Acta Psychiatrica Scandinavica* 85: 222–228.

KING, G. 1977. An evaluation of the effectiveness of a telephone counselling center. *American Journal of Community Psychology* 4: 75–83.

KOOCHER, G. P. 1973. Childhood, death and cognitive development. *Developmental Psychology* 9: 369–375.

LAU, E., and J. I. KOSBERG. 1979. Abuse of elderly by informal care providers. *Aging* September– October: 10–15.

LEENAARS, A., and D. LESTER. 1995. The changing suicide pattern in Canadian adolescents and youth, compared to their American counterparts. *Adolescence* 30(119): 539–547.

LEPINE, L. 1982. *Suicide among the Aged in Canada.* Ottawa (ON): Minister of Health and Welfare.

LESTER, D. 1983. Preventive effect of strict handgun control laws on suicide rates. *American Journal of Psychiatry* 140(9): 1259.

_____. 1984. *Gun Control: Issues and Answers.* Springfield (IL): Charles Thomas.

_____. 1988a. Research note on gun control, gun ownership, and suicide prevention. *Suicide and Life-Threatening Behaviour* 18(2): 176–180.

_____. 1988b. Youth suicide. *Adolescence* 23: 955–958.

LESTER, D., and A. T. BECK. 1974. Age differences in patterns of attempted suicide. *Omega* 5: 317–322.

LEVENSON, M., and C. NEURINGER. 1971. Problem-solving behaviour in suicidal adolescents. *Journal of Consulting and Clinical Psychology* 37(3): 433–436.

LIEBERMAN, M. A. 1983. Social contexts of depression. In *Depression in the Elderly*, eds. L. D. BRESLAU, and M. R. HAUG. New York (NY): Springer. pp. 121–123.

LOEBEL, J. P., J. S. LOEBEL, S. R. DAGER, B. S. CENTERWALL, and D. T. REAY. 1991. Anticipation of nursing home placement may be a precipitation of suicide among the elderly. *Journal of the American Geriatric Society* 39: 407–408.

LONETTO, R. 1980. *Children's Conceptions of Death*. New York (NY): Springer Publishing Co.

LONNQVIST, J. 1977. *Suicide in Helsinki. Monographs on Psychiatry*. Helsinki (Finland). Fennica.

LOPATA, H. 1973. Self-identity in marriage and widowhood. *The Sociological Quarterly* 14: 407–418.

MACMAHON, B., and T. F. PUGH. 1965. Suicide in the widowed. *American Journal of Epidemiology* 81(1): 23–31.

MARTTUNEN, M., H. ARO, and J. LONNQVIST. 1992. Adolescent suicide: Endpoint of long-term difficulties. *Journal of the American Academy of Child and Adolescent Psychiatry* 31(4): 649–654.

MATTER, D. E., and R. M. MATTER. 1984. Suicide among elementary school children: A serious concern for counsellors. *Elementary School Guidance and Counselling* 18: 260–267.

MCCALL, P. L. 1991. Adolescent and elderly white male suicide trends: Evidence of changing well-being. *Journal of Gerontology* 46(1): S43–51.

MCCARTNEY, J. R. 1978. Suicide vs. right to refuse treatment in the chronically ill. *Psychosomatics* 19(9): 548–551.

MCINTOSH, J. L. 1995. Suicide prevention in the elderly (age 65–99). *Suicide and Life-Threatening Behaviour* 25(1): 180–192.

MCINTOSH, J. L., J. F. SANTOS, R. W. HUBBARD, and J. C. OVERHOLSE. 1994. Elder suicide: Research, theory and treatment. Washington (DC): American Psychological Association.

MISHARA, B. L. and W. A. MCKIM. 1989. *Drogues et vieillissement*. Boucherville: Gaëtan Morin Éditeur.

MELEAR, A. 1973. Children's conception of death. *Journal of Genetic Psychology* 123: 359–360.

MILLER, M. 1978. Geriatric suicide: The Arizona study. *The Gerontologist* 18(5): 488–495.

MISHARA, B. L. 1995. An empirical investigation of children's understanding of suicide and death. Unpublished manuscript.

_____. 1996. Childhood conceptions of death and suicide: Empirical investigations and implications for suicide prevention. In *Suicide Prevention: A Holistic Approach*, eds. D. DE LEO and R. F. W. DIEKSTRA. Dordrecht, Netherlands: Kluwer Academic Press.

MISHARA, B. L., and R. KASTENBAUM. 1973. Self-injurious behaviour and environmental change in the institutionalized elderly. *International Journal of Aging and Human Development* 4(2): 133–145.

_____. 1980. *Alcohol and Old Age: Use and Abuse*. New York (NY): Grune and Stratton.

MISHARA, B. L., and R. RIEDEL. 1994. *Le Vieillissement*. 3rd ed. Paris (France): Presses Universitaires de France.

MOOS, R. 1979. *The Human Context: Environmental Determinants of Behaviour*. New York (NY): Wiley.

MORRISON, G. C., and J. G. COLLIER. 1969. Family treatment approaches to suicidal children and adolescent. *Journal of the American Academy of Child Psychiatry* 8: 140–153.

MOTTO, J. 1980. Suicide risk factors in alcohol abuse. *Suicide and Life-Threatening Behaviour* 10: 230–238.

MURPHY, G. E., and R. D. WETZEL. 1982. Family history of suicidal behaviour among suicide attempters. *Journal of Nervous and Mental Disease* 170: 86–90.

NAGY, M. 1948. The child's theories concerning death. *Journal of Genetic Psychology* 73: 3–27.

NATIONAL CENTER FOR HEALTH STATISTICS. 1988. *Vital Statistics of the United States Life Tables*. Hyattsville (MD): National Center for Health Statistics.

NATIONAL INSTITUTE ON AGING. 1987. *Personal Health Needs of the Elderly through the Year 2020.* Washington (DC): Public Health Service.

NELSON, F. L., and N. L. FARBEROW. 1980. Indirect self-destructive behaviour in the elderly nursing home patient. *Journal of Gerontology* 35(6): 949–957.

NORMAND, C., and B. L. MISHARA. 1992. The development of the concept of suicide in children. *Omega* 25(3): 183–203.

O'MALLEY, H. C., H. D. SEGEL, and R. PEREZ. 1979. *Elder Abuse in Massachussets: Survey of Professionals and Paraprofessionals.* Boston (MA): Legal Research and Services to the Elderly.

OFFORD, D. 1990. Social factors in the aetiology of childhood psychiatric disorders. In *Handbook of Studies on Child Psychiatry,* eds. B. J. TARGE, G. D. BURROWS, and J. S. AMSTERDAM. Netherlands: Elsevier Science Publishing Co. pp. 55–70.

OFFORD, D., BOYLE M., and RACINE, Y. 1989. *Ontario Child Health Study: Children at Risk.* Toronto (ON): Queen's Printer.

ORBACH, I., E. ROSENHEIM, and E. HARY. 1987. Some aspects of cognitive functioning in suicidal children. *Journal of the American Academy of Child and Adolescent Psychiatry* 26(2): 181–185.

ORBACH, I., GROSS, Y., GLAUBMAN, H., and BERMAN, D. 1985. Children's perception of death in humans and animals as a function of age, anxiety and cognitive ability. *Journal of Child Psychology and Psychiatry* 26: 453–463.

OSGOOD, N.J. 1985. *Suicide in the Elderly: A Practitioner's Guide to Diagnosis and Mental Health Intervention.* Rockville (MD): Aspen Systems Corp.

_____. 1992. Environmental factors in suicide in long-term care facilities. *Suicide and Life-Threatening Behaviour* 22: 98–106.

OSGOOD, N. J., and B. A. BRANT. 1990. Suicidal behaviour in long-term care facilities. *Suicide and Life-Threatening Behaviour* 20(2): 113–122.

PARKES, C. M. 1972. *Bereavement: Studies of Grief in Adult Life.* New York (NY): International Universities Press Inc.

PFEFFER, C. R. 1986. *The Suicidal Child.* New York (NY): The Guilford Press.

_____. 1990. Suicidal behaviour among children and adolescents: A clinical and research perspective. *The Yale Journal of Biology and Medicine* 63: 325–332.

PFEFFER, C. R., R. LIPKINS, R. PLUTCHIK, and S. MIZRUCHI. 1988. Normal children at risk for suicidal behaviour: A two-year follow-up study. *Journal of the American Academy of Child and Adolescent Psychiatry* 27: 34–41.

PFEFFER, C., G. KLERMAN, S. HURT, M. LESSER, J. PESKIN, and C. SIEFKER. 1991. Suicidal children grow up: Demographic and clinical risk factors for adolescent suicide attempts. *Journal of the American Academy of Child and Adolescent Psychiatry* 30(4): 609–616.

PFEIFFER, C. 1977. Psychopathology and social pathology. In *Handbook of the Psychology of Aging,* eds. J. E. BIRREN and K. W. SCHAIE. New York (NY): Van Nostrand Reinhold. pp. 650–671.

PHILLIPS, D. L., and L. L. CARSTENSEN. 1986. Clustering of teenage suicide after television news stories about suicide. *New England Journal of Medicine* 315(11): 685–689.

PIAGET, J. 1937. La construction du réel chez l'enfant. Neuchâtel, Switzerland: Delachaux et Niestlé.

PILLEMER, K., and D. FINKELHOR. 1988. The prevalence of elder abuse: A random sample survey. *The Gerontologist* 28(1): 51–57.

PLATT, S. 1984. Unemployment and suicidal behaviour. *Social Science and Medicine* 19: 93–115.

PODNIEKS, E., and K. PILLEMER. 1990. *National Survey on Abuse of the Elderly in Canada.* Toronto (ON): Ryerson Polytechnical Institute.

Poverty Profile, 1980–1990. 1992. A report by the National Council of Welfare. Minister of Supply and Services Canada, Cat. no. H67-1/4–1990E.

PRESTON, S. H. 1984. Children and the elderly: Divergent paths for America's dependents. *Demography* 21: 435–457.

QUÉBEC. SANTÉ QUÉBEC. (C. BELLEROSE, C. LAVALLÉE, L. CHÉNARD, and M. LEVASSEUR). 1995. *Et la santé, ça va en 1992–1993? Rapport de l'enquête sociale et de santé 1992–1993*, Vol. 1. Montreal (QC): Ministère de la Santé et des Services sociaux, Gouvernement du Québec.

RAIMBAULT, G. 1975. *L'enfant et la mort. Des enfants malades parlent de la mort: Problèmes de la clinique du deuil.* Toulouse (France): Privat.

RASCHKO, R. 1990. The gatekeeper model for the isolated, at-risk elderly. In *Psychiatry Takes to the Streets*, ed. N. L. COHEN. New York (NY): Guilford Press. pp. 195–209.

RICHMAN, J. 1986. *Family Therapy for Suicidal People.* New York (NY): Springer Publishing.

ROSENWAIKE, I. 1985. *The Extreme Aged in America: A Portrayal of an Expanding Population.* Westport (CT): Greenwood.

ROSOW, I. 1967. *Social Integration of the Aged.* New York (NY): Free Press.

ROURKE, B., G. YOUNG, and A. LEENAARS. 1989. A childhood learning disability that predisposes those afflicted to adolescent and adult depression and suicide risk. *Journal of Learning Disabilities* 22: 169–175.

SAKINOFSKY, I., and R. ROBERTS. 1987. The ecology of suicide in provinces of Canada, 1969–1971 to 1979–1981. In *The Epidemiology of Psychiatric Disorders*, ed. B. COOPER. Baltimore (MD): Johns Hopkins University. pp. 27–42.

SCHWEINHART, L. J., and D. P. WEIKART. 1988. The High/Scope Perry Preschool Program. In *Fourteen Ounces of Prevention: A Casebook for Practitioners*, eds. R. PRICE, E. COWEN, R. LORION, and J. RAMOS-MCKAY. Washington (DC): American Psychological Association. pp. 53–65.

SCHWEINHART, L. J., D. P. WEIKART, and M. B. LARNER. 1986. Consequences of three preschool curriculum models through age 15. *Early Childhood Research Quarterly* 1(1): 15–35.

SCHWEINHART, L. J., H. V. BARNES, D. P. WEIKART, W. S. BARNETT, and A. S. EPSTEIN, 1993. *Significant Benefits: The High/Scope Perry Preschool Study through Age 27.* Monograph no. 10 of the High/Scope Educational Foundation. Ypsilanti (MI): High/Scope Press.

SENDBUEHLER, J. M., and S. GOLDSTEIN. 1977. Attempted suicide among the aged. *Journal of the American Geriatric Society* 25: 245–248.

SHAFFER, D. 1974. Suicide in childhood and early adolescence. *Journal of Child Psychology and Psychiatry* 15: 275–291.

―――. 1988. The epidemiology of teen suicide: An examination of risk factors. *Journal of Clinical Psychiatry* 49: 36–41.

SHAFFER, D., and P. FISHER. 1981. The epidemiology of suicide in children and young adolescents. *Journal of the American Academy of Child Psychiatry* 20: 545–565.

SHAFFER, D., A. GARLAND, M. GOULD, P. FISHER, and P. TRAUTMAN. 1988. Preventing teenage suicide: A critical review. *Journal of the American Academy of Child and Adolescent Psychiatry* 27: 675–687.

SHAFFER, D., A. GARLAND, V. VIELAND, M. UNDERWOOD, and C. BUSNER. 1991. The impact of curriculum-based suicide prevention programs for teenagers. *Journal of the American Academy of Child and Adolescent Psychiatry* 30: 588–596.

SHAFFER, D., V. VIELAND, A. GARLAND, M. ROJAS, M. UNDERWOOD, and C. BUSNER. 1990. Adolescent suicide attempters: Response to suicide prevention programs. *Journal of the American Medical Association* 264: 3151–3155.

SHAFII, M., S. CARRIGAN, J. WHITTINGHILL, and A. DERRICK. 1985. Psychological autopsy of completed suicide in children and adolescents. *American Journal of Psychiatry* 142(9): 1061–1064.

SHULMAN, K. 1978. Suicide and parasuicide in old age: A review. *Age and Aging* 7(4): 201–209.

SILVERMAN, M., and R. FELNER. 1995. Suicide prevention programs: Issues of design, implementation, feasibility, and developmental appropriateness. *Suicide and Life-Threatening Behaviour* 25(1): 92–104.

SLOAN, J., F. RIVARA, D. REAY, J. FERRIS, M. PATH, and A. KELLERMAN. 1990. Firearms regulations and rates of suicide. *New England Journal of Medicine* 322: 369–373.

SMITH, K., and S. CRAWFORD. 1986. Suicidal behaviour among "normal" high school students. *Suicide and Life-Threatening Behaviour* 16(3): 313–325.

SPIRITO, A., J. OVERHOLSER, and L. J. STARK. 1989a. Common problems and coping strategies II: Findings with adolescent suicide attempters. *Journal of Abnormal Child Psychology* 17(2): 213–221.

SPIRITO, A., L. BROWN, J. OVERHOLSER, and G. FRITZ. 1989b. Attempted suicide in adolescence: A review and critique of the literature. *Clinical Psychology Review* 9: 335–363.

SPIRITO, A., B. PLUMMER, M. GISPERT, S. LEVY, J. KURKJIAN, W. LEWANDER, S. HAGBERG, and L. DEVOST. 1992. Adolescent suicide attempts: Outcomes at follow-up. *American Journal of Orthopsychiatry* 62: 464–468.

STACK, S. 1991. Social correlates of suicide by age. In *Current Concepts of Suicide*, ed. A. A. LEENAARS. New York (NY): Plenum. pp. 187–213.

STROEBER, M. S., and W. STROEBER. 1983. Who suffers more? Sex differences in health risks of the widowed. *Psychological Bulletin* 93: 279–301.

TIERNEY, R., R. RAMSAY, B. TANNEY, and W. LANG. 1991. Comprehensive school suicide prevention programs. In *Suicide Prevention in Schools*, eds. A. LEENAARS and S. WENCKSTERN. New York (NY): Hemisphere Publishing Corporation. pp. 83–98.

TISHLER, C. L., P. C. MCKENRY, and K. C. MORGAN. 1981. Adolescent suicide attempts: Some significant factors. *Suicide and Life-Threatening Behaviour* 11: 86–92.

TROVATO, F. 1992. A Durkheimian analysis of youth suicide: Canada, 1971 and 1981. *Suicide and Life-Threatening Behaviour* 22(4): 413–427.

VAN DER KOLK, B., C. PERRY, and J. HERMAN. 1991. Childhood origins of self-destructive behaviour. *American Journal of Psychiatry* 148(12): 1665–1671.

WASYLENKI, D. 1980. Depression in the elderly. *Canadian Medical Association Journal* 122: 525–532.

WEIKART, D. P., J. T. BOND, and J. T. MCNEIL. 1978. *The Ypsilanti Perry Preschool Project: Preschool Years and Longitudinal Results through Fourth Grade.* Monograph no. 3 of the High/Scope Educational Research Foundation. Ypsilanti (MI): High/Scope Press.

WHITE, J. 1994. After the crisis: Facilitating the suicidal student's return to school. *Guidance and Counselling* 10(1): 10–13.

WHITE, J., R. DYCK, G. HARRINGTON, A. AUBURN, and S. MEURIN. 1991. *Suicide Prevention in Alberta: Working towards Results.* Edmonton (AB): Alberta Health.

WORDEN, J. W. 1982. *Grief Counselling and Grief Theory: A Handbook for the Mental Health Practitioner.* New York (NY): Springer Publishing Co.

APPENDIX

SUICIDE IN THREE POPULATIONS—MAGNITUDE OF THE PROBLEM

Children

According to official statistics in Canada (Health Canada 1994) and the United States (National Center for Health Statistics 1988), children rarely commit suicide. Between 1950 and 1992 in Canada, not a single child under the age of five years was recorded as having committed suicide. During the same period, there were 18 reported suicides of children aged 5–9 years, which represents an annual in a suicide rate of 0.2 deaths per 100,000 population. In Canada, suicide rates for 10- to 14-year-olds increased from 0.1 per 100,000 population in 1951 (only one death) to 1.8 per 100,000 in 1992 (34 deaths). This is less than the rate of 12.9 per 100,000 per annum for the 15- to 19-year-olds.

Several researchers have suggested that the official statistics on children's suicides significantly underestimate the actual frequency of the phenomenon for younger ages (Cohen-Sandler, Berman, and King 1982; Matter and Matter 1984; Hoberman and Garfinkel 1988a; Pfeffer et al. 1988). For example, Pfeffer and colleagues (1988) found that 2 percent of a sample of preadolescents with no psychiatric history had made suicide threats, 1 percent had made a "mild" suicide attempt, and 8.9 percent had thought of suicide.

Other authors point to the fact that accidents are the number one cause of children's death in Canada and the United States, with the most common type of accidental death being children hit by cars. Winn and Heller (cited in Shaffer and Fisher 1981) observed that the majority of children who threatened to commit suicide were planning to die by throwing themselves in front of a moving car. Normand and Mishara (1992) found that running in front of a car was reported by 15 percent of a sample of Quebec grade school children as a possible means for people to commit suicide, and in a follow-up study Mishara (1996) reported that 12 percent of children in grades 1–5 said that intentionally being hit by a car is a means of committing suicide. Shaffer and Fisher (1981) observed that although no child had been reported committing suicide by being hit by a car in the United Kingdom, automobile deaths among children are a likely suicide method, and suicidal deaths by this method are not identified as such. Hoberman and Garfinkel (1988a) estimated that 15 percent of deaths that were actually suicides among people under age 20 in the United States had been classified as deaths by accident, homicide or undetermined causes and that this misclassification occurred more often for those below age 15.

A few studies have asked children if they had thought of suicide. Pfeffer asked 101 normal school-age children between the age of 6 and 12 whether they had ever thought of killing themselves. She found that 8.9 percent said they had thought of killing themselves and that another 2 percent said they had threatened or attempted suicide. Carlson, Asarnow and Orbach (1987) reported that 15.4 percent of normal children between ages 13 and 18 had suicidal fantasies. Mishara (1996) found that 13.8 percent of a sample of Quebec children in grades 1–5 reported that they had considered killing themselves.

The 1992–93 Quebec Health Survey (Québec. Santé Québec 1995) questioned a sample of 1,528 parents concerning suicide threats by their children 6–11 years old. In this random sample of Quebec households, 47 of the parents (about 3 percent) reported that their child had threatened to commit suicide. Although this constitutes a significant proportion of children having threatened to take their own lives, it is difficult to interpret the seriousness of the threats and the possible relationship between these threats and suicidal behaviour.

Adolescents

Completed suicide – Over the past three decades, the rate of completed suicide among youth has increased considerably, with the period between 1970 and 1980 showing a particularly dramatic rise in Canada and other parts of the world (Lester 1988b; Leenaars and Lester 1995). This worrisome trend is particularly evident among young males and is highlighted by the following figures: in 1962, the rate of suicide among Canadian males aged 15–19 was 5.1 per 100,000; in 1972, the rate for this age group had climbed to 13.8; and in 1982, it was up to 20.9 (Health Canada 1994). Since the 1980s it would appear that the rates for this age group may be starting to level out somewhat; in 1992, the rate of suicide among Canadian males aged 15–19 was 20.1 per 100,000 (Health Canada 1994).

Among young Canadian females, much less has changed. In 1962, the rate among females aged 15–19 was 1.3; in 1972, it rose to 4.2; by 1982, it was 3.1; and in 1992, the rate for this age group was 5.4 per 100,000 (Health Canada 1994). Among 20- to 24-year-olds, the rate of completed suicide in 1992 was 29.0 per 100,000 for men and 6.6 for women. The overall suicide rate in 1992 among Canadians of both sexes was 13.0.

Rates of completed suicide among young people from Inuit and First Nations communities are extremely high. The average suicide rate among Aboriginal youth aged 10–19 years for 1986–1990 was 37.0 per 100,000, which is well above the rate for the Canadian population as a whole (Canadian Institute of Child Health 1994).

Attempted suicide – It is difficult to obtain an accurate estimate of the extent of suicide attempts by young people for several reasons. First, many adolescents attempt suicide without anybody knowing about it, and the majority of attempters never receive any formal intervention (Smith and Crawford 1986). Second, even for those youths who do come to the attention of a helping professional or agency, no centralized registry exists to monitor the number of suicide attempts reported at hospitals, mental health clinics or school counsellors' offices. Survey data suggest that anywhere between 6 and 13 percent of adolescents have reported making a suicide attempt (Shaffer et al. 1991) and that for every adolescent death by suicide, there may be 50–100 attempts (Smith and Crawford 1986).

In 1991, 292 hospitalizations for self-inflicted injuries (suicide attempts) were reported for males aged 10–14, along with 2,299 hospitalizations for self-inflicted injuries for males age 15–19 (Choinière, Pickett, and Mishara, in press). This yields an attempt rate per 100,000 population per year of 15.75 for males 10–14 years old and 124.90 for males 15–19 years old. Young females were more often hospitalized for self-inflicted injuries: in 1991, there were 1,772 hospitalizations for females aged 10–14 and 5,331 hospitalizations for females aged 15–19, which yield annual attempt rates per 100,000 population of 100.59 for females 10–14 years old and 304.94 for females 15–19 years old. The mean number of days in hospital following a suicide attempt in Canada is 114 days (the median stay is 38 days). Young males, on the other hand, are hospitalized for briefer periods: their average stay is 33 days (median stay, 10 days). Hospitalization for self-inflicted injuries among young people aged 15–19 accounts for more than half of all injury-related days of hospitalization in Canada.

The Quebec Health Survey 1992–93 included a detailed investigation of whether participants in this representative population study had thought of killing themselves during the 12 months preceding the interview, as well as at any time in their life (Québec. Santé Québec 1995). They reported on suicidal ideation among participants aged 15–24 years. In the study, 7.5 percent of males and 8.4 percent of females aged 15–24 reported having thought of killing themselves in the 12 months preceding, and 10.9 percent of males and 12.9 percent of females said that they had considered suicide at some time in their lives. Comparisons with the same questions asked five years previously indicate increases in suicidal ideation in the 12 months preceding the interviews, from 5.6 in 1987 to 7.5 in 1992–93 for males and from 6.2 in 1987 to 8.4 in 1992–93 in females.

A slightly higher proportion of males (1.9 percent) than females (1.7 percent) aged 15–24 reported that they had attempted suicide in the 12 months preceding the study. In addition, 4.5 percent of males and 7.6 percent of females aged 15–24 said that they had attempted suicide at some time in their lives. The most common reported methods for the attempts were medications and other chemical substances (56.6 percent), followed by cutting veins (31.7 percent). In analyses of all age groups combined, suicidal ideation was more frequent (6.3 percent vs. 3.6 percent) when the respondent indicated an absence of at least one confidant with whom he could discuss problems. Furthermore, individuals who indicated that their level of social support was "poor" had much higher rates of suicidal ideation (9.6 percent) than those who rated their level of social support as "high" (2.6 percent).

Other significant yet sobering facts are related to the magnitude of the problem of suicidal behaviour among Canadian youth. For 1989–1991, suicide was the second leading cause of death, after motor vehicle accidents, for Canadians between the ages of 15 and 24 (Health Canada 1994). The number of potential years of life lost among Canadian teens aged 15–19 in 1989 was more than 15,000. The rate of hospitalization for suicide attempts among Canadian girls aged 10–14 was 81.5 per 100,000 and 17.0 for boys of the same age (Canadian Institute of Child Health 1994). Canadian adolescents, especially boys, are at greater risk of dying by suicide than their U.S. peers. During the 1980s, suicide rates for Canadian males age 15–19 were 50–60 percent greater then those of U.S. teens (Leenaars and Lester 1995).

The Elderly

Much attention has focused on suicide among the elderly over the past decade (McIntosh et al. 1994; Bille-Brahe, Jensen, and Jensen 1994; McIntosh 1995). Most published reports indicate that while the greatest number of suicides occur among adults aged 25–44, the highest rate of suicide occurs among older adults aged 65 years and over (Blazer, Bachar, and Manton 1986; McIntosh 1995). In Canada, the suicide rates among those aged 65 years and over have been declining since the mid-1980s to a rate of 13.7 per 100,000 population (compared with a rate of 13.2 for the nation). Subpopulations of older adults (the "young-old" aged 65–74 years, and the "old-old" aged 75 years and over), however, are distinct in terms of such factors as overall health, activity level and demographics (Rosenwaike 1985; McIntosh 1995) and may well have different rates of completed suicide. As shown in figure 1, suicide rates for young-old males have been increasing from the 1960s to the mid-1980s, before showing a dramatic decline to 1993. Old-old male suicide rates also increased from the 1960s to the mid-1980s but at faster rate and with a great deal more variability. As in the young-old males, rates declined for the old-old males from the mid-1980s to 1993, ending, however, with a slightly higher rate than young-old males by 1993.

Figure 1

Elderly suicide rate by selected age group, sex and census year: Canada*

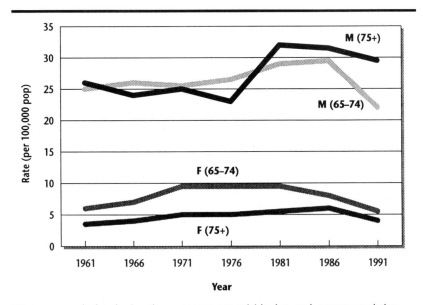

* Rates were calculated using three-year average suicide data and census population.

Suicide rates among young-old and old-old females also showed an increase from the 1960s to the mid-1980s and a decline to 1993. However, unlike the males, the young-old females tended, for the most part, to have suicide rates higher than old-old females. Note that suicide rates of young-old males are about 3–4 times higher than those of young-old females, whereas rates for the old-old male are 5–6 times higher than those for old-old females.

While the prevalence of completed suicide is high, especially among males, it is noteworthy that those over 65 years of age appear to engage in less nonfatal suicidal behaviour (attempted suicide) and report less suicidal ideation (cf. Blazer et al. 1986) than their younger counterparts. Hendin (1982) suggested that while the ratio of attempted suicides to actual suicides in the general population has been estimated at 10:1, it is estimated at closer to 1:1 among those over 55 years of age. Blazer and colleagues (1985), in a psychiatric epidemiology study, found that the frequency of suicidal thoughts and attempts occur less often in later life. More recently, findings from the 1992–93 Quebec Health Survey (Québec. Santé Québec 1995) revealed that about 8 percent of Quebecers reported having serious thoughts about suicide at some time in their lives. However, only 1.6 percent of persons aged 65 and over reported ever having considered killing themselves. The failure of a suicide attempt in older persons need not be due to lack of determination; rather, it may be due to poor planning, accidental discovery or poor coordination (Pfeiffer 1977; Sendbuehler and Goldstein 1977).

Living with a Disability in Canada: Toward Autonomy and Integration

JOHN LORD, ED.D.

Social Research Consultant
Kitchener, Ontario

PEGGY HUTCHISON, ED.D.

Associate Professor, Brock University
St. Catherines, Ontario

SUMMARY

A large number of Canadian citizens with disabilities experience many of the indicators associated with poor health—powerlessness, unemployment, social isolation, and poverty. This paper outlines some historical trends in systems and services designed for citizens with a disability, and considers the ways in which paradigms of disability have been shifting dramatically in the last two decades. Key conclusions from research and literature related to determinants of health are presented, along with a number of "promising community practices" that have been used to support people with a disability. Finally, policy implications for children and adults are proposed.

A study of historical perceptions can reveal a great deal about the barriers and health problems experienced by citizens with disabilities. The traditional dominance of professionals in the context of the medical model has been gradually giving way to a broadened view of disability and intervention. This trend is part of a paradigm shift in the disability field, which is focusing more and more on citizen control, independent living, empowerment, social networks and support, and community inclusion. Many of these elements can also be considered determinants of health, although this understanding is not usually a conscious one in disability movements or health policy.

The independent living movement in Canada has been vital in enhancing disability rights and finding alternative ways of providing community support.

The definition of independent living includes the concept that consumers can best define their own needs. The principles of consumer control and participation are critical to achievement of this goal. This paper identifies the positive results achieved by Independent Living Resource Centres and emphasizes the importance of promoting independent living beginning in childhood. The paper links new approaches to health and disability with the concepts of independent living.

Most funding for support of Canadians with disabilities goes to institutional care. Reallocation of resources from institutions to community support is a critical issue in disability policy. This paper outlines the results of research into the deinstitutionalization process and its impact on community living and quality of life. Family and consumer initiatives that enhance quality of life in the community are also described.

The segregation of citizens with disabilities has been costly, demeaning, and illness producing. The move toward inclusion in education, recreation, and community is a constructive trend in disability policy and practice. Research on the outcomes of inclusion is presented. Special emphasis is placed on relationships and social networks as an important avenue for integration of children with disabilities to become embedded in family and community life. Social networks are strongly linked to quality of life and health status.

"Experiencing control" is also a key determinant of health. Studies show that many citizens with disabilities lack personal control over the most basic aspects of their lives. Research on the process of empowerment illustrates the kind of support and resources that people may require to gain more control and participation. Empowerment principles for citizens with disabilities can be an important guide for policymakers and service organizations.

There are several other key conclusions from research and literature related to determinants of health. In order for children with disabilities to grow up with the same opportunities as nondisabled children, there must be a focus on ways to enhance family well-being. The paper explores a number of principles related to early intervention and individualized family support programs which can contribute to child and family well-being.

The paper includes some success stories and failures to illustrate the changing environment related to disability. These examples show the power of consumer and family control as well as the value of networking and mutual support. Other stories demonstrate new ways of working "in community", stressing the interdependence and collaboration required to maximize community involvement, empowerment, and positive health outcomes.

Finally, implications for health policy are outlined. Policies are needed to enhance individualized support for families who have a child with a disability, increase the community involvement of children with disabilities, reallocate resources from institutions to community in a way that builds family and consumer initiatives and provides direct funding to people with disabilities, and enhance independent living and the development of Independent Living Resource Centres.

TABLE OF CONTENTS

LIST OF TABLES

INTRODUCTION

A large number of Canadian citizens with disabilities experience many of the indicators associated with poor health—powerlessness, unemployment, social isolation, and poverty. This paper presents some historical trends in systems and services designed for citizens with a disability. It then outlines the ways in which paradigms of disability have been shifting dramatically in the last two decades. Key conclusions from research and literature related to determinants of health are presented, along with a number of "promising community practices" or success stories about ways to support people with a disability. Finally, policy implications for children, families, and adults are proposed.

Defining Disability

The World Health Organization (WHO) defines disability as "any restriction or lack (resulting from an impairment) of ability to perform an activity in the manner or within the range considered normal for a human being." Within this and most other acceptable definitions of disability, the focus is on limitation of performance or activities. Defined in this way, disabilities are not necessarily handicapping.

The major contribution of the WHO model of disability has been the conceptual distinction among three levels of disablement outcomes: 1) impairments (at the organic level), 2) disabilities (at the personal level), and 3) handicaps (at the societal level). However, some Canadian researchers have been critical of the model's implication of linear causation of disablement. Whiteneck and Fougeyrollas (1995) point out the importance of the environment in defining disability:

> The WHO model has emphasized disablement as originating with pathology, leading to impairment, which in turn produces disability, and finally handicap. While this conceptualization is well-grounded in the medical model, it fails to acknowledge the importance of the environment as a major contributor to the disablement process, acting to either restrict or facilitate the importance of the individual.

These authors note the importance of internal factors (impairments, abilities, disabilities) and personal identity, as well as environmental factors and their interaction in determining the degree to which a person with a disability is actually handicapped.

Disability in Canada

According to the last census, 13.2 percent of the population—over 3,300,000 Canadians—reported some level of disability (Statistics Canada

1988). Several other factors also contribute to the vital importance of disability as a health issue:

- Most Canadian families are touched by disability in one way or another.
- Disability is costly in Canada, where almost 250,000 people with disabilities were residing in health care institutions and homes for senior citizens in 1988.
- Some research indicates that people with disabilities are less likely to be employed and more likely to be poor, and often have limited social support. These factors, important determinants of health, will be discussed throughout the paper.

Statistics Canada data confirms that disability increases with age. The disability rate is 5.2 percent in the 0–14 age group, 5.7 percent for those 15–34, and 15.5 percent among those aged 35–64. Forty-five point five percent of people over 65 have a disability; further, 76 percent of those have multiple disabilities.

Of Canadian children with disabilities, the vast majority (99 percent) live in private households—in contrast with the situation in 1986, when approximately 2,400 disabled children resided in health care institutions. The emphasis in all provinces is to provide support for families so that children with disabilities can stay at home.

Employment figures help indicate the social and economic status of disabled adults. Of those aged 15–64 living in private households, 39.2 percent were employed in contrast to approximately 70 percent of nondisabled persons in this age group. Forty-nine point three percent of the total described themselves as "not in the labour force." While many of these people had never worked, the majority reported that their condition or health problem completely prevented them from working.

In the last two decades, our awareness of disability has increased dramatically for a number of reasons:

- Adults with disabilities have organized into consumer advocacy and support groups.
- Physical and mental disability are both included in the Canadian Human Rights Code and in the Charter of Rights.
- Families of children with disabilities have increasingly demanded that their children have the right to go to regular schools and participate in the community in the same way as other children.
- The aging of the population has brought about increased demand for facilities and support systems which can accommodate disabilities.

SHIFTING PARADIGMS OF DISABILITY

A Brief Look Back

A study of historical perceptions can reveal a great deal about the barriers and health problems experienced by citizens with disabilities. Three major trends have been evident during the past 150 years. The first is the establishment of "asylums" across Canada, beginning in the mid-1800s. Originally intended for the insane, these soon expanded to accommodate citizens with a wide variety of disabilities, as well as those marginalized for other reasons (Goffman 1961; Rothman 1981). During the next century, institutions played a central role in disability policy, even though most families kept their children with disabilities at home. The legacy of this period is still quite apparent, particularly in Quebec and Ontario where thousands of citizens with disabilities continue to live in institutions.

The second major trend was the development of service systems for a variety of disabilities which began in the 1950s. Typically, they fell under the jurisdiction of the health care system and were oriented toward treatment and rehabilitation. An extensive body of professional knowledge and expertise accumulated during this period. In fact, professional interventions were often seen as essential if people with disabilities were to be enabled to "adjust" and "cope" (Wright 1989). Although the focus was ostensibly on "community-based services", few of them were designed to help people with disabilities function as part of the community (Lord and Pedlar 1991).

The third trend has become significant only in the last 20 years, with the traditional dominance of the medical model in the disability field gradually giving way to a broadened view. Some critics have even described the former focus on rehabilitation and professionalization as "disabling" (McKnight 1995). As part of this paradigm shift, the disability field has increasingly focused on family and consumer control, independent living, individualized control over support funding, empowerment, social networks and support, self-help and natural aid, and community inclusion (Schwartz 1992). Many of these elements can also be considered determinants of health, although this understanding has not usually been a conscious one in disability movements or health policy. Access to valued community resources is a significant aspect of the emerging paradigm. The collective voice of citizens with disabilities has grown stronger as their active participation has increased in such areas as policy consultations, community planning, and consumer leadership in projects that provide support (Oliver and Zarb 1989).

Broadened View of Knowledge

The changing nature of knowledge in the disability field parallels a shift in our understanding of health. Just as we once thought of health primarily in terms of health services and individual health patterns, valid disability knowledge was for most of this century seen to be professionally based and clinically oriented. The notion that other sources of knowledge might contribute to our understanding of disability remained unarticulated for years. The new approach may be exemplified by the Canadian Mental Health Association document *Framework for Support*, which identifies four sources of knowledge relevant to disability: medical/clinical, social science, experiential, and customary/traditional (Trainor, Pomeroy, and Pape 1993).

The power and importance of experiential knowledge has perhaps been the most controversial part of the paradigm shift. Whether they express themselves through the "independent living movement" (Carpenter 1991) or through "consumer participation" efforts (Church 1995), people with disabilities are increasingly saying they can best determine their own needs, and insisting on the legitimacy of their own viewpoints and experience. Qualitative studies have illustrated the importance of listening to people with disabilities and their families in order to gain deeper understanding of people's needs, strengths, and dreams (Lincoln and Guba 1985; Lord, Hutchison, and Schnarr 1987). Significantly, this research has illustrated that consumers often have a different perspective on issues than do service providers or policy people.

Shift from Treatment to Promotion

Most community services and interventions on behalf of people with disabilities have been oriented toward assessment and treatment. As such, they have typically been designed to improve or "fix" the problems that the person or the family is experiencing. Such "deficit-oriented" interventions pay little attention to the contexts in which people are living (McKnight 1987).

More recent research and intervention has focused on the environment and the particular situation of the person involved (Albee 1981). It is increasingly being recognized that people exist in families and within a variety of social relationships, and that one of the most effective ways to assist people is to promote the capacity and functioning of those interactive systems. In some innovative family support programs, for example, the goal is to promote and strengthen individual and family capabilities in ways that promote function and effectiveness of the family as a unit (Dunst 1991). This move from treatment to promotion is not easy to put into practice, but recent research is giving growing evidence of its efficacy (Epp 1986; World Health Organization 1986).

Key Elements of the New Paradigm

A variety of writers have suggested that there is a paradigm shift occurring in the disability field (DeJong 1979; Lord and Hutchison 1993; McKnight

1990; Oliver and Zarb 1989; Schwartz 1992). The key elements in this paradigm shift are outlined in the following table. It is significant that many of these elements relate to determinants of health. The focus on enhancing social support networks, increasing the control of the person, and expanding community participation are all areas that have been shown to enhance health and well-being. In the next section of this paper, we identify the key conclusions from research and literature related to the historical and theoretical trends outlined above.

Table 1

Key elements: Old and new paradigms of disability

Old approach	New approach
Focus on systems and facilities	Focus on community and relationships
Deficit oriented	Strengths oriented
Management driven	Consumer driven
Service oriented	Support oriented
Individual must fit into program	Program tailored to individual
"Fix the person" attitude	Focus on person within social network
Passive clients	Participating consumers
Ad hoc or no planning	Short- and long-term planning
Professionally directed and controlled	Consumer directed and controlled

KEY CONCLUSIONS

Independent Living: Concept and Movement

Challenges to institutional, rehabilitative approaches to disability emerged in the 1970s. The rehabilitation paradigm was criticized for its control by professionals, its focus on deficits and remediation, and its treatment of people as dependent clients (Canadian Association for Independent Living Centres 1991; Schwartz 1992). During this period, independent living was introduced as an alternative to traditional services (DeJong 1979).

The concept of independent living reflects many of the attributes of the new disability paradigm. It maintains that the root of the problem lies in the environment—in segregation, discrimination and in an unwarranted dependency upon professionals and others (Carpenter 1991; Crewe and Zola 1984; Robinson 1991). It regards disability in a political and socio-logical context, not in isolation from power structures and social realities (Jongbloed and Crichton 1990). The sections which follow review the literature on independent living, its outcomes, its connections to health, and its implications for children.

The Concept of Independent Living

The independent living (IL) paradigm emphasizes that people with disabilities can best identify their own needs and lead productive lives in the community through self-help, empowerment, advocacy, and the removal of environmental, social and economic barriers (Crewe and Zola 1984; Lord 1991). IL is a central concept in the modern view of community support and the role of the consumer in support provision (Racino 1992). In Canada during the last decade, the language and direction of social policies and practices related to disability issues have begun to change as a result of these concepts (Dunn 1994).

Consumer advocacy groups were responsible for the initiation of the Canadian Association for Independent Living Resource Centres (CAILC) and its local affiliates (ILRCs). Now a major force in promotion of the IL concept, ILRCs offer individuals with disabilities a consumer-controlled, cross-disability, community-based model as an alternative to traditional rehabilitation services (Canadian Association for Independent Living Centres 1991; COPOH 1986; DeJong 1993; Enns 1991; MacPherson 1990; Valentine 1994; Winter 1993).

Consumer and Community Outcomes of Independent Living Resource Centres

Research on independent living identifies several outcomes associated with determinants of health. In Canada and the United States, ILRCs have been the vehicle for much of this research.

Giving People Control over Their Own Lives

Recent health research has identified the importance of people having control of their lives in the workplace, in families, and in the community (Frank and Mustard 1994; Marmot 1994). Within ILRCs, most directors, staffers, volunteers and members have disabilities themselves. This helps ensure consumer-controlled policy directions (Canadian Association for Independent Living Centres 1990).

In a recent study (Hutchison et al.1996), consumers reported that they are treated at ILRCs not as clients and disabled persons, but as valued citizens and full contributing members of the community. This promotes a sense of empowerment. Respondents spoke of the dignity and sense of control that results when they are both cared for and listened to with respect, when they have full access to information and when they can count on their ILRC for support even as they are encouraged to achieve more independence. Overall, consumers said that participation in the ILRCs gave them more control over their lives. These findings are echoed in other reports (Budde, Petty, and Nelson 1986; Carpenter 1991; Lord et al. 1992).

Helping People Maintain Connections in Their Communities

Social support is a strong indicator of health (Barrera and Ainlay 1983; Gottlieb 1985; House 1986; Lord and McKillop Farlow 1990; McIntyre 1987; Wyngaarden and Erikson 1988). There is also a growing recognition in the literature of the importance of increasing one's independence through building strong social networks (Hutchison and McGill 1992; Pedlar 1991; Seed and Montgomery 1989). Research indicates that ILRCs have a positive impact on people's sense of "community-connectedness". As individuals become empowered, participation in community life increases (Friedmann 1992; McKnight, 1987); in turn, the community becomes better educated and significant changes occur.

Building Skills and Confidence

Personal empowerment is characterized by increasing competence and confidence (Lord 1991). People with disabilities who are involved with ILRCs acquire a variety of tools, resources and skills which make it possible for them to achieve personal and career goals. Typical skills which may be developed include self-management, group facilitation, problem solving, writing and public speaking (Hutchison et al. 1996). ILRC consumers report a sense of accomplishment from volunteer activities, committee work, or participation in education sessions and peer support groups (Hutchison et al. 1996). People also experienced heightened self-esteem, as reflected in greater self-confidence and assertiveness. It appears that fostering consumer control and choice is a powerful way to build skills and promote autonomy (Canadian Association for Independent Living Centres 1990; COPOH 1986; Lord et al. 1992).

Despite feeling empowered at their ILRCs, however, people still felt devalued in their communities (Hutchison et al. 1996; Robertson 1991). Improvement in quality of life for people with disabilities requires not only skill development but also removal of environmental, social, and economic barriers (Carpenter 1991; Robinson 1991).

A preventive, consumer-controlled, community-based approach to health promotion and quality of life is seen as much more effective than traditional approaches in the long run (Wallerstein 1992; Watt and Rodmell 1988). ILRCs, for example, often support individuals who have been disempowered through social isolation, institutionalization, poverty and discrimination. For many of these people, disempowerment is accompanied by poor physical and mental health (Iso-Ahola 1994; Labonte 1994; Lord and McKillop Farlow 1990).

Implications of Independent Living for Children with Disabilities

A future of independent living has not always been a goal for children with disabilities and their families. Many people with disabilities live with their families of origin well into adulthood, continuing a pattern of physical, financial and emotional dependence.

In the past, many families overprotected their disabled children and failed to involve them as active participants in their schools, neighbourhoods and community groups. This not only contributed to inactivity and isolation among children, but also left them inadequately prepared to live independently as adults (Active Living Alliance for Canadians with Disabilities 1992).

While a trend toward social integration now exists, so do significant barriers. Children with poor motor skills often have difficulty being included (Evans and Roberts 1987; Watkinson 1994), while participation can become more demanding as a child gets older (Wall 1989). Meanwhile, a lack of participation while young has made many adults with disabilities more vulnerable to physical, health and emotional problems. Recent research shows that people with disabilities, especially women, are more likely to experience abuse than other citizens (CAILC 1995; Roeher Institute 1994).

The research suggests that parents—as well as all adults with disabilities who are successfully leading independent lives—bear a tremendous responsibility to provide support, modelling and encouragement to children with disabilities. Children must be gradually equipped with the skills, confidence, and social support they need to move toward an adult life of independence, confidence and community participation.

From Institutions to Community: Reallocating Resources

Research can offer valuable insights on deinstitutionalization— the process of moving from an institutional service system to a community service system. The impetus for deinstitutionalization in Canada has come from an understanding of the new paradigm discussed above, as well as from economic considerations. During the 1970s, voluntary advocacy associations and family groups began to call for the dismantling of large institutions. Although a major mental health facility closed in Saskatchewan in the 1960s, the first systematic institutional closures did not begin until the era of economic restraint in the early 1980s. During the next 10 years, many people with mild and moderate disabilities moved out of institutions. In 1986, at the time of the last Canadian census, 239,000 Canadians were living in institutions—a decline of almost 40,000 since 1980. The decline has continued steadily into the 1990s. Currently, some 200,000 Canadians are housed in institutions.

Institutionalization: Health and Family Dilemmas

Some criticisms of institutional life have focused on health-related issues, such as the lack of variety and nutritional value of institutional food, the rigid scheduling of meals to fit staff timetables, the inadequacy of dental and other ancillary care, the high incidence of smoking, the restriction of activity and the isolation from families, the community, and other residents. It has been noted that the "culture" of the institution—primarily, the custodial and medical environment—affects both residents and staff (Bogdan and Taylor 1982; Burstow and Weitz 1988; Gubrium and Buckroldt 1982; Hall 1983).

Despite such criticisms, there are many situations in which a family may have little choice but to institutionalize one of its members. For example, caregivers may fall ill; respite may be otherwise unavailable; families may break up; the community may lack adequate support systems, and specialized equipment or services may be available only at an institution (Lord, McGeown, and Ochocka 1993; Singer and Irvin 1991; Turbull, Brotherson, and Summers 1985; Willer and Intagliatea 1979).

Research on Outcomes

The outcomes of deinstitutionalization are varied. People living outside of institutions generally show a better quality of life than those within; still, their quality of life is not necessarily very high. In other words, when people move to the community with support, their living environments are less restrictive (Lord and Hearn 1987), many negative symptoms are reduced within two years (Anderson et al. 1993), more opportunities are available (Leff et al. 1994), and their social networks expand somewhat (Gollay et al. 1978; Hoffman 1993; Carling 1995). However, several authors caution that the advantages enjoyed by nondisabled citizens far outweigh those generally experienced by deinstitutionalized people with disabilities. In recent years, most Canadians leaving institutions have returned to communities where they are part of a formal human service system. According to Taylor, Biklen and Knoll (1987), research fails to show that community service systems necessarily enhance quality of life. That services are "community-based" does not necessarily mean that people have more control over their lives, or are truly connected with others in the community. The authors warn against the simplistic assumption that replacement of large institutions with smaller "community institutions" is a change for the better.

This dilemma is illustrated by recent Canadian research. One longitudinal study at the Centre for Research and Education (Lord and Pedlar 1991) revisited people who had left an institution four years previously. Although quality of life had improved for most of them, it was evident that the community services they relied upon possessed several "institutional" features. In other words, "in" the community did not mean "of" the community. With this understanding, the move from institutional to community-based services can best be seen not as an endpoint, but rather as part of the evolution toward supportive communities that will be truly empowering for citizens with disabilities (Nirje 1980; O'Brien 1987).

Costs, Reallocation and Community Living

It may cost as much as $15 to $20 million annually to operate large facilities—an expenditure which seems particularly huge in times of financial restraint. Several provincial governments have been reallocating institutional funds to community alternatives, especially in the area of developmental disabilities. In Newfoundland and British Columbia, for example, all such institutions have closed in recent years. Only in Ontario and Quebec are there significant numbers of people left in institutions. Deinstitutionalization has been slower and more cautious in the mental health area. Mental health advocates and consumer/survivors have called for a major reallocation of funds from psychiatric institutions to community mental health (Pape and Church 1987).

Research findings on the cost-effectiveness of deinstitutionalization have been somewhat mixed, at least partly due to differing social contexts and the complexity of the various disabilities (Canadian Council on Social Development 1985). In general, studies show that community living is somewhat less expensive for people with significant mental health problems (Carling 1990; Hallam et al. 1994; Lafave 1993; Leff et al. 1994). Lafave (1993) and his colleagues at the Brockville Psychiatric Hospital found that there were significant savings when a case manager was assigned responsibility for planning, monitoring and support for each individual.

In an extensive review of research in the developmental disability area, costs were shown to be slightly less for community-based efforts. However, the authors acknowledge that many of the studies under review had methodological problems and did not include hidden community costs. As more provinces embrace downsizing for economic reasons, they would do well to bear in mind the necessity of spending during the deinstitutionalization process itself to ensure that the necessary community infrastructures are in place.

The Canadian Mental Health Association (Pape and Church 1987) has conducted important research on the viability and effectiveness of strategies to reallocate resources from institutions to community support systems. Drawing lessons from the American and European experiences, researchers confirmed the importance of a comprehensive approach and found that the particular model chosen for reinvestment has a direct effect on costs.

The Process of Deinstitutionalization

Experience in Canada and the United States has produced some excellent research and documentation on the deinstitutionalization process, indicating the need for a comprehensive approach (Anderson et al. 1993; Carling 1995; Des Lauriers and Clair-Foyer 1982; Lord and Hearn 1987; McWhorter 1986). Individual planning approaches, parental and family involvement, worker retraining and individualized community service development are all part of the growing thrust towards a combined approach to deinstitutionalization and community integration.

Recent research shows that the most effective deinstitutionalization programs start with a focus on the individual and the goals the person wants to achieve. A personalized community support system evolves from the dreams, strengths, and preferences of the person and his social network. This is especially important for the many individuals who have weak social networks and who rely mostly on service staff for social support (McGeown 1993; O'Brien 1986; Taylor et al. 1987).

Leadership is required in all areas, including government policy and funding, family leadership, external advocacy, person-centred planning, and community integration strategies (O'Brien 1989; Pandiani et al. 1994). Consumer participation is an essential component in all aspects of the process (Church 1992).

People who remain in facilities throughout Canada despite extensive deinstitutionalization tend to be individuals with severe disabilities and complex needs. It is estimated that nearly 3,000 people with physical disabilities are living in chronic care hospitals because they are perceived to be "too severely disabled" to live in the community. This is a controversial issue in the disability field and in the literature. For example, in mental health, consumer/survivor groups and the Canadian Mental Health Association have strongly supported deinstitutionalization (Chamberlin 1978; Pape and Church 1987). On the other hand, some professional and family groups have been cautious about the prospect of people with severe chronic mental illness living in the community. The Ontario government, for example, spent about 80 percent of its 1993 mental health budget on institutional services and 20 percent on community-based services. The Ministry has now announced its intention to change this ratio to 40 percent for institutions and 60 percent for community services by 2003 (Ministry of Health 1993). Similar goals, which still leave a significant role for institutions, are held by other provinces.

There is more consensus in the area of developmental disabilities, especially with regard to large institutions. Many researchers have criticized institutional services and argue in favor of community living (Meyer, Peck, and Brown 1991; Taylor et al. 1987). Studies showing that appropriate supports can enable even people with the most severe disabilities to live in the community raise important policy questions (Taylor, Biklen, and Knoll

1987; Carling 1995). This emerging literature suggests that focusing on a continuum of services, placement, and "bricks and mortar" is no longer the only way to identify the most appropriate supports for people (Taylor 1988). By delinking housing and support, much more flexibility and creativity is possible.

As part of deinstitutionalization, significant efforts have been made towards increased family involvement with very positive results (Conroy and Bradley 1985; Gollay et al. 1978; Turnbull, Brothersm, and Summers 1985). As earlier work in British Columbia has demonstrated, even the most cautious families tend to become quite supportive of community alternatives when they are actively involved in the planning process for a son, daughter or sibling (Conroy and Bradley 1985; Lord and Hearn 1987). Family involvement also helps expand the person's social network and relationships. Many families have lost touch with their disabled relative or with the institution, and may require extensive outreach from those involved in the deinstitutionalization effort. Of course, it is not always appropriate to involve family, and this is why the principle of consumer preference is so critical. Many people who have been living in institutions have no family connections at all.

Consumer Initiatives

To ensure that deinstitutionalization does not simply lead to "more of the same" in the community, several thoughtful alternatives are now being demonstrated. Some of the most promising work has been done by the national office of the Canadian Mental Health Association. In its *Framework for Support*, the Association takes the position that too many resources are invested in formal systems and that a major shift is required to build the capacity of other sectors (Trainor, Pomeroy, and Pape 1993). Development of the consumer and family sectors and of community-based support systems will reduce the dominance of formal systems.

Three years ago, such arguments stimulated the Ontario government to begin funding consumer/survivor self-help and natural aid groups throughout the province. This Consumer/Survivor Development Initiative (CSDI) has been very well received by consumers. The initial evaluation showed that consumer/survivors felt more empowered and have had fewer days of hospitalization since the program's inception (Consumer/Survivor Development Initiatives 1993). The CSDI has also led to the development of a variety of other initiatives including peer support groups, community economic development, research activities and advocacy initiatives.

Inclusion and Participation in School, Recreation and Work

There is growing support for the idea that participation in the life of the community is essential for children's health and well-being. Children need strong social networks, full membership in their neighbourhood schools, and opportunities to participate in and contribute to community life (McKnight 1990; O'Connell 1988). Research shows that when these opportunities are lacking, children with disabilities become isolated, lonely, inactive, and vulnerable to physical and emotional problems (Bogdan and Taylor 1982; Gottlieb 1985; Lutfiyya 1988; Taylor 1988).

Relationships and Networks

Over the last decade, a great deal of literature on the friendships and relationships of children with disabilities has emerged. This relatively new awareness contrasts sharply with older approaches, which focused more on physical integration into community settings than on full inclusion in community life (Stainback et al. 1994). In the early days of integration, it was assumed that if people were integrated into the community, social relationships would naturally follow.

It is now known that many children with disabilities have weak social networks (Belle 1989). While family relationships are often strong, being without friends among one's peers results in loneliness and isolation (Lyons 1987, 1989). There is increasing awareness that disabled adults as well as children with disabilities often experience physical, emotional and behavioral problems as a result of segregation, loneliness and isolation from family, friends and community life (McGee et al. 1987). Thus, inclusion is increasingly acknowledged to be a complex concept which includes acceptance, friendship, and full participation (Eigner 1995; Hughes and Lyles 1994; Jacobsen and Sawatsky 1993; Lewis 1992). Concrete strategies are needed to ensure that children with disabilities are in the right places to meet people, and that supports for making and keeping friends are provided (Partin 1994; Pearpoint, Forest, and Snow 1992; Strully and Strully 1989).

Parents, teachers and children agree that numerous benefits follow when children with disabilities have friendships, especially with nondisabled peers. In learning how to be a friend, the child with disabilities gains access to everyday opportunities available to other children while becoming more sociable, self-confident, assertive, and willing to take risks. The benefits of improvement in communication skills gained in these relationships can extend well into adulthood (Heyne, Schleien, and McAvoy 1993; Giangreco et al. 1993; Perske 1988). For their part, nondisabled children stand to gain a strong sense of shared humanity, equity, fairness, acceptance and commitment along with increased confidence, self-awareness and self-esteem (Bogdan and Taylor 1982; Lusthaus, Gazith, and Lusthaus 1992; Peck, Donaldson, and Pezzoli 1990).

However, facilitating the development of friendships can be difficult and complex. Some adults are reluctant to take deliberate measures because they see friendship as a natural process, not to be interfered with (Hutchison

1990; Kishi and Meyer 1994). Children with behavioral problems may find they are not well accepted by peers (Breslau 1985; Mitchell 1982). Family stress may limit parents' capacity to initiate integration and support relationship development (Dunst et. al. 1988; Schilling and Schinke 1984). Children or adults who live in group homes often enjoy much less interaction within the neighbourhood and the community than those in family homes (Crapps and Stoneman 1989), and when children do participate in the community, the constant presence of a support worker or other adult can limit opportunities for peer-to-peer relationships (Hutchison and McGill 1992; Intagliatea, Crosby, and Neider 1981).

Inclusion in Education: Emerging Outcomes

There has been much debate over school integration in the past 10 years (Salend 1994; Winzer 1993). While many believe that parents and children have a right to choose integration, progress has been slow (Bailey 1994; Smith and Lusthaus 1994). Those who advocate integration feel strongly that it is an essential early intervention strategy which increases the likelihood of having an ordinary life as an adult (Stanley 1993).

Research has identified several key principles of successful school integration. Children should attend neighbourhood schools with their siblings; support, individualized goals and strategies for socialization are all essential; children should be in regular classrooms with age-appropriate peers; teachers need support to learn curriculum adaptations; and finally, consideration should be given to the benefits a teacher's aide might bring (Brown et al. 1989; Giangreco et al. 1993; Jackson 1993; Jacobsen and Sawatsky 1993; Kennedy and Itkonen 1994; Klassen 1994; Nevin 1993; Pearpoint, Forest, and Snow 1992; Putnam 1993).

Children in integrated settings have shown improved responsiveness to school routines and higher academic performance (Giangreco et al. 1993). They also enjoy greater opportunities for social and extracurricular activity (Lusthaus, Gazith, and Lusthaus 1992), get a chance to practice possible future roles (Bradley 1994), and increase their social skills, self-esteem and sense of belonging (Ministry of Education 1992).

Others also benefit from integration. Peers get an opportunity to develop tolerance and caring—important skills for future parents, service providers and community members (Stainback, Stainback, and Forest 1985; Stanley 1993). They learn about the need for mutual support and learn to appreciate each other's strengths (Biklen 1992). The earlier this process of integration begins, the greater the benefits (Gould 1994). Teachers experience greater confidence and a sense of pride, as well as an increased willingness to change teaching methods and learn from their students through such approaches as cooperative learning, peer tutoring and support circles (Brown et al. 1989; Giangreco et al. 1993; Gold 1994; Graden and Bauer 1991; Putnam 1993;

Salisbury, Palombaro, and Hollowood 1993; Zey 1990). Teachers also experience increased understanding of the importance of strong parent/teacher relationships (Stanley 1993).

However, barriers remain to the establishment of inclusive systems. Few school boards have policies on integration; segregated classes and segregated schools are still prevalent; training for teachers is limited; teaching assistants are being eliminated to save money; some parents feel that their children require specialized support that only segregated settings can give; parents and teachers commonly hold low expectations, and there is often concern that children with severe disabilities will adversely affect others in the same classroom (Bilken 1992; Davern and Schnorr 1993; Dyson 1994; Giangreco et al. 1993; Gould 1994; Grenot-Scheyer 1994; Guralnick, Connor, and Hammond 1995; Hamre-Nietupski et al. 1994; Hunt et al. 1994; Lewis 1992; Sharpe, York, and Knight. 1994; Sobsey, Dreimanis, and MacEwan 1993).

Participation in Recreational and Leisure Activities

The importance of spare-time activities, friendships and a sense of competence to people's overall satisfaction, quality of life and health has been well documented (Headey 1988). However, feelings of personal competence are especially elusive for people who are poor, socially isolated, unemployed or who live in substandard housing (Rosenfield 1992).

While leisure makes positive contributions to health and quality of life (Argyle 1987), it is not always a good thing. It is unhealthy when it leads to apathy, boredom and anxiety, or to excessive television watching, compulsive shopping, overexposure to the sun, overindulgence in alcohol, drug abuse or crime. All these are hallmarks of uprooted communities and lack of adequate value systems (Carruthers and Hood 1994; Csikszentmihalyi and LeFevre 1989). Youth and people with disabilities in particular are susceptible to such problems. If people are inadequately prepared and their leisure time is wasted or inappropriately used, poor health and quality of life can be the result (Walker 1994).

Well-spent leisure time brings many health benefits. The positive mood thus induced can improve the immune function (Folsom et al. 1985; Hull 1990). Constructive leisure activities produce "flow experiences"— challenging, skill-building experiences characterized by enjoyment, deep concentration, and a lowered awareness of the passage of time (Csikszentmihalyi 1990). Self-esteem, self-actualization and feelings of increased competence are enhanced through leisure participation, as has been convincingly demonstrated in the adventure therapy and outward-bound movements (Berman and Davis-Berman 1993). Leisure activities contribute to stronger social networks, which are also associated with better health. When people have friends, they are less isolated, less bored, less lonely and less dependent on professionals (Larsen, Mannell, and Zuzanek 1986). Leisure reduces stress by acting as a buffer between stressful life events and illness (Coleman and Iso-Ahola 1993). Finally, leisure contributes to self-determination by encouraging freedom of choice and a sense of control over one's life (Coleman 1990). The Active Living Movement in Canada recognizes all these connections and has been a preeminent force for change at both the individual and community levels (Caldwell and Smith 1988; Quinney, Gauvin, and Wall 1994).

Integration of people with disabilities into leisure activities has perhaps been less controversial than integration in other areas of life. Generally, the informality and flexibility of leisure pursuits is seen as conducive to integration. A growing amount of literature is focusing on the integration process and its benefits, strategies, and outcomes (Bullock and Howe 1991; Certo, Schleien, and Hunter 1983; Gold 1988; Heyne, Schleien, and McAvoy 1993; Lyons 1991; Morgan 1989; Pedlar 1992; Potschaske 1988; Sandys and Leaker 1987).

Community Contribution and Preparation for Work

Over the past decade, it has been shown that when people are denied opportunities to contribute in a meaningful way to society, their mental and physical well-being suffers (Canadian Mental Health Association 1984; Pedlar, Lord, and VanLoon 1989). This situation is especially common among the unemployed, retirees and older persons, people with disabilities who are considered unemployable, and youth. In addition, active participation in work-related decision making and control over one's own work have been identified as important determinants of health (Ochocka, Lord, and Roth 1994; Syme 1994).

While societal attitudes toward work have fluctuated, it is still generally accepted that meaningful work is a valued activity that should be accessible to anyone, including people who have disabilities (Hagner and Dileo 1993; Sandys and Leaker 1987). Proponents of work for disabled people have demonstrated that even those whose disabilities are quite severe can work in the community and make a positive contribution (Bellamy et al. 1988; Gardner et al. 1988). Researchers argue that it is devaluing to treat people with disabilities as trainees and clients in segregated, sheltered workshops rather than as employees in regular enterprises (Brown et al. 1991; Worth 1988).

People with disabilities experience a high rate of unemployment and are often seen as unemployable (Roeher Institute 1988). As a result, many live below the poverty level, subsisting on a fixed pension. Others find themselves living at home with their parents, in substandard housing, or in residential units specifically designed for people with hand-icaps. They experience not only the stigma of their particular impairment, but also that of being labelled permanently unemployable and poor. The close association among poverty, unemployment and poor health is well known (Bridge and Gold 1989).

In order to prepare people with disabilities for productive work in adulthood, there has been greater emphasis on prevention among children and youth with disabilities. School integration, cooperative work placements, school-to-work transition programs, part-time and volunteer jobs can all be of value. When expectations are high and development opportunities abundant, people are healthier and happier as children, youth and adults (Panitch 1988).

Researchers also contend that not all people with disabilities can or will be employed in the labour market. A combination of factors has been cited, including the nature and severity of a person's disability and difficult economic conditions (Browne, Connors, and Stern 1985; Revaud, Madiot, and Ville 1992). It is believed that the most severely disabled people would be unable to work and make a meaningful contribution even in a sheltered workplace, let alone in the community. The cost and effort of providing supports would far outweigh the benefits accruing to either the person or the community. Realistic alternatives to work could contribute significantly to the quality of life of people with severe developmental disabilities.

The current economic climate is also identified as a significant barrier to employment of people with developmental disabilities (McLoughlin et al. 1987). Society is becoming desensitized to hearing about unemployment rates of well over 10 percent. Employers and unions are seen as being resistant to the idea of hiring people with disabilities, particularly at a time when other workers are being laid off. If this trend continues, it will be increasingly difficult for those previously labelled "unemployable" to find work. People with disabilities, as well other citizens who are finding themselves with a large amount of discretionary time, can enhance their overall quality of life by pursuing a variety of nonwork alternatives (Reid 1990).

The argument is also put forth that people with disabilities—and all citizens—have the right to choose whether they wish to work (Farina 1982). While choosing to be unemployed often results in less income for the individual, many—such as stay-at-home parents, some older persons and some people receiving social assistance—have made that choice, at least temporarily (Guest 1985). Their reasons may include such factors as dissatisfaction with a former workplace, inadequate income from current position, a desire to raise children, or an interest in pursuing nonwork alternatives.

Enhancing Family Well-Being

Family and Disability

Parenting a child with a disability in our culture is filled with paradoxes and dilemmas (Turnbull 1985). Historical perceptions of disability cloud all efforts to raise one's child the same as other children. Support has typically been provided in professionalized, clinical settings. Adults with physical disabilities often remember a childhood characterized by "visits to the clinic" and "little involvement with other kids" (Lord 1991). Moreover, the family—supposed to be the site of nurturing and care—can also be a place of violence and risk, as demonstrated by recent Canadian data (Roeher Institute 1994). In short, researchers have identified a multitude of situations in which families may require support (Dunst et al 1988; Roeher Institute 1994).

Families whose children grew up in the 1950s and 1960s faced a very different situation from those raising young children in the 1990s. The threat of institutionalization has diminished and a variety of community-based family support options has emerged. These alternatives, while usually quite limited and poorly funded by governments, provide one of the most cost-effective ways to improve the determinants of health.

Advocacy by affected families has been a strong force for change in the paradigm of disability. As Simmons (1982) has pointed out, people with disabilities, unlike the organized working class, have a limited recorded history. Simmons emphasized that the political voice of people with developmental disabilities has been heard only since representations began to be made on their behalf after 1945 by interested groups and families. Families as advocates have also helped shape government policy and social change by presenting a vision of what could be possible for people with disabilities. Usually, their vision has been challenging and well ahead of existing policy. For example, the Canadian Association for Community Living *Vision 2000* paper proposed in 1980 that all children should have access to neighbourhood schools and regular classrooms. Similarly, families who have a loved one with a mental health problem have presented many briefs to government recommending that effective community support services be put in place.

Family Support: Elements in the Emerging Vision

Canadian families are increasingly diverse. Despite their structural differences, all families "need to be acknowledged, recognized, supported so that they can perform their many functions more effectively" (Vanier Institute on the Family 1992, 16). Industrial society has significantly changed the roles which families have to play in the culture. Because of the changing nature of families, according to the Vanier Institute on the Family (1992), every government has a family policy if only by default:

(It is) in the nature of modern industrial society (that) no government, however firm might be its wish, can avoid policies that profoundly influence family relationships. This is not to be avoided. The only option is whether these will be purposeful, intended policies or whether they will be residual, derivative, in a sense concealed ones (Moynihan 1986, 12).

Numerous family support principles, as distinct from other human service initiatives, can now be found in the literature (Center on Human Policy 1986; Hobbs et al. 1984; Dunst, Trivette, and Deal 1988). Examples include:

- Opportunities must exist for people to gain the skills they need to promote individual and family development.
- Mutually beneficial person-to-person linkages must be forged.
- Families need permission and encouragement to make informed decisions about themselves and their children.
- Families must have access to the resources, time, energy and information they need to perform child-rearing functions well.
- Partnerships and parent-professional collaboration helps families become more capable and competent.

Similarly, the Family Support Institute of Ontario, a parent-driven organization, has promulgated a set of six guiding principles for support of families who have a child with a disability:

- Family support programs must not be prescriptive, but flexible. Whatever it takes to meet a family's needs must be the basis of the program.
- Support must build on existing social networks.
- The program must maximize the family's control over the services and supports they receive.
- Family support includes the entire family.
- Family support must encourage the integration of individuals with disabilities into the community.
- Planners must bear in mind that all families, regardless of disability, need enduring family relationships.

Such principles are creating an emerging vision of family support. Increasingly, family support programs are oriented toward "empowerment." They try to provide the resources and supports that families need to enhance their own control and competence, and try to help them make the best use of the resources they have in collaboration with their communities. Dunst (1991) lists five critical questions for evaluating family support policy and practice.

1. Does the policy or practice enhance a sense of community amongst its members?
2. Does it promote the flow of resources and supports to and from the family?
3. Does it strengthen and protect the integrity of the family unit?

4. Does it operate according to the principle of empowerment, promoting the confidence of the family and of individual family members?
5. Does it encourage adoption of these principles for approaches to human service delivery in general?

Thus, the emerging vision of family support is a series of comprehensive, interdependent policies which enhance the determinants of health by giving families more control over their resources and networks. In turn, this enables them to support full participation of their disabled children in community and school life.

Individualized Funding and Family Support

In the last decade, there has been increased interest in the development of individualized funding programs to meet the support needs of people with disabilities and their families (Agosta 1989; Pape and Church 1987; Salisbury, Dickey, and Crawford 1987; Torjman 1991). In individualized funding initiatives, money goes from the government to the family either directly or through an agency. In either case, the individual needs of the family are used to determine what money and resources should be provided. Families make their own decisions about the services they wish to purchase.

Individualized funding programs are producing positive results. For example, the Review for Support Services for Ontario (Lord, Hutchison, and Farlow 1988) found that 78 percent of consumers favoured an independent living allowance. Similarly, there were positive outcomes demonstrated for families enrolled in the *Special Services at Home* program, sponsored by the Ontario government and the Ministry of Community and Social Services (Lord and Ochocka 1995). Table 2 shows the percentage of families who feel things have become better, stayed the same, or become worse since they began receiving funding with this program.

The most notable effect of the program was reduction in the mother's stress levels. This is consistent with research related to institutionalization, in which crises were often related to "the wearing down of the mother" (Bullock 1990; Lord and Hearn 1987).

Individualized family support programs, such as Ontario's *Special Services at Home*, provide a new and exciting approach for working with families and children with disabilities. Family-centred support services let families participate in and control critical issues which affect their lives. However, such programs are currently very limited in terms of scope and impact. In addition, families report problems such as lack of agency responsiveness and lack of appropriate services for purchase. There were also complaints that the system failed to recognize that not all families "wish to play such an empowered role" (Agosta 1989, 8).

Table 2

General family outcomes

Family togetherness						Family stress					
Worse	▮					Worse	▮				
Same	▬▬▬▬▬					Same	▬▬				
Better	▬▬▬▬▬▬▬					Better	▬▬▬▬▬▬▬▬				
	0	20	40	60	80		0	20	40	60	80

Quality of family life						Family participation in the community					
Worse	▯					Worse	▯				
Same	▬▬▬▬					Same	▬▬▬▬▬				
Better	▬▬▬▬▬▬					Better	▬▬▬▬▬▬				
	0	20	40	60	80		0	20	40	60	80

Empowerment, Control and Participation

Several fields of endeavour have begun to incorporate the language of empowerment. Health promotion, for example, is defined by the World Health Organization (1987, 1) as "the process of enabling people to increase control over, and to improve their health." In social work, empowerment is seen by some critics as an alternative to the professional control exercised by social workers and the systems within which they work (Freire 1985). And in the area of disability (and especially family support), there is a growing network of researchers and practitioners interested in the concept of empowerment (Dunst et. al. 1988; Rose and Black 1985.

The Process of Empowerment

We can begin to understand empowerment by examining the concepts of power and powerlessness. Power is defined by the Cornell Empowerment Group (1989, 1) as the "capacity of some persons and organizations to produce intended, foreseen and unforeseen effects on others."

At the individual level, powerlessness can be seen as the expectation that one's own actions will be ineffective in influencing the outcome of life events (Kieffer 1984). Rappaport notes that empowerment "conveys both a psychological sense of personal control or influence and a concern with actual social influence, political power and legal rights" (Rappaport 1987, 121). In this sense, empowerment can exist at three levels: the personal level, where empowerment is the experience of gaining increasing control and influence in daily life and community participation; the small group level, where it involves the shared experience, analysis and increasing influence of small groups on their own efforts and their community; and the community level, where it implies the optimal utilization of resources and strategies to enhance community control.

Recent research has focused on citizens with disabilities who have moved from a situation of powerlessness to one of participation and control. Five research themes have solidified our understanding of the need for new approaches to community services (de Boer 1992; Lord 1991; Lord and Hutchison 1993; Lord and McKillop Farlow 1990). Each is presented below.

Powerlessness

Most research on empowerment describes in great detail the anguish of feeling powerless. This feeling is the cumulative result of a series of experiences rather than of any single factor. For most people with disabilities, social isolation began early in life—at home, school, and in the community. As Foucault (1984) has pointed out, one of the cruelest myths experienced by people with disabilities is that their difference is somehow not socially acceptable.

A number of studies demonstrate that early intervention is an essential prevention strategy which can break the continuity of powerlessness from childhood to adult life (Cochran 1986; Dunst et al. 1988; Shipe 1984). The primary function of early intervention is to keep impairments or disabilities from becoming serious social handicaps.

Impetus for Personal Change

The transition toward personal empowerment is a continuous, individual process. For most people, change is not the result of a one-time concrete decision. Instead, it is motivated by a variety of factors that people can identify upon reflection. These factors or situations act as catalysts for empowerment, helping individuals to become aware of their own capacities and of alternatives to the experience of powerlessness. The main factors which participants identified as providing the impetus for change were:
- a crisis or "life transition";
- anger or frustration with things as they are;
- exposure to new information;
- realization of inherent strengths and capabilities;
- a change in context.

Support from Others

Personal supports are vital in expanding personal empowerment. Three main types of support were identified as being particularly significant: practical support, moral support, and mentoring. Most research participants identified at least one significant person as being important to their own personal empowerment.

Several studies have shown the correlation between social support and health. In summary, the intrinsic value of social connections is thought to reside in four basic characteristics: emotional concern and caring, practical aid, information sharing and social comparisons and appraisals (Barrera and Ainlay 1983; Gottlieb 1985; House 1986; Lord and McKillop Farlow 1990; McIntyre 1987; Wyngaarden and Erikson 1988). Most authors agree that relationships are "supportive" when they involve a two-way "flow" of valued resources between parties (House 1986; Lord and McKillop Farlow 1990; Wellman and Hall 1986). People with disabilities have a long history of experiencing social isolation and very small social networks. While disabilities themselves can make people vulnerable, lack of social connection puts them in double jeopardy and increases powerlessness.

An innovation in the disability field is the growth of strategies for building social support networks, including support circles and support clusters (see the "Success Stories" section, later in this paper). These strategies, often informal and always community oriented, provide a collective approach to vulnerability, and appear to contribute to a sense of security for the whole family as well as to the empowerment of the person with the disability. The importance of peers and mentors is also demonstrated by research into the self-help movement, which has grown remarkably during the last decade (see entire Special Issue of the Canadian Journal of Community Mental Health, fall 1995).

As people gain more control in their lives, they often attribute the change to themselves and to a small number of individuals or groups. The self-help movement among consumers with disabilities has made substantial contributions. Whether it be the independent living movement, the People First organization for citizens with a developmental disability, or consumer/survivor initiatives in mental health, the power of peer support, mentors, and self-help groups has had great impact in the areas of health and social well-being (see the "Success Stories" section, later in this paper).

Access to Valued Resources

Most people who experience powerlessness have access only to resources which they perceive as being "different"—specifically for "rehabilitation" or "welfare." Research shows that access to resources and opportunities that are valued by the community as a whole is important for people's empowerment. For example, getting a job is a pivotal point in people's lives, expanding their economic power and gaining them respect. Other examples of valued resources include independent housing, money and technical resources such as motorized wheelchairs.

Research participants have been highly critical of systems which are bureaucratic, congregating and controlling. Pinderhughes (1983) points out that service workers and systems too often see people as victims and keep them in inferior, powerless positions. Services that are of real value have common qualities: they are personalized, responsive, interactive and consumer controlled, providing a degree of self-reliance. Significantly, workers regarded as most "helpful" by participants were characterized in such terms as "a good listener", "an equal", "a guide", and a person "who really cares."

Participation

Participation significantly advances the process of empowerment by reducing isolation, increasing social interaction, building skills, giving the opportunity to experience a range of valued roles, and raising confidence (Lord and Hutchison 1993). As people gain in self-confidence, they seek more avenues for participation. "Getting involved" is a particularly important way for people to feel affinity with others (Bellah et al. 1985).

However, participation can be double-edged for people with disabilities. "Community participation" is an essential part of quality of life and health. There is also the "consumer participation" that is so often required to ensure that their voices are heard (Church 1995). While both kinds of participation can be empowering, consumer participation does not necessarily lead to increased control. Too often, consumers are expected to support service practices that are disempowering. While the idea of "consumer participation" is gaining support, some service providers still find the prospect unsettling and this can jeopardize plans for change (Church 1995).

Empowerment Principles for Community Work with People with Disabilities

Many organizations that support people with disabilities espouse the concept of empowerment, and principles for achieving it are increasingly being identified (Lord and Hutchison 1993; Dunst et al. 1988; Labonte 1990; Rose and Black 1985; Whitmore 1988). Interestingly, the central principles identified in the research focus on areas that are essentially determinants of health—shifting the focus of control to the person, enhancing social support, accessing valued resources, and facilitating participation. According to the research, these principles do not work singly, but only in concert with one another.

Consumer Initiatives and Health

For the past two decades, self-help initiatives by consumers with disabilities have played an active role in Canadian policy analysis. Strong national groups such as the Council of Canadians with Disabilities, People First, the Mental Health National Network, the Canadian Association of Independent Living Centres, and the Disabled Women's Network have done extensive research and policy analysis, and represent the consumer perspective on a number of issues. Substantive health-related issues that these groups have addressed include:

- social security reform, with a focus on the relationship between poverty and disability. Proposals have been made to ensure an adequate income and "safety net" for people with disabilities (Canadian Association for Independent Living Centres 1994; Council of Canadians with Disabilities 1995; Film Images Production 1995; Worth 1988);
- the issue of choice and control in treatment and services. For example, consumers have been active in mental health legislation reform (Consumer Survivor Development Initiatives 1996);
- the vulnerability of people with disabilities—particularly women—to sexual and physical abuse both in institutions and the community (Browne, Connors, and Stern 1985; Husien 1995; Code 1991; Maurice 1995; Roeher Institute 1994; Tomlinson 1995);
- the ethics regarding mercy killing, assisted suicide, reproductive technologies and compensation for forced sterilization (Advocacy Resource Centre for the Handicapped 1995);
- the physical, economic and social accessibility of education, employment and training, housing, and community participation.

SUCCESS STORIES

Special Services at Home: A Provincial Individualized Family Support Program

The Ontario *Special Services at Home* program (SSAH), initiated in 1982 to avoid the institutionalization of children with developmental disabilities, was expanded to include children with physical disabilities and, more recently, adults with developmental disabilities. The SSAH focuses on two broad areas: the personal development and growth of the family member with a disability, and relief and support for the family generally. In a typical SSAH intervention, a paid person comes into the family home and provides relief for the family by giving the parents and siblings a break. The worker may also provide one-to-one support, helping get the individual with a disability involved in community activities. Families apply for SSAH funding directly to the area government office in their community. Once an application is approved, the government provides funds to the family either directly or through an agency.

Actions on Nonmedical Determinants of Health

This individualized family support program addresses determinants of health in several ways. It helps keep children with disabilities out of institutions, where they are much more likely to suffer a deterioration in health. It provides resources directly to families to enhance their quality of life. Third, it helps integrate children with disabilities into community activities, increasing their capacity for expanded social networks and enhancing their control over their own lives.

Principles and values underlying the *Special Services at Home* program include:

- Children with disabilities have the right and should have the opportunity to remain with their families wherever possible.
- Families should have control over the resources that are used for their own support.
- Families' situations and needs are extremely varied, making it impossible for a single program to be effective. The individualized nature of SSAH is its key to success.

Reasons for the Initiative

Ontario is the only province in Canada with a comprehensive individualized family support program. Prior to its inception, there was tremendous growth in community services for people with disabilities and their families, including developmental programs, respite care, an assistive devices program, a benefit program for handicapped children and increased availability of family support workers. Despite the growth, family support advocates argued that these initiatives were too limited and "institutional" to be of real service for families.

Actors

Each area office of the Ministry appoints a SSAH officer, who invites applications from families who meet certain criteria. Following release of the initial program guidelines in 1984, an SSAH Family Coalition was formed to advocate for increased funding and changes to the program. Updated guidelines issued in 1991 reflected many of their concerns. Although formal power over the program remains with the Ministry of Community and Social Services, families that receive individualized funding do have a great deal of "control" over the resources they receive. In fact, the evaluation confirmed that this is the characteristic of the program that families most appreciate.

Evaluation

A major evaluation of SSAH by the Centre for Research and Education in Human Services in 1993 confirmed that the program's objectives were largely fulfilled. Outcomes reported by families were classified into four categories:
- those related to community integration;
- those related to family life;
- those related to skill and behavioral development;
- general outcomes.

Within these four areas, key findings included reduced family stress, avoidance of institutionalization, and increased integration into community recreation. Families credited several factors for the program's success, including its individualized nature. The motivation of workers was identified as critical to enhancement of family life. In summary, the program demonstrated that progressive policy and straightforward implementation can effectively meet individual and family needs.

The evaluation also demonstrated some unsettling aspects of the program, many attributable to its uneven implementation across the province. Some families, for example, had difficulty finding workers, and reported less satisfaction with the program for this reason. The remedy may lie in the development of a community infrastructure of informal family networks which can share information and pool workers.

Overall, the SSAH evaluation raises important questions for the implementation of similar individualized programs. Typically, human services for people with disabilities emphasize the "supply" side of delivery— in other words, they establish services and programs with particular criteria. The SSAH program, on the other hand, focuses on the "demand" side, giving consumers the ability to purchase the needed support. In theory, the consumer demand should "create" appropriate services. As the evaluation pointed out, however, some families could not obtain adequate support, either because of unavailability of workers or high worker turnover. This finding suggests that careful attention must be paid to both the "demand" and "supply" sides of the service system.

The executive summary and full evaluation report, entitled *Family Directed Support: Diversity, Hopes, Struggles, Dignity, Special Services at Home Evaluation*, is available in both French and English from the Ontario Ministry of Community and Social Services.

Replicability of the Initiative

Ontario's Family Support SSAH Alliance maintains that the program can be expanded to include adults with disabilities living independently, as well as those who live with a family. Certainly, the program's principles can be put to work in other provinces and with other populations. The extensive evaluation and other program-related documents would be helpful to others who are considering replicating the program. When combined with informal support mechanisms, an individualized program like this can have significant positive impact on the health determinants of families and individuals with disabilities.

Funding

The Ontario Ministry of Community and Social Services provides ongoing funding for SSAH, totalling $26 million in 1994. Interestingly, demand for the service did not accelerate until the early 1990s. The cost-effectiveness of the program was confirmed in 1993. Families can receive a maximum of $10,000, and the amount paid out by government is far less than it would be for the alternatives of group home or institutional placement. In addition, the evaluation confirmed that quality of life is much greater for individuals who stay at home and function as part of their community.

Support Clusters Network of Ontario: Building Partnerships and Enhancing Social Support

The Support Clusters Network of Ontario was originally a three-year demonstration project entitled the *Support Clusters Project*. The original project involved persons with complex disabilities—individuals with a "dual diagnosis" of developmental disabilities and mental health problems. Intervention was aimed at helping the individual indirectly, by working with his "cluster" of friends, family and professional supporters.

Actions on Nonmedical Determinants of Health

The goal was improvement in the quality of life and physical and mental health for everyone within the support network or cluster. The central values and principles underlying this intervention are:
- Support for supporters is essential for helping the person with complex disabilities.
- The disabled person must be regarded holistically, as an integral part of his social environment.
- The immediate goal is empowerment of the support cluster.
- Families, friends, and professionals can work in partnership to enhance quality of life for the disabled person and for each other.
- Education and learning help clusters be more effective.
- Research helps ensure ongoing learning and support for clusters.

Reasons for the Initiative

People with complex disabilities who are experiencing serious mental health problems often have other significant health difficulties. Despite the good intentions of all involved, present practice for service delivery can best be described as fragmented, insensitive and ineffective. According to research done for this project, it is not unusual for such citizens to be overmedicated, frequently hospitalized, and generally to have a poor quality of life.

As institutional closures continue across Canada, the responsibility for daily support of individuals with very complex and difficult disabilities falls increasingly upon a network of well-meaning but ill-prepared families and community service providers. Most initiatives in this area call for more services. However, the founders of the Support Clusters Network of Ontario believe that this solution seldom addresses the underlying problems. Those involved in the original demonstration project realized that people with a dual diagnosis required an intervention which would address their consumer health needs, reduce inequities in health status and demonstrate a cost-effective, community-based method of delivering services. The need for change became most apparent when the initial founders began to think of what was "actually needed" instead of focusing purely on "getting more services."

Actors

The group that originated the *Support Clusters Project* included service providers, family members and researchers, and had many of the qualities which are required by small groups that are initiating community change. Each member enjoyed wide credibility and extensive social networks in the community. Early meetings uncovered another reality: each member had personal motivations to find alternative ways to resolve serious issues for the community. Several members were "innovators", able to see beyond the traditional ways of doing things. The final spark to action was a funding opportunity from the Health Innovation Fund of Ontario.

Evaluation

The 1993 evaluation by the Centre for Research in Human Services, entitled *Support Clusters Project: Evaluation Report of the Research Demonstration Project,* is available from the Support Clusters Network of Ontario, c/o Canadian Mental Health Association, Waterloo Region.

The chief goal of the *Support Clusters Project*—to increase social support within the networks of people with a dual diagnosis—was achieved for

20 families and individuals over a three-year period. The evaluation identified several factors associated with successful support clusters:
- a balance between informal and formal support within the cluster;
- involvement of the person with a complex disability;
- the willingness and capacity of members to work together;
- an informal approach to group interaction;
- establishment of practical, useful goals;
- effective facilitation of the process;
- shared leadership and development of partnerships.

Families were extremely satisfied with the *Support Clusters Project*. Most reported a marked increase in their ability to cope with stress. In addition, families noted that their relationships with informal and formal supporters had strengthened. Many expressed a real—and novel—sense of control in their relationship with professionals. Cluster members, including professionals, agreed that the network helped them to deal with difficulties and stress. Many also reported greater understanding of the disabled person and his strengths as an individual and as a family member. Finally, the research found that effective, paid facilitators helped cluster members to work together toward common goals.

Some contradictions should be noted. Support clusters that reported a lack of success did not have a good balance of members, and experienced struggles with some of the institutional health sectors. This suggests that the support clusters approach, while a viable model, may be appropriate only for certain individuals and families. The need for professionals to "buy into" the intervention can be either a strength or a liability.

Replicability of the Initiative

In its three-year term, the *Support Clusters Project* produced some long-term change in the communities where it operated. For 20 support clusters, for example, 86 professionals and 75 informal supporters attended more than two cluster meetings. This extensive participation had a "ripple effect", with individual clusters affecting perhaps eight or ten different people. Many agencies identified the project as a beginning point for positive change in their organizations and communities, and expressed willingness to continue their involvement.

While this intervention can clearly be replicated with people with complex disabilities, it is still uncertain whether it can successfully be used with other populations, such as people with Alzheimer's or those with serious mental health problems. Nevertheless, it is currently being tried. So far, it appears that the principles themselves can be replicated in a variety of situations.

The legacy of the *Support Clusters Project* is the Support Clusters Network of Ontario, which provides education and training opportunities for people across the province who are interested in using the support clusters model.

Funding

The three-year *Support Clusters Project* was funded by the Health Innovation Fund of Ontario. Since that time a Support Clusters Network of Ontario has received three-year funding from the Trillium Foundation. In addition, the Ministry of Community and Social Services now funds a dual diagnosis consultant who uses this model in an agency in Kitchener. This kind of intervention could be more effectively developed with ongoing and secure funding; currently there is one year left in the second three-year funding period. Several of the originators of the *Support Clusters Project* have continued their involvement.

Circle of Friends/Support Circles

In 1983, the "Joshua Committee"—the first documented support circle—was formed around Judith Snow, a woman who is a quadriplegic (Forest and Snow 1983). Judith had been living in a chronic care hospital, and experiencing such loneliness, frustration and malnutrition that she felt ready to die. Toronto professor Dr. Marsha Forest visited the hospital with her students and immediately developed a bond with Judith. It took some time, but a circle of friends was developed and the group secured funding from an Order in Council to get Judith out of the hospital and into a home of her own. Judith has now fulfilled many of her dreams, including completing a master's degree in psychology, getting married, working, and teaching people about the importance of friends and circles. Through all the frustrations and struggle involved in community living, Judith has maintained strong support from her circle of friends (Pearpoint 1990). This model of support and friendship has been replicated all across Canada, the U.S. and Australia. The circle of friends has been of particular significance as a support system for school integration (Forest 1987; Pearpoint, Forest, and Snow 1992).

Circle of support programs have been developed in many parts of Canada, including Vancouver (Planned Lifetime Advocacy Network), Alberta (Personal Support Communities), Manitoba (Winnipeg Association for Community Living), and Ontario (New Frontiers, London; Extend-a-Family, Kitchener and Toronto; NABORS, Toronto).

Actions on Nonmedical Determinants of Health

Circles of support can make a significant contribution to social well-being, an important determinant of health.

Reasons for the Initiative

Circles of support or friendship may be initiated in situations such as the following:

- The complexity of the person's disability or situation requires a level of support and facilitation that cannot be left to chance.
- Lack of accessibility to appropriate community support is severely limiting the person's options and leading to frustration.
- Because of lack of human contact due to isolation or rejection, the person has developed behaviours that are disturbing to others, and which make participation in the community difficult.
- Decisions about the person's life have been based on stereotypes about the needs of people with that disability or particular behaviour, with the result that personal needs, goals and dreams are not fulfilled.
- The person has little or no self-confidence and has lost the motivation to become involved.
- The person lacks friends and is lonely and isolated.
- The person and his friends and family are frustrated with enforced dependence on existing services and lack of responsiveness from professionals (Hutchison and McGill 1992).

The support circle approach provides significant contrast to other models such as peer tutoring, "leisure buddies," and citizen advocacy, which are based on one-to-one volunteer models and seem to offer less potential for strengthening the person's social network and providing real friendships (Hutchison 1990; Snow 1989).

Actors

The makeup of circles of support varies according to the needs and desires of the person with a disability. Some circles are limited to family members, friends and potential friends. Others include a few trusted professionals from the person's life, such as a health care worker or teacher, who are there not because they are being paid, but because they have been invited to get involved with the person in a different and deeper way. Members are sometimes known to the person as individuals who may be willing to make a bigger commitment to the person's life. Sometimes circle members use their own personal networks to identify potential new members (Mount, Beeman, and Ducharme 1988).

Analysis of the Results

There has been extensive documentation of support circles and their strategies along with anecdotal evidence of their importance (Falvey et al. 1994; Forest 1989; Haring 1991; Perske 1988). However, very little research has been conducted directly. The one major study on circles (Gold 1994) made several interesting findings. The ethos of the group—that is, the ideals that pervade it—was quite strong. A circle tries to make its activities seem as natural and normal as possible, integrating the social and support aspects—in other words, members see no need to separate support from friendship. The results also indicate that friendship with the person is far more important to most circle members than the circle itself. Further research is obviously needed to complete this picture of the circle concept and the most natural ways for people to develop friendships and support (Shaffer and Anundsen 1993; Uditsky 1993). Overall, the idea of "constructed social support" appears to have a lot of merit for increasing health and friendships.

Gerstein Centre: Community Mental Health Crisis Support

Actions on Nonmedical Determinants of Health

The provision of community-based crisis services for persons who experience significant mental health problems is considered crucial. Alternatives to institutions are not only seen as less restrictive, but also more economical. The rise of community-based alternatives to hospitals has led to the development of several models including nonmedical crisis centres, home treatment services, respite services, and consumer-run safe houses. The Gerstein Centre in Toronto is an innovative nonmedical crisis centre, which aims at enhancement of consumer control and quality of life. Its principal objectives are:
  – to enable people, whenever possible, to remain in the community while receiving the support they need to get through their crisis;
  – to respond as soon as possible to people in crisis;
  – to encourage clients to work with staff to identify their needs and to decide upon an agreed plan of action;
  – to respect the individuality, dignity, ability and autonomy of those who use the services.

Reasons for the Initiative

In response to concerns about the welfare of people discharged from hospitals who suffer from serious mental health problems, coupled with a lack of appropriate services and accommodations, the city of Toronto established the Mayor's Action Task Force on Discharged Psychiatric Patients with Dr. Reva Gerstein as chair. In March 1984 the Task Force recommended the establishment of a nonmedical crisis service centre in the community. In May 1986, the Crisis Centre Subcommittee submitted a proposal for funding to the Ministry of Health following a lengthy consultation process which included clarification of the goals of the Centre and agreement on the ways to achieve those goals.

The Centre began operation in September 1989, initially providing a crisis line to the community and a mobile team. The residence opened in February 1990, providing 24-hour telephone, mobile and residential services.

Key Actors and Elements

The Gerstein Centre offers a 24-hour, seven-days-a-week crisis intervention service, usually initiated by self-referral through the crisis line number. Services are voluntary and nonmedical.

The Centre is staffed by community crisis workers with a broad range of experience. Services are free of charge and confidential. The staff is complemented by well-trained, committed volunteers who enhance the Centre's services by preparing in-house meals, publishing the Centre's newsletter *Leaflettes,* and offering telephone follow-up and support. Services include:

Telephone Crisis Intervention

Crisis workers are available 24 hours per day. Medical emergencies are not dealt with by the Centre. The goal is to help callers in crisis to work out effective ways of addressing their immediate problems.

Mobile Crisis Team

Staff can meet people in their own community through a mobile team visit which is arranged during the crisis telephone call. The meeting place can be where the person is calling from, or a mutually chosen convenient location.

Residential Crisis Intervention

The Centre has 10 residential crisis rooms for both men and women, with one wheelchair-accessible suite. A short stay at the Centre is intended to provide a safe, supportive environment to help people through a crisis. The staff share information and, where appropriate, refer individuals to other community supports and services.

Telephone Follow-Up and Support

Volunteers who have completed a thorough training program offer telephone support for people who have recently used the Centre's services. The volunteers maintain contact with individuals for about one month after they have used the crisis services.

At least one-third of the Centre's board of directors must be consumers. This nonprofit organization has demonstrated that a consumer-oriented approach to mental health crisis is workable and cost effective. The following table contrasts this approach with more traditional models.

Table 3

How the Gerstein Centre differs from more traditional models of crisis intervention

Gerstein Centre	Traditional settings and models
Self-referral and second-party referral	Professional referral (usually medical)
Strictly voluntary	Voluntary and involuntary
Client-centred approach; for example, if people prefer to be left alone while staying at the Centre, their wishes are honoured	Approach depends on worker's credentials (e.g., physician, social worker, nurse, therapist) and usually does not involve the client's stated needs and wishes
Credentials not required for staff. Staff includes qualified consumer/ survivors	Staffed by professionals with degrees and all appropriate credentials
Early intervention takes place on demand, with response tailored to the client's assessment of the crisis. No separation between intake and intervention	Intervention usually takes place only when an emergency stage has been reached, and there is usually a wait for admission
No diagnosis or formal psychosocial/ medical assessment	Formal assessment, diagnosis and treatment
Nonclinical approach	Clinical approach
Involves usual social supports when available	Person in crisis is generally kept isolated from the community
Home-like setting	Institutional setting
Usual routines encouraged—for example, the kitchen is always open, no set wake-up or lights-out times.	Routines depend on the setting— that is, "hospital rules" apply
No waiting list; no triage	Scheduled appointments, repeated assessments
Workers strive for relationship of equals with individuals in crisis, seeing each as a person rather than a "patient" or "client"	Clear differences between worker and person in crisis (e.g., patient/ therapist)
Interaction not limited by being defined as "professional" intervention; for example, practical assistance may be given through emergency fund	Mobile team allows interaction to take place where the person feels most comfortable

Table 3 (cont.)

Gerstein Centre	Traditional settings and models
Interaction usually limited to therapy, medication and treatment	Interaction is usually in formal setting (e.g., hospital emergency department, worker's office)
Supportive, practical approach	Formal therapy or counselling.
Unstructured setting—no designated activities, schedules, requirements Rules are based on safety and comfort of all	Structured setting
Open setting—person is encouraged to keep appointments and is otherwise free to come and go as needed	Usually closed setting—person cannot leave during the designated stay
Community connections encouraged	Person may be removed from community and may have to do without usual routines
Centre has transportation budget to allow people to make and keep appointments, etc.	Deemphasis on the community
Flat management—staff, users, board work together to make decisions	Usually hierarchical, top-down approach to policies, major decisions, protocols, etc.
All complaints responded to— consumer input is encouraged and listened to	Consumer usually does not have a forum—may be labelled "non-compliant" for complaining

Source: Barbara Fitchette, Gerstein Centre, unpublished.

Evaluation

Phillips Group (1991) indicates that the Gerstein Centre is an effective organization which is meeting the expectations of consumer/survivors, board members, staffers and, to a lesser degree, com-munity agencies. It provides a cost-effective service for consumers who would otherwise seek hospital admission. Statistical information confirms that those who use the Centre would have used hospitals in the past. Statements by consumer/survivors indicate that the Centre is preferable to hospitals. The net result is a service that costs less than hospitalization and provides crisis inter-vention in a manner preferred by many consumer/survivors. This is an exciting model that reflects the paradigm shift occurring in the disability field. Despite its cost-effectiveness (in comparison with hospitalization), the Gerstein Centre is an expensive community model. When deinstitutionalization occurs within a framework of reallocating resources to the community, innovative health alternatives such as this become possible.

POLICY IMPLICATIONS

The research presented here reflects a substantial criticism of many common practices. But as we think about policy implications, it is clear that "more of the same" will not contribute to the determinants of health. The paradigm shift that is occurring in the disability field has significant implications for the future of community supports and the health of Canadians with disabilities.

There are numerous implications to the conclusions that have been drawn from the review of research and literature presented. Obviously, given the extent of the field, it has been impossible to review all research and literature. There is, for example, an enormous body of literature on rehabilitation and traditional service systems which did not seem appropriate for this review. The studies selected describe new approaches which contribute to the determinants of health.

The following recommendations for policy consideration are based on several assumptions which have emerged from the research and literature analyzed in this paper. These assumptions include:

- Many people with disabilities live in poverty and have poor health status.
- It takes additional resources to enable children with disabilities to grow up in ways that allow them to lead full lives as adults.
- Most segregated service systems are dysfunctional and inappropriate for enhancing the health status of Canadians with disabilities.
- There are many policies and programs which currently act as disincentives for families and people with disabilities to take more control over their lives and become active participants.
- The decision-making ability and independence of people with disabilities depends on the personal supports that are made available to them, not on their disability or intellectual functioning.

We have classified our recommendations for policy action in four areas:

A. Policy changes that enhance individualized family support for families who have a child with a disability

1. Provide incentives for provinces to implement individualized family support programs.

Only Ontario currently has a comprehensive provincial family support program for families with physically and developmentally disabled children. Positive outcomes from the Ontario *Special Services at Home* program demonstrate the need for this type of initiative in every province. The federal government could provide incentives to the provinces by adjustments to future cost-sharing agreements.

2. Redistribute resources to ensure that families receive money and support directly.

Typically, governments provide block funding to agencies for the implementation of specific programs. Families increasingly have been asking for more control over the support they receive. Currently, several projects in Ontario and Alberta provide individualized funding for family support and for adults with disabilities. Other provinces need to learn from these initiatives and implement projects of their own to enhance family support and control. The federal government could play an important leadership role in coordinating these developments.

3. Promote, through demonstration projects and research, initiatives which foster health and improve determinants of health for children with disabilities and their families.

The fact that so many Canadian citizens with disabilities are poor, unemployed and vulnerable demands attention. Federal projects such as *Brighter Futures* and the *Community Action Program for Children* are excellent examples of national prevention-oriented demonstration projects. Subsequent funding of these pilot projects should be augmented to enable them to give greater attention to the lives of people with disabilities. There would need to be government collaboration with family and disability groups in the development of this initiative.

4. Provide more flexibility in the policy and support funding to families and individuals with disabilities, so that people are not penalized for working or for trust funds established on their behalf.

Most current funding to people with disabilities, such as the Family Benefits Allowance (FBA), penalizes families and individuals who acquire funds by other means, such as employment income or bequests. This dilemma keeps many people with disabilities in a perpetual state of poverty and welfare dependency. Governments at all levels need to collaborate to develop more flexible legislation. Similarly, change in tax policy could benefit Canadian families who have a child with a disability by enabling families to deduct more disability expenses.

B. Policy changes that enhance community involvement of children with disabilities

5. Seek to implement "zero admission" policies to institutions for children with disabilities.

Currently only three provinces (Newfoundland, British Columbia, and New Brunswick) have such policies for children with developmental disabilities. These policies have been part of the fairly rapid downsizing of large institutions in those provinces. This change requires that the development of community supports be ensured, including adequate respite for families and individualized family support programs. It must also recognize that not all families will be able to support a disabled relative at home. Small selected community residential services may be required for some individuals.

6. Implement educational policies that ensure children with disabilities will be included in their neighbourhood schools.

Although education is a provincial responsibility, it is important to recognize that the segregated and inadequate education of many children with disabilities contributes to poverty and poor health. The federal government could develop a task force to examine the U.S. experience with the American Disabilities Act (Baker 1990), legislation which has created constructive change for individuals with disabilities in education, housing, employment, recreation and community access.

7. Develop rehabilitation services to become more family centred.

Many children with physical disabilities spend a lot of time in rehabilitation. The family-centred approach, while recommended by experts, is quite rare in Canada and needs support to be fully developed. Funding for conferences and research would provide strong incentives for more provincial initiatives in this area.

8. Develop effective school-to-work transition programs for adolescents with disabilities.

Many youths with disabilities are unemployed and often considered "unemployable", which severely limits their independence and adversely affects health status (DeJong et al. 1989). Research shows that participation in school-to-work programs greatly improves the chances of finding employment. Such transition programs are particularly important at a time when employment equity programs are being reduced or eliminated.

C. Policy changes that reallocate resources from institutions to community in a way that builds family and consumer initiatives and provides direct funding to adults with disabilities

9.   Reallocate resources from the institutional sector so that individuals with disabilities have direct access to the funds they need for their support.

Typically, individuals leaving an institution receive support from an agency in the community. Their new living arrangement may or may not be one they choose. Projects in Alberta and British Columbia have vast experience with ensuring that the person coming out of the institution has control over the dollars needed for community living. Ontario now has three pilot projects looking at individualized funding. As we have noted, there are some dilemmas with this approach; nevertheless, it needs to be fully explored. The federal government could sponsor policy forums and research endeavours in this area.

10. Reallocate resources to fund consumer groups in such a way that consumer and family sectors can implement creative initiatives and build upon their strengths.

In some areas of disability, the bulk of funding goes to the institutional sector. The need to reallocate resources is widely recognized, but there is no agreement on how to do this. One promising approach is a "framework for support" (Trainor et al. 1993) that builds a community resource base of various stakeholders. National mental health forums in the last few years have been an important federal initiative in this area. More of this work, combined with adjustments to future cost-sharing arrangements, could help provinces develop their consumer and family sectors. At the moment, only Ontario has adopted such an approach in mental health; however, there is potential for this to develop in all provinces and across all disability areas.

D. Policy changes that enhance independent living and the development of Independent Living Resource Centres

11. Institute a national home ownership program for people with disabilities.

One of the significant challenges facing people with disabilities is the search for affordable, accessible housing. The Canadian Mortgage and Housing Corporation could provide incentives and guidelines for a national program of home ownership.

12. Assure continued financial support for Independent Living Resource Centres (ILRCs) across Canada that can provide education, peer support and information to people with disabilities and their families.

During the last five years, the federal government has funded more than 20 ILRCs, which has brought substantial benefit to consumers and communities. Continued federal support will give ILRCs the time they need to develop appropriate sustaining infrastructures in cooperation with their communities and provincial governments.

13. Support the principles of consumer participation at all levels of decision making (community, agency, system, government).

In the last decade, the participation of consumers with disabilities in program and policy decision making has increased dramatically. Nevertheless, many consumers say they are offered only a "token" role, and believe that the prospect of full consumer participation may be "unsettling" for professionals and bureaucrats (Church 1995). Leadership is required from all sectors to ensure that genuine consumer participation can occur at all levels of decision making. National consumer groups have much knowledge and experience to contribute in the areas of health and disability. Much more concerted effort is needed to develop partnerships with these groups, facilitating their involvement in program development, evaluation, and policy setting.

14. Remove barriers that limit access and choice in employment, education, and culture.

In some ways, this policy recommendation is the most important of all, and the most difficult to implement. Our culture rejects "differentness" in all kinds of ways. While the federal government's 10-year *Initiative on Integration* has made significant progress in removing barriers and raising awareness, this initiative is now ending. The Social Sciences and Humanities Research Council, for example, should continue its joint funding for research into integration. As another example, the federal government could develop a project with consumer groups and private enterprise, focusing on training and increased employment for people with disabilities. There are many other ways in which all sectors can contribute to the development of an inclusive society. This in turn will have enormous health benefits.

John Lord, *Ed.D., lives in Kitchener-Waterloo, Ontario where he is currently a social research consultant. He is also a research associate in the Faculty of Community Services at Ryerson Polytechnic University in Toronto. He is a founder, and was coordinator for more than a decade, of the Centre for Research and Education in Human Services in Kitchener. He had previously been a faculty member at Dalhousie University.*

Peggy Hutchison, *Ed.D., is an associate professor in recreation and leisure studies at Brook University, St. Catherines, Ontario. She teaches and does research related to inclusion, independant living, empowerment, and community development for people who are marginalized due to poverty, age, disability, gender, or ethnicity.*

BIBLIOGRAPHY

ACTIVE LIVING ALLIANCE FOR CANADIANS WITH A DISABILITY. 1992. *A Blueprint for Action.* Ottawa (ON).

ADVOCACY RESOURCE CENTRE FOR THE HANDICAPPED. 1995. *ArchTYPE.* Toronto (ON). AGOSTA, J. 1989. Using cash assistance to support family efforts. In *Support for Caregiving Families: Enabling Positive Adaptation to Disability,* eds. G. SINGER, and L. IRVIN. Baltimore (MD): Paul H. Brookes. pp. 189–204.

ALBEE, G. 1981. Politics, power, prevention and social change. In *Prevention through Political Action and Social Change,* eds. J. JOFFE, and G. ALBEE. Hanover and London: University Press of New England.

ANDERSON, J., D. DAYSON, W. WILLS, C. KOOCH, O. MOROGOLIUS, C. O'DRISCOLL, and J. LEFF. 1993. The TAPS Project 13: Clinical and social outcomes of long-term stay psychiatric patients after one year in the community. *British Journal of Psychiatry* 19: 45–56.

ARGYLE, M. 1987. *The Psychology of Happiness.* London: Methuen and Company.

BAILEY, L. 1994. Are we finally getting there? Integrating students with developmental disabilities. *ArchTYPE* 2: 4.

BAKER, D. 1990. *The Quest for Independence: Lessons from the Americans with Disabilities Act.* Toronto (ON): Advocacy Resource Centre for the Handicapped.

BARRERA Jr., M., and S. L. AINLAY. 1983. The structure of social support: A conceptual and empirical analysis. *Journal of Community Psychology* 11: 133–143.

BELLAH, R., R. MADSEN, W. SULLIVAN, A. SWIDLER, and S. TIPTON. 1985. *Habits of the Heart.* New York (NY): Harper and Row.

BELLAMY, G., L. RHODES, D. MANK, and J. ALBIN. 1988. *Supported Employment: A Community Implementation Guide.* Baltimore (MD): Paul H. Brookes.

BELLE, D., ed. 1989. *Children's Social Networks and Social Supports.* New York (NY): John Wiley.

BERMAN, M., and J. DAVIS-BERMAN. 1993. *Wilderness Therapy.* Dubuque (IA): Kendall-Hunt Publishing Company.

BIKLEN, D. 1992. *Schooling without Labels: Parents, Educators, and Inclusive Education.* Philadelphia (PA): Temple University Press.

BIRENBAUM, A., and H. COHEN. 1993. On the importance of helping families: Policy implications from a national study. *Mental Retardation* 21: 75–77.

BOGDAN, R., and S. TAYLOR. 1982. *Inside Out: Two First-Person Accounts of What It Means to Be Labeled "Mentally Retarded".* Toronto (ON): University of Toronto Press.

———. 1989. Relationships with severely disabled people: The social construction of humanness. *Social Problems* 36: 135–146.

BRADLEY, D. 1994. Moving into the mainstream. *The Educational Forum* 59: 81–91.

BRESLAU, N. 1985. Psychiatric disorder in children with physical disabilities. *Journal of the American Academy of Child Psychiatry* 24: 87–94.

BRIDGE, N. J., and D. GOLD. 1989. An analysis of the relationship between leisure and economics. *Journal of Leisurability* 16(2): 10–14.

BROWN, L., A. UDVARI-SOLNER, E. FRATTURA-KAMPSCHROER, L. DAVIS, C. AHLGREN, P. VAN DEVENTER, and J. JOGENSEN. 1991. Integrated work: A rejection of segregated enclaves and mobile work crews. In *Critical issues in the Lives of People with Severe Disabilities,* eds. L. H. MEYER, C. A. PECK, and L. BROWN. Baltimore (MD): Paul H. Brookes Publishing Co.

BROWN, L., E. LONG, A. UDVARI-SOLNER, L. DAVIS, P. VANDEVENTER, C. AHLGREN, F. JOHNSON, L. GRUENEWALD, and J. JORGENSEN. 1989. The home school: Why students with severe intellectual disabilities must attend the schools as their brothers, sisters, friends, and neighbors. *JASH* 14: 1–17.

BROWNE, S., D. CONNORS, and N. STERN. Ed. 1985. *With the Power of Each Breath : A Disabled Women's Anthology.* Pittsburgh (PA): Cleis Press.

BUDDE, J., R. PETTY, and C. NELSON. 1986. *Problems and Benefits Associated with Consumer Satisfaction Evaluation at Independent Living Centers.* Kansas (ON): University of Kansas Research and Training Center on Independent Living.

BULLOCK, A. 1990. Community care: Ideology and lived experience. In *Community Organization and the Canadian State,* eds. R. NG, G. WALKER, and J. MULLER. Toronto (ON): Garamond Press. pp. 65–82.

BULLOCK, C., and C. HOWE. 1991. A model therapeutic recreation program for the reintegration of persons with disabilities into the community. *Therapeutic Recreation Journal* 24: 7–17.

BURSTOW, B., and D. WEITZ. Eds. 1988. *Shrink Resistant: The Struggle against Psychiatry in Canada.* Vancouver (BC): New Star Books.

CALDWELL, L., and E. SMITH. 1988. Leisure: An overlooked component of health promotion. *Canadian Journal of Public Health* 79: 544–556.

CANADIAN ASSOCIATION FOR COMMUNITY LIVING. 1980. *Vision 2000.* Downsview (ON).

CANADIAN ASSOCIATION FOR INDEPENDENT LIVING CENTRES. 1990. *A Guide to Independent Living Centres.* Ottawa (ON).

_____. 1991. *Guidelines for Independent Living Centres in Canada.* Ottawa (ON).

_____. 1994. *A Time for Change: A Time for Choice.* Ottawa (ON).

_____. 1995. *Responding to Abuse: An Independent Living Approach.* Ottawa (ON).

CANADIAN COUNCIL ON SOCIAL DEVELOPMENT. 1985. *Deinstitutionalization: Costs and Effects. Report from an Invitational Symposium.* Ottawa (ON): C.C.S.D.

CANADIAN MENTAL HEALTH ASSOCIATION. 1984. *Work and Well-Being: The Changing Realities of Employment.* Toronto (ON).

CARLING, P. 1990. Major mental illness, housing, and supports: The promise of community integration. *American Psychologist* 45: 969–975.

_____. 1995. *Return to Community.* New York (NY): Guilford Press.

CARPENTER, S. 1991. The role of Independent Living Centres in the lives of Canadians: Colouring outside the lines. *Abilities* 35–36.

CARRUTHERS, C., and C. HOOD. 1994. Alcohol use in leisure. *Journal of Leisurability* 21: 3–12.

CENTER ON HUMAN POLICY. 1986. *A Statement in Support of Families and Their Children.* Syracuse (NY): Division of Special Education Rehabilitation, School of Education, Syracuse University.

CERTO, N., S. SCHLEIEN, and D. HUNTER. 1983. An ecological assessment inventory to facilitate community recreation participation by severely disabled individuals. *Therapeutic Recreation Journal* 17: 29–37.

CHAMBERLIN, J. 1978. *On Our Own.* Toronto (ON): McGraw Hill.

CHURCH, K. 1992. *Moving Over: A Commentary on Power Sharing.* Toronto (ON): Ministry of Health, Community Mental Health Branch.

_____. 1995. *Forbidden Narratives: Critical Autobiography as Social Science.* Luxembourg: Gorden and Breach Publishers.

COALITION AGAINST INSTITUTIONS AS COMMUNITY RESOURCE CENTRES. 1987. Institutions: New forms, new fears. Unpublished discussion paper. ON.

COCHRAN, M. 1986. The parental empowerment process: Building on family strengths. In *Child Psychology in Action: Linking Research and Practice,* ed. J. HARRIS. Brookline (MA): Croon Helm Publishers. pp. 12–33.

CODE, L. 1991. Special issue on women and disability. *Entourage* 6.

COLEMAN, D. 1990. An analysis of stress-buffering effects of leisure-based social support and leisure dispositions. Unpublished master's thesis. Maryland (MD): University of Maryland.

COLEMAN, D., and S. ISO-AHOLA. 1993. Leisure and health: The role of social support and self-determination. *Journal of Leisure Research* 25: 111–128.

CONROY, J., and V. BRADLEY. 1985. *The Pennhurst Longitudinal Study: A Report of Five Years of Research and Analysis.* Philadelphia (PA): Temple University Developmental Disabilities Center.

CONSUMER/SURVIVOR DEVELOPMENT INITIATIVES. 1993. *Report on Activities.* Toronto (ON): Ministry of Health.

_____. 1996. *Consumer Survivor Development Initiatives: Project Evaluation.* Toronto (ON): Ontario Ministry of Health.

COPOH. 1986. *Defining the Parameters of Independent Living.* Winnipeg (MB): COPOH.

CORNELL EMPOWERMENT GROUP. 1989. Empowerment and family support. *Networking Bulletin* 1: 2.

COUNCIL OF CANADIANS WITH DISABILITIES. 1995. *A Voice of Our Own.* Winnipeg (MB).

CRAPPS, J., and Z. STONEMAN. 1989. Friendship patterns and community integration of family care residents. *Research in Developmental Disabilities* 10: 153–169.

CREWE, N., and I. ZOLA. 1984. *Independent Living for Physically Disabled People.* San Francisco (CA): Jossey-Bass Inc.

CSIKSZENTMIHALYI, M., 1990. *Flow: The Psychology of Optimal Experience.* New York (NY): Harper Collins Publishers.

CSIKSZENTMIHALYI, M. and J. LeFEVRE. 1989. Optimal experience in work and leisure. *Journal of Personality and Social Psychology* 56: 815–822.

DAVERN, L., and R. SCHNORR. 1993. Public schools welcome students with disabilities as full members. In *Resources on Inclusive Education*, ed. K. HULGIN. Syracuse (NY): Research and Training Center on Community Integration. pp. 22–25.

DE BOER, M. 1992. Women and empowerment. Unpublished master's thesis. Waterloo (ON): Wilfrid Laurier University, School of Social Work.

DEJONG, G. 1979. Independent living: From social movement to analytic paradigm. *Archives of Physical Medicine and Rehabilitation* 60: 435–446.

_____. 1993. Three trends to look for in the American Independent Living movement in the 1990s. In *Independent Living: An Agenda for the '90s*, ed. A. NEUFELDT. Ottawa (ON): Canadian Association for Independent Living Centres. pp. 109–120.

DEJONG, G., A. BATAVIA, and R. GRISS. 1989. America's neglected health minority: Working-age persons with disabilities. *The Milbank Quarterly* 67: 311–351.

DES LAURIERS, G. and M. CLAIR-FOYER. 1982. Deinstitutionalization in action. *Canadian Journal of Mental Retardation* 32: 20–24, 30–36.

DUNN, P. 1990. The impact on the housing environment upon the ability of disabled people to live independently. *Disability, Handicap and Society* 5: 37–52.

_____. 1994. *Government Policy Innovations in Barrier-Free Housing, Accessible Transportation and Personal Supports.* Winnipeg (MB): National Independent Living Conference.

DUNST, C. J. 1991. *Family Support Principles: Checklists for Program Builders and Practitioners.* Family Systems Intervention Monograph 2(5). Morganton (NC): Western Carolina Center, Family Infant and Preschool Program.

DUNST, C., C. M. TRIVETTE, and A. G. DEAL. 1988. *Enabling and Empowering Families: Principles and Guidelines for Practice.* Cambridge (MA): Brookline Books.

DYSON, L. 1994. Social integration in an elementary school and its implications. *Exceptionality Education Canada* 4: 13–28.

EDGERTON, R. B. 1984. *Lives in Process: Mildly Retarded Adults in a Large City.* Washington (DC): American Association of Mental Deficiency.

EIGNER, W. 1995. The most effective means of combating discriminatory attitudes. *Inclusion International* 1: 2–3.

ENNS, H. 1991. Introduction to independent living. *Compass* 2: 1.

EPP, J. 1986. *Achieving Health for All: A Framework for Health Promotion.* Ottawa (ON): Minister of Supply and Services.

EVANS, J., and G. ROBERTS. 1987. Physical competence and the development of children's peer relations. *Quest* 39: 23–35.

FALVEY, M., M. FOREST, J. PEARPOINT, and R. ROSENBURG. 1994. *All My Life's a Circle.* Toronto (ON): Inclusion Press.

FAMILY SUPPORT INSTITUTE OF ONTARIO. n.d. Brochure. Toronto (ON).

FARINA, J. 1982. The eighth deadly sin. *Journal of Leisurability* 9: 12–14.

FILM IMAGES PRODUCTION. 1995. *Voices of Experience: Community Economic Development.* Toronto (ON).

FOLSOM, A., C. CASPERSEN, H. TAYLOR, D. JACOBS, R. LUEPKER, O. GOMEZ-MARIN, R. GILLUM, and H. BLACKBURN. 1985. Leisure time physical activity and its relationship to coronary risk factors in a population-based sample. *American Journal of Epidemiology* 121: 570–579.

FOREST, M. 1987. *More Education Integration.* Downsview (ON): G. Allan Roeher Institute.

———. 1989. *It's About Relationships.* Toronto (ON): Frontier College Press.

FOREST, M., and J. SNOW. 1983. The Joshua Committee: An advocacy model. *Journal of Leisurability* 10: 20–23.

FOUCAULT, M. 1984. The means of correct training. In *The Foucault Reader*, ed. P. RABINOW. New York (NY): Pantheon Books. pp. 188-205.

FRANK, J., and J. MUSTARD. 1994. The determinants of health from a historical perspective. *Daedalus: Journal of the American Academy of Arts and Science* 123: 1–19.

FREIRE, P. 1985. *The Politics of Education: Culture, Power and Liberation.* South Hadley (MA): Bergin and Garvey Publishers.

FRIEDMANN, J. 1992. *Empowerment: The Politics of Alternative Development.* Cambridge (MA): Blackwell.

GARDNER, J., M. CHAPMAN, G. DONALDSON, and S. JACOBSON. 1988. *Toward Supported Employment.* Baltimore (MD): Paul H. Brookes.

GIANGRECO, M., R. DENNIS, C. CLONINGER, S. EDELMAN, and R. SCHATTMAN. 1993. "I've counted Jon": Transformational experiences of teachers educating students with disabilities. *Exceptional Children* 59: 359–372.

GOFFMAN, E. 1961. *Asylums.* Garden City (NJ): Anchor at Doubleday.

GOLD, D. 1988. A look at Leisure Buddy programs. In *The Pursuit of Leisure*, eds. D. GOLD, and J. MCGILL. Toronto (ON): G. Allan Roeher Institute.

———. 1994. "We don't call it a 'circle'": The ethos of a support group. *Disability and Society* 9: 435–452.

GOLLAY, E., M. FREEDMAN, M. WYNGAARDEN, and N. KURTZ. 1978. *Coming Back: The Community Experiences of Deinstitutionalized Mentally Retarded People.* Cambridge (MA): Abt-Books.

GOTTLIEB, B. 1985. Social networks and social support: An overview of research, practice and policy implications. *Health Education Quarterly* 12: 6–22.

GOULD, A. 1994. The integration challenge: Kids with special need. *Today's Parent* E23–E24.

GRADEN, J., and A. BAUER. 1991. Using a collaborative approach to support teachers in inclusive classrooms. In *Curriculum Considerations in Inclusive Classrooms*, eds. S. STAINBACK, and W. STAINBACK. Baltimore (MD): Paul H. Brookes. pp. 85–100.

GRENOT-SCHEYER, M. 1994. The nature of interactions between students with severe disabilities and their friends and acquaintances without disabilities. *JASH* 19: 253–262.

GUBRIUM, J., and D. BUCKROLDT. 1982. *Describing Care: Image and Practice in Rehabilitation.* Cambridge (MA): Oelgeschlager, Gunn, and Hain Publishers Inc.

GUEST, D. 1985. *The Emergence of Social Security in Canada.* Vancouver (BC): University of British Columbia Press.

GURALNICK, M. J., R. T. CONNOR, and M. HAMMOND. 1995. Parent perspectives of peer relationships and friendships in integrated and specialized programs. *American Journal on Mental Retardation* 99: 457–476.

HAGNER, D., and D. DILEO. 1993. *Working Together: Workplace Culture, Supported Employment, and Persons with Disabilities.* Cambridge (MA): Brookline Books.

HALL, I. 1983. Playing for keeps: The careers of front-line workers in institutions for developmentally handicapped persons. Unpublished master's thesis. Waterloo (ON): University of Waterloo.

HALLAM, A., J. BEECHAM, M. KNAPP, and A. FENYO. 1994. The costs of accommodation and care: Community provision for former long-stay psychiatric hospital patients. *European Archives of Psychiatry and Clinical Neuroscience* 243: 304–310.

HAMRE-NIETUPSKI, S., J. HENDRICKSON, J. NIETUPSKI, and M. SHOKOOHI-YEKTA. 1994. Regular educators' perceptions of facilitating friendships of students with moderate, severe, or profound disabilities with nondisabled peers. *Education and Training in Mental Retardation and Developmental Disabilities.* pp. 102–117.

HARING, T. 1991. Social relationships. In *Critical Issues in the Lives of People with Severe Handicaps,* eds. L. MEYER, C. PECK, and L. BROWN. Baltimore (MD): Paul H. Brookes Publishing. pp. 195–217.

HEADEY, B. 1988. The life satisfactions and priorities of Australians. In *Australian Attitudes: Social and Political Analysis from the National Science Survey,* eds. J. KELLEY, and C. BEAN. Sydney, Australia: Allen and Unwin.

HEYNE, L., S. SCHLEIEN, and L. MCAVOY. 1993. *Making Friends: Using Recreation Activities to Promote Friendship between Children with and without Disabilities.* Minneapolis (MN): Institute on Community Integration, University of Minnesota.

HOBBS, N., P. R. DOKECKI, K. V. HOOVER-DEMPSEY, R. M. MORONEY, M. W. SHAYNE, and K. H. WEEKS. 1984. *Strengthening Families.* San Francisco (CA): Jossey-Bass.

HOFFMAN, B. 1993. *Psychiatry without Asylums: A Look at the Italian Mental Health System and Its Implications for Ontario.* General Hospital Psychiatric Services.

HOUSE, J. 1986. Social support and the quality and quantity of life. In *Research on the Quality of Life,* ed. F. ANDREWS. University of Michigan (MI): Survey Research Centre.

HUGHES, M. J., and S. K. LYLES. 1994. The meaning of friendship: Expectations and understanding of friendship of mainstreamed intellectually challenged students. *Exceptionality Education Canada* 4: 43–53.

HULL, R. 1990. Mood as product of leisure: Causes and consequences. *Journal of Leisure Research* 22: 99–111.

HUNT, P., F. FARRON-DAVIS, S. BECKSTEAD, D. CURTIS, and L. GOETZ. 1994. Evaluating the effects of placement of students with severe disabilities in general education versus special classes. *JASH* 19: 200–214.

HUSIEN, N. 1995. *Youth Speak Up! Youth Speak Out.* Ottawa (ON): Canadian Association of Independent Living Centres.

HUTCHISON, P. 1990. *Making Friends: Developing Relationships between People with a Disability and Other Members of the Community.* Downsview (ON): G. Allan Roeher Institute.

_____. 1994. Work and leisure: Paradoxes and dilemmas for people with developmental disabilities. *Journal on Developmental Disabilities* 3: 1–15.

HUTCHISON, P., and J. MCGILL. 1992. *Leisure, Integration and Community.* Toronto (ON): Leisurability Publications.

HUTCHISON, P., A. PEDLAR, J. LORD, P. DUNN, C. VANDETELLI, M. MCGEOWN, A. TAYLOR. 1996. The impact of Independent Living Resources Centres in Canada upon people with disabilities. *Canadian Journal of Rehabilitation,* spring.

ISO-AHOLA, S. 1994. Leisure lifestyle and health. In *Leisure and Mental Health,* eds. D. COMPTON, and S. ISO-AHOLA. Park City (UT): Family Development Resources Inc. pp. 42–46.

INTAGLIATEA, J., N. CROSBY, and L. NEIDER. 1981. Foster family care for mentally retarded people: A qualitative review. In *Deinstitutionalization and Community Adjustment of Mentally Retarded People,* eds. R. H. BRUININKS, C. E. MEYERS, B. B. SIGFORD, and K. C. LAKIN. Monograph no. 4. Washington (DC): AAMD. pp. 233–259.

JACKSON, J. 1993. Full inclusion at Helen Hansen Elementary School: It happened because we all value children. In *Resources on Inclusive Education*, ed. K. HULGIN. Syracuse (NY): Research and Training Center on Community Integration. pp. 161–168.

JACOBSEN, S., and D. SAWATSKY. 1993. Meeting the challenge of integrating students with special needs: Understanding, building and implementing integration as inclusion. *Canadian Journal of Special Education* 9: 60–66.

JONGBLOED, L., and A. CRICHTON. 1990. Difficulties in shifting from individualistic to socio-political policy regarding disability in Canada. *Disability, Handicap and Society* 5: 25–35.

KELLY, J. 1987. *Freedom to Be: A New Sociology of Leisure.* New York (NY): MacMillan Publishing Company.

KENNEDY, C., and T. ITKONEN. 1994. Some of the effects of regular class participation on the social contacts and social networks of high school students with severe disabilities. *JASH* 19: 1–10.

KIEFFER, C. H. 1984. Citizen empowerment: A developmental perspective. *Prevention in Human Services* 3(16): 9–35.

KISHI, G. S., and L. H. MEYER. 1994. What children report and remember: A six-year follow-up of the effects of social contact between peers with and without severe disabilities. *JASH* 19: 277–289.

KLASSEN, R. 1994. Research: What does it say about mainstreaming? *Education Canada* 34: 27–35.

LABONTE, R. 1990. Empowerment: Notes on professional and community dimensions. *Canadian Review of Social Policy* 26: 4–75.

_____. 1994. Community empowerment and fitness. In *Toward Active Living*, ed. H. QUINNEY, L. GAUVIN, and A. E. WALL. Windsor (ON): Human Kinetics Publishers. pp. 219–226.

LAFAVE, H. 1993. *A Service Consortium for People with Serious Mental Illness in Leeds and Grenville Counties.* Brockville: Canadian Mental Health Association.

LARSEN, R., R. MANNELL, and J. ZUZANEK. 1986. Daily well-being of older adults with friends and family. *Journal of Psychology and Aging* 1: 117–126.

LEFF, J., G. THORNICROFT, N. COXHEAD, and C. CRAWFORD. 1994. The TAPS Project 22: A five-year follow-up of long stay psychiatric patients discharged to the community. *British Journal of Psychiatry* 25: 3–7.

LEWIS, T. 1992. Rising expectations: Relationships and children with disabilities in the regular school system. *Entourage* 7: 3–6.

LINCOLN, Y.S., and E. G. GUBA. 1985. *Naturalistic Inquiry.* Newbury Park (CA): Sage Publications.

LORD, J. 1991. *Lives in Transition: The Process of Personal Empowerment.* Kitchener (ON): Centre for Research and Education in Human Services.

_____. 1994. *Genuine Partnerships: Challenges and Opportunities.* Winnipeg (MB): National Independent Living Conference.

LORD, J., and C. HEARN. 1987. *Return to the Community: The Process of Closing an Institution.* Kitchener (ON): Centre for Research and Education in Human Services.

LORD, J., and P. HUTCHISON. 1993. The process of empowerment: Implications for theory and practice. *Canadian Journal of Community Mental Health* 12: 5–22.

LORD, J., and J. OCHOCKA. 1995. Outcomes of an individualized family support program. *Journal of Leisurability* 22: 22–32.

LORD, J., and A. PEDLAR. 1991. Life in the community: Four years after the closure of an institution. *Mental Retardation* 29: 213–221.

LORD, J., P. HUTCHISON, and D. FARLOW. 1988. *Independence and Control: Today's Dream, Tomorrow's Reality. Review of Support Service Needs of Adults with Physical Disabilities in Ontario.* Toronto (ON): Ministry of Community and Social Services.

LORD, J., MCGEOWN, and J. OCHOCKA. 1993. *Family Directed Support: Diversity, Hopes, Struggles, Dignity.* Toronto (ON): Ministry of Community and Social Services.

LORD, J., and D. MCKILLOP FARLOW. 1990. A study of personal empowerment: Implications for health promotion. *Health Promotion* 29: 2–8.

LORD, J., A. SCHNARR, and P. HUTCHISON. 1987. The voice of the people: Qualitative research and the needs of consumers. *Canadian Journal of Community Mental Health* 6: 25–36.

LORD, J., M. MCGEOWN, A. TAYLOR, and S. YOUNG. 1992. *More Than Just Another Human Service.* Ottawa (ON): Canadian Association of Independent Living Centres.

LUSTHAUS, E., K. GAZITH, and C. LUSTHAUS. 1992. Each belong: A rationale for full inclusion. Unpublished manuscript. Montreal (QC): McGill University Press.

LUTFIYYA, Z. 1988. *Other than Clients: Reflection on Relationships between People with Disabilities and Typical People.* Syracuse (NY): Syracuse University.

LYONS, R. 1987. Friendship and loneliness: Challenges for the recreation profession. *Recreation Canada* 45: 8–15.

_____. 1989. The effects of acquired illness and disability on friendships. In *Advances in Personal Relationships,* eds. W. H. JONES, and D. PERLMAN. JAI Press.

_____. 1991. *Recreation Services for Persons with a Disability: Municipal Government Policy Guidelines.* Ottawa (ON): Canadian Parks and Recreation Association.

MACPHERSON, G. 1990. Are you ready for the revolution? *Canadian Journal of Rehabilitation* 3: 1.

MARMOT, M. 1994. Social differentials in health within and between populations. *Daedalus: Journal of the American Academy of Arts and Science* 123: 197–216.

MAURICE, L. 1995. *Prevention of Abuse against Elderly Citizens with Disabilities.* Ottawa (ON): Canadian Association of Independent Living Centres.

MCGEE, J. F., D. MENOLASCINO, HOBBS, and P. MENOUSEK. 1987. *Gentle Teaching: A Non-Aversive Approach to Helping Persons with Mental Retardation.* New York (NY): Human Science Press, Inc.

MCGEOWN, M. 1993. A conceptual framework for responsive social planning: Each other's future-case studies of the community living movement. Unpublished doctoral dissertation. Waterloo (ON): University of Waterloo.

MCINTYRE, E. L. G. 1987. Social networks and social work. *Social Work,* January.

MCKNIGHT, J. 1987. Regenerating community. *Social Policy* 17: 54–58.

_____. 1990. Beyond community services. Unpublished paper. Evanston (IL).

_____. 1995. *The Careless Society: Community and Its Counterfeits.* New York (NY): Basic Books.

MCLOUGHLIN, C., J. GARNER, and M. CALLAHAN. 1987. *Getting Employed, Staying Employed: Job Development and Training for Persons with Severe Handicaps.* Baltimore (MD): Paul Brookes Publishing Co.

MCWHORTER, A. 1986. *Mandate for Quality: Changing the System.* Vol. 3. Downsview (ON): National Institute on Mental Retardation.

MEYER, L., C. PECK, and L. BROWN. Eds. 1991. *Critical Issues in the Lives of People with Severe Disabilities.* Baltimore (MD): Paul H. Brooks.

MINISTRY OF EDUCATION. 1992. *Consultation Paper on the Integration of Exceptional Pupils.* Toronto (ON): Province of Ontario.

MINISTRY OF HEALTH. 1993. *Putting People First: The Reform of Mental Health Services in Ontario.* Toronto (ON).

MITCHELL, R. 1982. Social networks and psychiatric clients: The personal and environmental context. *American Journal of Community Psychology* 10: 387–401.

MITCHELL, D. and D. BRADDOCK. 1994. Compensation and turnover of direct care staff and developmental disabilities, residential facilities in the United States. *Mental Retardation* 32: 34–42.

MORGAN, L. 1989. Planning for inclusion and support by reviewing a delivery system. *Journal of Leisurability* 16: 8–12.

MOUNT, B., P. BEEMAN, and G. DUCHARME. 1988. *What Are We Learning about Circles of Support?* Manchester (CT): Communitas, Inc.

NEVIN, A. 1993. Curricular and instructional adaptations for including students with disabilities in cooperative groups. In *Cooperative Learning and Strategies for Inclusion*, ed. J. PUTNAM. Baltimore (MD): Paul H. Brookes Publishing Co. pp. 41–56.

NIRJE, B. 1980. The normalization principle. In *Normalization, Social Integration and Community Services*, eds. R. J. FLYNN, and K. E. NITSCH. Baltimore (MD): University Park Press. pp. 31–49.

O'BRIEN, J. 1986. *Discovering Community: Learning from Innovations in Services to People with Mental Retardation*. Georgia (GA): Responsive Systems Associates.

———. 1987. Embracing ignorance, error, and fallibility: Competencies for leadership of effective services. In *Community Integration for People with Severe Disabilities*, eds. S. TAYLOR, D. BIKLEN, and J. KNOLL. New York (NY): Teachers College Press.

———. 1989. *What's Worth Asking for? Leadership for Better Quality Human Services*. Syracuse (NY): The Centre on Human Policy, Syracuse University.

OCHOCKA, J., J. LORD, and D. ROTH. 1994. Workplaces that work: Successful employment for people with disabilities. *Journal on Developmental Disabilities* 3: 29–50.

O'CONNELL, M. 1988. *The Gift of Hospitality: Opening the Doors of Community Life to People with Disabilities*. Evanston (IL): Centre for Urban Affairs and Policy Research, Northwestern University.

OLIVER, M., and G. ZARB. 1989. The politics of disability: A new approach. *Disability, Handicap and Society* 4: 221–239.

PANDIANI, J., E. EDGAR, and J. PIERCE. 1994. A longitudinal study of the impact of changing public policy on community mental health attitudes. *Journal of Mental Health Administration* 21: 71–79.

PANITCH, M. 1988. Community college integration: More than just an education. *Entourage* 3: 26–32.

PAPE, B., and K. CHURCH. 1987. *Community Reinvestment: Balancing the Use of Resources to Support People with Mental Disabilities*. Toronto (ON): Canadian Mental Health Association.

PARTIN, M. 1994. Inclusion in the public schools: Strategies for parents. *JASH* 20: 4–7.

PEARPOINT, J. 1990. *From behind the Piano: The Building of Judith Snow's Unique Circle of Friends*. Toronto (ON): Inclusion Press.

PEARPOINT, J., M. FOREST, and J. SNOW. 1992. *Strategies to Make Inclusion Work: A Collection of Articles from the Centre for Integrated Education and Community*. Toronto (ON): Inclusion Press.

PECK, C.A., J. DONALDSON, and M. PEZZOLI. 1990. Some benefits nonhandicapped adolescents perceive for themselves from their social relationships with peers who have severe handicaps. *JASH* 15: 241–249.

PEDLAR, A. 1991. Supportive communities: The gap between ideology and social policy. *Environments* 1: 1–7.

———. 1992. Deinstitutionalization and normalization in Sweden and Ontario, Canada: Supporting people in leisure activities. *Therapeutic Recreation Journal* 26: 21–35.

PEDLAR, A., J. LORD, and M. VANLOON. 1989. *The Process of Supported Employment and Quality of Life*. Kitchener (ON): Centre for Research and Education in Human Services.

PERSKE, R. 1988. *Circles of Friends: People with Disabilities and Their Friends Enrich the Lives of One Another*. Burlington (ON): Welch Publishing Company Inc.

PHILIPS GROUP. 1991. *Evaluation of Gerstein Centre*. Toronto (ON): Philips Group.

PINDERHUGHES, E. 1983. Empowerment for our clients and for ourselves. Social casework. *The Journal of Contemporary Social Work* 64: 331–338.

POTSCHASKE, C. 1988. Characteristics of innovative services in Southern Ontario. *Journal of Leisurability* 15: 24–29.

PUTNAM, J. 1993. *Cooperative Learning Strategies for Inclusion: Celebrating Diversity in the Classroom*. Baltimore (MD): Paul H. Brookes Publishing Co.

QUINNEY, A., L. GAUVIN, and T. WALL. Eds. 1994. *Toward Active Living*. Windsor (ON): Human Kinetics Publishers.

RACINO, J. A. 1992. Life in the community: The independent living and support paradigms. In *Transition from School-to-Work for Youth and Adults with Disabilities*, eds. F. R. RUSCH, L. DESTEFANO, J. CHADSEY-RUSCH, L. A. PHELPS, and D. E.. SYZMANSKI. Sycamore (IL): Sycamore Publishing Co.

RAPPAPORT, J. 1987. Terms of empowerment/exemplars of prevention: Toward a theory for community psychology. *American Journal of Community Psychology* 15: 121–148.

REID, D. 1990. Leisure and recreation as an instrument for maintaining life quality during unemployment. *Journal of Leisurability* 17: 3–11.

REVAUD, J. F., B. MADIOT, and I. VILLE. 1992. Discrimination towards disabled people seeking employment. *Social Science Med.* 35: 951–958.

ROBINSON, R. 1991. Canadian Association of Independent Living Centres: Growing pains and empowerment. *Abilities* (summer):16–19.

ROEHER INSTITUTE. 1988. *Income Insecurity: The Disability Income System in Canada.* Downsview (ON).

———. 1994. *Violence and People with Disabilities.* Ottawa: Health Canada, Family Violence Prevention Division.

ROSE, S., and B. BLACK. 1985. *Advocacy and Empowerment: Mental Health Care in the Community.* Boston (MA): Routledge and Kegan Paul.

ROSENFIELD, S. 1992. Factors contributing to the subjective quality of life of the chronically mentally ill. *Journal of Health and Social Behavior* 33: 299–315.

ROTHMAN, D. 1981. *Social Control: Uses and Abuses of the Concept in the History of Incarceration.* Rice University Studies.

SALEND, S. 1994. *Effective Mainstreaming: Creating Inclusive Classrooms.* 2nd ed. Toronto (ON): Maxwell Macmillan Canada.

SALISBURY, B., J. DICKEY, and C. CRAWFORD. 1987. Service brokerage: Individual empowerment and social service accountability. *Entourage* 3: 26–31.

SALISBURY, C., M. PALOMBARO, and T. HOLLOWOOD. 1993. On nature and change in an elementary school. *JASH* 18: 75–84.

SANDYS, J., and D. LEAKER. 1987. The impact of integrated employment on leisure lifestyles. *Journal of Leisurability* (14:3) 19–23.

SAULNIER, K. 1982. Networks, change, and crisis: The web of support. *Canadian Journal of Community Mental Health* 1: 5–23.

SCHILLING, R. and S. SCHINKE. 1984. Personal coping and social support for parents of handicapped children. *Children and Youth Services Review* 6: 195–206.

SCHWARTZ, D.B. 1992. *Crossing the River: Creating a Conceptual Revolution in Community and Disability.* Pennsylvania (PA): Bookline Books.

SEED, P. and B. MONTGOMERY. 1989. *Towards Independent Living: Issues for Different Client Groups.* London: Jessica Kingsley.

SHAFFER, C., and K. ANUNDSEN. 1993. *Creating Community Anywhere: Finding Support and Connection in a Fragmented World.* New York (NY): G. P. Putnam's Sons.

SHARPE, M., J. YORK, and J. KNIGHT. 1994. Effects of inclusion on the academic performance of classmates without disabilities. *Remedial and Special Education* 15: 281–287.

SHIPE, D. 1984. Early intervention. In *Dialogue on Disability: The Service System*, eds. N. J. MARLETT, R. S. GALL, and A. WIGHT-FELSKE. Calgary (AB): The University of Calgary Press.

SIMMONS, H. 1982. *Asylums to Welfare.* Toronto (ON): National Institute on Mental Retardation.

SINGER, G., and L. IRVIN. 1991. Supporting families of persons with severe disabilities: Emerging findings, practices, and questions. In *Critical Issues in the Lives of People with Severe Disabilities*, eds. L. MEYER, C. PECK, and L. BROWN. Baltimore (MD): Paul H. Brooks. pp. 271–312.

SMITH, W., and C. LUSTHAUS. 1994. Students with disabilities in Canada. What rights do they have? *Education Canada* 4: 9, 44–47.

SNOW, J. 1989. Systems of support, a new vision. In *Educating All Students in the Mainstream of Regular Education*, eds. S. STAINBACK, W. STAINBACK, and M. FOREST. Baltimore (MD): Paul H. Brookes.

SOBSEY, D., M. DREIMANIS, and G. MACEWAN. 1993. Integration outcomes: Theoretical models and empirical investigations. *Developmental Disabilities Bulletin* 21: 1–14.

STAINBACK, S., W. STAINBACK, and M. FOREST. 1985. *Educating All Students in the Mainstream of Regular Education*. Baltimore (MD): Paul H. Brookes.

STAINBACK, S., W. STAINBACK, K. EAST, and M. SAPON-SHEVIN. 1994. A commentary on inclusion and the development of a positive self-identity by people with disabilities. *Exceptional Children* 60: 486–490.

STANLEY, P. 1993. Teachers involved in the mainstreaming of students with intellectual disabilities: Their goals, attitudes and beliefs. *NETWORK* 39: 44.

STATISTICS CANADA. 1988. *The Health and Activity Limitation Survey.* Ottawa (ON): Statistics Canada.

STRULLY, J. 1985. Being together: Living, learning, working and having friends in the community. *Canadian Journal on Mental Retardation* 35 (1): 24–28.

STRULLY, J., and C. STRULLY. 1989. Friendships as an educational goal. In *Educating All Students in the Mainstream of Regular Education*, eds. S. STAINBACK, W. STAINBACK, and M. FOREST. Baltimore (MD): Paul H. Brookes. pp. 59–68.

SYME, S. 1994. The social environment and health. *Daedalus: Journal of the American Academy of Arts and Science* 123: 79–86.

TAYLOR, S. 1988. Caught in the continuum: A critical analysis of the principle of the least restrictive environment. *JASH* 13: 41–53.

TAYLOR, S., D. BIKLEN, and J. KNOLL. Eds. 1987. *Community Integration for People with Severe Disabilities.* New York (NY): Teachers College Press.

TOMLINSON, D. 1995. *Responding to Abuse: An Independent Living Approach.* Ottawa (ON): Canadian Association of Independent Living Centres.

TORJMAN, S. 1991. Individualized funding in relation to the Canada Assistance Plan. In *The Power to Choose: An Examination of Service Brokerage and Individualized Funding.* North York (ON): G. Allan Roeher Institute. p. 16.

TRAINER, J., E. POMEROY, and B. PAPE. 1993. *Framework for Support.* Toronto (ON): Canadian Mental Health Association.

TURNBULL, A. P., M. J. BROTHERSM, and J. A. SUMMERS. 1985. The impact of deinstitutionalization on families and family systems approach. In *Living and Learning: The Last Restructured Environment*, eds. R. H. BRUININK, and K. C. LAKIN. Baltimore (MD): Paul H. Brookes.

UDITSKY, B. 1993. Natural pathways to friendships. In *Friendships and Community Connections between People with and without Developmental Disabilities*, ed. A. NOVAK AMADO. Baltimore (MD): Paul H. Brookes.

VALENTINE, F. 1994. *The Canadian Independent Living Movement: An Historical Overview.* Ottawa (ON): Canadian Association for Independent Living Centres.

VANIER INSTITUTE OF THE FAMILY. 1992. *Transitions: A Newsletter.* Ottawa (ON): Author.

WALL, E. E. 1989. The winds of change in school physical education: Community networking for a lifetime for active living. Paper presented at CAHPER Convention, Halifax (NS), October.

WALLERSTEIN, N. 1992. Powerlessness, empowerment and health: Implications for health promotion programs. *American Journal of Health Promotion* 6: 197–205.

WALKER, B. 1994. Shared perspectives: Substance abuse and disability. *Journal of Leisurability* 21: 27–29.

WATKINSON, E.J. 1994. Preparing children with mental disabilities for active living. In *Toward Active Living*, ed. H. QUINNEY, L. GAUVIN, and A. E. WALL. Windsor (ON): Human Kinetics Publishers. pp. 164–171.

WATT, A., and S. RODMELL. 1988. Community involvement in health promotion: Progress or panacea? *Health Promotion* 2: 359–367.

WELLMAN, B., and A. HALL. 1986. Social networks and social support: Implications for later life. In *Later Life: The Social Psychology of Aging*, ed. V. MARSHAL. Newbury Park (CA): Sage.

WHITENECK, G., and P. FOUGEYROLLAS. 1995. Environmental factors and ICIDH. Presented at ICIDH Meeting, Quebec City, September 18–22.

WHITMORE, E. 1988. Empowerment and the process of inquiry. A paper presented at the annual meeting of the Canadian Association of Schools of Social Work, Windsor, Ontario.

———. 1988. Participation, empowerment and welfare. *Canadian Review of Social Policy* 22: 51–60.

WILLER, B., and J. INTAGLIATEA. 1979. Crisis for families of mentally retarded persons including a crisis of deinstitutionalization. *British Journal of Mental Subnormality* 25, part 1, no. 48, pp. 38–49.

WINTER, M. 1993. The growth and development in independent living in America. In *Independent Living: An Agenda for the '90s*, ed. A. NEUFELDT. Ottawa (ON): Canadian Association for Independent Living Centres. pp. 121–136.

WINZER, M. 1993. *Children with Exceptionalities: A Canadian Perspective.* 3rd ed. Scarborough (ON): Prentice Hall Canada, Inc.

WOLFENSBERGER, W. 1983. Social role valorization: A proposed new term for the principle of normalization. *Mental Retardation* 21: 235–239.

WORLD HEALTH ORGANIZATION, HEALTH AND WELFARE CANADA, CANADIAN PUBLIC HEALTH ORGANIZATION. 1986. Ottawa Charter for Health Promotion. Proceedings from International Conference on Health Promotion, Ottawa, November.

WORLD HEALTH ORGANIZATION. 1987. Ottawa Charter for Health Promotion. *Canadian Journal of Public Health* 77: 1.

WORTH, P. 1988. Real jobs for real wages. *Entourage* 3: 41,49.

WRIGHT, D. 1989. Informal support and aging. Unpublished paper. Kitchener (ON).

WYNGAARDEN, K., and M. ERICKSON. 1988. Informal support networks among aging persons with mental retardation: A pilot study. *Mental Retardation* 26: 197–201.

ZEY, K. 1990. How to facilitate integration: A resource teacher's perspective. *Entourage* (autumn): 13–15.

Protecting and Promoting
the Well-Being of Family Caregivers

BENJAMIN H. GOTTLIEB, PH.D.

Department of Psychology
University of Guelph

SUMMARY

In the present era of deinstitutionalization and community integration, enormous pressures are being placed on families to render practical care and emotional support, and to identify and orchestrate community services on behalf of family members who suffer from chronic illnesses, disabilities, or age-related declines in functioning. In Western societies, women shoulder the bulk of the family care responsibility for both the older and younger generations, a responsibility that can severely strain their coping resources, place them at an economic disadvantage, curtail their freedom and independence, and jeopardize their mental health. Indeed, both the scholarly literature on family care of elderly persons and reports in the public media make it abundantly clear that numerous wives, mothers and daughters lack the community resources they require to render adequate care to their demented spouses or parents, children with disabilities, or family members who suffer from a medically complex chronic disease or disorder. Moreover, even those who temporarily gain access to needed community services tend to become exhausted and demoralized by the work entailed in coordinating and monitoring the services. In addition, they are typically dissatisfied with the type, duration, quality and extent of control they can exercise over the services they wrest from community agencies.

This paper begins by describing converging social, demographic and policy trends that have resulted in pressures to maintain disabled, ill and frail family members at home, including the deinstitutionalization movement, the aging of the population (including the workforce), pressures to effect early discharge of elderly persons from hospital and convalescent beds, and the shift from acute and infectious disease control to the management of chronic illness.

The next section offers a succinct review of the literature that elaborates on the demands and toll of caregiving and the factors that mitigate the stress and strain experienced by caregivers. Although unique coping challenges face each family caregiver, all family caregivers share some common hardships and vulnerabilities, whether they look after children with developmental disorders or chronic illnesses, adults with special needs, or frail or demented elderly relatives. Specifically, there is evidence that caregivers must deal with at least four sets of potentially stressful demands:

1. *the demands of rendering optimal care, which may involve providing assistance with both activities of daily living (e.g., grooming, bathing, using the toilet) and with instrumental activities of daily living (e.g., mobility inside and outside the home, shopping, household chores), as well as monitoring and managing medically complex illnesses;*
2. *the demands of managing difficult behaviours associated with the disability or illness, such as wandering, wakefulness at night, and aggressive or belligerent behaviours;*
3. *the challenges associated with identifying, securing, orchestrating and maintaining high-quality health and/or human services; and*
4. *the secondary repercussions or dislocations of caregiving that may disrupt, curtail, or preclude the caregiver's participation in other valued roles or spheres of life, including the opportunity costs of forgoing or reducing participation in the paid workforce.*

Family caregivers also share certain resources for resisting stress, including factors at the individual, group and community levels. Personal resources include the coping skills and personality assets of the caregiver, whereas group resources include the support of family members and peers. Community resources are by far the most complex and, often, intractable sources of stress resistance. They not only include the major health, social welfare and employer institutions, but also encompass the broader sociocultural and political currents that shape the responses of policymakers and the public to the needs of family caregivers.

Drawing on this tripartite classification of resources for resisting stress, this paper seeks to identify avenues that promise to protect and promote the well-being of family caregivers of elderly persons, adults with special needs, and children with disabilities and chronic illnesses. Specifically, it identifies a set of employer initiatives *and a set of* community service and support strategies, *examining the strength of the evidence and the criteria for their effectiveness. In addition, it sets out a framework of values for family support programs, and principles to guide the conduct of professional practitioners who serve these families.*

These sources of stress resistance are then used as a framework for organizing programs and services for family caregivers, producing two main classes of initiatives for resisting caregiver stress:

A. Employer initiatives *support family caregivers and reduce the conflict they face between their job and dependent care responsibilities. Such initiatives involve the implementation of a set of flexible work arrangements and certain types of family-friendly services and initiatives. In addition, evaluations conducted by the Families and Work Institute in New York and the Canadian Aging Research Network (CARNET) are presented in order to document the impact of these initiatives on employee morale and performance.*

B. Community service interventions *principally involve programs that marshal social support, respite services and family-centred, multifaceted case management and counselling on behalf of family caregivers of elderly persons, especially those affected by dementia. In addition, for caregivers of children with developmental disabilities or chronically ill family members, programs that offer skill training, respite and comprehensive family support are spotlighted. Equally important, the planning and delivery of these services must be guided by a value framework that underscores the importance of creating mutual aid networks among families with common needs, as well as equal status partnerships and shared responsibility between parents and professionals. Moreover, the protection of family integrity and the strengthening of family functioning depend on the injection of greater flexibility, coordination, choice, family control, and responsiveness in developing supportive service arrangements.*

The paper concludes with policy implications that feature a set of recommendations to alter provincial employment standards in order to provide improved leave and benefit provisions for employees with responsibilities for family care, and to extend maternity and parental leave provisions under the federal unemployment insurance legislation to employees with family care responsibilities. In addition, changes in tax legislation should be considered to offset the actual and opportunity costs associated with family care.

Implications for program planners and policymakers in the long-term and continuing care fields include the importance of implementing sustained rather than episodic interventions, including:

- *ongoing rather than time-limited support groups;*
- *provisions for early outreach to family caregivers in order to deliver to them continuous, generous, and flexible respite and daycare arrangements;*
- *phe need for innovative approaches that blend family (informal) and agency (professional) care without supplanting the contributions of family caregivers;*
- *phe broader implementation of multicomponent, family-centred programs of support and advocacy on behalf of family caregivers;*
- *further efforts to makes services more unified, flexible, continuous, responsive and accountable to families—especially families with members who have severe disabilities or chronic illnesses;*
- *incentives for the creation of grassroots organizations, like the B.C. Caregivers Associations, that can advocate for people with disabilities and their caregivers, the creation of registries of temporary, substitute caregivers; and*
- *more concerted efforts to evaluate the sufficiency and responsiveness of services.*

In the context of ongoing initiatives to achieve equity and productivity, and to recognize diversity in the workplace, efforts should be made to educate middle managers about the work-family interface, and to encourage employers and managers to find new ways of helping employees achieve a healthy balance between their work and home life responsibilities, including wider use of flexible work options, the development of family-friendly programs and services, and leave arrangements that are responsive to the needs of employees facing intensive short- or long-term family care demands. In addition, employers should examine opportunities for developing new public/private partnerships with local human services that specialize in dependent care.

TABLE OF CONTENTS

INTRODUCTION: TRENDS CONVERGING ON FAMILY CAREGIVING

A number of converging social, demographic, technological and policy trends are bringing greater pressure to bear on an ever-increasing number of families in which there is a member who requires help and support due to an illness, disease, or disability that has rendered him partially or wholly dependent on others. Although the nature of the help that is required may differ from one family to the next, and the resources available to meet the family member's needs may also differ, all the types of family care that are addressed in this paper call for sustained assistance due to the long-term or chronic nature of the disease, disability or dependency. In some instances there is the added threat of deterioration, with increased dependency over time, and even death. For example, the family caregivers of children who suffer from certain forms of cancer, cystic fibrosis, or liver disease must adhere to complex and time-consuming medical monitoring and treatment procedures, while also enduring a bleak prognosis. Similarly, those who care for elderly family members who suffer from Alzheimer's disease not only must provide assistance to compensate for their relative's loss of cognitive and behavioral functions, but also must come to terms with the future implications of this diagnosis.

Demographic trends make it abundantly evident that a larger number of Canadian families will be faced with decisions about whether and how to assume responsibility for the care of aged relatives who are no longer able to care for themselves or live independently. Largely due to declining fertility rates, the proportion of the population that is 65 years of age or older has almost doubled in the last 50 years, from 6.7 percent of the population in 1941 to 11.8 percent in 1991 (Vanier Institute of the Family 1994). However, it will rocket to approximately one-quarter of the Canadian population by 2031, with vast implications for social security payments, health care and family care. At the same time, if public policy continues to favour de-institutionalization and community integration of persons with severe intellectual, emotional, or physical disabilities, then an increasing number of families will be obliged to care for them, with implications for further development of an infrastructure of supportive family services. Moreover, even excluding children and the elderly, as well as all those persons with disabilities who reside in institutions, the disability rates in 1992 were 7.9 percent among persons aged 15–34, 13.7 percent among those aged 35–54, and 26.6 percent among those aged 55–64. Almost 20 percent of persons in the latter age group reported having a severe disability (Statistics Canada 1992b).

Among children 14 years of age and younger, 7 percent have a disability; but, in 1991, only 2.9 percent of these children had a severe disability (Statistics Canada 1992b). Chronic health problems make up by far the largest single category of children's disabilities. And this is where the impact of technology is being acutely felt. Conditions that were once life threatening or required prolonged hospital stays are now amenable to care at home because of the invention of portable medical monitoring and treatment devices that family caregivers can be taught to use. In short, medical technology has made it possible to implement policies that favour community-based rather than costly hospital-based care. And when the veil is removed from terms such as "community-based care" and "family care," it becomes evident that it is women—predominantly mothers, daughters and wives—who shoulder the bulk of the hands-on daily work of caring for ill and dependent children, spouses and parents.

Yet another powerful social trend intersects with women's extensive involvement in caregiving, adding considerable strain to their lives. This trend concerns women's increased participation in the labour force. In 1941, only about 4.5 percent of married women were in the labour force, whereas by 1992, 61.4 percent were employed, and fully three-quarters of mothers with children under 12 are now working for pay. And yet, research reveals that the division of labour between the two partners at home has been virtually unchanged over the years, with women continuing to spend significantly more time than their male counterparts engaged in housework and the care of children and elderly relatives (Baines, Evans, and Neysmith 1991; Marshall 1990).

Little wonder, then, that so many women experience high levels of conflict between their paid and unpaid work. In 1994 a national survey of over 2,000 Canadian adults revealed that more than a quarter of employed women felt that they did not have a good balance between their jobs and time with their family, and about 20 percent felt that their difficulties trying to balance their job and family demands had limited their career advancement (Angus Reid Group 1994). More relevant to the concerns of this paper, the percentage of employed women who are having trouble balancing these two spheres of their life is even higher among those who have significant child care and/or elder care responsibilities (CARNET 1994).

Finally, the present era of deinstitutionalization and community integration has seen enormous pressures being placed on families to provide practical care and emotional support, and to identify and orchestrate community services on behalf of loved ones who suffer from severe intellectual, emotional, or physical disabilities. It is now widely recognized that neither families nor communities have received the preparation needed to cope with the challenges of caring for persons with severe handicaps. There have been numerous barriers to full participation and quality care of these persons, ranging from physical obstacles in the built environment to psychological obstacles preventing acceptance of persons who were "differently abled." Moreover, community support systems are underdeveloped, not only in terms of delivering the resources needed to sustain families, but also in terms of enabling families to realize their vision of community living.

AIMS AND PLAN OF THE PAPER

This position paper critically reviews numerous programs and initiatives that have been implemented on behalf of the family caregivers of elderly persons, adults with special needs, and children with disabilities and chronic illnesses. It spotlights programs that have demonstrated successful ways of mobilizing resources on behalf of family caregivers, using these resources to protect and promote the caregivers' health and well-being. In addition, it features initiatives that show great promise as preventive interventions, either because caregivers have expressed enthusiasm about a particular way of tendering support, or because the initiative represents an innovative and responsive partnership between families and the institutions and agencies of the community.

In addition, the paper addresses the value bases of programs that support families, and the criteria for determining the acceptability and success of family-focused interventions and services. The paper concludes with a set of policy implications that arise from the programs, values and evaluation data examined.

FAMILY CAREGIVERS: DEMANDS, COSTS AND HEALTH DETERMINANTS

The Demands of Caregiving

Although unique coping challenges face family caregivers who look after children with developmental disorders or chronic illnesses, adults with special needs, and frail or demented elderly relatives, they share some common hardships and vulnerabilities, as well as some resources for dealing with stress. On the former score, there is evidence that caregivers must deal with at least three stressful demands:
- the demands of rendering optimal care, which may involve providing assistance with both activities of daily living (e.g., grooming, bathing, using the toilet) and instrumental activities of daily living (e.g., mobility inside and outside the home, shopping, household chores);
- the demands of managing difficult behaviours associated with the disability, illness, or chronic conditions, such as wandering, socialization with peers, and aggressive or belligerent behaviours; and
- the secondary repercussions or dislocations of caregiving that may disrupt, curtail, or preclude the caregiver's participation in other valued roles or spheres of life. This third demand calls attention to the special impact of caregiving on employment, a subject that is separately addressed in the intervention section of this paper.

In addition to these stressors, which are common to all three types of family caregiving, there are unique stressors facing each caregiving context.

For example, many parents of children with chronic illnesses and severe disabilities must grapple with the impact of the child's condition on their marriage and on other family members, particularly siblings. In addition, there are the stressors associated with relating to and negotiating with the medical and human service systems, and with the child's school. In contrast, family caregivers of elderly persons affected by dementia face the special challenge of coming to terms with wholesale changes in the personality and role functioning of their relative, and even more profoundly, coping with the loss of their relationship with a significant attachment figure. Finally, those who care for an adult who suffers from chronic mental illness or from a condition that impairs normal role functioning must deal with the stigma that attaches to their relative and with the burden of having to monitor and supervise their relative around the clock.

In Canada, a significant number of families contain a member who requires both informal and professional care due to a disability or chronic illness. According to the Health and Activity Limitation Survey (Statistics Canada 1992a), 4.2 million Canadians or 15.5 percent of the population reported some level of disability. By age group, disability affects 7 percent of children under 15 (although only 2.9 percent of children with any disability had a severe disability), 14 percent of adults between 35 and 54, and 46.3 percent of those over 65. It is noteworthy that 93.7 percent of those with disabilities live in the community. For the population of people with disabilities as a whole, the most prevalent disability affects mobility (limited ability to walk, move or stand), whereas for children the most prevalent disabilities are chronic health problems such as diabetes and asthma.

The work of caregiving for children with medically complex conditions and severe disabilities is enormous, involving the need to provide assistance with every activity of daily living, including play and mobility in the home and community. In addition, many families must administer medication and specialized medical procedures and treatments, regularly monitor medical conditions (e.g., blood, respiration, urine), and handle challenging behaviours. Challenging behaviours include self-injurious and repetitive behaviours, wandering, and socially offensive behaviours. And beyond all of these direct demands, there is the larger impact on the family and on other spheres of the caregivers' lives, such as employment and continuing education. Further complicating this picture are both the economic costs and deprivations occasioned by the child's needs, and the relative paucity of informal and formal sources of support. For example, in one recent survey of a national U.S. sample of families with children who had severe disabilities, 30.4 percent reported that they received no assistance from any relative outside the household, 32.6 percent reported that they received no help from any professional, and 16.3 percent said they had no one to turn to in a crisis. In fact, many of the principal caregivers—almost always mothers—reported that family members pulled away when they recognized the long-term prognosis, or pressured the caregiver to institutionalize the child (Knoll 1992).

Regrettably, the harsh reality today is that most families with a child who needs virtually round-the-clock supervision, special technology, and supportive services report that they find themselves in a world of bureaucrats and service agents who are socially and often culturally distant, speak a language that is incomprehensible, operate according to procedures and policies that serve their agency's needs rather than the needs of the intended beneficiaries, and are loathe to allow families the control over their lives that they need to serve their childrens' best interests. Whether trying to care for an adolescent with diabetes or haemophilia, an infant who is dependent on medical technology, a child who has a degenerative or life-threatening disease, or a child with a major intellectual, physical, or behavioral disability, all too often family members find themselves stretched to the limit, depleted of their financial resources, and nearing the breaking point.

Perhaps the most dramatic and poignant examples of the desperation that besets families who are denied the resources to care for their children with disabilities are the recent deaths of a Hamilton, Ontario woman and her disabled son. The two died of carbon monoxide poisoning in an apparent murder-suicide after the family was denied further funding under the Special Services at Home program. In addition, there is the case of a Saskatchewan farmer, Robert Latimer, who was convicted of murdering his disabled 12-year-old daughter. Moreover, in a meeting held as recently as December 1994, the Deputy Minister of Community and Social Services of Ontario told a group of parents who were caring for their children with severe disabilities at home that they should call the Ministry if they knew of anyone who was contemplating suicide or murder.

The Costs of Caregiving: Effects on Morbidity and Employment

Although many individual and situational factors come into play in determining the nature and extent of the adverse effects of caregiving, there is abundant evidence that family caregivers' physical and psychological stamina are depleted over time, compromising their physical and psychological health. For example, in the gerontology field, a large number of mainly cross-sectional studies show an increased prevalence of psychiatric and somatic symptomatology among caregivers of persons with dementia when compared to control groups or to age- and gender-based population norms (Schulz, Visintainer, and Williamson 1990; Schulz et al. 1995). There is even evidence that caregiving has an adverse effect on immune system functioning. Compared to a demographically matched sample of noncaregivers, Kiecolt-Glaser et al. (1987) found that those caring for a relative with Alzheimer's disease had significantly lower percentages of total

T-lymphocytes and helper T-lymphocytes, as well as significantly lower helper/suppressor cell ratios. Finally, across all caregiving contexts, there is evidence that strain and morbidity are increased when the recipient of care expresses disruptive, aggressive, or bizarre behaviours.

Similarly, research on the caregivers of children with mental handicaps and life threatening illnesses reveals their increased risk of psychiatric and somatic illness (Avison et al. 1993). Mothers of chronically ill children have been reported to have a high occurrence of depressive symptoms, stemming in part from feelings of loneliness and disappointment. In many instances, loneliness results from the tendency of the father/husband to withdraw, and even to blame the mother/wife for venting her fears and anxieties. Based on interviews with mothers of children who had serious illnesses, Gottlieb and Wagner (1991) report that these mothers had to feign stoic and effectively neutral styles of coping with their children's illnesses in order to maintain their husbands' involvement and support. Moreover, the extra effort entailed in putting on such a false show of toughness added to the considerable burden they already shouldered, and ultimately left them feeling alienated from their husbands. Aside from these interspousal tensions, the mothers typically suffer from chronic fatigue and anxiety about their children's future.

Among the most far-reaching dislocations engendered by caregiving is its impact on the caregivers' involvement in the labour force, in terms of their entry to and exit from the labour force as well as the morale, productivity, and career mobility of those caregivers who do hold jobs. Although many employers have now recognized that it is in their own best interest to assist employees with child care responsibilities by providing some measure of job flexibility and certain information and referral services, they have only recently begun to acknowledge that many workers have exceptionally demanding home life responsibilities—especially single parents, elder care providers and employees who care for children and adults with special needs. Moreover, many Human Resource departments have revised benefit plans and work schedules that were originally designed in an era when there was only one breadwinner in the family, and when women stayed at home.

A number of recent studies have examined the prevalence of elder care responsibilities among the workforce, and the impact of these responsibilities on employees and their work (Brody et al. 1987; Neal et al. 1993; Scharlach and Boyd 1989; Stone, Cafferata, and Sangl 1987). There is evidence that employees who shoulder elder care responsibilities forego employment or curtail their job involvement by reducing their hours (Gibeau, Anastas, and Larson 1987) or by taking temporary periods of leave (Scharlach and Boyd 1989; Stephens and Christianson 1986). For example, based on a national U.S. sample of caregivers of frail elderly persons, Stone, Cafferata and Sangl (1987) report that 14 percent of wives, 12 percent of daughters, 11 percent of husbands, and 5 percent of sons attributed their exit from their jobs to the demands of caring for an elderly relative. In addition, they found that 21 percent worked fewer hours, 18.6 percent took time off without pay, and almost 30 percent rearranged their work schedule. Moreover, findings from the National Hospice Study reveal that, of 1,445 primary caregivers, fully one-third terminated employment to assume care responsibilities (Muurinen 1986). Based on their review of several studies, Scharlach, Lowe and Schneider (1991) report that 9–28 percent of caregivers state that they retired early, quit work, or took an extended leave of absence in order to care for an elderly relative.

Whereas these studies testify to the impact of elder care on the termination, reduction and rescheduling of employment, other studies reveal that employees' involvement in elder care can affect their ability to meet their job responsibilities and to advance at work. Stone and Short (1990) found that primary caregivers (those who report that they have the major care responsibility for an elderly relative), and those caring for relatives with the greatest impairment and need for care, were more likely to take unpaid leaves, reduce their work hours and rearrange their work schedules. As for on-the-job performance, Neal et al. (1993) report that the number of hours of care predicted work interruptions, as measured by the number of telephone calls from or about the recipient of care. In addition, a recent Canadian study of 1,419 employees, each of whom provided assistance to an elderly relative by helping them with at least one activity of daily living or at least two instrumental activities of daily living revealed that those who assisted more impaired elderly relatives, those who had to deal with crises affecting their relative's health, and those who were involved in orchestrating community services on their relative's behalf were at greater risk of experiencing more family interference with work, more stress and more personal and job costs. The personal costs included reduced time for continuing education, volunteer work and leisure activities, whereas the job costs involved missed meetings or training sessions, the need to decline business travel, extra projects, or promotions, and the inability to attend job-related social events that were scheduled outside regular work hours (Gottlieb, Kelloway, and Fraboni 1994).

The Determinants of Caregivers' Health and Well-Being

Although the caregiving literature has emphasized the heightened risk of psychological distress and physical illness among caregivers as a function of the multiple burdens and demands they face, only a small minority experience serious emotional illness. This suggests that the majority of caregivers possess certain *resources for resisting stress*, reducing their vulnerability. The literature on the psychosocial determinants of mental and physical health suggests that these resources fall into three classes, including factors at the individual, group and community levels.

Personal resources include the coping skills and personality assets of the caregiver, including such dimensions of self-concept as self-esteem and self-efficacy. Whereas self-esteem is allied with feelings of self-worth, self-respect and self-acceptance, self-efficacy refers to confidence in one's ability to influence or control the forces affecting one's life. The latter construct has particularly important implications for caregivers because it may equip them to wrest the resources they need from schools, social agencies and medical practitioners, and give them confidence in their ability to master other critical environmental events (Silver, Bauman, and Ireys 1995). One's sense of self-efficacy may influence another set of personal resources, namely problem- and emotion-focused coping efforts (Lazarus and Folkman 1984). That is, people who have confidence that they can fulfil desired goals are more likely to engage in such problem-focused coping efforts as confronting people who stand in the way, logically analyzing problems and generating alternative solutions, and seeking practical and emotional support. In short, health protection is afforded by the interaction between dispositional coping resources and specific situationally grounded coping efforts (Wheaton 1983).

Group resources include the support of family members and peers. There is little question that the practical help, cooperation and accommodations provided by immediate family members, particularly those in the same household, are of enormous value to the principal caregiver. They not only reduce stress by sharing the work of caregiving, but also mitigate feelings of isolation and demoralization. Moreover, by filling in for the caregiver to allow for periods of respite, and by acknowledging and validating the caregiver's competence and commitment, supporters can shore up the caregiver's mental health and feelings of self-efficacy. In addition, the support of peers who are in similar stressful circumstances can be of unique value to caregivers because of its normalizing function and because of the insights about new ways of coping and managing illness that are generated through the process of mutual aid. In short, there is a strong fabric of evidence documenting the health-protective and health-promoting impact of both received and perceived support from kith and kin (Gottlieb 1989).

From an intervention perspective, there is broad consensus that it is more feasible to modify and mobilize resources at the group level than at the individual level. This is because personality traits are relatively stable and resistant to change, whereas social support is an environmental resource that can be marshalled, specialized, intensified, or redirected. However, it is important to acknowledge that individual difference variables, such as extraversion and social self-esteem, may influence the success of support interventions, and that some person-focused interventions hold more promise than others. On the latter score, psychoeducational programs that teach caregivers practical behaviour and stress management skills have shown greater success than initiatives directed toward changing basic personality characteristics. Such skill training strategies are represented among the "success stories" spotlighted in this paper.

Finally, *community resources* are by far the most complex and vexing sources of stress resistance because they include not only the major health, social welfare and employer institutions, but also the broader sociocultural and political contexts that shape the responses of the public and policymakers to the needs of family caregivers. Because the work of caregiving is so onerous, and because families can only continue to care for their own as long as they have a durable safety net of basic health, financial and human services, concerted efforts must be made to engineer *systems of shared care* that fully acknowledge the partnership and covenant between citizens and their governments. This is why intervention at the community level must concurrently address both the values and the tangible resources affecting the well-being and survival of families carrying excess burdens due to a disability, chronic illness or disease, or age-related dependency of one or more members.

STRATEGIES TO PROTECT AND PROMOTE THE WELL-BEING OF FAMILY CAREGIVERS

Employer Initiatives for Workers with Family Responsibilities

Recognizing the extent to which caregiving responsibilities can spill over into the workplace, creating unwanted turnover and productivity losses, and recognizing the productivity gains and morale boost that can result from family-friendly programs and policies, many companies are now proactively designing new initiatives aimed at reducing the work-family conflict experienced by caregiving employees. In addition, it is expected that these progressive initiatives will increase loyalty and give the company a competitive edge in recruiting "bright-collar" workers who, since they would receive the same financial compensation regardless of where they worked, choose jobs based on issues of job flexibility and job-family balance (Galinsky, Bond, and Friedman 1993).

What sort of initiatives have been introduced? They can be divided into two classes, one comprising flexible or alternative work arrangements, and the other consisting of information, referral and direct services, such as emergency elder care, support groups, family life seminars, telephone hotlines, caregiver fairs, personal elder care and child care counselling, and paid leave days for family responsibilities. The flexible work arrangements are designed to make it easier for working caregivers to meet both their job and home obligations, and include flexitime, telecommuting, job sharing, compressed work weeks, part-time employment with prorated benefits, and a variety of extended unpaid leave arrangements with job guarantees after the period of leave has ended.

Employers who now recognize that, when it comes to the hours and location of work, "one size does not fit all", and who no longer subscribe to the belief that simply showing up at work is a valid measure of productivity and motivation, have created procedures and practical guidelines for managers and employees to negotiate the terms of flexible work arrangements. Some have created parallel career ladders for part-time employees. For example, the Royal Bank has developed a series of brochures that not only describe the mechanics of different types of work arrangements, but also address the personal skills they call for (e.g., the ability to work unsupervised and to be self-motivated, for those considering work-at-home arrangements) as well as the pros and cons of each work option. Similarly, through its *Work and Lifestyles* program, the CIBC has delivered materials to every branch manager, informing them of the procedures and conditions for granting flexible work arrangements to employees and instructing them to give every consideration to such requests.

Data gathered by Watson Wyatt, a management consulting firm, reveal that larger companies and companies with a greater proportion of female workers have initiated more work and family programs (Watson Wyatt Memorandum 1995). In their national survey of 777 Canadian companies, they found that more than three-quarters of the responding companies offered one or more family-friendly benefits, such as dependant care services or flexible work arrangements or family life seminars. However, among 60 percent of the companies, they also found an ominous degree of scepticism on the part of senior management that the programs made business sense. Furthermore, they found that more than half of the responding companies believed that employees needed to make a choice between family and the possibility of moving up the corporate ladder.

What are these companies actually doing to help employees balance their work and family lives? The Watson Wyatt survey indicates that the bulk of the assistance takes the form of information and referral (I and R) programs rather than direct services. Flexible hours are the most prevalent form of flexible work arrangement—not those options that permit caregivers to spend more time with a dependant who requires more assistance, like job sharing and telecommuting. Specifically, the survey found that, while 28 percent of the responding companies offered child care I and R services, and 23 percent offered elder care I and R, no more than 7 percent of the companies provided any form of direct child care service and less than 1 percent provided any form of direct elder care service, such as subsidizing elder care costs or access to off-site or on-site daycare. In short, most of the assistance took the form of education, information and referral, leaving the employee with the time-consuming and complex work of actually accessing and orchestrating direct services.

When examined closely, the most prevalent flexible work options were actually quite rigid. For example, flexible hours were tightly constrained to a one- or two-hour window at the start and end of the day, employees being required to be on the job during certain core hours. Moreover, all of the responding companies (56 percent) that did offer such individualized start and stop times indicated that employees had to adhere to the hours they had initially selected. This leaves questions about the flexibility of the arrangement, especially for employees who are on call when crises occur at home or when routine medical monitoring and treatment are required at certain daily intervals. For these employees, greater flexibility in hours of work, job sharing, or telecommuting would be much more desirable. However, the survey found that only 29 percent of companies permitted some form of job sharing or telecommuting. And, even in these companies, only certain categories of employees were eligible to work at home (usually middle management).

Finally, perhaps the most vexing and worrisome findings of the survey concerned the attitude of senior managers toward these family-friendly initiatives, since these views reflect the norms of the corporate culture. Only 15 percent of the responding companies offered any training to managers or directed any communication to them about the importance of helping employees to achieve a healthy work-family balance. Only 5 percent of companies tied managers' performance evaluation and compensation to their flexibility with respect to their subordinates' family responsibilities. Perhaps more important, members of middle management see those in senior management putting in 60- to 80-hour weeks and never see them using flexible work options. Hence, the unspoken message is that flexible work options are only for those who are not serious about moving up on the career ladder. In fact, when asked about the main obstacles to work and family programs, 10 percent of the responding companies mentioned employee concern about career advancement, 48 percent mentioned cost containment, 42 percent stated that senior managers do not consider the issue important, 46 percent stated there was no competitive pressure on them to initiate any programs, and 42 percent stated that managers' concerns about scheduling precluded implementation of flexible work options. However, since these findings are based on one individual's perceptions of the obstacles (the HR representative who replied to the survey), rather than on the actual opinions of managers and employees, they may not accurately reflect the real obstacles or the extent of endorsement of these obstacles by members of the company's workforce.

Evaluation of Employer Initiatives

Despite widespread claims for and against the benefits of work-family programs, there have been almost no rigorous evaluations of their impact on productivity, morale, recruitment, retention, or absenteeism of employees. At best, companies have periodically surveyed employees to inquire about their satisfaction with initiatives, and at worst, they have either failed to gather feedback from employees or selectively canvassed the opinions of high utilizers or favourable managers. The exceptions have been two studies, one a U.S. study of Johnson and Johnson's *Balancing Work and Family Program*, and the other a Canadian study of the CIBC's *Work and Lifestyles Program*.

Conducted by the Families and Work Institute in New York City, the evaluation of Johnson and Johnson's program was based on two comprehensive surveys of J&J employees at four companies in 1990, just after the program was introduced, and again in 1992. Almost 2,500 employees responded each time, yielding a large and statistically reliable (although not necessarily representative) sample. The program itself must be considered a model of progressive action on the work-family front because the package of initiatives spanned child care and elder care resource and referral services, on-site child development centres, flexible work schedules, various leave arrangements for family responsibilities, and management training "…to help them understand the business case for work-family policies and help them implement effective work-family practices" (Families and Work Institute 1993).

The most significant findings of the study had far less to do with rates of utilization of specific services than with a fundamental change in the corporate climate and with the perceived costs of using family-friendly programs and work arrangements. Specifically, the data revealed that in 1992, 51 percent of the respondents strongly agreed with the statement "My supervisor is helpful to me when I have a routine family or personal matter," whereas only 36 percent had strongly agreed with that idea two years earlier. Similarly, the number of employees who said that they paid a price for using flexible time and leave policies fell from 44 percent, when the program was first announced, to 32 percent, two years after the program's implementation. Equally impressive are the findings that the new programs and policies figured prominently in employees' decisions to stay at the company, and to recommend it to others, whether or not they had actually availed themselves of the initiatives. In short, the mere introduction of work and family programs communicates to all employees that they are working in a setting that cares about and views as legitimate employees' responsibilities off the job. Moreover, the sheer availability of these initiatives reduces apprehensions in the same way that perceived support has been found to moderate stress. Letting employees know there is a safety net and flexible work options also builds loyalty and reduces turnover.

The second study was conducted by a team of investigators affiliated with CARNET: The Canadian Aging Research Network. It systematically compared the performance and morale of employees using conventional work arrangements at the CIBC with those who had entered flexible work arrangements. One of the strengths of the study was that data were collected not only from the employees themselves, but also from their managers (Barham et al. 1995). The key finding of the study was that there were no differences in productivity, morale, or work-family balance as a function of the type of work arrangement an employee had. Instead, these outcomes were affected by whether or not employees were working in the type of arrangement that they personally desired, presumably because it suited their needs for balance between their job and family responsibilities. That is, no differences were found in these outcomes for employees who were working in conventional versus alternative work arrangements, or for employees in different types of alternative work arrangements. For example, there were no significant differences in employees' own ratings and in their managers' ratings of the quality of customer service for employees in flexible work arrangements versus those in conventional arrangements.

The chief determinant was whether employees wanted to work in the schedule they had; those who wanted to be in a different work arrangement gave significantly worse ratings to their relations with coworkers and their manager, and experienced more interruptions at work than those who were in the arrangement they wanted. Equally important, in terms of their attitudes, those who were satisfied with their present work arrangement had significantly higher levels of job satisfaction, decreased work-family conflict and stress, and they perceived their managers, coworkers and the company as a whole as significantly more supportive than those who wished to change their job arrangement. Equally important from the employer's perspective, those who were unhappy with the fit between their lifestyle and their job arrangements were significantly more likely to intend to leave the organization.

Key Conclusions Regarding Employer Initiatives

What are the implications of the above findings regarding the recent developments and research on employer responses to the needs of workers with family responsibilities? First, as mentioned earlier, people at all levels of the organization need to "buy into" policies and practices that afford flexibility when work and family demands clash. The business case for these new initiatives and the cultural norms in which they are embedded needs to be clearly articulated. There should be sessions that allow managers to compare solutions to the predicaments of individual employees and *link work-family issues to the broader themes of equity, diversity and productivity.* Through discussion, managers must come to understand that equity does not mean doing the same thing for everyone, but being consistently fair to everyone. Managers must adopt a "can do" stance toward employees who request a change in their work arrangement, the default response being to grant the request unless there are compelling business reasons not to do so.

Managers must also formulate certain procedures for negotiating and contracting with employees who choose alternative arrangements, building in periodic appraisals of the arrangement in terms of its effects on coworkers, managers themselves, and the employee's job performance and ability to meet their home life demands. These agreements must also provide certain guarantees to employees regarding job security, fringe benefits and career progress.

Flexibility regarding work-family issues must be built in as a criterion in managers' performance evaluations, with data collected from annual employee morale surveys as the basis for judging managers' performance in this respect. For example, at the Bank of Montreal, employees are regularly surveyed about whether they have requested and been denied a flexible work arrangement. If so, the manager responsible for the decision is approached and efforts are made to ensure that company policy is administered consistently. In short, regardless of the number of new programs and services that are introduced, unless all levels of management internalize the business case for flexibility and serve as models of flexibility, a fundamental shift in the culture of the organization will not occur. As Johanne Totta, the Bank of Montreal's vice president of Employee Programs and Workplace Equality observed: "The success of our program rests on how we have integrated it into the fabric of our organization, from training to performance, and from communication to continuous performance."

The second implication of the above findings is that, for employees who experience longer periods of relatively onerous caregiving demands at home, leave policies must be put in place that provide job guarantees at the end of the leave. In the United States, legislation has recently been passed requiring employers to provide such unpaid leave for a period of up to 12 months, although it has not yet been evaluated. In Canada, only a handful of employers provide such a leave arrangement. Therefore the majority of caregivers have little choice but to compromise the care they offer to a family member, lose their jobs, or pass on the care of their relative to another family member or to an institutional authority.

Third, especially in the present economic climate, since it is doubtful that employers will offer direct services such as day programs and emergency child care or elder care services to employees with heavy caregiving responsibilities, *new public/private partnerships need to be formed* with local service providers. Employers may provide small grants to agencies to allow them to expand their service to accommodate more clients, or lend their expertise at no charge to assist with an agency's budgeting or accounting operations, in return for the agency partially or wholly subsidizing service costs to the company's employees. In addition, several employers in a local community may form an elder care consortium or work-family council, thereby combining their resources to address a shared, high-priority work-family issue, such as sponsoring an intergenerational day program that serves employees with either child care or elder care needs. The point is that caregivers with more onerous home life responsibilities do require more than information and referral services; they require practical assistance with the work of caregiving!

Fourth, even information and referral services need to be carefully examined. In too many cases these services amount to little more than a brief phone call to an 800 number serviced by the staff of an Employee Assistance Program (EAP)—people who know little about the quality of programs in different locales, their admission requirements, the availability of spaces/beds and the costs. Moreover, since EAP firms are inevitably concerned about profitability, basing their fees on estimates of the number of employees who will require service and the amount of time that can be devoted to each employee, there are often severe constraints on the quantity and continuity of assistance given to employee clients. Too often, callers receive little more than an empathetic response from the phone counsellor, followed by a mailed package of information that may include a "quick and dirty" self-assessment instrument with unknown diagnostic precision. What they need instead is *assistance in negotiating the service system* and identifying and procuring the resources they require for their particular caregiving situation.

Finally, since work-family initiatives are primarily restricted to large, nonunionized organizations in which the majority of employees are female— such as banks, insurance companies, hospitals and government ministries— *concerted efforts must be made to spur small employers to initiate family-friendly programs and flexible work arrangements*. Moreover, although some flexible work options cannot be made available to some employees (such as telecommuting for employees in the manufacturing sector) other alternative work arrangements can be made, including compressed work weeks, job sharing and family leave. These initiatives are not costly, but they do require a sea change in managers' attitudes and behaviours; they are ways of working differently and working smarter so that productivity is maintained while employee job and home life satisfaction are optimized.

Community Service and Support Strategies

The second main class of resources for resisting caregiver stress involves a range of service and support initiatives focused on providing accessible and acceptable support, respite, and multifaceted, family-focused case management and counselling services. Each of these initiatives is discussed separately, with careful attention paid to effectiveness and successful implementation.

Programs in Support of the Family Caregivers of Elderly Persons

Before detailing some of the most promising interventions on behalf of family caregivers of the elderly, it should be noted that rigorous evaluation of programs has been relatively recent and a diversity of programs have been evaluated. For example, even though support groups have been offered to caregivers for at least 15 years, controlled evaluations of this intervention strategy have only appeared in the past five years. This is also the case for individual or family counselling, respite services, case management, skills training and various combined approaches. One implication of this is discussed by Bourgeois, Schulz and Burgio (1996), who recently reviewed the intervention literature and observed that:

> Direct comparisons between individual studies are difficult to make because structural details (such as target population, frequency and duration of intervention, content of intervention, peer versus professional intervention agents, home- or community-based treatment, outcome measures, level of analysis) vary widely across studies (9).

It is premature to draw any firm conclusions about programs that "work" for caregivers. This is because demonstration and pilot projects have not been examined long enough to determine whether or not their results can be replicated or generalized.

Psychoeducational support in a group context, *respite,* and *multifaceted, family-focused case management and personal counselling* have been the three most popular initiatives that have been extended on behalf of the family caregivers of elderly relatives. Moreover, these interventions have largely been offered to the caregivers of persons with dementia because it is widely acknowledged that their burdens and dislocations are the most severe and far reaching.

Although initiatives like those described below have been offered in many locales throughout Canada, the particular programs presented here are research demonstration projects that were implemented by academically based investigators. These investigators received grant and/or private foundation funding that included monies for the evaluation component.

Support Groups

Two recent reviews of the literature reveal that support groups alone have not proved effective in ameliorating the mental health of caregivers, at least not on the basis of existing measures of psychiatric symptomatology or quality of life indicators (Lavoie 1995; Toseland and Rossiter 1989). On the basis of their review of 29 studies of support groups for caregivers of elderly persons, mainly caregivers of relatives with AD, Toseland and Rossiter (1989) conclude that:

> Clinical impressions and participants' self-reports of satisfaction with support groups have been confirmed by rigorous studies, but caregivers' feelings of burden, levels of stress, and sense of well-being are not (446).

They observe that the studies show no evidence that support groups can help caregivers to cope with or alleviate stress associated with specific problems in providing care, reduce the risk of psychological disturbance, or increase access to or use of community and/or informal resources.

Two studies by Hebert and his colleagues at the Centre for Research in Gerontology and Geriatrics of the Hôpital d'Youville in Sherbrooke, Quebec are typical of the findings of even the most rigorously designed support group interventions. In the first study, caregivers of persons with dementia were randomly assigned either to a support group that met for two hours a week for eight weeks or to a group which was referred to the informal monthly meetings of the Alzheimer's Society (Hebert et al. 1994). Then measures of burden, psychiatric symptoms, use of health services, and knowledge of AD were taken at entry, after the eight–week intervention, and after eight months. Despite the fact that the support group sessions featured development of behaviour management skills, information about AD, discussion of the emotional impact of the disease on the caregiver, and stress management techniques, there was only one significant difference between the groups, namely increased knowledge about the disease among the support group members. Moreover, a second study designed along the same lines found that the support group did not prolong the length of community tenure of the person with AD (Hebert et al. 1995).

Recognizing these null effects, Toseland and Rossiter (1989) suggest that improvements should be made in the measurement of support group outcomes, shifting them from global mental health measures to specific measures of behavioral functioning. They also suggest that more attention should be paid to composing groups in ways that reflect differences in the needs and risk status of different subgroups of caregivers (e.g., employed daughters versus retired husbands). In addition, Toseland and Rossiter (1989) observe that most support groups terminate too early; typically, participants want to continue meeting after the last formal session has ended. This suggests that the group process is attractive to participants even though it does not seem to exert any significant impact on the standard measures used by researchers to date. In turn, it suggests either that researchers need to rethink these outcomes or that they need to extend the life of the support group and then examine the outcomes that resulted after increasing the "dosage" in this way. In addition, Lavoie (1995) suggests that researchers need to make an effort to align the group's focus with the perceived wants and goals of the participants, and then measure the attainment of these goals on a person-by-person basis.

What, then, can be concluded about the value of support groups for family caregivers? Can this mode of intervention be considered a "success story"? First, it must be recognized that support groups are not universally attractive, and that they require a modicum of social skills, self-confidence, and an orientation toward monitoring and airing rather than repressing one's stressful feelings. Second, even among those who are motivated to attend, when standard measures are used, support groups have not proved their effectiveness in alleviating caregivers' (subjective) burden, mitigating feelings of anxiety or depression, or dealing more effectively with the practical demands and behavioral disturbances of the recipient of care. Third, evidence based on consumer satisfaction suggests that support groups are valuable because the participants gain a sense of being understood by others, learn to accept feelings such as anger more naturally, and feel less alone.

Finally, from a logistical standpoint, support groups pose barriers for people who live in rural or remote locations because of the time and effort involved in meeting on a face-to-face basis. The alternative is telephone support groups, one example being Goodman and Pynoos' (1990) program in which networks of four or five caregivers were established to discuss issues related to the care of a relative with Alzheimer's disease (AD). However, in comparing the effects of the telephone support group with those produced among a group of caregivers randomly assigned to listen to a lecture series on the subject of AD, Goodman and Pynoos found no differences in the two groups' information gain, or in their perceptions of or satisfaction with social support. More important, those assigned to the peer telephone support group actually gained less emotional support from family and friends than those who listened to lectures over the phone. This suggests that the support group supplanted the natural network, a possibility which, depending on one's perspective, could be an asset or a risk. On one hand, it may have introduced new peer contacts who could offer more specialized, stress-relevant support than the natural network members. On the other hand, it could have caused the participants to neglect or even reject the help of their own networks, with ominous implications for their responsiveness once the support group ends.

Respite Services

In terms of standard outcome measures, respite programs have fared much like support groups, and therefore cannot be considered successful as a stand-alone intervention for family caregivers (Bourgeois, Schulz, and Burgio 1996). In the most rigorous evaluation of respite services, Lawton, Brody and Saperstein (1989) used a randomized experimental and control group to determine whether respite provided by informal or formal sources at home or at a centre over a period of a year had any impact on the caregivers' well-being (subjective burden, depressive symptoms, general mood/affect, self-rated physical health) or on the length of the demented relative's community tenure. Respite made no difference in the proportion of persons with dementia who remained in the community after 12 months, even though those elderly persons whose caregivers had been assigned to the respite intervention spent a significantly greater number of days in the community (as opposed to the hospital) than members of the control group. Nor did respite have any appreciable (statistically significant) impact on the caregivers' well-being. In addition, within the respite group, the amount of respite received had no effect on the well-being of the caregivers.

Despite these null effects, the authors offer several important observations, with implications for future program design, about the pattern of respite use and caregivers' satisfaction with the respite. Echoing the findings for support groups, they state that the high level of consumer satisfaction with the respite time received is important per se, and that it may be unrealistic to expect the effects of respite to spill over into other sectors of caregiver well-being or to delay long-term placement. In addition, they note that the caregivers needed time, education and encouragement before they were prepared to avail themselves of respite, and most only sought it when they were in crisis or very late in the caregiving process. In fact, the modest effects of respite may be due to the relatively small average amount of respite time that caregivers actually take. Across studies, even when respite was subsidized or free, only a small minority of caregivers sent their relatives on a daily basis, the majority using no more than about 10 days per year (Lawton, Brody, and Saperstein 1989).

The findings of the latter study concur with the results of Gottlieb and Johnson's (1995) recent study of the impact of several centre-based respite programs in Ontario on the mental health of 103 family caregivers of persons with dementia. They, too, found that respite was an instance of "too little, too late" since, at the time when the relatives were enrolled, half the caregivers who did avail themselves of respite had already placed their relative's name on a waiting list for long-term care. Moreover, after approximately five months, almost half of the caregivers had either placed their relative or dropped out of the respite program for other reasons. At this time, the remaining 58 caregivers were experiencing a small but statistically significant reduction in levels of anxiety, somatization and stress. There was no reduction in depressive mood, life satisfaction, or perceived physical health.

The findings of these two studies, together with evidence that centre-based respite programs actually add to rather than diminish the work of caregiving because of the time and effort involved in preparing the relative to attend and then receiving the relative back home, suggest that the following steps must be taken to make respite a more powerful and attractive preventive service intervention:

- Information about respite programs ought to be conveyed to caregivers as soon as a diagnosis of probable dementia is made, ideally through the caregivers' contacts with the family physician, who is typically the first professional to be consulted.
- Transportation arrangements must be available so that this burden does not fall on the caregiver.

- Program hours must be flexible enough to accommodate the needs of employed caregivers. For those caregivers who are disturbed at night due to their relative's wakefulness, some provision ought to be made for at least one or two overnight stays per week.
- Screening of caregivers and their relatives for respite programs ought to distinguish between those caregivers who see the program as a stepping stone to long-term care and those who are seeking the relief they need to continue in the caregiving role.
- Respite programs need to establish a balance between providing direct service provision to caregivers (e.g., through counselling, support groups, education and assistance with long-term care planning) and allowing them time to themselves, free of any involvements that pertain to the care they provide.

Multicomponent Interventions

There have been a number of comprehensive, multicomponent intervention studies that combine peer support, individual counselling and community services in the hope that a scattershot strategy will be more effective than any single mode of intervention. For example, Ferris and his colleagues (1987) offered 41 caregivers of AD patients individualized attention that included private counselling, referral to appropriate agencies, home visits, family meetings, telephone consultation and support groups. They found a significant reduction in caregiver depression, anger, insomnia and anxiety as well as differences in the rates of institutionalization between those participating in the intervention and a control group of caregivers. Unfortunately, in this and other comprehensive programs (e.g., Mohide et al. 1990; Montgomery and Borgatta 1989; Seltzer, Irvy, and Litchfield 1987), analyses of the effectiveness of the individual components were not performed, leaving uncertainty about which ingredients of the package deserve replication and which could be eliminated in order to effect cost savings.

Because of its recognition for providing "...the most compelling evidence for the effectiveness of classical treatment" by the Committee on Aging of the Group for the Advancement of Psychiatry (1994, 268), Mittelman and her colleagues' comprehensive program of counselling and support for the spouse-caregivers of persons with dementia deserves special attention (Mittelman et al. 1993, 1995). The program was structured around formal counselling sessions, two of which were with the caregiver alone and four with the family. All counselling sessions took place within four months of intake and were focused on problems that had been identified during initial evaluation. Hence, in addition to the broad goals of educating family members about dementia, improving understanding and communication between the caregiver and family members, and reducing conflict about the sharing of responsibilities in the household, the counsellors addressed the specific problems of individual families. These problems included concerns about the caregiver's relationship with their spouse, feelings of inadequacy and guilt, and anxieties about the future. The counsellors' interventions included:

- role playing ways of preventing or responding to the demented family members' problem behaviours;
- encouraging the caregiver to seek paid and/or unpaid help; and
- providing information about and practical assistance in obtaining a variety of community services.

A second major component of the program commenced after the four months of counselling, and involved participation in an open-ended support group composed of AD caregivers. However, ad hoc counselling and crisis intervention were still provided when problems arose, and counsellors facilitated new arrangements for assistance and services to the caregiver when needed.

The results of the program revealed that, within one year, only 10.7 percent of the demented relatives of the caregivers who had received the program required nursing home placement, compared to 23.3 percent of those persons with dementia whose caregivers had been randomly assigned to a usual support condition. Further analyses revealed that younger spouse-caregivers were more likely to place their demented spouses in nursing homes than older caregivers, perhaps because they were more involved than older caregivers in other valued life spheres. In addition, the more assistance needed by the relative with activities of daily living, the greater the likelihood of placement.

More recently, Mittelman et al (1995) have reported that this supportive intervention package had a statistically significant impact on the spousal caregivers' depressive symptomatology. However, it is noteworthy that depressive affect did not decline significantly until eight months after the program was implemented. At the four-month measurement interval, the intervention had had no effect on levels of depressive mood—the size and significance of the effect increased after eight and twelve months. In fact, by the 12-month follow-up, treatment group membership accounted for 23 percent of the variance in depression, after controlling for baseline levels of depressive symptoms. In sum, not only did this multifaceted program of family and personal counselling plus support group participation reduce placement, but it also mitigated the depressive effect associated with the continuing care of demented relatives. For these reasons, this study marshals rigorous and compelling evidence for the effectiveness of a family-centred counselling and support intervention in reducing rates of nursing home placement and significantly lowering depression.

The study's limitations are that it fails to identify the exact components of the intervention or the intensity that may be responsible for the observed beneficial effects. That is, since many different kinds of assistance were provided to the caregivers, it is impossible to determine which elements of the package should be retained and which can be dropped. This limitation, in turn, conceals the mechanisms that may be at work in reducing caregiver depression. The positive impact could be attributable to the reduction of family conflict over the relative's care, the training the caregivers received in techniques of managing and interacting with their relatives, or improvements in the family's cohesion and participation in the care of the relative. The knowledge yield of this program is also limited by the absence of any information about the costs associated with the provision of the counselling, and how these costs compare to the costs of nursing home placement over the same time period. Perhaps costs could be reduced by substituting peer counsellors for the four professional family counsellors with either master's degrees or Ph.D.s—as long as the peer counsellors had the skill and authority to engage in family counselling and crisis intervention, and to identify and mobilize services.

Like many other demonstration projects, funding for the program was provided through a grant from the National Institute of Mental Health (NIMH) in the United States to the Aging and Dementia Research Centre of New York University's Medical Centre. Subject recruitment for the research program was made easier by the fact that all caregivers of patients with dementia were required, as a routine aspect of their clinical evaluation at the Centre, to complete a comprehensive questionnaire. In addition, the staff of the Centre already had established a rapport with almost half the study participants. Additional respondents were recruited through collaboration with the Alzheimer's Association of New York City and with other local day centres and agencies that serve elderly persons in New York City. Finally, since the study has not been replicated and was limited mostly to white spousal caregivers, its external validity and general relevance have not been established.

More generally, this intervention points to the probable *superiority of multicomponent strategies over stand-alone strategies of assisting family caregivers.* The particular blend of peer support, individualized family counselling, crisis intervention and advocacy, combined with the deployment of a dedicated team of service providers who actively reached out to caregivers by visiting them in their homes, is indeed a commendable but expensive formula for shoring up family care of the elderly.

Programs in Support of Family Caregivers of Persons with Developmental Disabilities and Chronic Illnesses

Family Support Initiatives

In Canada and the United States, relative to the scope and intensity of their needs, the caregivers of persons with pervasive developmental disabilities and chronic illnesses receive little by way of services. That is, when *family* support services are viewed apart from services designed to meet the care needs of the child, one is left with the impression of an impoverished service environment. Moreover, the bulk of those services that are extended to the caregiver or family have typically been arranged and delivered by a parent advocacy or self-help organization, not by the government. For example, such services are provided by the Association of Relatives and Friends of the Mentally Ill, the Autism Society, the Family Support Institute (a network of parents of individuals with disabilities with offices in several Canadian provinces), Friends of Schizophrenics, and many other informal and not-for-profit organizations.

In literature that addresses strategies of shoring up the well-being of family caregivers of persons with pervasive developmental disabilities and chronic illnesses, particular psychosocial interventions are not typically featured as they are in the literature on caregiving to the elderly. Instead, the emphasis is placed on *a broad set of principles or values that ought to guide practice. As well, a comprehensive range of family supportive resources are identified that need to be made accessible to families in a flexible and proactive manner.* A responsive and effective service delivery system is chiefly characterized by the following three hallmarks:

– a focus on the entire family;
– flexibility, coordination, choice, family control and responsiveness in service arrangements; and
– a focus on mobilizing and strengthening informal sources of community support.

An emphasis must be placed on the provision of functional supports to enhance community integration, quality of life and individualization of services. In addition, increased efforts should be made to interweave formal and informal networks of support so as to create a system of *shared care.*

In the United States, pilot or demonstration projects on behalf of families in which one individual has a developmental disability have involved the following components:

1. a financial subsidy in the form of a line of credit that families have as their due with no strings attached, recognizing that the care of a child with a disability far exceeds the cost of raising a child who does not have any disabilities;

2. establishment of a Parent Advisory Council to guide and inform the pilot planning;

3. provision of core services: a range of basic and supplementary services (see below);

4. deployment of a case manager: someone who links families to local human resources, both formal and informal, in a individualized fashion, and who is committed to empowering and supporting the family and engaging members in long-range planning.

A review of state initiatives with respect to services on behalf of families with a member who has a developmental disability identified the following ingredients of a comprehensive system of family support (Knoll et al. 1992):

- Core services:
  - respite and child/adult daycare;
  - recreation;
  - family counselling;
  - support groups;
  - sibling groups;
  - parent training;
  - in-home services: homemaking, attendant care, home health care;
  - environmental adaptations: adaptive equipment, home and vehicle modifications;
  - information and referral;
  - advocacy;
  - transportation.
- Developmental services:
  - behaviour management;
  - speech therapy;
  - occupational therapy;
  - physical therapy;
  - nursing.
- Case management/service coordination.
- Financial assistance:
  - discretionary cash subsidy;
  - allowances;
  - vouchers and tax credits.

This is not to say that all families will make use of all services, but that such services must be available and easily accessible, ideally through a single source.

Based on a set of four case studies of initiatives in the United States designed to focus on the needs of families with a child who had a developmental disability, Ellison et al. (1992) offer the following lessons, which they learned from key informants:

1. Emphasize the importance of listening to the caregivers before designing services.
2. Regularly schedule evaluations of programs to ensure that they stay responsive.
3. Deploy staff who are trained in a family-centred service model.
4. Coordinate, if not unify, services.
5. Ensure that services are flexible and that there is continuity of service providers.
6. Ensure that there are abundant opportunities and settings for the expression of informal support among families.

In addition, programs and public policies directed toward families of children with developmental disabilities and chronic illnesses need to adhere to a set of guiding values that reflect the following points:
- All children, regardless of disability, belong with families and need enduring relationships with adults.
- Family support services must be based on the principle "whatever it takes."
- Family supports should build on existing social networks.
- Family supports should maximize the family's control over the services they receive.
- Family supports should support the entire family.
- Family supports should encourage the community integration of people with disabilities (Taylor et al. 1989).

In sum, to be effective and responsive, programs and policies for the caregivers of persons with developmental disabilities and chronic illnesses must be broadly conceived. A review of the literature suggests that no single intervention program can successfully meet the needs of the principal caregivers in these families.

What follows is an examination of one demonstration program that shows great promise as a means of blending informal and professional support on behalf of the caregivers of children with disabilities. In addition, skills training and respite initiatives are highlighted because of their central role in mitigating the stress experienced by family caregivers of persons with developmental disabilities.

Family Clusters: A Promising Intervention Strategy

A recent Canadian demonstration project offers a novel and promising strategy of mobilizing support from both professional and informal sources on behalf of families with a member who has received a dual diagnosis, consisting of both a developmental disability and a mental health problem. Equally important, the strategy has had a significant impact on the families' service providers and the organizations they represent.

Reasons for and Values Underlying the Initiative

The *Support Clusters* project was based on several premises regarding the wants, needs and goals of families in which there was an individual with a dual diagnosis:
- First, it was based on the recognition that these families were having great difficulty coping with the multiple needs and demands they faced, partly because services were either undeveloped or hard to access, and partly because there was no coordinated response to the family's needs from professionals and informal sources of support.

- Second, there was a strong conviction that, in order to render continuing support to the person with the dual diagnosis, the key supporters needed to gain support themselves. Hence, the support cluster was invented as a mechanism for ensuring that the principal supporters gained the resources they needed.
- Third, the project was grounded in an ecological model of practice designed in recognition of the complex system of social influences in which people are embedded. The practical implication of this model was that intervention needed to take into account the interdependence among all the actors in a network; intervention with one person necessarily has radiating effects on other people with whom that individual is linked.
- Fourth, the project was founded on an ideology of empowerment, which in this instance translated into full participation by families in all aspects of the project, beginning with their choice of people to invite into their cluster meetings and ending with their decisions about how to evaluate the project's impact and whether to maintain their cluster after the demonstration had ended.
- Fifth, the project was committed to breaking down communication barriers between professionals and families, giving them a chance to get to know one another as people and to collaborate on ways of building a mutually satisfying support network.
- Finally, the project was structured in a way that would optimize learning about the intervention itself. This was accomplished by creating three six-month cycles or "rounds" of clusters, with the second and third phases incorporating lessons gained from the previous phase of intervention.

Actors

Prior to the intervention, a group of six concerned citizens in the Kitchener-Waterloo area came together to discuss ways of meeting the many needs of families in which someone had received a dual diagnosis. The group had recently reviewed the results of a needs assessment of such families, undertaken by the District Health Council, and were committed to finding an innovative and family-inclusive strategy of serving those needs. In addition, based on a review of the literature, the group determined not to take an enhanced service system approach because they did not feel that this would result in more durable or robust support for the labelled persons and their families or in meaningful influence and control for the families themselves.

The possibility of receiving funding from the Ontario government's Health Innovation Fund spurred the group to formulate the *Family Clusters* proposal, and once funds were granted, a new steering committee was formed. It began the arduous work of translating the concepts and values (inclusion, empowerment, systems framework, support for the supporters)

into practical intervention manoeuvres, using nominal groups to clarify goals and implementation steps. In fact, the project's final report states that, after the project's first year, most of the steering committee members attributed progress in project design to the process that occurred in the nominal groups. Moreover, they generally agreed that six major factors contributed to the project's forward movement:
- articulating a set of common values and ideology;
- convening the key stakeholders and helping them to communicate;
- drawing in people with commitment, including the project staff;
- drawing in a diverse set of participants, including families and professionals;
- creating a nonjudgmental milieu for the clusters; and
- having faith in the participatory process and in one another's flexibility.

In sum, the goals of the *Support Clusters* project were to increase the quantity and family focus of social support, enhance cluster members' sense of competence and control, and provide a mechanism for more effective service coordination and communication among all the parties significant in the family's life. With minor modifications, the strategy for creating and developing support clusters involved three main steps:

1. staff assistance to families (the person with the dual diagnosis and/or the principal caregiver) in identifying the significant figures of the support network, including both informal sources (kith and kin) and professional helpers;
2. inviting the chosen network members to an initial orientation meeting so that the project's general goals and processes could be explained, and so that the invitees could determine whether they wished to become members of the support cluster; and
3. staff facilitation of support cluster meetings held to identify key support issues and strategies to meet cluster members' support needs.

Evaluation

Evaluation of the project proceeded through the use of numerous types of information (observation of the group process, surveys, telephone and in-person interviews, case studies of clusters, focus groups with service providers) collected from numerous sources (steering committee and cluster members) at several points in time (before, immediately after and six months after a cluster was initiated). This comprehensive and sensitive data collection process yielded numerous insights about the process, including factors that enhanced and hindered cluster development, and about the outcomes for the person with the dual diagnosis label and his family. On the latter score, the 20 (focal) individuals with the dual diagnoses reported that they had developed closer personal relationships with the members of their cluster and resolved conflicts with particular family members. However, the benefits to relationships varied depending on the extent of participation of the focal individual in the cluster. Some cluster members felt that the focal individual's presence in the group derailed them from supporting the supporter because of the need to respond to the focal individual's own support needs.

However, the intervention had a pronounced positive impact on the principal family supporters or caregivers of the person with a dual diagnosis. They reported decreased stress and dissatisfaction with community services, and increased ability to cope with stress—a finding that testifies to the stress-buffering function of social support. Decreased stress was associated not only with the provision of emotional and practical support by cluster members, but also by the perception that the cluster was ready to render support when called upon. In addition, stress reduction was predicated on the caregivers' ability to share decision making and responsibility with others. As one sibling of a person with a dual diagnosis observed: "The cluster members see the needs and come up with their own ideas, but before they didn't want to infringe on your privacy—so this opened a door." Many families reported that they had developed new skills through their involvement in the clusters, such as time management and problem prevention skills, improved ability to communicate confidently with professionals, and greater competence in expressing their needs for, and actually seeking out, support. In addition, in almost every cluster, family members reported that they felt better understood by professionals and more effectively supported by them. The latter impression was validated by interviews with the professionals who were members of the clusters, many of whom reported greater appreciation of the person and familiarity with his family life context.

Analysis of the Results and Replicability

The project's ability to draw in large numbers of potentially critical supporters is indeed impressive. Across the 20 clusters, each of which lasted for at least six months, there were 89 informal supporters and 106 professionals representing 52 different agencies. The model's appeal to professionals is borne out by the fact that several joined more than one cluster. Equally important, the project had an impact at the agency level. Interviews with 11 professionals from four agencies (two social service and two health agencies) revealed that they were more prepared to become involved with people who had dual diagnoses because the cluster was available as a resource, that the needs of this underserved group would receive more attention from the agency, and that the cluster model was a potentially useful strategy of serving people with other types of disabilities. Finally, perhaps the best testimony of the success of the project is the fact that 9 of the 20 clusters continued to meet after their formal six-month termination point.

There are some caveats regarding this program and its evaluation. First, the outcome data are somewhat limited by exclusive reliance on the self-reports of the participants. No standardized and psychometrically sound outcome measures were adopted, and there was virtually no follow-up of the study's impact, especially on the principal caregivers. Second, more concerted efforts need to be made to involve the family's informal network, and to empower them to assert their needs for both formal services and informal support. Third, more systematic attention needs to be devoted to assessing the impact of the intervention on agency practices and norms, as well as on staff training. Finally, the initiative has not yet been replicated elsewhere or in different stressful caregiving contexts.

Funding

Funding was obtained through a grant provided by the Government of Ontario's Health Innovations Fund.

Skill Acquisition through Group Support or Caregiver Training

A strategy of assisting family caregivers of children with disabilities that contrasts highly with the one described above is to equip them with the skills required to manage problem behaviours. Essentially, this approach is didactic in nature, professionally driven, and aimed at improving the caregivers' coping skills rather than broadening their base of support. The following two reports suggest that, although both group and individually focused skill training are relatively effective, they do not lighten the caregivers' burdens, but help them to deal with the burdens more successfully.

An example of psychoeducational group support is described in a report by Schultz et al. (1993) who formed several groups, composed of 12 parents each, that met for two hours per week over a period of six weeks. The parents all had children with intellectual impairment. Topics of discussion included family dynamics, loss and grief, communication and conflict resolution skills, resource utilization, stress management and relaxation skills. The conceptual model on which the group was predicated emphasized the development or refinement of personal coping skills and the mobilization of social support as ways of moderating stress. Consequently, the outcome measures focused largely on the parents' mental health, gauging it with the 28-item version of the General Health Questionnaire. Using a control group that was matched on relevant demographic variables, marital happiness, social support, and the occurrence of life events, outcome data were collected 12 months after the group sessions ended. The results revealed a significant reduction of emotional distress among members of the "treatment" group. Participants reported high levels of satisfaction with virtually all aspects of their group experience, with two exceptions: 30 percent felt that the groups ended too soon, and 20 percent expressed a desire for a stronger focus on the acquisition of new skills, mainly stress management, relaxation tech-niques, and assertiveness training so they could gain more confidence in their interactions with professionals.

An example of a more explicit skill-oriented training program is described by Hawkins and Singer (1989) who instructed parents of moderately
and severely handicapped children in ways of managing stress. The participants attended two-hour classes once a week for 8 weeks, each group being
composed of 8–10 participants and two leaders—a licensed clinical psychologist and a certified special educator. While the parents attended these
group sessions, their children were cared for by the staff of a respite agency.

The sessions focused on stress management skills, explaining why they
should be learned, presenting examples of situations in which they could
be used, practicing them in class, and completing homework assignments
involving their practice in naturally occurring situations. The actual skills
taught included:
- self-monitoring: keeping track of the specific antecedents of stressful
  feelings so that appropriate coping skills can be deployed;
- relaxation: progressive muscle relaxation;
- cognitive modification: monitoring and altering negative or irrational
  self-talk, and replacing it with more positive responses; and
- social support: keeping track of both the frequency and satisfaction of
  interactions with others, and then setting goals and developing strategies
  of gaining more support.

Evaluation of the training revealed that, compared to a group of parents
randomly assigned to a waiting list control group, the participants had
significantly lower scores on the state and trait scales of the State Trait Anxiety
Inventory, and on the Beck Depression Inventory. In addition, interviews
conducted between six months and a year after the last class revealed that all
parents continued to use some of the stress management techniques. Although
the parents reported that their lives were no less stressful, partly because their
children continued to manifest numerous problems, they felt better able to
cope with the stress. Many parents recommended preceding the stress management training with training in behaviour management skills.

Respite and Substitute Care

No other service is demanded as much as respite by families that have onerous
caregiving responsibilities. Several initiatives have been developed to provide
relief and support to family caregivers of persons with developmental
disabilities. One novel Canadian initiative deserves special mention because
of its creativity and longevity.

A program called Associate Family Care, originated by parents and
advocates of children with handicaps in British Columbia, pays families to
take a child with severe or multiple handicaps out of an institution and care
for him on a long-term basis in their own homes. In addition, the program
has made a respite service available to these family associates, provided by
other families that are trained and paid to serve this function. Through a

careful process of screening and selection, associate families are matched with children, approved by the biological parents, and trained (with respect to diet, medication, mobility, lifting, personal care, recreation and education) to care for the child. Wherever possible, the biological parents remain involved in planning for their child's care. Meanwhile, a multidisciplinary team comprehensively assesses the child's needs and, together with the natural and associate parents, develops an individualized plan that sets out the services, care requirements, goals and objectives for the child and family. Moreover, these plans are regularly reviewed once the child is in the community, and the child's care is regularly monitored by a service coordinator. To date, the program has not been subjected to a formal evaluation.

Yet another option for providing respite to these families is to identify other families in the community who are willing to provide short-term care and support on a regular basis. In England, Wales and Northern Ireland, an organization called *Shared Care* was formed in 1989 by social workers from seven regions of the United Kingdom. Essentially, families that are interested in providing respite are recruited, screened and matched to families desiring respite, and the two families are assisted by a social worker to make arrangements that are mutually convenient. Shared Care pays the respite providers for their work, and serves as a national coordinating body that sets standards, provides consistency in policies and practices, holds an annual conference, distributes a newsletter and generally promotes the whole concept of family-based short-term care.

In Ontario, a similar function is filled by the Extend-a-Family organization, although the primary emphasis of its family-matching service is not respite but the integration of children with developmental disabilities into the community through regular episodes of friendly companionship with a volunteer (unpaid) host.

And finally, a national self-help and advocacy organization called the Family Support Institute consists of a network of parents of persons with disabilities who exchange mutual aid and resource information about family support strategies. Through a system of mentor families, called Resource Parents, families that need support or information, especially families that have recently experienced the deinstitutionalization of their child, are linked to other families and to appropriate services (Romance 1988). In addition, the organization conducts member surveys, writes proposals for funding needed services (e.g., for respite care), and issues a newsletter. A recent sampling of the newsletters includes articles on what to tell a teacher about a child with a disability, how to start up a parent group, where to purchase special equipment, and how to build a support network around a child. The Family Support Institute also serves as a collective voice for families, lobbying and presenting briefs to policymakers and attempting to reorient the service delivery system toward a more "family-directed" approach to practice.

Schemes to Provide Payment to Family Caregivers

For a variety of reasons—principally the high cost of institutional care for dependent seniors—provincial governments of Quebec, Nova Scotia and New Brunswick have experimented with different payment-for-care schemes. Before detailing how these schemes operate, important distinctions should be drawn between those that involve direct compensation to family caregivers and those that provide compensation indirectly. Indirect compensation usually takes the form of a tax deduction or credit, whereas direct compensation involves payment to the caregiver for services purchased or provided by the caregiver. Such direct compensation may take the form of a token payment with strict eligibility requirements, as in Nova Scotia, or an hourly wage, as in Scandinavia (Keefe and Fancey 1992).

As of 1978, Quebec provided direct funding to persons with handicaps so that they could purchase the home care and personal services they wanted. Although this scheme puts care receivers "in the driver's seat," granting them greater choice and control over services, there is no provision for quality control of the services purchased because the providers are often untrained lay people who accept lower wages than professionally trained home care providers. Moreover, there is a potential for exploiting women by paying them low wages outside the legal framework that governs employer-employee relations. Thus, the providers were often paid "under the table," with no contributions to unemployment insurance or pension. Nevertheless, from the viewpoint of the service purchasers, the direct funding mechanism was highly satisfactory (Levesque and Prevost 1992).

In Nova Scotia and New Brunswick, where so many people live in rural areas and where the economy is relatively depressed, immediate family members who provide care to dependent elderly relatives receive direct cash compensation for their labour. In Nova Scotia, local municipalities are involved in cost sharing and managing the *Home Life Supports Program*, as well as in determining families' eligibility for the compensation. The latter criteria include income and level of care needed. Evaluation of the scheme showed that the amount of compensation was quite low, averaging $356.42 a month, and paying for services and equipment needed rather than compensating family caregivers for their time. Moreover, some proportion of the caregivers were women who had left or foregone paid employment at a much higher rate of compensation. In addition, the evaluation found that levels of stress and burnout were actually higher among the caregivers who received compensation, compared to those who were employed outside the home and used public home support services (Keefe 1994).

In New Brunswick there are two different financial compensation schemes, one that provides up to $400 per month to family members or care recipients with proven financial need and need for assistance with activities of daily living, and one that provides up to $1,100 per month to the care recipient for the purchase of services that the client and a social worker determine are needed. According to this scheme, known as the *Single Entry Pilot Project*, family members are ineligible for cash compensation. Neither program has been subject to formal evaluation.

According to Stryckman and Nahmiash (1994), these payment-for-care schemes reduce the cost of caring for the elderly because the care recipient can hire almost anyone he chooses, eliminating the costs of case management, administration and expensive and often unionized para-professional workers. The schemes also give the care recipient greater control over the choice of services, while theoretically making the providers more directly accountable to the care recipient. In addition, payment-for-care schemes promise relief (in principle), from the perspective of those who have complained that women's domestic work is devalued, and that caregiving necessitates large out-of-pocket and hidden opportunity costs (Fast et al. 1995). However, evaluation of the Nova Scotia scheme suggests that the compensation received by caregivers simply reconfirms women's historic status as underpaid and exploited domestic labourers, especially considering the number of hours that they devote to their caregiving responsibilities. Under these schemes, they have no job security and no retirement plan or other fringe benefits. Moreover, from the perspective of the care recipients, although direct payment gives them a greater say in the amount and types of services they can purchase, there are few quality controls on the service providers because many of them operate outside the formal service delivery network.

Payment-for-care schemes also carry the spectre of supplanting the natural support system, and even inducing families that would otherwise be disinclined to care for their aged relatives to apply for payment and then to render inferior or custodial care to them. Government policymakers also worry about the runaway costs that might result from wide-scale implementation of payment-for-care schemes, and therefore would insist on including some strategy of means testing in any legislation. As for indirect compensation, critics argue that those with low incomes would reap virtually no benefit from an additional tax deduction, and that a system of tax credits for the purchase of services would defer reimbursement so long as to preclude their purchase.

In short, family caregivers must be adequately compensated. They must be compensated for the purchase of services and equipment at a rate that offsets their cost. They must also be paid for their time at a rate that fully reflects the value of their domestic labour as well as the opportunity costs foregone on the open market. Until this happens, payment-for-care schemes will meet with criticism from the majority of potential users and will be rejected by the remaining minority. From the perspectives of policymakers and professionals in the long-term care field, these schemes also create serious problems in maintaining service quality and integrity, erode professional and union standards and control of services, and threaten, if enlarged, to become a burden on the public coffer (Keefe and Fancey 1992).

POLICY IMPLICATIONS

Throughout this paper, numerous suggestions have been offered regarding ways of strengthening, augmenting, or specializing the psychosocial and community resources of family caregivers. Of the initiatives reviewed, few have proved effective in moderating caregiver stress and reducing burden, or in augmenting or maintaining well-being. For example, despite their popularity and widespread implementation by community agencies, support groups have not had any measurable impact on the mental health or morale of the caregivers of persons with dementia. Nor have respite programs been proven effective on empirical grounds. Only multifaceted and individualized family-focused interventions have shown evidence of ameliorative effects, although the example discussed in this paper has not been replicated or subjected to a cost-benefit analysis. It appears that this multifaceted program is very expensive, and in the absence of data revealing which components of the program are necessary in order for it to be effective and which can be dropped, there is as yet no way of streamlining the program to make it more cost efficient. One possible avenue to cost reduction is to attempt to train lay counsellors to provide support to families in lieu of the highly paid professionals that were used by Mittelman et al. (1995), and then evaluate program outcomes and costs.

Recognizing the cross pressures faced by caregivers in their efforts to balance paid employment with the unpaid work of caregiving, many employers have initiated "family-friendly" programs aimed at harmonizing these two spheres, and improving morale and productivity. However, these are entirely voluntary efforts, and are largely restricted to workplaces that include sizeable numbers of women who occupy clerical and white-collar positions.

At both the *federal and provincial levels*, new legislation could be introduced that would go a great distance toward alleviating the pressures on family caregivers who are employed, and fully recognizing their value to society. Specifically, as proposed by Nora Spinks (1996), the president of Canadian Work and Family Services, the following legislative initiatives should be considered:

- At the federal level, the provision for maternity leave under Canada's Unemployment Insurance Program should be expanded to become a "family care leave." Any employees who have the responsibility of caring for family members who are seriously ill, dying, adopting, experiencing major flare-ups of chronic health conditions, and/or recovering from hospitalization would be entitled to the same leave provisions as those taking maternity and parental leaves. The government should convene panels of experts and family caregivers in diverse contexts to identify the types of family care responsibilities that would make someone eligible for family care leave, and the (medical or compassionate) documentation that is needed to obtain such leave. The leave itself should offer all the financial provisions and job protections that are currently available to those taking maternity leave. Family care leave should be equally available to men and women and to full-time and part-time employees.

- At the provincial level, legislation should be prepared to alter employment standards to permit individuals to obtain an unlimited period of unpaid leave in order to provide care to a family member in need. Such leave should be granted with careful documentation of the circumstances requiring family care and with specific job guarantees upon return to the workplace. Such legislation has already been passed in the United States, but as yet there has been no rigorous evaluation of its impact on employers and employees. The lessons learned from implementation in the United States should be considered when introducing legislation in Canada.

- At present only Saskatchewan has introduced legislation requiring employers to provide full benefits to permanent part-time employees. Elsewhere in Canada, the practice that is most prevalent (although not universal) is to pay only statutory benefits, and deny permanent part-time employees the supplemental benefits received by their full-time counterparts. In consideration of the fact that women far outnumber men in the ranks of part-time employees—opting for part-time employment precisely because of their family care responsibilities—it is these supplemental health benefits that most part-time employees say would be most valuable.

- By virtue of an amendment to employment standards in Quebec and British Columbia (the latter effective as of November 1, 1995) a Family Responsibility Leave was created that provides for up to five days of paid leave per employment year for employees who must meet responsibilities for:
  - the care, health, or education of a child who is in the employee's care;
  - the care or health of any other member of the employee's immediate family (spouse, parent, guardian, grandparent, sibling, grandchild) or anyone who lives with the employee as a member of his family.

Townson (1988) defines family responsibility leave as:

The right to take a certain number of days off each year for such family-related responsibilities as…accompanying a child or an elderly or disabled family member to a medical appointment, making alternative care arrangements for family members when their regular caregivers are sick, attending a child's school or daycare centre to meet with teachers or caregivers, and similar family needs (24).

Such legislation should be adopted in every province. It effectively creates a more equitable situation for caregivers by reducing or removing managerial discretion in responding to employee requests for periods of a day's leave to handle family responsibilities. It also means that employees do not have to deceive their managers about the reasons for their absence, nor do they have to draw on their allotment of sick or vacation days to attend to these family demands.

- Federal tax legislation ought to be introduced allowing employers to make contributions (e.g., daycare subsidies) toward the care of employees' dependent family members, without such contributions being treated as a taxable benefit. In the United States, as part of a flexible benefit plan, many employers create a dependent care spending account for their employees, with the monies being exempted from employee income.

- New legislation should be introduced that provides tax relief and possible subsidies to caregivers (most of whom are women) in recognition of their home labour and the opportunity costs they incur. This legislation should be introduced after careful review of the financial and personal impacts of existing payment-for-care schemes in Canada and abroad.

Steps should be taken to encourage *workplaces, especially small businesses,* to offer greater flexibility to employees and to cooperate and share the costs of implementing information and referral programs for employees with dependent care responsibilities. In addition, the following initiatives should be considered by employers in both the public and private sectors:

- Employers should develop a better understanding of the links among work-family issues and the broader themes of equity, diversity and productivity.

- Employers should examine opportunities for developing new public/private partnerships with local human services that specialize in dependent care.

- Employers need to sensitize senior managers to work-family issues and encourage senior managers to partake in flexible work arrangements themselves in order to set an example.

- Sensitivity to and greater flexibility in addressing work-family issues should be factors which are incorporated in the performance evaluations of managers.

- Employers should ensure that, in evaluating the performance of the EAP providers with whom they contract, adequate provision is made for follow-through services for family caregivers.

For *program planners and policymakers in the long-term and continuing care fields,* the following considerations should be taken into account:

- Respite programs must be easily accessible and more responsive to the needs of employed caregivers. Especially for the caregivers of persons with dementia, respite services must be marketed earlier and their use should be actively encouraged by family physicians. Greater flexibility in program hours is needed, along with the provision of educational and skill-training services for caregivers—especially those who must cope with behavioral difficulties associated with their dependent's disease or disability. A range of respite services, including day programs, domiciliary services and short-term institutionally based vacation care should be made available to fit varying circumstances and preferences of caregivers. Transportation should be provided by the program.

- Support groups alone have yet to prove their value. In the future, these groups should be held for a longer period of time, ideally becoming self-sustaining mutual aid groups after the professional leadership withdraws. In addition, support groups should offer caregivers behavioral skill training. The focus of each group should be guided by the specific needs that the participants bring to the group rather than by a preestablished curriculum imported by the professional.

- Generally, multicomponent, family-centred strategies have proved superior as a means of responding to the needs of caregivers and their families, especially when all components of the program are accessible through, and unified by a single consistent gatekeeper who is available in crises and advocates on the family's behalf. Such programs ought to be more broadly implemented.

- The training of staff who serve families with a disabled or dependent should underscore the importance of adopting a family-centred service model. In addition, staff should be guided by a broad set of principles or values that emphasize flexibility, coordination, choice, family control, and responsiveness in service arrangements;

- More concerted efforts need to be made to coordinate, if not unify, services through a single point of access; services must be flexible and changes of service providers should be avoided, for continuity.

- A program of small grants should be provided to grassroots consumer and advocacy organizations so that they can extend their reach to other families and involve them in mutual aid activities.

- Incentives should be provided to develop registries of substitute caregiving families, modelled on the Shared Care organization in the United Kingdom and the Associate Family Care program in British Columbia.

- The *Support Clusters* strategy of serving families by enlarging and integrating their fund of professional and informal supporters ought to be further disseminated and evaluated. It should be applied to contexts other than families with a member who has received a dual diagnosis. For example, it should be tested among families caring for elderly relatives and families caring for children with chronic illnesses and developmental disabilities.

Benjamin H. Gottlieb *is a professor in the Department of Psychology at the University of Guelph. He obtained a joint Ph.D. in psychology and social work from the University of Michigan, and is a fellow of both of the American and Canadian Psychological Associations. Dr. Gottlieb has authored and edited several volumes on the subject of coping and social support, of which the most recent is* Coping with Chronic Stress *(1997).*

BIBLIOGRAPHY

ANGUS REID GROUP. 1994. *The State of the Family in Canada*. Ottawa (ON): Vanier Institute of the Family (120, Holland Ave., Suite 300, Ottawa, K1Y 0X6).

AVISON, W., J. TURNER, S. NOH, and K. SPEECHLEY. 1993. The impact of caregiving: Comparisons of different family contexts and experiences. In *Caregiving Systems: Informal and Formal Helpers*, eds. S. ZARIT, L. PEARLIN, and K. W. SCHAIE. Hillsdale (NJ): Erlbaum.

BAINES, C., P. EVANS, and S. NEYSMITH. Eds. 1991. *Women's Caring: Feminist Perspectives on Social Welfare*. Toronto (ON): McClelland and Stewart Inc.

BARHAM, E., B. GOTTLIEB, K. KELLOWAY, and M. GIGNAC. 1995. *An Evaluation of the CIBC's "Work and Lifestyles" Initiative*. Guelph (ON): University of Guelph, Gerontology Research Centre.

BOURGEOIS, M., R. SCHULZ, and L. BURGIO. 1996. Interventions for caregivers of patients with Alzheimer's Disease: A review and analysis of content, process, and outcomes. *International Journal of Aging and Human Development* 43: 35–92.

BRODY, E., M. H. KLEBAN, P. T. JOHNSEN, C. HOFFMAN, and C. B. SCHOONOVER. 1987. Work status and parent care: A comparison of four groups of women. *The Gerontologist* 27: 201–208.

CARNET: THE CANADIAN AGING RESEARCH NETWORK. 1994. *Work and Family: Survey Findings*. Guelph (ON): University of Guelph, Gerontology Research Centre.

CENTRE FOR RESEARCH AND EDUCATION IN HUMAN SERVICES. 1993. *Support Clusters Project: Evaluation Report of a Research Demonstration Project*. Waterloo (ON): Centre for Research and Education in Human Services.

COMMITTEE ON AGING, GROUP FOR THE ADVANCEMENT OF PSYCHIATRY. 1994. Impact of Tacrine in the care of patients with Alzheimer's Disease. *American Journal of Geriatric Psychiatry* 2: 285–289.

DUNST, C., C. TRIVETTE, A. STARNES, D. HAMBY, and N. GORDON. 1993. *Building and Evaluating Family Support Initiatives*. Baltimore (MD): Paul H. Brookes.

ELLISON, M., H. BERSANI, JR., B. BLANEY, and E. FREUD. 1992. Family empowerment: Four case studies. In *Emerging Issues in Family Support*, eds. V. J. BRADLEY, J. KNOLL, and J. M. AGOSTA. Washington (DC): American Association on Mental Retardation.

EVERS, M. PIJL, and C. UNGERSON. Eds. 1994. *Payments for Care: A Comparative Overview*. Vienna, Austria: Avebury Publishers.

FAMILIES AND WORK INSTITUTE. 1993. *An Evaluation of Johnson and Johnson's Work-Family Initiative*. New York (NY): Families and Work Institute.

FAST, J., D. WILLIAMSOM, N. KEATING, and L. OAKES. 1995. The hidden costs of eldercare: Development of a taxonomy. Poster presented at the annual meeting of the Canadian Association on Gerontology, Vancouver (BC).

FERRIS, S. H., G. STEINBERG, E. SHULMAN, R. KAHN, and B. REISBERG. 1987. Institutionalization of Alzheimer disease patients: Reducing precipitating factors through family counseling. *Home Health Care Services Quarterly* 8: 23–51.

GALINSKY, E., J. BOND, D. FRIEDMAN. 1993. *The National Study of the Changing Workforce*. New York (NY): Families and Work Institute.

GIBEAU, J. L., J. L. ANASTAS, and P. J. LARSON. 1987. Breadwinners, caregivers and employers: New alliances in an aging America. *Employee Benefits Journal* 12: 6–10.

GOODMAN, C., and J. PYNOOS. 1990. A model telephone information and support program for caregivers of Alzheimer's patients. *The Gerontologist* 30: 399–404.

GOTTLIEB, B.H. 1989. *Social Support Strategies: Guidelines for Mental Health Practice*. Newbury Park (CA): Sage.

GOTTLIEB, B.H ., and J. JOHNSON. 1995. Impact of day programs on family caregivers of persons with dementia. Guelph: University of Guelph, Psychology Department (in-house technical report).

GOTTLIEB, B. H., and F. WAGNER. 1991. Stress and support processes in close relationships. In *The Social Context of Coping*, ed. J. ECKENRODE. New York (NY): Plenum.

GOTTLIEB, B. H., E. K. KELLOWAY, and M. FRABONI. 1994. Aspects of eldercare that place employees at risk. *The Gerontologist* 34: 815–821.

HAWKINS, N. E., and G. H. SINGER. 1989. A skills training approach for assisting parents to cope with stress. In *Support for Caregiving Families*, eds. G. SINGER, and L. IRVIN. Baltimore (MD): Paul H. Brookes.

HEBERT, R., G. LECLERC, G. BRAVO, D. GIROURD, and R. LEFRANCOIS. 1994. Efficacy of a support group programme for caregivers of demented patients in the community: A randomized controlled trial. *Archives of Gerontology and Geriatrics* 18: 1–4.

HEBERT, R., D. GIROURD, G. LECLERC, D. BRAVO, and R. LEFRANCOIS. 1995. The impact of a support group programme for care-givers on the institutionalisation of demented patients. *Archives of Gerontology and Geriatrics* 20: 129–134.

KEEFE, J. 1994. *Shared Care: The Organization of Home Care and Family Caregiving*. Halifax (NS): Mount St. Vincent University Centre on Aging.

KEEFE, J., and P. FANCEY. 1992. Financial compensation or home help services: Examining differences among program recipients. Paper presented at the annual meeting of the Canadian Association on Gerontology, Edmonton (AB).

KIECOLT-GLASER, J., R. GLASER, C. DYER, E. SHUTTLEWORTH, P. OGROCKI, and C. SPEICHER. 1987. Chronic stress and immune function in family caregivers of Alzheimer disease victims. *Psychosomatic Medicine* 49: 523–535.

KNOLL, J. 1992. Being a family: The experience of raising a child with a disability or chronic condition. In *Emerging Issues in Family Support*, eds. V. J. BRADLEY, J. KNOLL, and J. M. AGOSTA. Washington (DC): American Association on Mental Retardation.

KNOLL, J., S. COVERT, R. OSUCH, S. O'CONNOR, J. AGOSTA, and B. BLANEY. 1992. Supporting families: State family support efforts. In *Emerging Issues in Family Support*, eds. V. J. BRADLEY, J. KNOLL, and J. M. AGOSTA. Washington (DC): American Association on Mental Retardation.

LAVOIE, J-P. 1995. A critical review of the impact of support groups for family caregivers. *Canadian Journal on Aging* 13: 23–41.

LAWTON, M. P., E. BRODY, and A. R. SAPERSTEIN. 1989. A controlled study of respite service for caregivers of Alzheimer's patients. *The Gerontologist* 29: 8–16.

LAZARUS, R. S., and S. FOLKMAN. 1984. *Stress, appraisal and coping*. New York (NY): Springer.

LEVESQUE, P. and C. PREVOST. 1992. *Rapport final sur le projet pilote "L'autonomie c'est la vie"*. Montreal (QC): NIC.

MARSHALL, K. 1990. Household chores. *Canadian Social Trends* 16: 18–19.

MITTELMAN, M. S., S. H. FERRIS, G. STEINBERG, E. SHULMAN, J. MACKELL, A. AMBINDER, and J. COHEN. 1993. An intervention that delays institutionalization of Alzheimer's Disease patients: Treatment of spouse-caregivers. *The Gerontologist* 33: 730–740.

MITTELMAN, M. S., S. H. FERRIS, E. SHULMAN, G. STEINBERG, A. AMBINDER, J. MACKELL, and J. COHEN. 1995. A comprehensive support program: Effect on depression on spouse-caregivers of AD patients. *The Gerontologist* 35: 792–802.

MOHIDE, A., D. PRINGLE, D. STREINER, J. JILBERT, G. MUIR, and M. TEW. 1990. A randomized trial of family caregiver support in the home management of dementia. *JAGS* 38: 446–454.

MONTGOMERY, R., and E. BORGATTA. 1989. The effects of alternative support strategies on family caregiving. *The Gerontologist* 29: 457–464.

MUURINEN, J. M. 1986. The economics of informal care: Labour market effects in the National Hospice Study. *Medical Care* 24: 1007.

NEAL, M. B., N. J. CHAPMAN, B. INGERSOLL-DAYTON, and A. C. EMLEN. 1993. *Balancing Work and Caregiving for Children, Adults and Elders*. Newbury Park (CA): Sage Publications.

ROMANCE, E. 1988. Families supporting families. *Entourage* 3: 26–31.

SCHARLACH, A. E., and S. L. BOYD. 1989. Caregiving and employment: Results of an employee survey. *The Gerontologist* 29: 382–387.

SCHARLACH, A. E., B. F. LOWE, and E. L. SCHNEIDER. 1991. *Eldercare and the Workforce: Blueprint for Action.* Toronto (ON): Lexington Books.

SCHULZ, R., P. VISINTAINER, and G. WILLIAMSON. 1990. Psychiatric and physical morbidity effects of caregiving. *Journal of Gerontology: Psychological Sciences* 45: 181–191.

SCHULZ, R., A. T. O'BRIEN, J. BOOKWALA, and K. FLEISSNER. 1995. Psychiatric and physical morbidity effects of dementia caregiving: Prevalence, correlates, and causes. *The Gerontologist* 35: 771–791.

SCHULTZ, C., N. SCHULTZ, E. BRUCE, K. SMYRNOS, L. CAREY, and C. CAREY. 1993. Psychoeducational support for parents of children with intellectual disability: An outcome study. *International Journal of Disability, Development and Education* 40: 205–216.

SELTZER, M., J. IRVY, and L. LITCHFIELD. 1987. Family members as case managers: Partnerships between the professional and informal support networks. *The Gerontologist* 27: 722–728.

SILVER, E. J., L. J. BAUMAN, and H. T. IREYS. 1995. Relationships of self-esteem and efficacy to psychological distress in mothers of children with chronic physical illnesses. *Health Psychology* 14: 333–340.

SPINKS, N. 1996. Personal communication.

STATISTICS CANADA. 1992a. *Health and Activities Limitation Survey.* Ottawa (ON): Statistics Canada.
_____. 1992b. Persons with disabilities in Canada. *The Daily,* October 13. Ottawa (ON).

STEPHENS, S. A., and J. B. CHRISTIANSON. 1986. *Informal Care of the Elderly.* Lexington (MA): Lexington Books.

STONE, R. I., and P. F. SHORT. 1990. The competing demands of employment and informal caregiving to disabled elders. *Medical Care* 28: 513–526.

STONE, R., G. L. CAFFERATA, and J. SANGL. 1987. Caregivers of the frail elderly: A national profile. *The Gerontologist* 27: 616–626.

STONE, R. I., and P. F. SHORT. 1990. The competing demands of employment and informal caregiving to disabled elders. *Medical Care* 28: 513–526.

STRYCKMAN, J., and D. NAHMIASH. 1994. Payments for care: The case of Canada. In *Payments for Care: A Comparative Overview,* eds. A. EVERS, M. PIJL, and C. UNGERSON. Vienna, Austria: Avebury Publishers.

TAYLOR, S., J. KNOLL, S. LEHR, and P. WALKER. 1989. Families for all children: Value-based services for children with disabilities and their families. In *Support for Caregiving Families,* eds. G. SINGER, and L. IRVIN. Baltimore (MD): Paul H. Brookes.

THE VANIER INSTITUTE OF THE FAMILY. 1994. *Profiling Canada's Families.* Ottawa (ON): Vanier Institute of the Family.

TOSELAND, R. W., and C. M. ROSSITER. 1989. Group interventions to support family caregivers: A review and analysis. *The Gerontologist* 29: 438–448.

TOWNSON, M. 1988. *Leave for Employees with Family Responsibilities.* Ottawa (ON): Women's Bureau, Labour Canada.

WATSON WYATT MEMORANDUM. 1995. *1995 Canadian Work and Family Survey Report.* Vancouver (BC): Watson Wyatt Worldwide.

WHEATON, B. 1983. Stress, personal coping resources, and psychiatric symptoms: An investigation of interactive models. *Journal of Health and Social Behavior* 24: 208–229.

Improving Dying in Canada

PETER A. SINGER, M.D., MPH, FRCPC
DOUGLAS K. MARTIN, PH.D.

University of Toronto Joint Centre for Bioethics

SUMMARY

Because everyone dies, the issues around death and dying are relevant to every Canadian. The public stereotype of dying is a patient hooked up to a machine, in pain, and out of control. In this discussion paper, we explore the goals of social policy with respect to death and dying; describe three specific strategies for care at the end of life; examine in detail success stories related to palliative care and advance care planning; and propose a comprehensive strategy for improving dying in Canada.

Three separate strategies have been developed to address the issue of death and dying: palliative care, advance care planning, and euthanasia/assisted suicide. Palliative care *"as a philosophy of care is the combination of active and compassionate therapies intended to comfort and support individuals and families who are living with life-threatening illness" (Ferris 1995).* Advance care planning, *which may contain written advance directives, is a "process of communication among patients, their health care providers, their families, and important others regarding the kind of care that will be considered appropriate when the patient cannot make decisions" (Teno, Nelson, and Lynn 1994).* Euthanasia *is "a deliberate act undertaken by one person with the intention of ending the life of another person to relieve that person's suffering where that act is the cause of death," and* assisted suicide *is "the act of intentionally killing oneself with the assistance of another who provides the knowledge, means, or both" (Senate of Canada 1995). Since palliative care and advance care planning are legal in Canada, while euthanasia and assisted suicide are not, the former two are examined in detail in this report.*

We examine success stories related to palliative care and advance care planning to illustrate how they could be put to better use in Canada. These examples include the Centre to Improve Care of the Dying at George Washington University Medical Centre; the Department of Bioethics and Pastoral Care, VITAS Healthcare Corporation; the palliative care module of the Comprehensive Guide for the Care of Persons with HIV Disease *developed by Mount Sinai Hospital and Casey House Hospice as part of the National AIDS Strategy of Health Canada; the Ontario Substitute Decisions Project; and the Advance Care Planning Research Program of the University of Toronto Joint Centre for Bioethics.*

Evidence from the literature and these examples demonstrates that there are no clearly articulated goals of social policy in Canada with respect to death and dying. Clarification of these goals is urgently needed. Paradoxically, the determinants of health framework (i.e., physical, psychological, social, cultural, economic) provides a useful conceptual tool to help clarify the goals of social policy in Canada with regard to death and dying. Once the social policy goals are clear, it can be determined whether available approaches (palliative care, advance care planning, and the possibility of legalized euthanasia/assisted suicide) are sufficient, and what proportion of resources should be devoted to each. It will then be important to articulate the appropriate role of government in addressing the various goals of social policy. Both government and private individuals and groups have important and complementary roles to play in the development of social policy approaches to the issue of death and dying in Canada. Government has the ability to enact legislation, to fund needed development and evaluation projects, and to disseminate information to the public. By contrast, private individuals and groups have expertise in the development and evaluation of tools and programs. With regard to private individuals and groups, there is a need to involve both front-line health workers/ consumers and academic researchers. Interdisciplinary or even transdisciplinary research is particularly needed into the complex phenomenon of death and dying and policy responses to it.

A federal/provincial strategy to improve the dying of Canadians is needed. This report makes three recommendations:

1. *Set social policy goals with respect to death and dying.*
2. *Develop a coherent research strategy to evaluate ways of achieving these goals.*
3. *Develop a coherent education strategy to disseminate the results of the research.*

The approach suggested in this report provides a way for government in collaboration with private individuals and groups to respond to the public's concerns and fears, and to improve dying in Canada.

TABLE OF CONTENTS

FIGURE

LIST OF TABLES

KEY CONCLUSIONS FROM THE LITERATURE

Death and Dying

What should be the goal of social policy in Canada with regard to death and dying? This question is where any reasoned discussion on issues related to death and dying must start. Palliative care, advance care planning, and euthanasia/assisted suicide are all potential policy responses. But what goals are they intended to achieve? How do they address the fundamental policy question: How do we want to die? Examinations of death and dying are ancient and modern, complex and simplified, and span a wide variety of sources. This section will merely provide snippets of this literature to illustrate some of its richness and texture.

A familiar biblical passage comes from Solomon's book, *Ecclesiastes:* "For everything there is a season, and a time for every matter under heaven: a time to be born and a time to die; a time to plant, and a time to pluck what is planted, ..." (Eccles. 3:1,2). This statement implies the need to accept death as part of the natural order. However, some people are not at all prepared to accept death. For many, death is the enemy. The concept of fighting death is perhaps most artfully expressed in Dylan Thomas' poem, *Do Not Go Gentle unto That Good Night:*

> Do not go gentle unto that good night,
> Old age should burn and rave at close of day;
> Rage, rage against the dying of the light.

Ramsey has provided a more complex interpretation of this conflict:

> So the grandeur and misery of man are fused together in the human reality and experience of death. To deny the indignity of death requires that the dignity of man be refused also. The more acceptable in itself death is, the less worth or uniqueness ascribed to the dying life (Ramsey 1974).

The psychosocial aspects of dying are captured in Tolstoy's *The Death of Ivan Ilych.* Any serious student of social policy related to death and dying is well advised to read this story. For instance, the following passage illustrates both the physical weakness and the psychosocial loneliness of the dying:

> Ivan Ilych was still sitting in the same position in the armchair.
> "Gerasim," he said when the latter had replaced the freshly-washed utensil. "Please come here and help me." Gerasim went up to him. "Lift me up. It is hard for me to get up, and I have sent Dimitri away."
> Gerasim went up to him, grasped his master with his strong arms deftly but gently, in the same way that he stepped—lifted him, supported him with one hand, and with the other drew up his trousers and would have

set him down again, but Ivan Ilych asked to be led to the sofa. Gerasim, without an effort and without apparent pressure, led him, almost lifting him, to the sofa and placed him on it.

"Thank you. How easily and well you do it all!"

Gerasim smiled again and turned to leave the room. But Ivan Ilych felt his presence such a comfort that he did not want to let him go.

Further insight regarding the needs of the dying are provided by the following passage:

> ...what most tormented Ivan Ilych was that no one pitied him as he wished to be pitied. At certain moments after prolonged suffering he wished most of all (though he would have been ashamed to confess it) for someone to pity him as a sick child is pitied. He longed to be petted and comforted. He knew he was an important functionary, that he had a beard turning grey, and that therefore what he longed for was impossible, but still he longed for it.

Perhaps the best-known psychological theory of death and dying is that of Elisabeth Kübler-Ross, enunciated in her book, *On Death and Dying* (Kübler-Ross 1969). Kübler-Ross described five stages of the dying process: 1) denial and isolation, 2) anger, 3) bargaining, 4) depression and 5) acceptance. She describes a patient in the final stage, acceptance, as follows:

> ...(H)e will reach a stage during which he is neither depressed nor angry about his "fate." He will have been able to express his previous feelings, his envy for the living and the healthy, his anger at those who do not have to face their end so soon. He will have mourned the impending loss of so many meaningful people and places and he will contemplate his coming end with a certain degree of quiet expectation. He will be tired and, in most cases, quite weak. He will also have a need to doze off, to sleep often and in brief intervals... Acceptance should not be mistaken for a happy stage. It is almost void of feelings. It is as if the pain had gone, the struggle is over, and there comes a time for "the final rest before the long journey" as one patient phrased it (112–113).

Daniel Callahan, in his controversial book *Setting Limits*, defines a tolerable death as the individual event of death at that stage in a life span when a) one's life possibilities have on the whole been accomplished; b) one's moral obligations to those for whom one has had responsibility have been discharged; and c) one's death will not seem to others an offense to sense or sensibility or tempt others to despair and rage at the finitude of human existence (Callahan 1987).

These few excerpts from a vast literature may leave us wondering how so subtle a phenomenon can be addressed by the relatively blunt tool of democratic social policy. We might be tempted to ignore death and leave dealing with death in the private sphere. However, as sociologist Peter Berger points out, death is the essential feature of life. We must develop means of coping with death because to neglect it is to neglect one of the few universals around which life is constructed (Berger 1967).

Since death is a universal, a constant upon which we build our society, our social policy should not ignore issues in death and dying. But do we have enough information on how to deal with the experience of dying in our society?

In February 1996, the Council on Scientific Affairs of the American Medical Association published a report on "Good Care of the Dying Patient" prepared by Joanne Lynn and Joan Teno of the Centre to Improve Care of the Dying at the George Washington University Medical Centre (Council on Scientific Affairs 1996).[1] The primary conclusion of this report was that "the information base for good care of the dying patient is inadequate at this time to support effective policy decisions." Because the report provides a fine summary of many important issues with regard to death and dying, we will repeat some of the report's conclusions here:

- Most people probably die in hospital, but the actual rates are unclear.
- The illnesses that shape dying now are mostly cancer, heart and vascular disease, other degenerative organ failures and central nervous system dysfunction.
- The majority of cancer patients experience pain, but the rates of pain in persons who are dying of diseases other than cancer is not well described.
- There is a low rate of serious pain in systems of care that emphasize pain management.
- Other symptoms during the dying process include shortness of breath, depression, loss of cognitive function, fatigue, hiccoughs, mouth sores, skin breakdown, constipation, urinary retention, nausea and itching.
- Many dying persons will contemplate suicide.
- The present ability to design systems of care for dying persons based on scientific research is limited.
- Even though the contemporary model for optimal decision making requires that decisions reflect patient preferences and values, the role of patient preferences regarding death has been studied very little (see description of SUPPORT study in the section on advance care planning).

How are we then to "cope" with dying? What should be the goal of social policy in Canada with regard to death and dying? Palliative care, advance care planning and euthanasia/assisted suicide are responses to these questions. But are they appropriate or effective responses? Do they provide us with good social policy on issues of death and dying? In the next sections we will examine each of these three policy responses individually.

---

1. See "Success Stories."

Palliative Care[2]

Definition of Palliative Care

Palliative care as a philosophy of care is the combination of active and compassionate therapies intended to comfort and support individuals and families who are living with life-threatening illness. During periods of illness and bereavement, palliative care strives to meet physical, psychological, social and spiritual expectations and needs, while remaining sensitive to personal, cultural and religious values, beliefs and practices. Palliative care may be combined with therapies aimed at reducing or curing the illness, or it may be the total focus of care.

Palliative care is planned and delivered through the collaborative efforts of an interdisciplinary team including the individual, family, and caregivers. It should be available to the individual and his family at any time during the illness trajectory and bereavement.

While many caregivers may be able to deliver some of the therapies that provide comfort and support, the services of a specialized palliative care program may be required as the degrees of distress, discomfort and dysfunction increases.

Integral to effective palliative care is the provision of opportunity and support for caregivers to work through their own emotions and grief related to the care they are providing.

Philosophy of Palliative Care

The features of the palliative care philosophy include:
- When living with a life-threatening illness, and especially when dying, every individual has the right to participate in informed discussion about health care resource options, and to choose the best possible option to maximize the quality of his life.
- Palliative care strives to meet the physical, psychological, social and spiritual needs of individuals and families, with sensitivity to personal, cultural and religious values, beliefs and practices. It includes supportive interventions at the direction of the individual, whether or not the individual is receiving antidisease therapy.
- Care should be delivered in a person-focused, family-centred environment.
- The patient has a right to information and services from an interdisciplinary team of appropriately trained professionals and volunteers, who receive continuing palliative care education and evaluation.

---

2. The initial parts of this section are adapted, with permission, from Ferris et al. (1995).

Principles of Palliative Care

The principles of palliative care include:

- *Holistic care* is provided to meet the physical, psychological, social and spiritual expectations and needs of the person and his family with sensitivity to personal, cultural and religious values, beliefs and practices.
- The *unit of care* consists of the individual and his family.
- *Information is a right.* It is the individual's right to be informed about his disease, potential treatments and outcomes, appropriate resources and options. The family and caregiver(s) also have a right to this information, while respecting the individual's right to confidentiality.
- *Choice is a right.* Decisions are made by the individual and family in collaboration with caregivers, while respecting the level of participation desired by the individual and family. The individual's and family's choices for care, settings of care and information sharing are respected within the limits of available resources.
- *Access to care and information.* Individuals and families have timely access to information and palliative care services whenever they need and are prepared to accept them. Information and care is provided in a language they can understand. Essential palliative care services are available 24 hours a day, 7 days a week.
- *Equal availability of services without discrimination.* Services are equally available to all regardless of age, gender, national and ethnic origin, geographical location, race, colour, language, creed, religion, sexual orientation, diagnosis, disability, availability of a primary caregiver, ability to pay, criminal conviction, or family status.
- *Ethics and confidentiality.* Care is provided in accordance with principles of ethics, including confidentiality.
- *Interdisciplinary team.* Care is provided by an interdisciplinary team of caregivers working collaboratively with the individual and family
- *Continuity of care.* A coordinated, continuous plan of care incorporating minimal duplication is maintained across all settings of care, from admission of the individual to bereavement support for the family

Evolution of the Palliative Care Concept

Palliative care evolved from the management of persons living with cancer. It developed from the ideology that cancer could be beaten: that treatment usually starts with a period of active and aggressive therapy, followed by a cure or period of remission, and ultimately by a transition to palliative care. In many ways, this original perception of palliative care, with its assumptions about the timing of services, has been an impediment to care and the development of care delivery models for people living with other life-threatening conditions such as HIV/AIDS.

The current trend is to involve the broad range of palliative care services when the individual is first diagnosed with a life-threatening illness. These interventions can range from provision of information about palliative care services to work on advance planning or anticipatory grief issues with the person having the life-threatening conditions and his family.

The shift in conceptualization of palliative care has now been adopted nationally and internationally (Scott 1992; World Health Organization 1990). It is one of the important insights that HIV/AIDS has given to the delivery of health care. However, the conceptualization of palliative care continues to evolve due to the tensions inherent in balancing investigation, diagnosis and treatment versus measures directed solely at palliative comfort.

Evaluation of Palliative Care Programs

Historically, palliative care was designed around the needs of dying cancer patients. In 1991, the Cancer 2000 Task Force, with representation from all national and provincial bodies involved in cancer control, stated that palliative care is an effective and efficient method for dealing with advanced disease and the needs of the dying. The Task Force made 117 recommendations for increasing the prevalence and effectiveness of palliative care (Cancer 2000 Task Force 1992). Those recommendations included:

- A reordering of cancer control priorities so that palliative care and the control of suffering is viewed as the essential fourth phase of cancer control.
- A radical shift in the allocation of cancer resources so that the control of suffering receives a just and equitable share.
- A detailed measurement of the burden of cancer suffering and the effectiveness of palliative care in relieving this burden.
- A major shift of resources into home care and the establishment of palliative care units–in-the-home projects.
- Government reimbursement to families for lost income and expenses incurred in providing home care.
- Accreditation of cancer centres and health care facilities based on the ability to relieve pain and provide palliative care.
- The development of at least 16 regional palliative care centres in Canada to act as teaching, research, and consultation units for an entire health region and to act as a base for specialized palliative home care.
- The development of a compulsory and tested palliative care curriculum in all health care professional schools.
- The development of palliative care as a certified specialty in both nursing and medicine.
- Restrictions on the use of therapies and investigations that have little proven benefit and a reallocation of their funding to pain relief and palliative care.

- An end by the National Cancer Institute of Canada to its neglect of this field and the assumption of a proactive stance towards palliative care research.
- A revision of the Canadian Cancer Society's cure-oriented and death-denying policy and adoption of a strong focus on the control of suffering in both public education and fundraising.

The Task Force Report also helped to provide a framework within which coordination of cancer control could take place (Margolese and Adair 1992). According to the chair of the Task Force, the recommendations have received little concrete attention and any changes that have been made have been superficial (Scott 1994).

The definition of palliative care most often used in the current literature comes from the World Health Organization: "The active total care, by a multi-professional team, of patients whose disease is not responsive to curative treatment. Control of pain, of other symptoms and of psychological, social and spiritual problems is paramount. The goal of palliative care is achievement of the best quality of life for patients and their families" (World Health Organization 1990). Because this description includes nonphysiological objectives such as the best social, psychological and spiritual quality of life, it is difficult to define and measure "good" palliative care. In fact, it may be that current trends toward evidence-based medicine and quantitative program evaluation may threaten palliative care programs where validity cannot be measured and justified in this way (James and Macleod 1993). In a recent survey, 88 percent of palliative care workers welcomed an audit of their programs (Higginson 1995). However, they did not specify how they thought effectiveness should be measured. Palliative care is characterized by its willingness to explicitly involve patients in setting care goals and treatment regimens. This patient-centred approach means that patterns of care may vary with each patient, making it difficult to objectively evaluate the quality of care at either an individual or a programmatic level.

To date, the effectiveness of palliative care programs has not been well documented. Three evaluations that are reported leave us with more questions than answers about the effectiveness of palliative care programs:

- Parkes (1980) evaluated a home care program, finding that both its home care team and family caregivers were required to provide increased levels of care and experienced increased stress. As a result, patients were more likely to consider themselves a burden and accept care reluctantly. However, families associated home visits by nurses with "peace of mind."
- Kane et al. (1984) evaluated cases of people receiving hospice care and those receiving conventional care. There was no significant difference between the two with respect to measurements of patients' pain, symptom relief, activities of daily living and affect. There was also no difference in overall costs. Patients and families did report being more satisfied with hospice care, but for unspecified reasons.

- Greer et al. (1986) reported the findings of the U.S. National Hospice Study. Measures of quality of life included pain, symptoms and satisfaction with care. The author concluded that there were no differences in measures of quality of life between hospice and non-hospice patients.

Educational Issues

Undergraduate medical curricula have been found wanting in terms of the effort spent preparing future physicians to participate in palliative care. Specifically, physicians are not trained adequately in controlling symptoms common to dying patients, including pain and breathlessness (Twycross and Lack 1983; Mason and Fenton 1992). It has been noted that the "certainty" which is instilled in future physicians during medical training may be incompatible with the goals of palliative care (Atkinson 1984; Fox 1957).

Because palliative care is patient-centred, professionals must spend more time with patients in order to involve them in making decisions. This places emotional demands on professionals who may be more comfortable distancing themselves from their dying patients in order to protect their own psyche. Currently, professionals are not prepared by their training to deal with these greater emotional demands (Mason and Fenton 1992). This is one reason that many professionals do not cope well with providing ongoing palliative care.[3]

Service Issues

The needs of terminally ill people are complex and wide ranging, requiring multiprofessional teams. However, a multidisciplinary approach to patient care—professionals from different disciplines, each working toward discipline-specific objectives—will not achieve the goals associated with patient-centred care. Instead, palliative care professionals must work towards *interdisciplinarity*—professionals from different disciplines working to achieve the same patient-defined goals (Melvin 1980). In this environment the division of professional roles becomes uncertain and the structure of palliative care challenges the hierarchy of traditional medical care (Meyer 1993). One attempt to bring professionals to a interdisciplinary working relationship is the *Unite the Team!* interactive software package, which requires caregivers to work together, using the diversity of their strengths to solve palliative care problems (University of Glasgow 1993).

One feature of palliative care programs that has been singled out for praise is the movement to involve nonprofessional volunteers in providing

---

3. For one attempt to address this issue, see "Success Stories"—*VITAS Healthcare Corporation*: Department of Bioethics and Pastoral Care.

care. Volunteers play an important role in meeting the social and emotional needs of the dying, especially when professional staff cannot (Brazil and Thomas 1995). Volunteer involvement has a twofold benefit. First, volunteers help palliative care programs meet more needs of more patients within already constrained budgets (Mount 1992). Second, volunteers can reintroduce 'caring' into a system that emphasizes 'treating' (Fraser and Adair 1989). Volunteers can provide care for people who have no one else. Some palliative care programs have been criticized for assuming that each dying person has a circle of loved ones who will work with the palliative care professionals to meet the dying person's care needs. Smith (1994) writes, "The assumption that everyone has someone to turn to when they are dying is a form of class prejudice." The availability of volunteers may help to overcome this bias.

A patient-centred approach requires that health care professionals spend a great deal of time interacting with patients to elicit their involvement in articulating care goals. The increased time demands on professionals who care for dying patients may be interpreted as a demand for more staffing resources than may be available. Currently, Canadian health care policy allocates resources according to a battlefield-type triage, giving highest priority to dying people who can be saved—often only at great expense, with the aid of complicated technology—and lowest priority to the needs of those who are dying and cannot be saved (Roy 1995). But this method of allocating health care resources has perpetuated "the lie that more research and more technology conquers death" (Scott 1994). Resource limitations do not need to endanger palliative care programs if a central attitudinal change can be engineered. In fact, palliative care costs can be more than offset by an attitudinal change in resource priorities which would see more resources allocated to palliative care and less to expensive high-tech medical interventions in incurable and dying patients. However, this type of change must fit within a context of a widespread attitudinal change that infiltrates general practice, hospital practice, home care, professional organizations, academic health science centres, undergraduate and graduate training towards research and, of course, governmental policies (Dossetor 1994).

Advance Care Planning[4]

What is Advance Care Planning?

Advance care planning (ACP) is a "process of communication among patients, their health care providers, their families, and important others

---

4. Reproduced from Singer P. A., G. Robertson, and D. J. Roy. Bioethics for clinicians VII: Advance care planning. *Can. Med. Assoc. J.* 1996, 155: 1689–1692.

regarding the kind of care that will be considered appropriate when the patient cannot make decisions" (Teno, Nelson, and Lynn 1994). ACP may contain written advance directives (ADs) (Advance Directives Seminar Group 1992; Emanuel 1993). Completed by a person when he is capable, the AD is used at a time when the person has become incapable. ADs indicate *who* a person would want to make treatment decisions on his behalf, and/or *what* treatments a person would or would not want in various situations.

Ethics

ACP is a strategy to ensure the norm of consent is still operative and respected when sick persons are no longer able to discuss their treatment options with physicians and thereby exercise direct control over the course of their care. The norm is grounded in the principle of self-determination/respect for autonomy, a classic expression of which is Justice Benjamin Cardozo's 1914 statement: "Every human being of adult years and sound mind has the right to determine what shall be done with his own body" (cited in Faden, Beauchamp, and King 1986, 123). The traditional ethical basis of ACP is the principle of respect for autonomy. Autonomy can be defined as the "capacity to think, decide and act ... freely, and independently and without ... hindrance" (Gillon 1986, 60).

The principle of self-determination places high value on individual liberty and reflects the fundamental belief or world view that individuals are sovereign and are not to be subjected to others, be they strangers, family members, neighbours, health care professionals or authorities of the state, in governing matters relating to their own bodies and life plans. Restraints on individual liberty are justifiable, according to the argument of John Stuart Mill, only when the exercise of liberty threatens harm to others (Mill 1987).

A quite different view of human life emphasizes the interdependence of human beings and casts doubt on the notion that people really are Mill's sovereign selves (Gray 1993, 52). Moreover, there are people living in cities across Canada who belong to cultures that emphasize the close integration of family, and even of a belief community, in medical decision making about a sick relative or community member.

There should be nothing in principle, of course, that would limit the usefulness of ACP to those who hold to an individualistic world view. This is particularly true if ACP also rests on the principle of respect for persons. Persons deserve respect, whatever their world views may be. ACP recognizes that the human dignity of sick people suffers diminishment when they cannot command respect for their considered and cherished intentions.

It is illusory to think that ACP will prevent all clinical-ethical uncertainties and conflicts. People themselves may change between the time they write ADs and the time comes for implementation of these ADs.

Moreover, proxies may be uncertain whether sick people really are in the situation described in the AD. Others, in their ADs, may have requested life-prolonging interventions that now, at the time for their implementation, are totally unrealistic.

One should consider that the dying person's biography, even in its final stages, is still emerging as the dying person—biologically and personally—reacts to and confronts treatments, care and quite new experiences and events. When communication is working as it should, the clinical community around the bedside of a gravely ill or dying person enters into the dying person's biography, and the dying person becomes a part of the biography of those giving care.

Law

The provinces of British Columbia (Representation Agreement Act 1993), Manitoba (The Health Care Directives and Consequential Amendments Act 1992), Newfoundland (Advanced Health Care Directives Act 1995), Nova Scotia (Medical Consent Act 1989), Ontario (Consent to Treatment Act 1992; Substitute Decisions Act 1992), and Quebec (Civil Code of Quebec) have legislation supporting the use of ADs (the B.C. law has not yet been proclaimed). ADs are given various names in provincial legislation, including representation agreement (B.C.), health care directive (Manitoba), advance health care directive (Newfoundland), consent agreement (Nova Scotia), power of attorney for personal care (Ontario), and mandate in the event of inability (Quebec). The laws vary with respect to the scope of ADs, who may serve as a proxy, witnessing requirements, procedures for activating an AD, etc. Even when there is no legislation, legal decisions such as the Malette case suggest that ADs may still be legally valid (*Malette v. Shulman* 1990; *Airedale NHS Trust v. Bland* 1993).

Policy

The Canadian Medical Association has endorsed a policy supporting ADs (CMA Policy Summary 1992). Some hospitals and long-term care facilities have policies regarding ADs (Rasooly et al. 1994; Choudhry et al. 1994).

Empirical Studies

Key findings from empirical studies can be summarized briefly as follows:
- Doctors and patients have positive attitudes towards ADs (Kelner and Bourgeault 1993; Lo, McLeod, and Saika 1986; Shmerling et al. 1988; Frankl, Oye, and Bellamy 1989; Teno et al. 1990; Stolman et al. 1990; Gamble, McDonald, and Lichstein 1991; Emanuel et al. 1991; Joos et al. 1993; Pfeifer et al. 1994; Molloy, Guyatt, et al. 1991). For example,

85 percent of Ontario family physicians favoured the use of ADs, (Hughes and Singer 1992) and 62 percent of medical outpatients wanted to discuss their life-sustaining treatment preferences (Sam and Singer 1993).

- Only 12 percent of Ontarians and 10 percent of Canadians have completed an AD form (Singer et al. 1993; Singer, Choudry, et al. 1995).
- People change their preferences over time (Danis et al. 1994; Emanuel et al. 1994), so ADs should be updated.
- Culture plays an important role in ACP (Caralis et al. 1994; Blackhall et al. 1995).
- ACP programs are associated with increased AD completion, but there is a ceiling on the rate of completed AD forms. These studies are detailed below (table 1).

Although these studies show that ACP programs are associated with increased AD completion, they do not address key issues in program design, such as participants, interventions, and outcome measures. Previous studies have generally examined ACP programs in the context of health care institutions. However, most of the potential participants in ACP live in the community. Previous studies have generally not compared the effectiveness of different AD forms, or of counselling. Yet the first questions faced by those who want to develop an ACP program is which type of form they should use, and whether they should provide only AD forms, or whether they should also provide a video and the services of a trained facilitator to assist people in their ACP. Previous research has primarily used the rate of completion of AD forms as the marker of effective ACP.

There are few studies about substitute decision making for incapable persons with or without ADs or ACP. The following studies suggest that much more work is needed before patients' documented preferences are consistently followed (table 2).

Finally, the effect of ADs on health care costs is controversial (Molloy and Guyatt 1991; Molloy et al. 1992; Chambers et al. 1994; Teno, Lynn, et al. 1994; SUPPORT Principal Investigators 1995), but the largest and most recent randomized trial does not support the notion that ADs decrease health care utilization or costs (SUPPORT Principal Investigators 1995).

Table 1

Empirical studies

Author(s)	Design	Participants	Intervention	Outcomes
Sachs et al. 1992	RCT	Geriatric clinic outpatients	AD + MD initiated discussion vs. control	No difference in documentation of AD or physician discussion in patient chart at 6 mos. (15% for experimental group vs. 10% for control)
High 1993	RCT	Community-dwelling seniors	Different ADs ± meeting vs. control	Increase in completed AD by self-report in moderate information plus meeting group (25% to 50%)
Rubin et al. 1994	RCT	Seniors discharged from hospital	AD vs. control	More completed ADs documented in patient chart in AD group (1.5% vs. 0.4% in controls)
Reilly et al. 1995a	RCT	Patients discharged from hospital	Educational brochure and encouragement	12.3% completed proxy documents. No difference between intervention and control groups
Hare and Nelson 1991	NRC	Internal medicine outpatients	AD vs. AD + MD initiated discussion vs. control	More completed ADs documented on patient charts after 4 mos. in AD/discussion group (11.5% vs. 0% for AD alone and control groups)
Holley et al. 1993	Cohort	Hemodialysis unit	AD + discussion	Increase in completion of AD (13% to 37%) after 6 mos. by self-report
Silverman et al. 1995	Cohort	Hospitalized patients	AD + assistance	In hospital, 24% had discussions and 2% completed an AD. Within 6 mos. after discharge, 39% had discussions and 15% completed an AD

Table 1 (cont.)

Author(s)	Design	Participants	Intervention	Outcomes
Markson et al. 1994	Cohort	Home care and nursing home patients	AD + MD education	In home care, 21% approached and 13% completed AD. In nursing home, 100% approached and 90% completed AD
Luptak and Boult 1994	Cohort	Geriatric clinic	AD + counselling	71% completed AD
Cohen-Mansfield, Droge, et al. 1991	Cohort	Hospitalized patients	AD	11.5% completed AD after 3 mos.
Cohen-Mansfield, Rabinovich, et al. 1991	Cohort	Long-term care residents	AD	25% completed AD
Emanuel et al. 1993	Time series	Hospitalized patients	Patient Self-Determination Act	Significant increases in advance care planning (60.9% vs. 72.6%) and general discussions with proxies (61% vs. 73%). No increase in written ADs (19% vs. 25.5%), discussions between patients and physicians (13.6% vs. 17.1%) or discussion with proxies about specific treatment preferences (33.6% vs. 33.2%)
Reilly et al. 1995b	Time series	Hospitalized patients	Phase 1: Education to physicians; Phase 2: promoted new AD form; Phase 3: control	Proportion of inpatients with completed AD, as documented on chart by physician, significantly higher in intervention phase (62.5%) than in education phase (23.6%) or control phase (25.3%)

Table 2

Other studies

Author(s)	Design	Participants	Intervention	Outcomes
Danis et al. 1991	Prospective cohort	Nursing home residents	Completed ADs placed in medical record	Care was consistent with wishes in 75% of events; not affected by presence of written AD
Morrison et al. 1995	Retrospective chart review	Geriatric hospital patients	Review charts for documentation of patient's AD status	14 (26%) incapable patients had AD recognized in chart; AD influenced care in 12 (86%) of these cases
SUPPORT Principal Investigators 1995	RCT	Hospitalized adults with life-threatening illness	Trained nurse had multiple contacts with patient, family, physician and hospital staff to facilitate ACP	No improvement in patient-physician communication or physicians' knowledge of their patients' wish not to be resuscitated. No change in utilization or cost variables

Euthanasia/Assisted Suicide[5]

Introduction

In a recent Special Senate Committee report, *euthanasia* is defined as "a deliberate act undertaken by one person with the intention of ending the life of another person to relieve that person's suffering where the act is the cause of death" (Senate of Canada 1995). According to the report, euthanasia can fall into one of three categories:
- *voluntary*—where the act is undertaken in accordance with the wishes of a competent individual or a valid advance directive;
- *nonvoluntary*—where the act is done without knowledge of the individual's wishes whether he is competent or not; or
- *involuntary*—where the act is done against the wishes of a competent individual or a valid advance directive.

Assisted suicide is defined in the same report as the act of "intentionally killing oneself with the assistance of another who provides the knowledge, means, or both."

Euthanasia and assisted suicide have been the subject of a long-standing ethical and legal debate (Senate of Canada 1995; Emanuel 1994a, 1994b; Fins 1994; Bloch 1994). Proponents have argued that euthanasia and assisted suicide should be available to certain individuals in certain circumstances, as a way of allowing them to maintain control in the dying process and of preventing suffering (Humphrey and Wickett 1986). Opponents of euthanasia and assisted suicide, on the other hand, have argued for main-taining the illegal status of these acts on various grounds, including religious (Pope John Paul II 1995) and secular (Kass 1990) views of the sanctity of life, the difficulty anticipated in trying to keep euthanasia and assisted suicide within clear guidelines (for example, stipulating that it must be "voluntary", or limited to certain stages of "terminal" illness), and the view that euthanasia and assisted suicide are unnecessary to address such issues as avoidance of suffering, fear of dying and fear of being dependent or becoming a burden on loved ones (Sachs et al. 1995)—in short, all those issues commonly thought to lead to requests for euthanasia or assisted suicide in the first place.

Although euthanasia and assisted suicide are practiced openly in the Netherlands, this is possible only by agreement on the part of the judiciary not to prosecute participating physicians if they adhere to existing guidelines (Gevers 1995). On May 25, 1995 Australia's Northern Territory became the first jurisdiction to formally decriminalize assisted suicide in legislation (Northern Territory of Australia 1995). Similar legislative initiatives have recently been struck down in Washington State (Washington State Initiative

---

5. The contribution of James V. Lavery, M.Sc., to the writing of this section is acknowledged.

1991), and passed in a referendum but subsequently suppressed by court injunction in Oregon (Oregon's Death with Dignity Act 1995).

In March and April of 1996, two U.S. Federal Appeals Court decisions brought U.S. social policy one step closer to legalized euthanasia and assisted suicide. The Ninth Circuit Federal Appeals Court struck down a 130-year-old Washington State statute criminalizing assisted suicide. The Court found that requesting assistance in dying is a constitutionally protected liberty interest, and that the law in question, by constraining that liberty unnecessarily, violated the Fourteenth Amendment of the U.S. Constitution. The Second Circuit Federal Appeals Court declared unconstitutional a similar New York statute. The Second Circuit Court determined that terminally ill patients who could not kill themselves because of physical disability were subject to discrimination not present for similarly situated patients who were capable of killing themselves. Therefore, the statute in question criminalizing assisted suicide violated the U.S. Constitution's equal protection clause.

Several sections of the Criminal Code of Canada relate to euthanasia and assisted suicide. These include Section 14, which states that no individual may consent to have death inflicted on him; Section 215, regarding the duty to provide the necessaries of life; Sections 216 and 217, regarding undertaking acts dangerous to life; Section 226, regarding accelerating death; Section 241, regarding counselling or aiding suicide; Section 245, on administering a noxious thing; Section 246, on overcoming resistance to commission of offence; and Section 430 regarding mischief (Ogden 1994b). Recently, euthanasia and assisted suicide became pressing public policy issues in the wake of the Supreme Court decision in the case of Sue Rodriguez (*Rodriguez v. British Columbia* 1993). In a five to four ruling by the Supreme Court of Canada, the young woman who was afflicted with amyotrophic lateral sclerosis was refused in her bid to receive openly the assistance of a physician in ending her life. Ms. Rodriguez died in 1993, reportedly after receiving the assistance of a willing physician.

On June 6, 1995, a Special Senate Committee struck after the *Rodriguez* decision reported the findings of its 16-month study (Senate of Canada 1995). The Senate Committee report addresses a wide variety of issues related to euthanasia and assisted suicide. In particular, individual chapters of the report are dedicated to palliative care, pain control and sedation, withholding and withdrawing life-sustaining treatment, and advance directives (Senate of Canada 1995). Among its recommendations, the Senate Committee report highlights the need for further research into how many people are requesting euthanasia and assisted suicide, why they are being requested, and whether alternatives exist that might be acceptable to those who are making the requests (Senate of Canada 1995).

The lack of empirical information about euthanasia and assisted suicide is not a newly identified problem. Dr. Alvin Novick, editor of the journal

AIDS and Public Policy, has made repeated appeals for research in the area of euthanasia and assisted suicide:

> Assisted death is the unspoken theme of AIDS and many patients and loved ones are sufficiently engaged, damaged, fulfilled, or interested to become part of the real dialogue. Are we resisting doing the necessary research because it will be too difficult? Is any serious research easy? (Novick 1995).

Empirical Studies

While Canadians are polarized with respect to their views on euthanasia and assisted suicide (Senate of Canada 1995), support for these measures has been growing steadily over the past decade. Gallup polls in 1989, 1991 and 1992 showed that more than three-quarters of adult Canadians support euthanasia and assisted suicide in principle (Bozinoff and Macintosh 1989, 1991; Bozinoff and Turcotte 1992). However, there is considerable variability in attitudes regarding the circumstances in which euthanasia and assisted suicide should be employed. In a recent Canadian public opinion poll, 66 percent of respondents considered euthanasia acceptable where there is a poor likelihood of recovery in a terminally ill patient, while 78 percent disapproved of it if the patient was likely to recover (Singer, Choudry, et al. 1995). A similar survey in Edmonton found that 65 percent of respondents supported euthanasia for patients experiencing severe pain and terminal illness, but 65 percent were opposed to it for an elderly disabled person who feels he is a burden on relatives. Seventy-five percent were opposed to euthanasia for an elderly person with poor life satisfaction, and 83 percent were opposed to euthanasia for an elderly person with minor physical ailments (Genius, Genius, and Chang 1994). In Holland, euthanasia and assisted suicide have been practiced openly since 1966, and since then public opinion has steadily become more permissive (van der Maas et al. 1995).

Studies of the attitudes and practices of physicians and nurses reveal that slightly more than half of these professionals support euthanasia and assisted suicide *in principle,* though levels of support change dramatically according to the circumstances of the proposed recipient—following a trend similar to that of public opinion. The illegality of euthanasia and assisted suicide also appear to have a inhibitory effect on the willingness of physicians and nurses to endorse or participate in euthanasia and assisted suicide (Backman et al. 1996; Kuhse and Singer 1988, 1992; Lee et al. 1996; Pijnenborg 1994; Slome et al. 1992; Searles 1995).

Information is available from the Dutch experience regarding *what* decisions are being made in this relatively permissive environment (van der Maas et al. 1996; Hendin, Rutenfrans, and Zylica 1997; Emanuel 1994a; Jochemson 1994). For the most part, euthanasia and assisted suicide in

Holland most often involve cancer patients (83 percent) who have good insight into their disease and prognosis (100 percent) and who make strong, explicit, repeated requests (96 percent) for euthanasia and assisted suicide to their physicians (van der Maas et al. 1992). The most commonly cited reason for requesting euthanasia in Holland was to avoid "unworthy" dying (van der Maas et al. 1992).

Only one published study has used qualitative methods to study euthanasia and assisted suicide (Ogden 1994a). Ogden conducted interviews with 18 persons living with HIV/AIDS (PHAs) and 17 individuals who had been involved in a total of 34 acts of euthanasia and assisted suicide of PHAs. The study provides a description of persons who have participated or may participate in euthanasia and assisted suicide, along with their relevant attitudes and personal experiences. Eighty-three percent of the PHAs reported that euthanasia and assisted suicide were options for them personally. Within this group, 53 percent had already taken steps to plan their deaths. In general, these plans were developed cooperatively with friends, family members, and physicians. Ogden's study documents the comments of the participants regarding issues such as control, suffering, fear and stigmatization, clearly establishing these concepts as elements in the phenomena of euthanasia and assisted suicide.

Summary of Key Conclusions from the Literature

- Death and dying are complex phenomena which involve not only physical aspects but also psychological, social, and cultural considerations.
- Palliative care programs are thought to be effective at controlling pain in the context of cancer care; however, knowledge is limited regarding its effectiveness with respect to other outcomes and outside the context of cancer.
- Advance care planning programs increase the rate of completed AD forms, but there appears to be a ceiling on this rate. Knowledge regarding the effect of advance care planning programs on other outcomes is limited.
- Although there is a clear trend towards support for legalized euthanasia and assisted suicide in the United States, Australia and the Netherlands, euthanasia and assisted suicide are illegal in Canada at this time
- Overall, there is insufficient information on which to base informed social policy decisions with respect to death and dying and the strategies needed to improve the process of dying in Canada.

SUCCESS STORIES

The *Centre to Improve Care of the Dying*: George Washington University Medical Centre[6]

Actions on Nonmedical Determinants of Health

The goals of the *Centre to Improve Care of the Dying* focus directly on nonmedical determinants of health. The goals are to raise awareness of the psychosocial needs of people who are dying and to influence the way society, the health care system and health care providers are equipped to meet those needs. The underlying value that drives this initiative is the belief that all people should be able to live well before death. People should be comfortable and comforted in their dying and should be able to live meaningfully.

The goals are met through a series of projects designed to highlight the needs of the dying. The Centre's staff are engaged in gathering data from multiple sources and assembling a basic description of the dying process, including material answering the questions: What are the priorities of dying patients? What do the dying need to live well? A proportion of the Centre's work is devoted to disseminating information to the public, with the belief that the public can shape the necessary changes to health care systems.

Reasons for the Initiative

The Centre's director, Dr. Lynn, has spent much of her career caring for dying people and working in hospice settings. In that time she has observed that the needs of the dying have largely been ignored by both professional and lay media and by the education system that shapes upcoming health care providers. Her commitment and energy were largely responsible for the establishment of the *Centre to Improve Care of the Dying* in September 1995. Her efforts have attracted support from other professionals as well as private funding foundations.

Actors

The research work for this project has been conducted by members with a personal commitment to the goals of the Centre—many having gone through the dying experience with loved ones. They include five full-time faculty members who have expertise in medicine, epidemiology, public policy, education and public health. In addition, the Centre employs a full-time staff of four. The Centre also consults with many other professionals

---

6. All information for this section comes from an interview with Joanne Lynn, M.D., director of the *Centre to Improve Care of the Dying*.

from a wide range of backgrounds. The Centre hopes to add three more members in the near future with expertise in economics, administration and public information/relations.

Analysis of the Results

Although it is too early to judge the effectiveness of the program, tangible results can be cited. The Centre's members have written several publications including two compilations of data related to dying: *Sourcebook on Dying* written for professionals and *Handbook for Mortals* written for the public. In addition, members have appeared on public media. The Centre is hosting a policy symposium in 1996. Dr. Lynn is a principal investigator on the Study to Understand Prognoses and Preferences for Outcomes and Risks of Treatments (SUPPORT)—a large initiative funded by the Robert Wood Johnson Foundation to improve end-of-life decision making and reduce the frequency of a mechanically supported, painful, and prolonged process of dying. Several other projects are well under way.

Replicability of the Initiative

The director assumes that the model is replicable and is certain that many of the individual projects are replicable. Since a major thrust of the Centre is to disseminate information to the public, she feels the Centre should be replicated in a few major cities. A major obstacle to the project has been the discomfort people feel when discussing issues related to dying. Any similar venture will need to work to overcome this discomfort.

Funding

The Centre's primary source of funding is individual project grants from eight private foundations spawning approximately 36 different projects. The Centre received minimal start-up help from its home institution, but does not receive government funding. The projected annual budget for a staff of 12 plus visiting scholars is approximately $1.5 million.

Evaluation

Evaluation reports do not exist because the Centre is so new. A formal evaluation will be difficult because of the Centre's fluid structure, however, each individual project is evaluated by its particular funding agency. The director is assembling a large multidisciplinary steering committee that will meet annually to reflect on the directions and priorities of the Centre.

VITAS Healthcare Corporation: Department of Bioethics and Pastoral Care[7]

VITAS Healthcare Corporation is a for-profit proprietary company that operates 30 hospices in 12 states caring for approximately 5,000 patients and families per day and providing bereavement counselling for approximately 20,000 families. VITAS is the largest hospice organization in the United States, and employs approximately 3,600 staff.

Actions on Nonmedical Determinants of Health

The Department of Bioethics and Pastoral Care focuses on caring for all people. Two primary values underpin the activities of the department: 1) patients and families come first; and 2) we take care of each other. This means that all activities of the corporation's staff and volunteers are oriented toward meeting the needs of the patients and families they serve. It also means that the corporation acknowledges that the staff who serve the patients are people too, and that they also require emotional and psychospiritual care. One goal of the organization is to cultivate and maintain a "moral community" in which there is opportunity for patients, families, staff and management to voice concerns openly and confidentially, and know that the concerns will be addressed in a meaningful way. This is achieved through the activities of a corporate ethics committee (concerned with policy issues), and the activities of local and regional clinical ethics committees (concerned with staff and patient care issues).

Reasons for the Initiative

The need for moral direction for VITAS arose out of the moral vision of the corporation's cofounders: a Methodist minister and a nurse. This vision reflected a great respect for the principle of caring for all people in a comprehensive way. The need for a moral direction and vision was also underscored by an event that took place in 1990: the media raised questions about the management of VITAS which created a climate of anxiety for staff throughout the corporation. Although no impropriety was ever found, this event led the heads of the corporation to focus greater attention on ethics and to provide the opportunity for staff members to discuss their concerns. That same year the corporation developed the Department of Bioethics and Pastoral Care and, later, the ethics committee structure. The ethics committees are groups of individuals that have diverse interests and

---

7. The source of information for this project is an interview with Dr. Richard Fife, vice-president of Bioethics and Pastoral Care, *VITAS Healthcare Corporation* (based in Miami, Florida).

experiences; the collective wisdom of these groups is channelled toward meeting the corporation's care goals. The committees take seriously their obligation to educate themselves about the issues they face and then to educate staff and the public they serve. In general, hospices are not required to have ethics committees and, typically, only those affiliated with hospitals do. VITAS is an important exception.

Actors

The department receives important support from the corporation's CEO who initiated it and hired Dr. Fife as vice-president in charge of the department. The department has no staff per se, but an organization of committees that deal with the ethical and psychospiritual issues that arise. The corporate ethics committee is made up of 12 upper-level managers and five community representatives. The community representatives are selected from major ethics programs and hospice organizations around the country and bring a variety of expertise to the committee's deliberations. The eight local and regional ethics committees have approximately 20 members each and include both staff and community representation. The com-munity representatives are selected for their skills and reflect the racial and cultural communities they serve.

At the hospice level, individual care teams are always staffed with social workers to help patients with emotional and psychosocial issues, and with chaplains to help people deal with psychospiritual issues.

Analysis of the Results

The corporate ethics committee has dealt with several important policy issues affecting care provided for patients. For example, the committee responded to the Patient Self-Determination Act by establishing a clear policy regarding the provision of CPR within the hospices and documenting people's wishes for CPR. Currently, in response to staff concerns, they are focusing their attention on policy regarding assisted suicide. The clinical ethics committees support the staff and formally address three to four difficult patient cases per year. One observation of interest is that the better the job the clinical ethics committees do educating staff to deal with emotional and psychospiritual problems "at the bedside," the fewer the cases they tend to address at the committee level.

An important component of Dr. Fife's work is to provide ongoing support—both emotional and financial—on a discretionary basis for staff who are experiencing particular psychospiritual or financial problems. This is a concrete way of implementing the second of the corporation's foundational values: We take care of each other. In addition, he is responsible for education of committee members.

Attrition and turnover of committee members are obstacles the department continually faces. Each committee (all members) takes part in a one-year training course to prepare them for their responsibilities. The goal of the training is to create a "moral community" that can deal effectively with care issues. In addition, members are taught a structured method for case analysis that is based on the 'Ethic of Care' model arising from feminist moral theory. This fits well with the overall corporate mentality which is largely feminist in orientation (75–80 percent of the corporation's staff are female). When committee members leave and are replaced, a new education cycle is needed and this sets back the process considerably. Another obstacle is the enormity of the communication task. It is difficult to communicate effectively and efficiently to thousands of staff, patients and families about the committees and the help they can provide. Dr. Fife has developed information packages that are given to each patient upon admission in order to orient and inform the patient about the committees and the care they provide.

Replicability of the Initiative

Dr. Fife believes that the team approach to patient care can be replicated within the context of a "moral community" that addresses the concerns of the staff, the patients and the families. The method for case analysis is currently replicated for each cycle of committee education and can be replicated elsewhere. However, it is much easier to replicate the methods than it is to duplicate the "moral community" and the climate of moral openness which has taken several years of constant cultivation to develop and maintain.

Funding

VITAS is a for-profit corporation which garners its income from Medicare, Medicaid and private insurance reimbursements. VITAS has an annual operating budget of approximately $200 million. The annual operating budget of the Department of Bioethics and Pastoral Care is approximately $1 million. This money comes directly out of the corporation's profits, and funds the work of the Bioethics and Pastoral Care Department, the one-year training for ethics committees, the expenses related to the functioning of the committees and the various efforts at staff and public education. Some of the corporation's profits are also diverted to provide hospice care to people who otherwise could not afford it—so-called "charity" cases.

Evaluation

There is no formal means of evaluating the work of the hospices or the work of the ethics committees. The corporate ethics committee evaluates the functioning of the clinical ethics committees by gathering information about their activities and addressing the concerns expressed by the clinical committee members, the staff and the patients. Each clinical ethics committee holds an annual retreat at which they evaluate their own activities of the previous year. In response to requests from staff and patients, the corporation's research department is in the process of developing a new instrument that can be used to evaluate the quality of the hospice care.

The *HIV Palliative Care Module*[8]

Actions on Nonmedical Determinants of Health

The palliative care module affects several nonmedical determinants of health, including physical, psychological, social, cultural and economic nonmedical determinants. This broad scope is inherent in the definition of palliative care (see above). The aim of the *HIV Palliative Care Module* project was to produce a brief resource guide for service providers, caregivers, patients and families to be used in addressing the physical, psychological, social and cultural aspects of living with a life-threatening illness, including dying and bereavement. The goals of the project were to relieve suffering on the part of dying patients, to empower service providers and others by providing useful information, and to confront directly the marginalized position of HIV/AIDS in the context of palliative care.

The process was as follows. In early 1994, a partnership was established between Mount Sinai Hospital and Casey House Hospice in order to commence the project. In March 1994, a two-day National Working Group meeting was held with funding from Health Canada to bring together people from 20 organizations to discuss the possibility of producing the palliative care module. Following the meeting, a proposal was written for the palliative care module, and in July 1994 Health Canada agreed to fund the project. Subsequently, a coordinator was hired, and lead expert authors were selected and contacted about the project. Between August and November 1994, the lead expert authors produced and revised drafts of various sections of the module. Between November 1994 and February 1995, the evolving drafts of the modules were sent to the reviewers and tested in focus groups. The final document was printed in March 1995 and launched on April 10, 1995 by the federal Minister of Health.

---

8. The sources of information for this success story are *A Comprehensive Guide for the Care of Persons with HIV Disease, Module 4: Palliative Care*, and an interview with one of the editors of the module, Dr. Frank Ferris (palliative medicine physician, Mount Sinai Hospital).

Reasons for the Initiative

The situation before the initiative was characterized by lack of knowledge on the part of service providers, caregivers, patients, and families about palliative care, especially in the context of HIV/AIDS. There was also a sense of marginalization of HIV/AIDS in the context of palliative care, and many palliative care programs did not treat people with HIV/AIDS. The initiative attempted to address this situation through collaboration and networking among many organizations and individuals concerned with palliative care and HIV/AIDS.

The need for change was recognized by the experiences of those involved. For example, Dr. Frank Ferris, a front-line worker providing palliative care, observed that large numbers of people with HIV/AIDS were not receiving adequate palliative care.

Actors

The actors included Dr. Ferris, a palliative care physician at Mount Sinai Hospital, and John Flannery, a nurse by training, from Casey House. They were assisted by the project coordinator, Helen McNeil. Members of the Executive Committee of the National Working Group played an active role in the project. For instance, Michel Morissette assisted greatly in the writing and in the French translation; Wayne Moore brought the important perspective of a person living with HIV/AIDS to the work; Gail Flintoft provided major input into the psychosocial chapters; and David Kuhl wrote much of the section on pain management. The National Working Group itself brought together representatives of 17 organizations. In addition, the 29 lead expert authors, 43 resource people, and 26 reviewers listed on the booklet all made major contributions to the publication. Finally, Gerry Bally from Health Canada served as a very effective liaison on the part of the funding organization. The module was a collaborative effort unparalleled in Dr. Ferris' experience.

Analysis of the Results

According to Dr. Ferris, the goals of the project were achieved. The evidence supporting this claim is that the booklet is the resource the group had intended to develop, and that 15,000 copies of the booklet have been distributed through the AIDS Clearing House of the Canadian Public Health Association in just over 6 months (an additional 25,000 copies are available). Feedback from service providers has been positive.

The keys to the success of this project were the motivation and dedication of the scores of people who participated in the work, as well as the political "buy in" of the 17 organizations that were part of the project from inception. The availability of the booklet free of charge was also viewed as an important facilitator of the dissemination effort.

Replicability

The general approach should be replicable in the general area of palliate care, although this might be unnecessary because the information in the module is applicable to non-HIV/AIDS palliative care contexts. The approach should also be replicable by any other group working to produce educational materials through a consensus-building process.

Funding

Funding was provided by the AIDS Care, Treatment and Support Unit under the National AIDS Contribution Program of the National AIDS Strategy of Health Canada. It was provided in two phases: a development grant of about $20,000 to support the initial National Working Group conference and proposal writing; and a subsequent grant of $478,000 for the project itself.

Evaluation

There are plans for an external evaluation to be conducted by the Canadian Palliative Care Association.

The Ontario *Substitute Decisions Project*: Power of Attorney for Personal Care[9]

Actions on Nonmedical Determinants of Health

In 1992 the Ontario Legislature passed the Substitute Decisions Act, Consent to Treatment Act and Advocacy Act. Proclamation of these acts was delayed to permit implementation (the acts ultimately came into force on April 3, 1995 and were repealed or substantially amended in March 1996). The goal of the *Substitute Decisions Project* (SDP), based in the office of the Public Guardian and Trustee (a part of the Ministry of the Attorney General) was to

---

9. The sources of information for this success story are the Substitute Decisions Act, interviews with staff of the Office of the Public Guardian and Trustee (Jacqueline Connors, senior communications coordinator and Trudy Spinks, legal counsel) and the author's own experiences. The mandate of the *Substitute Decisions Project* was to implement the Substitute Decisions Act. The distribution of Power of Attorney for Personal Care forms, the focus of this success story, was only one aspect of the *Substitute Decisions Project*.

implement the Substitute Decisions Act. Although implementation of the Substitute Decisions Act raised many issues, including assessment of capacity, this success story will focus on that part of the project related to the distribution of Power of Attorney for Personal Care (PAPC) forms.

The project proceeded in five stages:
- consultation (with staff in the ministries of Health, Attorney General, and Citizenship; advocacy groups; legal experts; medical experts);
- examination of options re PAPC forms (the decision was that government should not "be in the business of endorsing other people's products" so a decision was made that the government would draft its own forms);
- drafting of PAPC forms;
- review by the Interim Advisory Committee of the SDP (which raised concerns about the accessibility of the language in the PAPC form that were subsequently addressed); and
- communication and distribution of forms, starting April 1994.

The primary value underlying the SDP was personal choice. The perceived problem was that Ontarians had no legally recognized ability to make personal care (including health care) choices regarding who would make decisions and what decisions would be made on their behalf in the event of incapacity. The Substitute Decisions Act provided legal mechanisms for people to assert these personal choices in advance of incapacity, and the SDP aimed to implement these mechanisms and make them accessible. Although it was not explicitly recognized at the time, although the PAPC component of the SDP affects all nonmedical determinants of health (i.e., physical, psychological, social, cultural, and economic), it is probably most focused on the social determinants of health.

Reasons for the Initiative

The situation before the Substitute Decisions Act was characterized by: lack of legal vehicles for decision making in advance of incapacity; lack of information and misinformation regarding the legal vehicles that did exist; and lack of access to information and forms. The project attempted to solve these problems through disseminating information and providing forms.

The catalysts for change included the impending proclamation of the act, heightened public interest in PAPCs related to media coverage of the act, and misinformation related to the act. Although the project had always planned to disseminate PAPCs, this process was sped up in response to perceived misinformation in the media related to financial powers of attorney.

The need for change was recognized primarily as a result of public inquiries to ministry staff. The public wanted to know whether the government would be providing PAPC forms. These public inquiries took the form of telephone calls and letters to the PGT and Ministry of the Attorney

General, radio and television phone-in shows, and questions raised by the audience during speaking engagements. The need was also recognized by PGT staff from their interactions with advocacy groups (including seniors groups), the medical and legal communities, and the media. Some members of the medical and legal community expressed the contrary view that the government should not distribute PAPC forms.

Actors

The actors included MPPs, civil servants, the legal community and the Interim Advisory Committee of the SDP. Even those who were not enthusiastic about the distribution of PAPC forms, such as some members of the legal community, participated because they wished to have a voice.

Analysis of the Results

The goal of this aspect of the SDP was to educate people about their (impending) ability to complete a PAPC. It would then be up to the individual to decide whether to complete a form, and which form to complete.

PGT staff judged the project to have been a success. The evidence on which this claim is based is as follows:
- *Telephone calls to the Ministry and PGT*: In March, 1994, ministry staff were receiving 35,000 telephone calls per month, and they were almost all negative. The PAPC kits were introduced in April 1994. By January 1996, ministry staff were receiving only 110 calls per month and these were requests for the PAPC kit or for more information.
- *PAPC kit requests*: Since April 1994, the PGT's office has distributed a total of 2.4 million PAPC kits (including 100,000 in seven languages other than English). Every major Canadian bank has ordered PAPC kits. Several large public sector unions and private companies have sent the kits to all their employees.
- *Feedback from MPPs*: MPPs have ordered many kits for their constituents, and report that their constituents are satisfied.

The primary factor deemed responsible for the success of this initiative was the accessibility of the kits. In particular, the elimination of any financial barrier (the kits were distributed without charge to the consumer) was viewed as a crucial factor in the success of the initiative.

Replicability of the Initiative

Changes to provincial legislation were a key element of this project. A perceived deadline for proclamation of the Substitute Decisions Act fuelled much of the change. By implication, this initiative is likely adaptable to other jurisdictions, but perhaps not to other times; it may require the stimulus of impending proclamations of relevant legislation.

Funding

Funding for this project was provided by Ontario taxpayers. The Office of the PGT has declined to provide information regarding funding of this project at this time.

Evaluation

There was no formal evaluation of this project. Informal evaluative measures are detailed above in the section "Analysis of Results." Therefore, it is unknown how many of the 2.4 million PAPC forms distributed were completed, what type of PAPC forms were ultimately completed, how many people sought legal assistance in completing PAPC forms, and how many forms were completed correctly. Whether and to what extent distribution of PAPCs improved Ontarians' understanding of PAPCs is also unknown. Formal evaluations were not carried out because the primary objective was education, not completed forms and because informal indications, especially the number of PAPC requests, were that the project had been successful at its educational goals. Formal evaluation strategies were planned, but the provincial elections and the change in government that followed has delayed implementation.

Advance Care Planning Research Program: The University of Toronto Joint Centre For Bioethics[10]

Actions on Nonmedical Determinants of Health

Although this project likely affects all determinants of health, its primary influence is most likely on the psychological and social determinants of health. The *Advance Care Planning Research Program* promotes two main goals: achieving a sense of control and relieving loved ones of the burden of decision making. The project was fuelled by the motivation to develop new knowledge through research, and to disseminate this knowledge through research transfer in order to benefit Canadians.

Reasons for the Initiative

Prior to this project, there were several unknowns with respect to advance care planning in Canada (Advance Directives Seminar Group 1992). First,

---

10. The source of information for this success story is the authors' experiences.

although the attitudes of U.S. physicians and patients had been studied, there were scanty data on the attitudes of Canadian physicians and patients, and the policies of Canadian health care facilities with regard to advance directives. Second, very little work had been done with respect to tailoring advance directives to a person's actual disease. Finally, although quantitative studies had examined attitudes, there was a paucity of qualitative research leading to a fundamental understanding of the phenomenon of advance care planning in practice.

The project attempted to solve these problems through scholarly research. In the first phase, several surveys were conducted which confirmed that physicians and patients had positive attitudes towards advance directives but tended not to complete written advance directive forms (Hughes and Singer 1992; Sam and Singer 1993; Singer, Choudhry, and Armstrong 1993; Singer, Choudhry, et al. 1995). As well, the prevalence and content of policies regarding advance directives and life-sustaining treatment in Canadian hospitals and long-term care facilities was documented (Rasooly et al. 1994; Choudhry et al. 1994).

In the second phase of the project, the concept of disease-specific advance directives was described, and disease-specific advance directives were developed and evaluated in the context of dialysis, HIV/AIDS, and cancer (Singer 1994). Dialysis patients did not prefer the dialysis advance directive over the generic University of Toronto Centre for Bioethics Living Will, but the study yielded important insights about the greater influence of health states as opposed to treatments in determining a patient's preferences as recorded in an instruction directive (Singer, Thiel, et al. 1995). People living with HIV preferred the HIV advance directive over the generic Centre for Bioethics Living Will (Singer et al., in press). Testing of the cancer advance directive is currently under way (Berry and Singer 1995).

In the third phase, a new model of advance care planning was described (Singer, Martin, et al., in press). Traditional discussions of advance directives focus on preparing for incapacity, autonomy, advance directive forms, and the role of physicians in advance care planning. However, an examination of the phenomenon of advance care planning in practice in the context of dialysis revealed that people emphasize preparing for death, relationships, communication, and the role of close loved ones in advance care planning. Therefore, the assumptions on which many advance care planning programs have been based are flawed, and the new model suggests new directions for advance care planning programs (Singer 1995)

The catalysts for change included a supportive academic environment. The need for change was recognized though a careful assessment regarding the unknowns of advance care planning. This was not a single event that occurred at the beginning of this research program, but rather a process of continuous discovery as the research unfolded.

Actors

The research program was led by Dr. Singer, but many others were involved. The project has been supported by faculty from other disciplines, including behavioral science, philosophy, anthropology and law. Moreover, much of the actual research has been conducted by graduate students and research fellows.

Analysis of the Results

This research program has been a success as measured by the publications and research grants it has generated. The program has also been a success in terms of research transfer. Since 1992, almost 100,000 copies of the Centre for Bioethics Living Will have been distributed. In response to requests, the Centre has distributed over 33,000 copies of the Living Will directly to the public, health providers, lawyers and health care facilities.

Replicability of the Initiative

There is no need to replicate this initiative in other jurisdictions of Canada, since the knowledge gained through the research conducted at the University of Toronto can be generalized. The model of an interdisciplinary research team could be replicated for other social phenomena.

Funding

The research was funded primarily through research grants from the Ontario Ministry of Health, the Institute for Clinical Evaluative Sciences in Ontario, the National Health Research and Development Program, the Physicians' Services Incorporated Foundation, and the Agency for Health Care Policy and Research. All funding is temporary and project related. Revenues from the sale of living wills and videos have been used to support the costs of dissemination, and will be used to fund further research.

Evaluation

Each project was evaluated at the level of research grant funding by a peer review agency and/or publication of the results in a peer reviewed journal. Thus, each individual project has been the focus of considerable evaluative scrutiny. The overall program of research per se has not been evaluated.

POLICY IMPLICATIONS

Social Policy Goals Require Articulation

The first conclusion from the literature and success stories is that there are no clearly articulated goals of social policy in Canada with respect to death and dying. The three policy responses identified in this report—palliative care, advance care planning and euthanasia assisted suicide—have been pursued largely independently. A major contribution of the Senate Committee Report, June 1995, was to bring these issues together in one policy document. However, the Senate Committee Report still focuses on these three broad policy responses rather than on the social policy goals. Clarification of these goals is urgently needed.

Often a nation's social policy in a particular area is led by one significant issue, after which, other issues become significant. Policy is then assembled piecemeal, often with no coherent overall strategy and unsatisfying results. Policy regarding issues in death and dying are no different. In the United States, decisions to forgo treatment, beginning with the 1976 case of Karen Quinlan, was the early driving force behind the development of social policy around end of life. This was followed by a trend towards state-by-state living will/advance directive legislation. More recently, euthanasia/assisted suicide has become prominent with legislative initiatives in California, Washington, and Oregon, as well as through the work of Dr. Jack Kevorkian and the very recent appeal court decisions in the Second and Ninth Circuits. In the Netherlands, euthanasia/assisted suicide was historically the first issue addressed in-depth by national social policy. The Dutch are now beginning to address issues in palliative care and advance care planning.

In Canada, policies around palliative care, advance care planning and euthanasia/assisted suicide are progressing independently in the typical piecemeal approach that often leads to unsatisfying results. A coherent strategy is needed to address death and dying issues as a comprehensive whole, thus providing a framework within which individual issues can be located and developed.

Sufficiency of Available Approaches

As can be seen from the success stories documented here, there are no well-articulated criteria to evaluate the "success" of the stories. This observation should not be surprising given that establishing criteria for success follows logically *after* the objectives for the programs and the overall policy goals in which they are situated are set. Once the social policy goals are clear, the available approaches—palliative care, advance care planning, and the possibility of legalized euthanasia/assisted suicide—can be reviewed in the context of the social policy goals. It will then become apparent whether complementary approaches are needed, or whether the available social policy responses are sufficient to address the goals.

Role of Government

It will be important to articulate the appropriate role of government in addressing the various goals of social policy. Simply claiming that a given objective is an important social policy goal with respect to death and dying in Canada does not lead to the conclusion that it should be the responsibility of government to provide the means to ensure that this objective is met. For instance, we might decide that the availability of financial powers of attorney and wills are important in terms of the economic determinants of health with regard to death and dying. Traditionally, however, these financial vehicles have been provided in the private sector by lawyers, and the role of government has been limited to enacting legislation recognizing the legitimacy of such private action.

A comparison between two of the success stories addresses precisely this point. Advance care planning addresses the psychological and social determinants of health. In the Ontario government's *Substitute Decisions Project*, the government not only enacted enabling legislation, but also provided information to the public regarding powers of attorney for personal care and distributed without charge to the consumer power of attorney for personal care forms (as well as financial power of attorney forms). By contrast, the University of Toronto Centre for Bioethics distributed its "Living Will" for a $5 charge as a "nonprofit" activity (the funds were deposited into a research account and support further research on advance care planning). In many lawyers' offices, these documents are drawn up for clients as a for-profit activity. Is the distribution of power of attorney for personal care forms an appropriate role for government? The astonishing success of government in distributing 2.4 million of its PAPC forms, compared to 100,000 forms distributed by the University of Toronto Joint Centre for Bioethics, underscores the superiority of government in the area of dissemination. But is government well situated to develop the best products for distribution?

Role of "Private" Individuals and Groups

In contrast to the predominantly governmental approach in Ontario's *Substitute Decisions Project*, other success stories illustrate the potential of private individuals and groups. The *Centre to Improve Care of the Dying* conducted the SUPPORT study, which shed important new light on the effectiveness of advance care planning. The *VITAS Healthcare Corporation* has been very innovative in addressing not only the care of the dying, but also the care of those who care for the dying. The *HIV Palliative Care Module* illustrates the power of collaboration among front-line workers committed to developing a useful resource in their area. The University of Toronto *Advance Care Planning Research Project* has shown that some of the assumptions upon which advance care planning programs are based are incorrect. An advance care planning program developed with this research in mind has a better chance of being effective, and research itself can be focused on evaluating different advance care planning programs. The success stories illustrate the potential of the private sector, including both academics and front-line health workers, to develop and evaluate programs in the area of death and dying.

Public/Private Partnerships

The success stories, in the context of the key findings from the literature, illustrate that both government and private individuals and groups have important and complementary roles to play in the development of social policy approaches to the issue of death and dying in Canada. Government has the ability to enact legislation in an area such as advance care planning.[11] As illustrated by the *HIV Palliative Care Module*, and the University of Toronto *Advance Care Planning Research Program*, government also has the ability to fund needed development and evaluation projects. Finally, as illustrated by Ontario's *Substitute Decisions Project*, and to a lesser extent by the *HIV Palliative Care Module*, government has superior dissemination powers. By contrast, as shown by the *HIV Palliative Care Module*, the University of Toronto *Advance Care Planning Research Program* and the *Centre to Improve Care of the Dying*, private individuals and groups, both academics and front-line health workers, have expertise in the development and evaluation of tools and programs.

The abilities of government and private individuals and groups is complementary. The experience reviewed suggests that private/public partnerships represent a promising model for social policy in the area of death and dying in Canada. The Ontario government's *Substitute Decisions Project* is a triumph of dissemination, but the program was not informed by the wealth of research in the health care literature with regard to advance care planning. The University of Toronto *Advance Care Planning Research Program* illustrates the potential of scholarly approaches to this area, but its success at dissemination was meagre by comparison to the *Substitute Decisions Project*.

---

11. The recent history of the Advocacy Act, Consent to Treatment Act and Substitute Decisions Act in Ontario highlights the need to do this in consultation with front-line workers, but a full development of this point is beyond the scope of this report.

Need to Involve Front-Line Health Workers and/or Consumers

The *HIV Palliative Care Module* was developed largely by front-line health workers. In the University of Toronto *Advance Care Planning Research Program,* research on the HIV advance directive was done in close collaboration with both front-line health workers (at the Toronto Hospital Immunodeficiency Clinic) and a consumer group (the AIDS Committee of Toronto). These linkages with front-line workers and consumers were pivotal to the success of these initiatives. The *VITAS Healthcare Corporation* has very successfully collaborated with their front-line caregivers to create a "moral community" in which issues related to the care of the dying can be addressed.

Need to Involve Academic Researchers

The involvement of academic researchers in the *Centre to Improve Care of the Dying* and the University of Toronto Joint Centre for Bioethics were pivotal to the success of that initiative. Probably, some blend of research and front-line worker/consumer involvement is ideal; that is, within the public/private partnerships there should be a partnership between researchers and front-line health workers/consumers. The exact mix would depend on the state of knowledge in a particular area. If knowledge is well developed perhaps a primary front-line approach would be preferable. If the state of knowledge is not well developed, perhaps more of a research approach would be needed.

Need for Multimethod Research

The University of Toronto experience suggests that complex social phenomena, like issues in death and dying, cannot be adequately understood with quantitative research alone. Complementary quantitative and qualitative approaches are needed. Quantitative studies can provide a description of the phenomena of death and dying, but qualitative methods such as grounded theory can help explain how and why the phenomena occur. Grounded theory is "a general methodology for developing theory that is grounded in data systematically gathered and analyzed" (Strauss and Corbin 1994, 273). It is particularly well suited to examine phenomena that are "conceptually dense" and involve social processes (reciprocal changes in patterns of action/interaction and in relationship with changes of conditions either internal or external to the process itself). Therefore, grounded theory is the appropriate methodology to explore, in depth and in context, the complex phenomena of death and dying (Berkwits and Aronowitz 1995). Qualitative methods have been recognized as a promising approach to bioethics (Hoffmaster 1992).

Need for Interdisciplinary Research

A lesson from the University of Toronto Joint Centre for Bioethics and the *Centre to Improve Care of the Dying* experiences is the need for inter-disciplinary or even transdisiplinary research on the complex phenomenon of death and dying, and policy responses to it. This conclusion also follows from the relationship between the social policy goals in the area of death and dying and the determinants of health framework. It is useful here to differentiate multidisciplinary, interdisciplinary and transdisciplinary research (Rosenfeld 1992). In multidisciplinary research, researchers work in parallel or sequentially from a disciplinary-specific base to address a common problem. In interdisciplinary research, researchers work jointly but still from a disciplinary-specific basis to address a common problem. In transdisciplinary research, researchers work jointly using a shared conceptual framework drawing together disciplinary-specific theories, concepts and approaches to address a common problem. As a practical matter, inter-disciplinary research is difficult to do, but research networks have been used with some success to foster interdisciplinary research. Two federal granting programs in Canada—the SSHRC Networks and the Networks of Centres of Excellence—have experience with research networks. The MacArthur Foundation has published a booklet about its experience with research networks (Kahn 1993).

Recommendations

There are three concrete steps that can advance this discussion into actions that help address the issues faced by dying Canadians:

1. Set social policy goals.
2. Develop a coherent research strategy to evaluate ways of achieving these goals.
3. Develop a coherent education strategy to disseminate the results of the research.

These steps are illustrated in figure 1.

With feedback from administrators, professionals and the public, the process allows for continuous quality assurance and permits all parties to influence the social policy process.

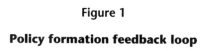

Figure 1

Policy formation feedback loop

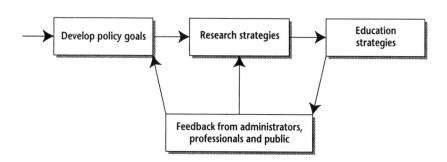

1. Set Social Policy Goals

The next step in social policy with regard to death and dying is to clarify the goals of social policy, and the appropriate role for government with respect to these goals. Health Canada, in collaboration with the provincial and territorial ministers of Health, should convene a conference to explicitly address this question. The conference should include interdisciplinary and interprofessional representation, strong consumer involvement, and representatives from palliative care, advance care planning, and euthanasia/ assisted suicide communities. Formal consensus-building methods (such as the Delphi technique) should be used to facilitate the process.

The determinants of health framework provides a useful conceptual tool to help clarify the goals of social policy in Canada with regard to death and dying (Evans and Stoddart 1990; Renaud 1993). A first attempt to articulate goals based on the determinants of health framework might include those listed in table 3.

Once the goals are clarified, Health Canada and the provincial ministries of Health should develop a targeted and cohesive program of funding, supporting and disseminating these goals. The program should have defined objectives and milestones, and it should be time limited. The program should foster interdisciplinary approaches, and collaborations among researchers, front-line health workers, and government policymakers. The program itself should provide an evaluative framework, flowing from the articulated goals of social policy, by which the success of the individual initiatives can be measured. It should be based on a two-pronged approach involving research and education strategies.

Table 3

Social policy goals vs. determinants of health framework

Determinant of health	Goals
Physical	• Controlling pain • Optimizing physical functioning
Psychological	• Fostering a sense of control (likely related to the social science concept, "control of destiny" [Syme 1994]) • Eliminating fear and anxiety
Social	• Strengthening relationships • Providing opportunities for social contact (avoiding isolation)
Cultural	• Providing a process that is consistent with cultural beliefs and "rituals" • Providing access to spiritual guidance and comfort and ensuring freedom for spiritual practices
Economic	• Fostering the ability to use planning tools (e.g., powers of attorney, wills, etc.) • Avoiding impoverishment due to illness

2. Develop a Coherent Research Strategy

Once the social policy goals are well articulated, Health Canada and the provincial Health ministries should collaborate with the federal research funding councils in developing a coherent research strategy designed to examine the systemic, policy, institutional, clinical and educational changes needed to achieve the goals. Currently, none of the federal research funding councils earmarks funds for research targeted directly at improving the care of the dying. Since funding opportunities are key to driving the research agenda, funds should be designated to examine efficient, effective and ethical ways of translating the policy goals into care practice at both the micro (clinical) and macro (system and institutional) levels.

Many important issues in end-of-life care remain poorly addressed by research, including questions such as:

• What are the physical, psychological, spiritual and social needs of the dying?
• What systems and structures are necessary to meet the needs of the dying?
• What care do people expect to receive when dying and how does this correspond to the care they actually receive? What effect does this correspondence, or lack of correspondence, have on well-being?

- How do health care professionals care for the dying? Are there alternative strategies that would better meet the needs of the dying?
- What type of care are health care professionals prepared to provide? How can education strategies be adapted to prepare professionals to meet the needs of the dying?
- How can palliative care programs be meaningfully evaluated?
- How effective are existing palliative care programs?
- How can advance care planning programs be meaningfully evaluated?
- How do current health care resource allocation policies correspond to the needs of the population and to the dying?
- What are the long-term social implications of decriminalizing euthanasia/ assisted suicide?
- Can effective advance care planning and palliative care adequately address the needs of the dying and so render euthanasia/assisted suicide moot?

The research agenda should include an effort to develop new models of health care delivery that are better suited to meet the needs of the dying. The models could address any or all of resource allocation decisions, institutional, organizational and clinical restructuring, financing and/or reimbursement strategies. These models should be tested according to well-established, rigorous, time-limited, program evaluation strategies.

In 1993, the U.S. Institute of Medicine (IOM) convened a committee to consider the merits of conducting a full-scale study of care near the end of life (Committee for a Feasibility Study on Care at the End of Life 1994). Subsequently, the IOM has undertaken the full study entitled *Approaching Death: Decision Making and Appropriate Care.* The goals of the project are to:

- examine the state of knowledge about clinical, legal and other important aspects of care for patients with life-threatening medical problems;
- evaluate methods for measuring outcomes, predicting survival and functional status, determining patient and family preferences, and assessing quality of care;
- identify organizational, financial and other factors that impede or promote high-quality care for patients approaching death; and
- recommend steps that policymakers, practitioners and others can take to improve care for those with terminal illnesses, and increase agreement on what constitutes appropriate care.

This study, which will be completed in 1997, may help to further define a research strategy with respect to the end of life.

3. Develop a Coherent Education Strategy

Education should be seen as an issue in research dissemination—another segment in the policy formation feedback loop.

Policy symposia can be used to transmit and translate research findings to both governmental and institutional administrators. Scholars who have done high-quality work relative to the social policy goals should be provided with fora to disseminate research findings and simultaneously engage in dialogue with policymakers.

Education standards for issues in death and dying should be set by the relevant bodies for the undergraduate and postgraduate professional education of health professionals (e.g., Association of Canadian Medical Colleges, College of Family Physicians of Canada, Royal College of Physicians and Surgeons of Canada in the case of physicians). These standards would be consistent with the social policy goals and incorporate the pertinent research findings.

A public education campaign using public media, community agencies and institutional public relations should be conducted to keep the public abreast of policy discussions and decisions (thus enabling them to provide input). Public education would also help shape the public's expectations of the care available to them from the "system" so that individuals can best formulate their own advance care plan for end-of-life care.

CONCLUSIONS

The public stereotype of dying is a patient hooked-up to a machine, in pain, and out of control. Social policy must respond to this image by improving dying in Canada. Palliative care, advance care planning, and euthanasia/assisted suicide are social policy responses to the problems of dying in Canada. Unfortunately, the overall goals of social policy with regard to death and dying in Canada have never been articulated. Although it may seem paradoxical, this paper recommends that policymakers think of improving the process of dying in Canada as a natural aspect of the nation's "health." This conceptual shift is facilitated by the determinants of health framework which provides a coherent way to approach social policy related to death and dying in Canada. This report makes three recommendations:
 1. set social policy goals with respect to death and dying;
 2. develop a coherent research strategy to evaluate ways of achieving these goals; and
 3. develop a coherent education strategy to disseminate the results of the research.

The approach suggested in this report provides a way for government, and private individuals and groups, to respond to the problems, and to improve dying in Canada.

Peter A. Singer, *M.D., MPH., FRCPC, is the Sun Life chair in bioethics and director of the University of Toronto Joint Centre for Bioethics. He is also an associate professor of medecine and practices internal medicine at The Toronto Hospital. He studied internal medicine at the University of Toronto, medical ethics at the University of Chicago, and clinical epidemiology at Yale University. He is a National Health Research scholar of Health Canada, and has published extensively on medical ethics.*

Douglas K. Martin, *Ph.D., is research associate at the University of Toronto Joint Centre for Bioethics. He studied bioethics at the University of Toronto.*

BIBLIOGRAPHY

ADVANCE DIRECTIVES SEMINAR GROUP. 1992. Advance directives: Are they an advance? *Canadian Medical Association Journal* 146: 127–34.

Advanced Health Care Directives Act, SN, 1995, c.A–4.1.

Airedale NHS Trust v. Bland [1993] A.C. 789 (H.L.).

ATKINSON, P. 1984. Training for certainty. *Social Science and Medicine* 19(9): 949–56.

BACKMAN, J. G., K. H. ALCSER, D. J. DOUKAS, R. L. LICHTENSTEIN, A. D. CORNING and H. BRODY. 1996. Attitudes of Michigan physicians and the public toward legalizing physician-assisted suicide and voluntary euthanasia. *New England Journal of Medecine* 334(5): 303–309.

BERGER, P. 1967. *The Sacred Canopy, Elements of a Sociological Theory of Religion*. New York (NY): Doubleday.

BERKWITS, M., and R. ARONOWITZ. 1995. Different questions beg different methods. *Journal of General Internal Medicine* 10: 409–410.

BERRY, S. R., and P. A. SINGER. 1995. Development and evaluation of a cancer living will. *Clinical and Investigative Medicine* 18(suppl.): B11A.

BLACKHALL, L. J., S. T. MURPHY, G. FRANK, V. MICHEL, and S. AZEN. 1995. Ethnicity and attitudes towards patient autonomy. *Journal of the American Medical Association* 274: 820–825.

BLOCH, S. D. 1994. Patients' requests to hasten death: Evaluation and management in terminal care. *Archives of Internal Medicine* 154: 2039–2047.

BOZINOFF, L., and P. MACINTOSH. 1989; Monday, July 24. Dramatic increase in support for euthanasia. *The Gallup Report (Canada)*. Toronto (ON): Gallup.

_____. 1991; November 7. Three in four Canadians favour legalized euthanasia. *The Gallup Report (Canada)*. Toronto (ON): Gallup.

BOZINOFF, L., and A. TURCOTTE. 1992; November 23. Majority of Canadians continue to support legalized euthanasia. *The Gallup Report (Canada)*. Toronto (ON): Gallup.

BRAZIL, K., and D. THOMAS. 1995. The role of volunteers in a hospital-based palliative care service. *Journal of Palliative Care* 11(3): 40–42.

CALLAHAN, D. 1987. *Setting Limits: Medical Goals in an Aging Society*. New York (NY): Simon and Shuster.

CANCER 2000 TASK FORCE. 1992. *The Proceedings of Cancer 2000*. Toronto (ON): Canadian Cancer Society.

CARALIS, P. V., B. DAVIS, K. WRIGHT, and E. MARCIAL. 1994. The influence of ethnicity and race on attitudes toward advance directives, life-prolonging treatments, and euthanasia. *Journal of Clinical Ethics* 4: 155–165.

CHAMBERS, C. V., J. J. DIAMOND, R L. PERKEL, and L. A. LASCH. 1994. Relationship of advance directives to hospital charges in a medicare population. *Archives of Internal Medicine* 154: 541–547.

CHOUDHRY, N. K., J. MA, I. RASOOLY, and P. A. SINGER. 1994. Long-term care facility policies on life-sustaining treatments and advance directives. *Journal of the American Geriatric Society* 42: 1150–1153.

Civil Code of Québec. Article 11.

CMA POLICY SUMMARY. 1992. Advance directives for resuscitation and other life-saving or sustaining measures. *Canadian Medical Association Journal* 146: 1072A.

COHEN-MANSFIELD, J., J. A. DROGE, and N. BILLING. 1991. The utilization of the durable power of attorney for health care among hospitalized elderly patients. *Journal of the American Geriatric Society* 39: 1174–1178.

COHEN-MANSFIELD, J., B. A. RABINOVICH, S. LIPSON, A. FEIN, B. GERBER, S. WEISMAN, and L. G. PAWLSON. 1991. The decision to execute a durable power of attorney for health care and preferences regarding the utilization of life-sustaining treatments in nursing home residents. *Archives of Internal Medicine* 151: 289–294.

COMMITTEE FOR A FEASIBILITY STUDY ON CARE AT THE END OF LIFE. M. J. FIELD. Eds. 1994. *Summary of Committee Views and Workshop Examining the Feasibility of an Institute of Medicine Study of Dying Decision Making and Appropriate Care.* Washington (DC): Institute of Medicine.

Consent to Treatment Act, SO, 1992, c. 31.

COUNCIL ON SCIENTIFIC AFFAIRS, AMERICAN MEDICAL ASSOCIATION. 1996. Good care of the dying patient. *Journal of the Americal Medical Association* 275: 474–478.

DANIS, M., J. GARRETT, R. HARRIS, and D. L. PATRICK. 1994. Stability of choices about life-sustaining treatment. *Annals of Internal Medicine* 120: 567–573.

DANIS, M., L. I. SOUTHERLAND, J. M. GARRETT, et al. 1991. A prospective study of advance directives for life-sustaining care. *New England Journal of Medicine* 324: 882–888.

DOSSETOR, J. 1994. Ethics of palliative care in the context of limited resources: An essay on the need for attitudinal change. *Journal of Palliative Care* 10(3): 39–42.

EMANUEL, E.J. 1994a. Euthanasia: Historical, ethical, and empiric perspectives. *Archives of Internal Medicine* 154: 1890–1901.

———. 1994b. The history of euthanasia debates in the United States and Britain. *Annals of Internal Medicine* 121: 793–802.

EMANUEL, E. J., D. S. WEINBERG, R. GONIN, L. R. HUMMEL, and L. L. EMANUEL. 1993. How well is the Patient Self-Determination Act working? An early assessment. *American Journal of Medicine* 95: 619–628.

EMANUEL, L. 1993. Advance directives: What have we learned so far? *Journal of Clinical Ethics* 4: 8–15.

EMANUEL, L. L., M. J. BARRY, J. D. STOECKLE, L. M. ETTELSON, and E. J. EMANUEL. 1991. Advance directives for medical care—a case for greater use. *New England Journal of Medicine* 324: 889–895.

EMANUEL, L. L., E. J. EMANUEL, J. D. STOECKLE, L. R. HUMMEL, and M. J. BARRY. 1994. Advance directives: Stability of patients' treatment choices. *Archives of Internal Medicine* 154: 209–217.

EVANS, R. G., and G. L. STODDART. 1990. Producing health: Consuming health care. *Social Science and Medicine* 31: 1347–1353.

FADEN, R., T. L. BEAUCHAMP, and N. M. P. KING. 1986. *A History and Theory of Informed Consent.* New York (NY): Oxford University Press.

FERRIS, F. D., J. S. FLANNERY, H. B. MCNEAL, M. R. MORISSETTE, R. CAMERON, G. A. BALLY. Eds. 1995. The interrelationship of palliative care and HIV/AIDS. In *A Comprehensive Guide for the Care of Persons with HIV Disease, Module 4: Palliative Care.* Toronto (ON): Mount Sinai Hospital/ Casey House Hospice.

FINS, J.J. 1994. The physician-assisted suicide debate: An annotated bibliography of representative articles. *Journal of Clinical Ethics* 5: 329–340.

FOX, R. 1957. Training for uncertainty. In *The Student Physician*, ed. R. K. MERTON. Cambridge (MA): Harvard University Press.

FRANKL, D., R. K. OYE, and P. E. BELLAMY. 1989. Attitudes of hospitalized patients toward life-support: a survey of 200 medical inpatients. *American Journal of Medicine* 86: 645–648.

FRASER, R., and W. ADAIR. 1989. Volunteers and patient support. *J. Palliat. Care* 5(2): 52–55.

GAMBLE, E. R., P. J. MCDONALD, and P. R. LICHSTEIN. 1991. Knowledge, attitudes and behavior of elderly persons regarding living wills. *Archives of Internal Medicine* 151: 277–280.

GENIUS, S. J., S. K. GENIUS, and W. C. CHANG. 1994. Public attitudes toward the right to die. *Canadian Medical Association Journal* 150: 701–708.

GEVERS, S. 1995. Physician-assisted suicide: New developments in the Netherlands. *Bioethics* 9: 309–312.

GILLON, R. 1986. *Philosophical Medical Ethics.* Toronto (ON): John Wiley and Sons.

GRAY, J. 1993. *Beyond the New Right.* London and New York: Routledge.

GREER, D. S., V. MOR, J. N. MORRIS, S. SHERWOOD, D. KIDDER, and H. BIRNBAUM. 1986. An alternative in terminal care: Results of the National Hospice Study. *Journal of Chronic Disease* 39: 9–26.

HARE, J., and C. NELSON. 1991. Will outpatients complete living wills? A comparison of two interventions. *Journal of General Internal Medicine* 6: 41–46.

HENDIN, H., C. RUTENFRANS, and Z. ZYLICA. 1997. Physician-assisted suicide and euthanasia in the Netherlands: Lessons from the Dutch. *Journal of the American Medical Association* 277(21): 1720–1722.

HIGGINSON, I. 1995. What do palliative staff think about audit? *Journal of Palliative Care* 11(3): 17–19.

HIGH, D. M. 1993. Advance directives and the elderly: A study of intervention strategies to increase use. *Gerontologist* 33: 342–349.

HOFFMASTER, B. 1992. Can ethnography save the life of medical ethics? *Social Science and Medicine* 35: 1421–1431.

HOLLEY, J. L., S. NESPOR, and R. RAULT. 1993. Chronic in-center hemodialysis patients' attitudes, knowledge and behavior toward advance directives. *Journal of the American Society of Nephrology* 3: 1405–1408.

HUGHES, D. L., and P. A. SINGER. 1992. Family physicians' attitudes towards advance directives. *Canadian Medical Association Journal* 146: 1937–1944.

HUMPHREY, D., and A. WICKETT. 1986. *The Right to Die: Understanding Euthanasia.* New York (NY): Harper & Row.

JAMES, C. R., and R. D. MACLEOD. 1993. The problematic nature of education in palliative care. *Journal of Palliative Care* 9(4): 5–10.

JOCHEMSON, H. 1994. Euthanasia in Holland: An ethical critique of the new law. *Journal of Medical Ethics* 20: 212–217.

JOOS, S. K., J. B. REULER, J. L. POWELL, and D. H. HICKAM. 1993. Outpatients' attitudes and understanding regarding living wills. *Journal of General Internal Medicine* 8: 259–263.

KAHN, R. L. 1993. *The MacArthur Foundation Program in Mental Health and Human Development: An Experiment in Scientific Organization.* Chicago (IL): MacArthur Foundation.

KANE, R .L., J. WALES, L. BERNSTEIN, A. LEIBOWITZ, and S. KAPLAN. 1984. A randomized controlled trial of hospice care. *Lancet* 1: 890–894.

KASS, L. R. 1990. Death with dignity and the sanctity of life. *Commentary* 89: 33–34.

KELNER, M. J., and I. L. BOURGEAULT. 1993. Patient control over dying: Responses of health care professionals. *Social Science and Medicine* 36: 757–765.

KÜBLER-ROSS, E. 1969. *On Death and Dying.* New York (NY): MacMillan.

KUHSE, H., and P. SINGER. 1988. Doctors' practices and attitudes regarding voluntary euthanasia. *Medical Journal of Australia* 148: 623–627.

———. 1992. Euthanasia: A survey of nurses attitudes and practices. *Australian Nurses Journal* 21: 21–22.

LEE, M. A., H. D. NELSON, V. P. TILDEN, L. GANZINI, T. A. SCHMIDT, and S. W. TOLLE. 1996. Legalizing assisted suicide: Views of physicians in Oregon. *New England Journal of Medicine* 334(5): 310–315.

LO, B., G. A. MCLEOD, and G. SAIKA. 1986. Patient attitudes to discussing life-sustaining treatment. *Archives of Internal Medicine* 146: 1613–1615.

LUPTAK, M. K., and C. BOULT. 1994. A method for increasing elders' use of advance directives. *Gerontologist* 34: 409–412.

Malette v. Shulman. 1990. 72 OR 2d 417 (Ont. CA).

MARGOLESE, R. G., and W. K. ADAIR. 1992. Cancer 2000: The need for coordination. *Journal of Palliative Care* 8(1): 9–12.

MARKSON, L. J., J. FANALE, K. STEEL, D. KERN, and G. ANNAS. 1994. Implementing advance directives in the primary care setting. *Archives of Internal Medicine* 154: 2321–2327.

MASON, C., and G. FENTON. 1992. How successful is teaching on terminal care? *Medical Education* 18: 394–400.

Medical Consent Act, RSNS, 1989, c. 279.

MELVIN, J. L. 1980. Interdisciplinary and multidisciplinary activities and the ACRM. *Archives of Physical and Medical Rehabilitation* 61: 379–380.

MEYER, J. 1993. Lay participation in care: A challenge for multidisciplinary teamwork. *Journal of Interprofessional Care* 7(1): 57–66.

MILL, J. S. 1987. *On Liberty.* Harmondsworth, Middlesex , U.K.: Penguin Classics.

MOLLOY, D. W., and G. GUYATT. 1991. A comprehensive health care directive in a home for the aged. *Canadian Medical Association Journal* 145: 307–311.

MOLLOY, D. W., G. GUYATT, E. ELEMAYHEU, and W. E. MCILROY. 1991. Treatment preferences, attitudes toward advance directives and concerns about health care. *Humane Medicine* 7: 285–290.

MOLLOY, D. W., M. URBANYI, J. R. HORSMAN, G. H. GUYATT, and M. BEDARD. 1992. Two years experience with a comprehensive health care directive in a home for the aged. *Annals of the Royal College of Physicians and Surgeons of Canada* 25: 433–436.

MORRISON, R. S., E. OLSON, K. R. MERTZ, and D. E. MEIER. 1995. The inaccessibility of advance directives on transfer from ambulatory to acute care settings. *Journal of the American Medical Association* 274: 478–482.

MOUNT, B. 1992. Volunteer support services: A key component of palliative care. *Journal of Palliative Care* 8(1): 59–64.

NORTHERN TERRITORY OF AUSTRALIA. 1995. *Rights of the Terminally Ill Bill.* Passed in the Legislative Assembly of the Northern Territory on May 25th.

NOVICK, A. 1995. Some thoughts on AIDS and death. *The Journal of Clinical Ethics* 6(1): 91–92.

OGDEN, R. D. 1994a. *Euthanasia, Assisted Suicide and AIDS.* Pitt Meadows (BC): Perrault & Goodman.

_____. 1994b. The right to die: A policy proposal for euthanasia and aid in dying. *Canadian Public Policy* 20: 1–25.

Oregon's Death with Dignity Act (Ballot Measure 16), 1995.

PARKES, C. M. 1980. Terminal care: Evaluation of an advisory domiciliary service at St. Christopher's Hospice. *Postgraduate Medical Journal* 56: 685–689.

PFEIFER, M. P., J. E. SIDOROV, A. C. SMITH, et al. 1994. The discussion of end-of-life medical care by primary care patients and their physicians: A multicenter study using structured qualitative interviews. *Journal of General Internal Medicine* 9: 82–88.

PIJNENBORG, L. 1994. Nationwide study of decisions concerning the end of life in general practice in the Netherlands. *British Medical Journal* 309: 1209–1212.

POPE JOHN PAUL II. 1995. *The Gospel of Life (Evangelium Vitae): The Encyclical Letter on Abortion, Euthanasia, and the Death Penalty in Today's World.* New York (NY): Random House.

RAMSEY, P. 1974. The indignity of "Death with Dignity". *Hastings Center Studies* 2: 47–62. Reprinted in *On Moral Medicine: Theological Perspectives in Medical Ethics*, eds. S. E. LAMMERS, and A. VERHEY. Grand Rapids (MI): William B. Eerdmans Publishing Co. pp. 185–196.

RASOOLY, I., J. V. LAVERY, S. UROWITZ, et al. 1994. Hospital policies on life-sustaining treatments and advance directives in Canada. *Canadian Medical Association Journal* 150: 1265–1270.

REILLY, B. M., M. WAGNER, J. ROSS, C. R. MAGNUSSEN, L. PAPA, and J. ASH. 1995a. Promoting completion of health care proxies following hospitalization. *Archives of Internal Medicine* 155: 2202–2206.

_____. 1995b. Promoting inpatient directives about life-sustaining treatments in a community hospital. *Archives of Internal Medicine* 155: 2317–2323.

RENAUD, M. 1993. The future: Hygeia versus Panakeia. *Health and Canadian Society* 1: 229–249.

Representation Agreement Act, S.B.C., 1993, c. 67.

Rodriguez v. British Columbia (Attorney General). File no. 23476. 1993: May 20; 1993: Sept. 30.

ROSENFELD, P. L. 1992. The potential transdisciplinary research for sustaining and extending linkages between health and social sciences. *Social Science and Medicine* 11: 1342–1357.

ROY, D. J. 1995. Is humanity too costly a place to keep open? *Journal of Palliative Care* 11(3): 3–4.

RUBIN, S. M., W. M. STRULL, M. F. FIALKOW, S. J. WEISS, and B. LO. 1994. Increasing the completion of the durable power of attorney for health care: A randomized, controlled trial. *Journal of the American Medical Association* 271: 209–212.

SACHS, G. A., C. B. STOCKING, and S. H. MILES. 1992. Empowerment of the older patient? A randomized controlled trial to increase discussion and use of advance directives. *Journal of the American Geriatric Society* 40: 269–273.

SACHS, G. A., J. C. AHRONHEIM, R. A. RHYMES, L. VOLICER, and J. LYNN. 1995. Good care of dying patients: The alternative to physician-assisted suicide and euthanasia. *Journal of the American Geriatric Society* 43: 553–562.

SAM, M., and P. A. SINGER. 1993. Canadian outpatients and advance directives: Poor knowledge, little experience, but positive attitudes. *Canadian Medical Association Journal* 148: 1497–1502.

SCHNEIDERMAN, L. J., R. KRONICK, R. M. KAPLAN, J. P. ANDERSON, and R. D. LANGER. 1992. Effects of offering advance directives on medical treatments and costs. *Annals of Internal Medicine* 117: 599–606.

SCOTT, J. F. 1992. Palliative Care 2000: Mapping the interface with cancer control. *Journal of Palliative Care* 8: 13–16.

――――. 1994. More palliative care? The economics of denial. *Journal of Palliative Care* 10(3): 35–38.

SEARLES, N. 1995. Silence doesn't obliterate the truth: A Manitoba survey on physician-assisted suicide and euthanasia. Prepared for the Manitoba Association for Rights and Liberties.

SENATE OF CANADA. 1995. *On Life and Death: Report of the Special Senate Committee on Euthanasia and Assisted Suicide.*

SHMERLING, R. H., S. E. BEDELL, A. LILIENFEL, et al. 1988. Discussing cardiopulmonary resuscitation: A study of elderly outpatients. *Journal of General Internal Medicine* 3: 317–321.

SILVERMAN, H. J., P. TUMA, M. H. SCHAEFFER, and B. SINGH. 1995. Implementation of the patient self-determination act in a hospital setting. *Archives of Internal Medicine* 155: 502–510.

SINGER, P. A. 1994. Disease-specific advance directives. *Lancet* 344: 594–596.

――――. 1995. Advance directive fallacies. *Health Law in Canada* 16: 5–9.

SINGER, P. A., S. CHOUDHRY, and J. ARMSTRONG. 1993. Public opinion regarding consent to treatment. *Journal of the American Geriatric Society* 41: 112–116.

SINGER P. A., G. ROBERTSON, and D. J. ROY. Bioethics for clinicians VII: Advance care planning. *Can. Med. Assoc. J.* 1996, 155: 1689–1692.

SINGER, P. A., S. CHOUDHRY, J. ARMSTRONG, E. M. MESLIN, and F. H. LOWY. 1995. Public opinion regarding end of life decisions: Influence of prognosis, practice and process. *Social Science and Medicine* 41: 1517–1521.

SINGER, P. A., E. C. THIEL, I. SALIT, W. PLANAGAN, and C. D. NAYLOR. In press. The HIV-specific advance directive. *J. Gen. Intern. Med.*

SINGER, P. A., D. K. MARTIN, J. V. LAVERY, E. C. THIEL, M. KELNER, and D. C. MENDELSSOHN. In press. Reconceptualizing advance care planning from the patient's perspective. *Arch. Intern. Med.*

SINGER, P. A., E. C. THIEL, C. D. NAYLOR, R. M. A. RICHARDSON, H. LLEWELLYN-THOMAS, M. GOLDSTEIN, C. SAIPHOO, P. R. ULDALL, D. KIM, and D. C. MENDELSSOHN. 1995. Life-sustaining treatment preferences of hemodialysis patients: Implications for advance directives. *Journal of the American Society of Nephrology* 6: 1410–1417.

SLOME, L., J. MOULTON, C. HUFFINE, R. GORTER, and D. ABRAMS. 1992. Physicians' attitudes toward assisted suicide in AIDS. *Journal of Acquired Immune Deficiency Syndrome* 5: 712–718.

SMITH, G. 1994. Palliative care in Toronto for people with AIDS: The impact of class on poor PWAs. *Journal of Palliative Care* 10(2): 50.

STOLMAN, C. J., J. J. GREGORY, D. DUNN, and J. L. LEVINE. 1990. Evaluation of patient, physician, nurse and family attitudes toward do not resuscitate orders. *Archives of Internal Medicine* 150: 653–658.

STRAUSS, A., and J. CORBIN. 1994. Grounded theory methodology: An overview. In *Handbook of Qualitative Research*, eds. N. K. DENZIN, and Y. S. LINCOLN. Thousand Oaks (CA): Sage. pp. 273–285.

Substitute Decisions Act, SO, 1992, c. 30.

SYME, S. L. 1994. The social evironment and health. *Daedalus* 123: 79–86.

TENO, J. M., H. L. NELSON, and J. LYNN. 1994. Advance care planning: Priorities for ethical and empirical research. *Hastings Center Report* Nov.–Dec. (suppl.): S32–36.

TENO, J., J. FLEISHMAN, et al. 1990. The use of formal prior directives among patients with HIV-related disease. *Journal of General Internal Medicine* 5: 490–494.

TENO, J. M., J. LYNN, R. S. PHILLIPS, et al. 1994. Do formal advance directives affect resuscitation decisions and the use of resources for seriously ill patients? *Journal of Clinical Ethics* 5: 23–30.

The Health Care Directives and Consequential Amendments Act, SM, 1992, c.33.

THE SUPPORT PRINCIPAL INVESTIGATORS. 1995. A controlled trial to improve care for seriously ill hospitalized patients: The Study to Understand Prognosis and Preferences for Outcomes and Risks of Treatment (SUPPORT). *Journal of the American Medical Association* 274: 1591–1598.

TWYCROSS, R., and LACK, S. A. 1983. *Symptom Control in Far-Advanced Cancer: Pain Relief.* London: Pitman.

UNIVERSITY OF GLASGOW. 1993. *Unite the Team!* London: University of Glasgow, University of Dundee.

VAN DER MAAS, P. J., L. PIJNENBORG, and J. J. M. VAN DELDEN. 1995. Changes in Dutch opinions on active euthanasia, 1966 through 1991. *Journal of the American Medical Association* 273: 1411–1414.

VAN DER MAAS, P. J., J. J. M. VAN DELDEN, L. PIJNENBORG, and C. W. N. LOOMAN. 1992. Euthanasia and other medical decisions concerning the end of life. *Health Policy* 22: 44–45.

VAN DER MAAS, P. J., G. VAN DER WAL, I. HOVERKATE et al. 1996. Euthanasia, physician-assisted suicide, and other medical practices involving the end of life in the Netherlands, 1990–1995. *New England Journal of Medicine* 335: 1609–1705.

WASHINGTON STATE INITIATIVE 119. 1991. *A Voluntary Choice for Terminally Ill Persons: Death with Dignity.*

WORLD HEALTH ORGANIZATION. 1990. *Expert Committee Report: Cancer Pain Relief and Palliative Care.* (Technical report series 804.) Geneva, Switzerland.

Labour Adjustment Policy and Health: Considerations for a Changing World

TERRENCE SULLIVAN, PH.D.
OKURI UNEKE, PH.D.
JOHN LAVIS, M.D., PH.D.
DOUG HYATT, PH.D.
JOHN O'GRADY

Institute for Work & Health

SUMMARY

In response to the forces of globalization, technological innovation, and trade agreements, most Western countries have experienced and continue to experience significant economic restructuring. Within the Organization for Economic Co-operation and Development (OECD) area, these changes have increased unemployment; rapidly changed skill requirements, and lowered the demand for unskilled labour; widened the income gap and the number of the working poor; and increased long-term unemployment, self-employment, part-time work and temporary employment. In Canada, these forces, coupled with a large national debt, have led to fiscal restraint by all levels of government, with associated cuts in social welfare spending. All of these changes affect the health of populations. What is the best way to understand these consequences? What practical considerations can Canada entertain to buffer the health consequences of labour market changes as we make adjustments to the new competitive order?

These changes flowing from globalization, technological innovation and trade agreements must be understood in a population health context. The state of the economy and labour market conditions are linked, and they directly and indirectly affect the health and well-being of both working and nonworking people. National income and its distribution, which depends in part on the value-added trade of goods and services on international markets, are associated with effects on health status of the population. National prosperity also influences health through the social environments in which people live and work. Health conditions become less favourable with declining income and with lower occupational and social status; thus people in disadvantaged circumstances encounter more risk factors and health hazards. There is evidence that widening social inequalities adversely affect national mortality and morbidity rates. Active labour adjustment strategies may buffer these adverse consequences.

A number of different types of initiatives could improve labour adjustment, and some of these initiatives have taken place with health in mind. The steel and electronics manufacturing industries in Canada provide an example of a national initiative. The Ontario Training and Adjustment Board (OTAB) and the Health Sector Training and Adjustment Program (HSTAP) in Ontario provide examples of regional labour adjustment programs. The development of the OTAB was actively supported by the Premier's Council on Health Strategy, a multistakeholder policy advisory group. However, labour adjustment mechanisms seem unable to do much for the long-term unemployed, and some comprehensive income assistance program seems necessary to assist these people.

Sweden and the Netherlands have gone further to make the link between state labour adjustment programs and health. Swedish and Dutch social policies target health inequities, but the two countries organize and execute their programs in different ways.

The impacts of labour adjustment programs on population health presents a challenge to policymakers. Cross-sectoral collaboration may encourage health-sensitive adjustment mechanisms and policies, such as geographic and sectoral adjustment agencies. Adjustment strategies leave at least partially unaddressed the issue of unemployment and maldistribution of work. Strategies for reducing working time are worthy of consideration.

There exist a number of barriers to a focus on health outcomes in labour adjustment, most notably the weak institutional role of health in public policymaking. Social reporting and policy indicators (e.g., a social GDP indicator) are needed to improve the analysis of the social costs of labour market experiences, such as of unemployment. More innovative research and multistakeholder processes are also needed.

TABLE OF CONTENTS

APPENDICES

LIST OF FIGURES

LIST OF TABLES

INTRODUCTION

In recent years, economic restructuring has become a striking feature of advanced economies in response to the three forces of globalization, rapid technological innovation, and trade agreements (Banting et al. 1995; Drache and Boyer 1996). These forces have driven a host of transnational changes involving firms in cross-border trade, foreign direct investment (FDI, which refers to the acquisition of real assets by nonresidents), product development, financing, production, marketing, sales and warehousing. Workers around the world now live in economies that are partly or fully integrated into the world market for goods and capital (World Development Report 1995).

As Lavis (1996) has argued, these forces appear to have altered how firms deal with their workforces and their demand for labour. For example, part-time hiring gives firms versatility and keeps down the cost of employee benefit. Retaining a core of long-term staff and hiring full-time workers on short-term contracts accommodates the volatility of open international markets. The nature and organization of available jobs is also changing. Demanding more from experienced workers can increase productivity, and contracting out can reduce overhead.

These changes have made a substantial impact on the domestic labour market beyond normal business cycle changes. They increase unemployment and polarize the labour market. Labour market polarization is characterized by a simultaneous decline in middle-income jobs and growth in both high-skill, high-wage jobs and low-skill, low-wage jobs (Banting et al. 1995).

Recent research on the determinants of health underscores that, like globalization and labour market changes, national prosperity has both macroeconomic and microeconomic effects on the health of populations (Frank and Mustard 1994; Evans, Barer, and Marmor 1994, Fogel 1993). Canadian federal and provincial governments are beginning to adopt this perspective (Canadian Federal, Provincial and Territorial Advisory Committee on Population Health 1994). Given that labour force changes can affect health, firms and governments become concerned with the amount of unemployment and how it affects health. Market strategies to enhance survivability and profitability in the competitive international environment are developed to benefit those firms that adopt them. Social losses are borne, not by the firms, but by workers, particularly the unemployed and their families, and by society as a whole (Lavis 1996). The workforce in Canada will not remain active and healthy unless government, business and labour cooperate to improve the labour market outcomes.

The first section of this paper, "Literature Review," highlights globalization, labour market trends in Canada, the link between health and unemployment, and the relationship between income and health. The section "Success Stories" provides examples of successful regional and national adjustment programs that have the potential to buffer some adverse labour market effects on health. The section "Policy Considerations" discusses geographic and sectoral adjustment processes, including working time and the distribution of work. It also addresses how the institutional legacy of health care can impede health improvement through labour adjustment policy, and what can be learned from the case studies. The final section, "Conclusions and Recommendations," concludes the paper with some policy recommendations.

LITERATURE REVIEW

Globalization

Globalization reflects the strategies of companies to exploit competitive advantages in international markets, to use favourable local inputs and infrastructure, and to locate in final markets (OECD 1995). Capital mobility and technological change have been the major forces driving global integration. International transport, communication and trade are easier today because political and ideological conflicts that partitioned the economic world for decades have eased. The changing attitude of developing countries is also important in reversing their failed import substitution–based development. These global influences have affected labour markets, and are affecting employment in the advanced economies of the OECD.

Canada has some unique labour market trends, but it shares many with other OECD countries. Between 1989 and 1991, Canada experienced a negative net employment change (table 1). In 1994, Canada's employment rate of 10.4 percent was surpassed only by those of France and Italy (table 2). Throughout the OECD, the relative importance of employment in manufacturing declined while employment in services increased (appendix 1). This shift to service sectors arises partly from changes in consumption patterns, trade and technology, reflecting how service-type activities formerly carried out within the industrial sector are increasingly being contracted out (OECD 1995). Two-thirds of all OECD jobs are now service sector jobs, although variations between countries exist (appendix 3). Canada and the United States have higher service sector employment—wholesale and retail trade, particularly in restaurants and hotels—than any other region.

These jobs are generally low skilled and low paid. Canada and the United States also have more employees in high-skilled and high-paid finance, real estate and business service sectors. Other OECD employment trends include the following:
- growth in self-employment, part-time work and temporary employment;
- unemployment caused by rapid changes in skill requirements because jobs and job seekers do not match—in the 1980s, employment grew faster in white-collar jobs (professional, administrative, managerial,

Table 1

Job gains and job losses for selected OECD countries
Average annual rates as a percentage of total employment

Country	Period	Gross job gains	Gross job losses	Net change
Canada	1989–1991	13.4	– 16.5	– 3.1
Denmark	1983–1989	16.0	– 14.5	– 5.2
France	1989–1992	13.7	– 13.9	– 0.2
Germany	1983–1990	9.0	– 7.5	1.5
Italy	1989–1992	11.8	– 11.9	– 0.1
New Zealand	1987–1992	15.7	– 19.8	– 4.1
Sweden	1989–1992	12.6	– 16.1	– 3.5
United Kingdom	1989–1991	8.0	– 6.4	1.6
United States	1989–1991	12.6	– 11.1	1.4

Source: Excerpts, OECD Jobs Study, 1995, Part I, p.17.

Table 2

Unemployment rates (%) in selected OECD countries, 1985–1994

	1985	1986	1987	1988	1989	1990	1991	1992	1993	1994
Canada	10.5	9.6	8.9	7.8	7.5	8.1	10.4	11.3	11.2	10.4
Australia	8.3	8.1	8.1	7.2	6.2	6.9	9.6	10.8	10.9	9.7
France	10.5	10.6	10.8	10.3	9.6	9.1	9.6	10.5	11.9	12.7
Germany	7.2	6.6	6.3	6.3	5.7	5.0	4.3	4.6	5.8	6.5
Japan	2.6	2.8	2.9	2.5	2.3	2.1	2.1	2.2	2.5	2.9
Italy	6.0	7.5	7.9	7.9	7.8	7.0	6.9	7.3	10.3	11.4
Netherlands	9.6	10.0	10.0	9.3	8.6	7.5	7.1	7.2	8.8	–
Sweden	2.8	2.6	2.2	1.9	1.6	1.8	3.1	5.6	9.3	9.6
U.K.	11.2	11.2	10.3	8.6	7.3	7.0	8.9	10.1	10.5	9.6
United States	7.2	7.0	6.2	5.5	5.3	5.5	6.7	7.4	6.8	6.1

Source: Monthly Labour Review, U.S. Department of Labour, November 1995, p. 141.

clerical and sales) and slowed or even declined in blue-collar jobs (transport, manufacturing and labour);
– rising levels of educational attainment, and decline in demand for low-skilled workers;

- rising workforce participation rates for women, especially in the public sector;
- wider wage gaps and a decline in real wages for low-skilled workers; and
- rising incidence of long-term unemployment.

Labour Market Trends in Canada

As in most OECD countries, unemployment trends in Canada have worsened in the last decade (Betcherman 1996). Statistics Canada figures show that Canada experienced a negative change in the annual average labour force participation rates between 1990 and 1995 (table 3). Over this five-year period, the most significant change occurred among men aged 15 to 24 and, to a lesser extent, among men aged 25 to 54. Women aged 25 to 54 maintained relatively stable rates, while women aged 15 to 24 stayed in school longer, which explains their lower participation rates. Table 4 shows that unemployment declined in 1995, but not as much as 1994. For example, monthly employment gains totalled 382,000 in 1994, but only 88,000 in 1995. There were also 36,000 employment losses in the goods sector in 1995, compared with 200,000 gains in 1994. The entire service sector recorded 112,000 employment gains in 1995, and 177,000 in 1994. The 1995 decline in unemployment rates came from a combination of employment growth and a drop in labour force participation. As well, the 1994 employment gains were in full-time work, but those in 1995 were mostly in part-time employment. (Appendix 2 provides detailed data on 1994 full-time and part-time employment by sex and age, Canada and provinces.) In 1995, adult women's employment increased by 48,000, 69 percent of it part time. Youth full-time employment dropped by 48,000 in 1995, and part-time employment rose by 16,000. The private sector generated most of this employment growth, particularly in the goods and services sectors. Self-employment increased as professional services were contracted out. With higher borrowing costs and government cutbacks, public sector employment grew only marginally (Statistics Canada 1996).

To understand the link between unemployment and health, one must understand the extent of unemployment in Canada. In March 1993, the highest unemployment rate since World War II—12.3 percent (1,696,000 unemployed)—was recorded. The official definition of unemployment covers only people who have actively sought work in the previous four weeks, a definition which excludes two large groups that constitute the "hidden unemployed" (Jackson 1992, 1987; Deveraux 1992).

The first of these groups, excluded in unemployment figures, comprises those who want work and are available for work (428,000 in March 1993), but did not seek it in the previous week because of personal or family responsibilities, illness or discouragement, or because they were awaiting replies to job applications (Akyeampong 1992). The second group, those

Table 3

Annual average labour force participation rates

	1990	1991	1992	1993	1994	1995	% point change 1990–1995
Men	76.3	75.1	74.0	73.5	73.3	72.5	– 3.8
15–24 years	71.4	69.1	67.0	65.5	65.2	63.9	– 7.5
25–54 years	93.3	92.5	91.6	91.6	91.4	91.0	– 2.3
55 and over	37.4	36.0	35.2	34.0	34.0	32.6	– 4.8
Women	58.7	58.5	58.0	57.8	57.6	57.4	– 1.3
15–24 years	67.0	65.5	63.6	61.5	60.6	60.4	– 6.6
25–54 years	75.7	76.0	75.6	76.0	75.7	75.9	0.2
55 and over	17.3	16.9	17.0	17.0	17.2	16.5	– 0.8

Source: Dumas, C. Statistics Canada. *Perspectives on Labour and Income* (spring 1996, 13).

Table 4

Annual average unemployment rates by province

	1994	1995	% point change
Canada	10.4	9.5	– 0.9
Newfoundland	20.4	18.3	– 2.1
Prince Edward Island	17.1	14.7	– 2.4
Nova Scotia	13.3	12.1	– 1.2
New Brunswick	12.4	11.5	– 0.9
Quebec	12.2	11.3	– 0.9
Ontario	9.6	8.7	– 0.9
Manitoba	9.2	7.5	– 1.7
Saskatchewan	7.0	6.9	– 0.1
Alberta	8.6	7.8	– 0.8
British Columbia	9.4	9.0	– 0.4

Source: Dumas, C. Statistics Canada. *Perspectives on Labour and Income* (spring 1996, 14).

underemployed, comprises part-time workers who are available for full-time work (705,000 in March 1993).

This group is described as the "underemployed," or relatively unemployed. If unemployment figures included these two groups, the "real" unemployed would increase to 2,829,000, or 20 percent of the labour force (Jin et al. 1995). A comparison of 1994 OECD unemployment rates (table 2) shows that Canada, France and Italy reported the highest rates of unemployment.

Due to shifts in employment structure, the Canadian labour market is increasingly characterized by the following features:

- An increasing shift to service employment. Services account for 72.6 percent of employment in Canada, and Canada has the highest service sector employment growth of the 21 high-income OECD countries (OECD 1995a, b).

- Polarization between knowledge workers (the intellectual, cultural and business elite), who are mobile and independent, and service workers, who are immobile and dependent (Drucker 1993). This implies changes in skill requirements as well as polarization of the occupational structure, with the loss of middle-income jobs and growth in jobs paying either very low or very high wages (Betcherman 1996). In particular, the wages of new entrants to the labour force have dropped (Banting et al. 1995; Banting 1995).

- Growth of long term unemployment (figure 1) and nonstandard employment. Many firms now use a core of long-term employees, hiring extra workers only when necessary (Heisz 1995). To cut labour costs, especially payroll taxes, many employers have resorted to reducing their workforce, buying readymade, and contracting out.

- Rising wage dispersion and labour market inequality, driven by growing inequality in working time. More workers are working part time, and are working longer than 35 to 40 hours per week (Morissette et al. 1995).

- Wage stagnation. The average worker's real earnings have remained the same since the 1970s, but average real income for families has declined in the 1990s (Banting 1995; Betcherman 1996).

For employers, this shift increased flexibility but, from a societal perspective, it has increased economic insecurity and labour market–based inequality. In Canada, the effect of globalization on national policy responses has been coloured by total debt (Banting 1995), resulting in a loss of control over fiscal policy. The most immediate labour market consequence of Canada's current debt-driven social policy is a downward effect on social transfers. Wolfson (1996) demonstrated how social transfers can buffer the dispersion of earnings in Canada. His analysis did not include the dispersion of earnings that will probably follow the major social transfer cuts consequent to the Canada Health and Social Transfer, the changes to unemployment insurance, or the provincial actions to reduce social assistance payments that will follow. Canada's downward fiscal adjustments are affecting the unemployed and the unskilled—the least financially secure. However, social transfer cuts are reducing spending in areas that have traditionally buffered the effects of the business cycle and of labour market shifts.

Figure 1

Relative duration of unemployment spells
Proportion of unemployed having duration in the indicated ranges

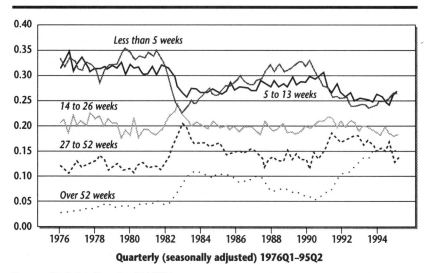

Quarterly (seasonally adjusted) 1976Q1–95Q2

Source: Statistics Canada, CANSIM.

Labour Market Changes, Unemployment and Health

In health and social science discourse, employment (that is, paid work) is recognized as a vital determinant of health. Regular, adequately paid employment basis does much to determine an individual's standard of living. Because it establishes social status and provides a sense of self-worth, identity, and opportunities for personal growth and self-actualization, employment significantly influences the mental, physical and social well-being of individuals and the population. Conversely, loss of employment usually means the loss of these benefits and, therefore is likely to have detrimental effects on health (Jin et al. 1995).

To understand the impact of unemployment on health, one must look at regional variations in unemployment within the Canadian jurisdiction. Table 3 shows that, in 1995, despite a drop in the labour force participation rates, unemployment was still high, reaching double digits in Quebec and the Atlantic Provinces. Newfoundland registered the highest unemployment rate of 18.3 percent, down from 20.4 percent in 1994. Ontario and the Western Provinces maintained single-digit rates within the two-year period.

The drastic changes in the labour market, resulting in high levels of unemployment, part-time work, and job insecurity, are likely to have adverse effects on population health. We highlight the health impact of unemployment at two levels: political jurisdiction (local, regional and national) and individual. (For a comprehensive review of the literature, including effects of unemployment on other family members, see Avison 1996.)

Political Level

Most studies have found a link between unemployment and a range of health outcomes, across various methodologies. In aggregate studies, a country, province or municipality is the unit of analysis. The independent variable is typically an economic indicator, such as the unemployment rate, per capita gross domestic product, or average household income. The dependent variables are population-based health outcomes, such as total mortality rate, infant mortality rate, suicide rate, deaths due to cardiovascular diseases, rates of admission to hospital (Brenner 1973, 1987a,b,c; Catalano 1991; D'Arcy and Siddique 1985). Although Brenner pioneered studies in this area, his work has been correctly criticized for not accounting for trends in education, income, occupation, housing status, nutrition and medical treatment (Joyce 1989; Gravelle et al. 1981; Eyer 1977). D'Arcy and Siddique's analysis of the Canada Health Survey was limited because it was cross sectional and, therefore, could not suggest the direction of causation.

Using time series analysis for Canada from 1950 to 1977, Adams (1981) found an inverse relationship between unemployment levels and overall mortality rates. Adams offered several possible explanations for this: 1) faulty assumptions concerning the intervening period between increases in unemployment and increases in mortality rates; 2) the moderating effect of unemployment insurance; 3) the lower risks of work-related deaths for the unemployed; 4) the reduction in mortality risks caused by the decline in alcohol and tobacco consumption related to lack of employment income; and 5) the confounding of the unemployment-mortality link by adverse population health outcomes that arise from income inequalities. The evidence supporting the unemployment-mortality relationship seems generally consistent. Recent large cohort studies in Denmark, Finland and Italy (Martikainen 1990; Iversen et al. 1987; Costa and Segman 1987) show a positive association between unemployment and overall mortality rates.

Heart disease and suicide are the causes of death most studied. The belief that unemployment induces stress and therefore increases the risk of heart disease is directly connected to the interest in cardiovascular diseases (Kasl and Cobb 1970; Kasl et al. 1975). An aggregate study in Australia reported positive associations between unemployment and death from heart disease (Bunn 1979). Adam's 1981 Canadian study also showed a positive correlation between unemployment and death from heart disease, despite the inverse relation with overall mortality rates. Adams suggests that heart disease occurs mainly among older adults, and that lack of jobs compels older workers to leave the labour force, thus increasing their unemployment rate.

A positive association between unemployment and suicide rates has been reported in several Western countries. Platt (1984) found that those who had committed or attempted suicide experienced greater unemployment, job instability or occupational problems. Unemployed British men, Finnish men, Danish men and women had suicide rates of 1.6, 1.9 and 2.5 times greater, respectively, than those of the general population of their respective countries (Moser et al. 1987; Iversen et al. 1987; Martikainen 1990). In a more recent study, Morrel and colleagues (1993) found a strong association between unemployment and suicide among young male adults in Australia and in Canada, France, and the United States, but weak associations in Sweden, former West Germany and Japan. These last three countries traditionally have low youth unemployment rates, and unemployed people in Sweden and the former West Germany were supported by generous state welfare programs, while those in Japan were supported by strong family networks.

However, nonlongitudinal studies (Platt 1984) did not show a consistent association between unemployment and suicide. There are some problems associated with the unemployment-suicide link. First, other factors may contribute to suicide: for example, mental illness can predispose people both to unemployment and suicide. Second, the relation to unemployment may be underestimated because suicide is generally underreported and suicide deaths are frequently attributed to other causes. The availability of firearms and cultural attitudes toward suicide may also affect the relation. However, economic hardship or loss of livelihood may contribute to suicide (Jin et al. 1995). The evidence from time series aggregate studies shows a positive relationship between unemployment and total mortality rates in most populations (Avison 1996).

Individual Level

Moser and colleagues (1986,1987) provided evidence of a positive association between unemployment and mortality rates. They reported that mortality rates among unemployed British men were greatest in regions with sustained periods of high unemployment. In Canada, Grayson conducted two cross-sectional studies of the impact of factory closures (SKF Canada Limited and Canadian General Electric) on the reported health of laid-off employees and their spouses. In the first study, Grayson (1985) indicated that stress attributed to plant closure was significantly associated with reported ill health, especially among those over 40. In the second study, Grayson (1989) found that, even 27 months after the factory closed, about 50 percent of former workers and spouses ranked the stress caused by job loss as greater than or equal to divorce. The former CGE workers and spouses also reported more physical ailments than Ontario respondents to the Canada Health Survey, even after adjusting for age, sex, education, and employment status. Whether aggregate or individual data are examined, there is ample evidence to support the conclusion that unemployment is a significant risk factor for health problems (Avison 1996).

A recent longitudinal cohort study in London, England to assess the effect of anticipating job change or loss on self-reported health status for middle-aged male and female white-collar civil servants provided evidence that anticipation of job loss affects health even before employment status changes. Ferrie and colleagues (1995) allowed the same individuals to be followed from job security into the "anticipation phase."

In addition to the decline in self-reported health status, fear of job change or loss might lead to increased incidence of illness and use of health care services. Compared to the employed and the general population, the unemployed tend to perceive a greater need for health care services and to use them more often (Linn et al. 1985; Kasl et al. 1975). They report more visits to hospitals, clinics and doctors as their unemployment period lengthens (Kasl et al. 1975). Similarly, health care providers report having more unemployed as their patients during economic downturns (Fortin 1984). Analyses of the Canada Health Survey show that about one of every six unemployed, compared to one of every 13 employed persons, sought admission to hospital in the preceding year. The unemployed reported an average of 3.4 telephone calls and visits to their doctors in the previous year, compared to 2.55 for the employed (D'Arcy 1986; D'Arcy and Siddique 1985). In a U.S. study, Linn and colleagues found that unemployed veterans visited their doctors in the previous six months five times more than the employed veterans. The link between unemployment and increased use of health care services is moderated by the extent to which health services are, for example, sensitive to fee barriers (as in the United States), or free but limited by policy (as in Canada).

Employment, Relative Wage Levels and Health

Relative wage is related to health in at least two ways. The poor suffer more from almost all health conditions and die from them sooner. Increasing polarization in the labour market and growing long-term unemployment means that Canada's national health status may change. The relative disadvantage of those without money and jobs gives new meaning to Riddell's 1986 assertion that labour adjustment has large-scale benefits (overall export-led growth in Canada), but also concentrated costs (growth of long-term unemployment and labour market polarization). Moreover, income distribution may have important emergent effects on population health.

Cross-national comparisons of OECD health trends suggest that unequal income distribution may explain variations between populations in life expectancy at birth (Wilkinson 1992, 1995). A comparison of 18 industrialized countries from 1950 to 1985 examined variations in income distribution, infant mortality and unemployment compensation (Wennemo 1993). The study showed that the degree of income inequality was significantly associated with the rate of infant mortality. High rates of family benefits have been associated with relatively lower rates of infant mortality (Whitehead 1995). Conversely, high unemployment coupled with inadequate social security benefits have been linked to high infant mortality rates (Wennemo 1993). Le Grand (1987) found that income distribution was related to life expectancy in 17 developed countries. Flegg (1982) reported that income inequality was related to national infant mortality among 59 developing countries.

Most recently, variations in life expectancy at birth within OECD countries has been associated with inequalities in regional income distribution. Two independent studies in the United States (Kaplan et al. 1996; Kennedy et al. 1996) have argued similarly that income distribution and life expectancy are closely associated in all of the 50 states. Although contentious, these findings suggest that overall national health status in advanced economies is influenced by income distribution inequities, and this effect does not seem to be driven only by the most disadvantaged segments of the population. Not only do these findings highlight the potential of labour market policies, they also point to the potential effects of social and tax policies on income inequality.

Given the relationship between employment and health, what adjustment mechanisms would ensure better and more equitable adjustment in an increasingly polarizing labour market?

SUCCESS STORIES

First, one must explore the role of industry and government in creating adjustment policy and mechanisms. At the national level, we present examples of sectoral adjustment mechanisms in the steel and electronics manufacturing industries. At the regional level, we discuss the activities of the Ontario Training and Adjustment Board (OTAB) and the Health Sector Training and Adjustment Program (HSTAP) two agencies that deal with training Ontario workers and help them adjust to economic changes. For international comparison, we also discuss initiatives in Sweden and the Netherlands that tackle health inequalities stemming from social and economic factors.

Sectoral Adjustment Mechanisms

In the 1980s, geographic and sectoral agencies emerged in response to the overall economic restructuring caused by increased international competition, new trade agreements, rapid technological innovation, and rising skills requirements. Sectoral-based agencies supported by business and labour deal directly with adjustment problems in specific industries. They are a promising strategy for industry-specific economic restructuring in Canada. In Canada, there are two types of sectoral agencies: government bodies that advise business and labour and bodies that work to influence government policy in specific areas. In the latter case, the agenda of these organizations is developed by business and labour; the government's role is essentially supportive (CLMPC 1992). In our examples, we examine four sectoral agencies: Canadian Steel Trade and Employment Congress (CSTEC), the Sectoral Skills Council (SSC), the OTAB and the HSTAP.

The Canadian Steel Trade and Employment Congress (CSTEC)

One of Canada's best-known national sectoral organizations, the CSTEC is a joint initiative of the Canadian wing of the United Steel Workers of America (USWA) and Canada's major steel companies. It originated at the May 1985, Sault Ste. Marie conference of USWA and steel company representatives who met to discuss labour adjustment, trade issues and the future of the steel industry. Incorporated under federal charter in May, 1988, the CSTEC received $20 million from Employment and Immigration Canada to provide labour market services. The most important activity of the CSTEC is its "downside adjustment" programs for displaced steel-workers. The agency formed an Employment and Adjustment Committee comprising equal numbers of business and labour representatives from the steel industry to design the program. The program was implemented in companies by HEAT (Helping Employees Adjust Together) teams of CSTEC employees and counsellors from the steel industry, and by local project committees. The programs include job search assistance, training, career counselling, relocation assistance, advice on starting a business, job referral and meeting rooms. The CSTEC adjustment model includes bipartite structure, strong emphasis on retraining, and sectoral design to meet the special problems of the industry.

By 1991, the CSTEC had assisted 18 projects involving 2,900 workers. The employment rate of workers in the CSTEC metal group was significantly better (7 percentage points lower) than that of the non-CSTEC metal control group. CSTEC participants were also much more satisfied with the assistance they received than participants in other adjustment programs. The CSTEC model is considered successful because of several factors: the more individual attention provided by CSTEC HEAT teams, the HEAT team members' personal knowledge of the steel industry, the active involvement of USWA, and the CSTEC's less bureaucratic, more user-friendly and flexible approach. Two key questions are: whether the CSTEC model should and could be implemented in other sectors; and whether the CSTEC downside adjustment (reducing job opportunities in the sector) model can be extended to upside adjustment (increasing jobs in the sector), technological change, skills shortages and changing workplace practices.

The Sectoral Skills Council (SSC)

Unlike the CSTEC, which deals with downside adjustment, the SSC focuses on upside adjustment. Both business and labour in the electronics manufacturing industry realized that the sector did not devote enough resources for upgrading workers' skills. The SSC established the Sectoral Training Fund to finance the increased training and retraining of workers in the electronics manufacturing industry. Although training is an upside adjustment, the program also includes a downside component—emphasis on portable skills.

Currently, Ontario is the only province using the Skills Training Fund. Sixteen firms, 25 workplaces and four nonunionized shops participate in the Fund. A total of 7,500 workers are covered, comprising 8 percent of the electronics industry's total employment in Ontario. There are four types of funded training programs:

- Type I – portable skills that are not specific to an employer;
- Type II – general education and training that is not restricted to current job requirements;
- Type III – employee group-directed training, such as seminars and union-sponsored training, that permits workers to contribute to the entire training process; and
- Type IV – contingency for plant closures, and involving training laid-off workers in counselling and referral skills so they can help colleagues deal with adjustment problems.

Overall, Canadian sector councils have been good for both business and labour. In contrast to the general experience at the workplace and aggregate economy level, where labour and management often clash, the sectoral initiatives have laid the foundation for new, effective forms of joint decision making. Although these adjustment mechanisms have clear labour market objectives, they have the potential to buffer the negative health effects of unemployment caused by restructuring.

The Ontario Training and Adjustment Board (OTAB)

The OTAB, established by legislation in September 1993, is the largest provincial labour force development board in Canada. Following a recommendation by the Premier's Council in its 1990 report, *People and Skills in the New Global Economy,* the OTAB was created to strengthen the skills of Ontario workers, by groups directly involved in training and adjustment (OTAB *Annual Report* 1994). The OTAB works with the Ontario Ministry of Education and Training, Human Resources Development Canada, and the Canadian Labour Force Development Board. The OTAB and its partners have launched 25 local boards across Ontario to improve community training and adjustment programs (CLFDB *Matters* 1995; OTAB *Annual Report* 1994).

The OTAB directs, advises and funds six types of training and adjustment programs. First, it offers programs with a number of objectives: to help workers, organizations communities understand, manage and anticipate changes resulting from labour market shifts; to help organizations and communities with planning, feasibility studies, market research and product development; and to help workers learn skills that will lead to new opportunities. Second, the OTAB offers on-the-job and in-school apprenticeships that lead to certification in recognized skilled trades. Not only do apprenticeship programs and services help workers, they also encourage young people, women, members of visible minorities, people with disabilities and Aboriginal people to learn skilled trades. Third, the OTAB offers literacy and numeracy programs for people who want to gain the literacy, communication, math and sciences skills required by today's increasingly technical workplace. Fourth, the OTAB offers individual employment counselling on career choices, job search techniques and work opportunities, and on-the-job training opportunities for people on social assistance. Fifth, the OTAB provides workplace training and consulting services that help employers and industry organizations to identify training needs and solutions, and foster joint employer-employee decision making. Sixth, the OTAB has several initiatives, including sectoral training agreements that provide a framework for entire industries and *Skills OK*, which promotes skilled trades to young people.

The Health Sector Training and Adjustment Program (HSTAP)

Provincial governments have several reasons for restructuring the health care system. Our understanding of the determinants of health has changed, shifting emphasis to the social environment; health care services are less institution based and more community based; and there is intense pressure to control costs and reduce apparent oversupply of hospital beds. Ontario has made some dramatic health changes in a short time. The government identified improved management, decreased duplication of services, increased efficiency, and a shift from inpatient to outpatient care as key components of hospital sector restructuring (HSTAP *Subsector Profiles* 1994), and rationalization of hospitals as the primary strategy to meet these objectives. In the proposed rationalization, 20,000 Ontario health sector employees may be laid off over the next three years (Coutts 1996). Labour adjustment is one of the most important concerns facing this labour-intensive sector. This dramatic scale of labour adjustment is also a significant concern in provinces where regionalization is the reform technique of choice (Sullivan 1996).

Since its inception in 1992, the mandate of the HSTAP has expanded to include enhancing the job security of health sector employees. To achieve this objective, the HSTAP uses a proactive labour adjustment strategy that includes adjustment and training, job retention research, and redeployment and jobs registry programs. The adjustment and training program is organized under START (Supports to Aid Restructuring and Training). It consists of a variety of exit, adjustment, and training incentives to help organizations with redeployment, while reducing layoffs and maintaining or improving services to clients. START seeks reorganization with as few layoffs as possible. Since October 1994, the HSTAP prevented 132 layoffs by offering employees training that helped them move into other positions at their facility (HSTAP 1995b). The training was offered under the Training to Prevent Layoff Program which was expanded to become START.

This program offers skills assessment to determine who could be reskilled or redeployed, and information workshops on early retirement. Also, adjustment counselling was provided for those considering voluntary exit or job sharing. This kind of labour adjustment plan enables those willing to retire to do so, and ensures that those who stay get the training they need. This program brought employers and unions together through their joint committees to organize proactive training for those whose employment was at risk (HSTAP 1995a).

The HSTAP used the Training to Prevent Layoff Program to develop a comprehensive job retention strategy. The strategy propelled a survey conducted by the University of Toronto Centre for Industrial Relations which surveyed all health sector transfer payment agencies for demographic information about their workforce, and identified training needs. The survey results were compiled and analyzed in 1995–1996. The organizational data that were gathered will serve as a planning tool for the HSTAP.

The Redeployment and Jobs Registry has been modified to meet the needs of the HSTAP: clients' records were updated and a job placement and coding system were developed. A job-matching system was established, and job matching began April 1, 1995. The procedure is as follows:

- All organizations post vacancies with the HSTAP and notify the HSTAP of laid-off employees.
- Within seven days, the HSTAP matches the vacancy with employees on the Registry.
- The HSTAP refers up to five qualified candidates to the employer, who interviews the candidates.
- After interviewing, the employer fills out an evaluation form confirming that a referred candidate was hired or explaining why no referred candidates were hired.
- The HSTAP evaluates the Jobs Registry, using the evaluation forms and data from the Registry.

By September 1995, 90 health workers had been hired through the Jobs Registry (HSTAP 1995a). The HSTAP offers up to $5,000 to cover associated training costs for people hired from the Registry. Overall, the HSTAP has provided 3,500 employees with adjustment counselling, relocation and training assistance. Despite the plan to adjust everyone in the workplace, layoffs may still be required. Hence, the labour adjustment planning process continues into the last stage, known as "adjusting after layoff." The Employee Support Program offers adjustment counselling, education and training, the Jobs Registry, and relocation assistance (HSTAP 1995c). Ontario is not the only province trying to support job security in the health sector, but as a unique sectoral adjustment mechanism, the HSTAP is worthy of further study.

Sweden: Social Adjustment and Health Inequalities

In Sweden, social welfare initiatives and legislation have been used extensively to rectify inequalities in infant mortality and ill health associated with the social environment (Whitehead 1995). The response to infant mortality during the Depression included housing programs and extensive support for women and children. In recent decades, the gap between social groups has narrowed, due to the effect of decreases in infant mortality for the population as a whole (Dahlgren and Diderichsen 1986; Leon et al. 1992). It has been argued that equitable income distribution policies and extensive social welfare support for families with children account for this decline (Wennemo 1993).

In Sweden, the strategic approach to ill health and the workplace stems partly from the traditional, corporatist strategies among government, business and labour (Whitehead 1995). The government has sup-ported extensive workplace and labour force research, and has passed legis-lation based on the findings of this research to improve psychosocial as well as physical workplace conditions. Through the Swedish Working Life Fund, Sweden offers businesses financial incentives to improve workplace conditions to comply with legislation (Whitehead 1995). In 1987, the manual workers' unions set up a five-year health program to improve health promotion opportunities in the workplace, in response to research showing higher mortality risks among manual occupational classes (Lundberg 1991; quoted in Whitehead 1995). On a broader scale, a concerted effort has been made to assess the health impacts of all public policies. The National Institute of Public Health was set up to develop and organize intersectoral health policies at national, county and local levels.

The Swedish corporatist approach has always involved cooperation between business and labour in policymaking. This cooperation, which began at the local level, now extends to every level of government. The National Labour Market Board, which is in charge of general labour market matters (including training), seeks advice from an advisory council with strong representation from business and labour organizations. The national board establishes guidelines, sets operational goals, and oversees the activities of the county boards.

The 24 county boards are the regional equivalent of the national board. Their responsibilities include decision making on subjects such as the creation of relief jobs. Like the national board, the regional boards have advisory councils with strong representation from business and labour. County boards delegate local affairs to local employment service committees, which include representatives from local governments as well as business and labour organizations.

The National Labour Market Board is currently facing its greatest challenge in almost half a century. Since the 1990s, unemployment rates have risen significantly in Sweden; the official unemployment rate was 1.5 percent in 1990; 2.7 percent in 1991; 5.2 percent in 1992; and rose to 8 percent by 1995. In an attempt to reverse this trend, the National Labour Market Board and its parent organization, the Labour Market Administration, have applied several proactive measures, including counselling, skills training, youth training and government employment programs. These measures have been preferred over income replacement payments.

Other initiatives, such as Working Life Services, a self-financing operation that sells vocational rehabilitation services to social insurance firms, provide services at the regional level. Intensive counselling and vocational rehabilitation are also provided at 100 agencies called Employment Institutes that operate through the county boards to serve those with special physical and mental needs. Measures to promote employment of the disabled are also given priority, and employers are given grants to purchase working aids.

Although the unemployment rate depends on economic decisions and factors operating inside and outside the country, the National Labour Market Board and its various agencies, by helping to fill vacancies, upgrading workers' skills, and providing reemployment training, are working to prepare the Swedish labour force for today's and tomorrow's market. Sweden is a small state, about the size of Ontario, so its multilevel adjustment approaches are relevant to the Canadian situation.

The Netherlands: Enlightenment Value of Research on Inequalities

The Netherlands, partly in response to the *Black Report* and the *WHO Health for All* strategy, has adopted a systematic research and consensus-building approach (Whitehead 1995). In 1987, the Ministry of Welfare, Public Health and Culture, in cooperation with the Scientific Council for Government Policy, united policymakers from political parties, business and labour organizations, and health care professions to formulate initiatives based on available evidence concerning health inequities. This result was a Five-Year Research Program by the Ministry to inform policymaking, to be carried out by the Dutch universities. Studies determined the nature and scope of the country's social inequalities in health, and made cross-country comparisons. Some small demonstration projects were undertaken to assess how trends in inequalities might be halted at the local level.

In addition to the research initiatives, the Scientific Council for Government Policy hosted a consensus conference, which concluded that health inequalities required an integrated, interdisciplinary approach by government agencies as well as statutory and nonstatutory organizations. They agreed that an integrated approach was needed to assess the impact of all major policies on the health of disadvantaged segments of the population. The program was extended until 1997, with a focus on policy development and related research. Thus, the approach in the Netherlands has been slow, careful analysis, based on integration and consensus building (Mackenbach 1994).

The Five-Year Research Program in the Netherlands has yielded remarkable results at two levels. First, the program has generated information regarding health inequities. A high-level committee was established with representatives from the government and the research community, as well as a scientific secretariat. The committee contacted research groups, organized review procedures for research proposals, and wrote reports. A documentation centre helped collect and distribute the available information on socioeconomic inequalities in health. Second, researchers and policy entrepreneurs armed with research evidence have generated wide publicity for health inequities, which has prompted several policy actions. For example, the government has initiated interdepartmental working groups to develop specific proposals for intersectoral action, and inner-city redevelopment programs to reduce socioeconomic health inequalities. The recommendations of the committee addressed the effects of the program on national health policy in non-health-related areas like income support and labour policy. The second Five-Year Research Program and the subsequent policy decisions should provide a clearer picture of the impact on non-health-related areas (Mackenbach, February 14, 1996, personal communication).

The Dutch experience may suggest strong enlightenment roles for both national and provincial councils, and associated health research organizations. If stakeholders have genuine political influence, the multistakeholder environments of the councils may help integrate economic objectives. Similarly, sustained strategic research on health inequities might stimulate integrated state-level policy by spreading ideas beyond the confines of government.

POLICY CONSIDERATIONS

Adjustment Processes

Adjustment Agencies and the Social Safety Net

Business, labour and government all recognize the importance of sectoral initiatives in economic restructuring. The CSTEC and the SSC are considered successful models for downside and upside adjustment, respectively. Effective sectoral agencies can affect economic restructuring and adjustment by:

- fostering trust based on mutual desire and ability to resolve labour-management problems, leading to labour-management cooperation (perhaps, beginning with immediate concerns such as training and expanding to issues such as the introduction of new technology);
- developing and delivering labour market programs more effectively, such as the CSTEC and the SSC;
- improving the development and implementation of public policy by providing joint advice and recommendations to government; and
- laying a sectoral-level foundation for broader, bipartite initiatives to satisfy the interests of business and labour.

The experience of sector councils in Canada in the past 10 years reveals several principles essential for successful sectoral initiatives. These principles as outlined by CLMPC (1992) include: equality of business and labour, avoidance of collective bargaining issues, joint decision making based on mutual recognition of concerns, strong workplace links, provision of adequate resources, and realistic expectations of the labour market partners for the outcome of the initiative (CLMPC 1992). Although the SSC has not been evaluated yet, there are indications that it is strongly supported by its industry association and participating unions, and that interest in the Sectoral Training Fund is growing.

Although sector councils offer significant potential to facilitate the economic and adjustment process, they can be hindered by inconsistencies between business and labour initiatives and national programs (e.g., tax policy, trade policy, resource management), by their inability to move beyond training issues, or by the scarcity of policy levers available to business and labour at the sectoral level.

Some sectoral problems require policy solutions that lie beyond the scope of business and labour in that particular sector. Organizations like the OTAB can foster adjustment across sectors, but the integration of adjustment efforts across the public and private sectors is incomplete and warrants further development.

Adjustment mechanisms accelerate the pace of adjustment and promote flexibility in a smaller labour force. Such mechanisms, however, do not appear sufficient to reduce the numbers of long-term unemployed (figure 1) and typically low-skilled workers whose jobs are threatened. Many of these workers are older or trained in old industries, and may not be able to learn the skills they need to compete. For these workers, active, redistributive social programs that permit some income replacement may be necessary (Betcherman 1996), if only to minimize income inequality.

The percentage of the unemployed who received regular UI benefits has declined sharply since 1988 (see figure 2). The decline resulted from benefit cuts and the tightening of eligibility requirements. However, those denied access to UI benefits go on social assistance. Thus, since the mid-1980s, welfare cases per 100 persons in the labour force continued to rise, even after unemployment began to fall.

Figure 2

Percentage of unemployed in receipt of regular UI benefits

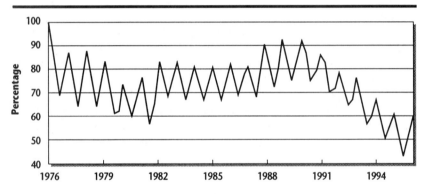

Source: Statistics Canada, CANSIM, Matrices 2074 and 5075.

As a result, Canada entered the 1991 recession with a welfare ratio higher than it was at the end of the previous recession (O'Grady 1995). Despite the scale of Canada's debt problem and the social spending cuts made necessary by today's smaller consolidated federal-provincial transfers, the federal and provincial governments may be compelled to find ways to minimize the social and health consequences of our labour market realities.

Special Features of the Health Sector

The health sector has features that distinguish it from other public sectors and from the private sector, and which affect the labour adjustment process. In this section, we highlight these features to illustrate the special problems of the health sector, which is being significantly restructured, and does not trade like other sectors on international markets (Evans 1996).

The health sector accounts for approximately 5.5 percent of jobs in Canada (Purchase 1996). It is large, labour intensive and diverse. It accounts for almost one-third of public sector employment and employee compensation accounts for 75 to 80 percent of the health budget (Haiven and Wetzel 1995; Gunderson and Hyatt 1996). Occupations within the sector vary, from less-skilled service jobs to highly segregated occupations, with discrete scopes of professional practice. Cutbacks in public spending have tremendous (and unequal) implications for health care employees and their unions.

Unlike the United States, Canada has mainly public sector, not-for-profit health care. Therefore, health care is subject to political budget decision pressures rather than market pressures, although there are shifts toward the latter. Cost reduction measures disproportionately affect women, who not only dominate occupations like nursing and home care, but also are disadvantaged as institutional services are shifted to community and family care.

Significant restructuring is occurring in the health care delivery system (Gunderson and Hyatt 1996). Five main actions affect labour adjustment: decentralization to regional and local health boards (occurring in nine of ten provinces); shifting of hospital services to communities and families; emphasizing prevention rather than treatment; emphasizing the cost-effectiveness of technology and information systems for providing and administrating health services; and emphasizing dwindling health resources and the need for cost restraint. These issues mean that service delivery will be organized differently and hence working conditions and pay will change.

The health sector is highly unionized—the unionization rate is double that of the economy as a whole. For example, in Ontario, unionized health care workers range from 20 percent in community health and support to more than 80 percent in nursing homes and public health (Cairns et al. 1993). The health care sector also has a proliferation of bargaining units, with many unions representing them. With conflicting interests jostling for power and remuneration, industrial relations in the health sector can be adversarial.

Dispute resolution procedures vary from province to province (Haiven 1995). For example, Alberta, Ontario and Prince Edward Island prohibit strikes and require binding arbitration, while Saskatchewan and Nova Scotia allow strikes and bargaining over the designation of essential employees who may not strike. The other provinces allow a restricted right to strike for nondesignated essential service employees, with designations determined by legislation or regulation. Although strikes are less common in the health sector than in other public sectors (Ponak and Thompson 1994), they have occurred even in jurisdictions where strikes are prohibited (Haiven 1995; White 1990).

Finally, although downsizing and cost reduction measures are being imposed, the health sector has prospects for growth. Health demands will change as the baby boomers age (Denton and Spencer 1975; Foot 1996). This growth will be double edged: it will make cost restraint difficult, and it will compel the adoption of labour adjustment strategies to anticipate needs. This implies training and adjustment geared to the needs of an aging population.

Labour adjustment is crucial to the success of restructuring, but it is affected by the powerful employment interests currently steering the sector (Evans 1996). To reform health care and maintain quality of patient care, the process of restructuring human resources must be given careful attention. Unfortunately, it is not receiving such attention from most provincial governments. Human resource plans that target the supply, compensation and distribution of professionals are essential to achieve cost-effective, high-quality care at manageable costs.

Hours of Work—Job Sharing

In addition to adjustment processes—which have little (short-term) effect on unemployment and some aspects of working conditions—policy initiatives aimed at regulating hours of work offer potential. These initiatives can include reductions in the standard work week, increased annual vacation, increased job-sharing schemes, increased access to sabbaticals, and early retirement (Reid 1987, 1995; World Labour Report 1994, Donner et al. 1994). To assess the long-term effects of these measures on employment, their effects on labour and capital costs must be evaluated. The application of each criterion can lead to opposite conclusions. For example, should the reduced work week or increased annual vacation take place with or without full wage compensation?

If employers provide full wage compensation, the cost of hourly labour will increase, as will final demand. A significant increase in the cost of labour may cause the competitive position of firms to decline in the long run, thereby reducing employment, while increased final demand causes a short-term employment increase. A shorter work week may result in lower capital utilization, leading to higher capital cost per hour worked. This cost could be offset if workers accepted shift work, which might increase the operation time of capital goods. To counteract this, employers might resort less frequently to overtime.

Reid's 1995 analysis of Statistics Canada's Work Reduction Survey provides evidence of the potential for job creation through voluntary work reductions. Table 5 summarizes work reduction options. Employees' preference for a work week reduced by 19.7 percent translates into 370,000 potential full-time jobs, a 3.9 percent increase in employment. A 15.9 percent reduction translates into 174,500 potential full-time jobs or a 1.8 percent increase in employment. Employees' preferences for an unpaid increase in their annual vacation (21.8 percent of employees selected that option) translates into a 5.5 percent reduction in work time and 118,400 potential full-time jobs. Similarly, employees' preferences for various self-funded sabbaticals (16 percent of employees selected that option) translated into 133,200 potential full-time jobs, a 1.4 percent increase in employment.

Table 5

Job creation potential for Canada: Summary of work reduction options

Work reduction options	% Reduction in work time	No. of employees selecting options	% Employees selecting options	Potential full-time jobs created	% Full-time jobs created
Reduced work week	19.7	1,896,000	19.8	370,000	3.9
Reduced work Day	15.9	1,079,400	11.3	174,500	1.8
Incr. annual vacation	5.5	2,096,000	21.8	118,400	1.2
Self-funded sabbatical	8.8	1,534,400	16.0	133,200	1.4
One or more options	–	2,953,500	30.7	–	8.3

Source: Reid, F., Working Less and Enjoying It More, a paper for the National Forum on Family Security (1995).

The actual number of new jobs created through voluntary work reduction may differ from the potential indicated by the survey data for various reasons. For example, if the employer responds to a reduction in work time by increasing the hours of part-time employees or the overtime of full-time employees, there may be fewer new jobs created than the calculated potential. Although work sharing does not eliminate the unemployment problem, the distributional effects can significantly alleviate the impact of unemployment.

In Europe, some studies have estimated the long-term effects of a reduced work week on employment. A study in France, which assessed the impact of reducing the work week from 40 to 39 hours, estimated that employment would increase by only 0.2 to 0.4 percent. As a result of national studies and experiments, like those in Belgium and France, governments tend to prefer a bargained reduction of work hours negotiated at the firm or industry level (World Labour Report 1994).

Job sharing is designed to reduce unemployment in a specific work group by reducing hours of work, including overtime. It is an option under the Skills Investment Program of the Canadian Jobs Strategy intended to maintain employment during economic downturns (Graves and Dugas 1993). The government encourages job sharing out of concern for the social costs of inequities.

Job-sharing arrangements are, however, most effective when settled between employers and employees. The 1994 *OECD Jobs Study* suggested that:

> ...legislated across-the-board work sharing addresses the unemployment problem not by increasing the amount of economic activity, but through rationing gainful work. Enforced work sharing never succeeded in cutting unemployment significantly, not least because of worker resistance to reduced income. The 'cure' must be distinguished from voluntary negotiations between workers and firms over more flexible working time arrangements, which can lower costs and lead to higher employment (45).

Job sharing attempts to avert layoffs by redistributing a fixed amount of work within the work unit by reducing the work week of all employees in that unit. UI benefits partially compensate for wages lost to the reduction of regular working hours. Employers must maintain the affected employees' benefits during the job-sharing program (Graves and Dugas 1993).

The program largely achieves its objective at the level of individual workers. In 1989–1990 and 1990–1991, the program avoided layoffs, although less than 25 percent (43,200 out of 177,800) of total program participants could be seen as people who would have been laid off without the program. Job sharing postponed layoffs for 29 percent of participants, who were laid off at the end of the program, 75 percent of them permanently. Sixty-four percent of potential layoffs can be said to have been averted by the program (Graves and Dugas 1993).

In the Graves and Dugas (1993) study, job sharing was reported to have cushioned participants from some of the negative financial effects associated with layoff, and enabled participants to maintain higher social, psychological, mental and physical well-being than those who were laid off. The income of program participants was reduced by 19 percent, compared with 47 percent for those laid off who collected UI benefits. There is evidence that the program benefitted employers. Participating firms realized a short-term profit as they expended $800 to $1,800 less per layoff than those firms laying off workers. There is also evidence that participating firms return to full production sooner than firms that lay off, but there is no evidence of a long-term effect on profitability or productivity. The costs of unemployment-induced stress on health care, social and employment services were also avoided, another potential benefit of the programs.

However, there are indications that participating firms are less likely to train employees than firms that lay off employees. This raises the concern that firms facing fundamental structural problems may prefer "stay-the-course" solutions that hinder or delay more appropriate adjustment strategies, especially in the context of globalization, rising skill requirements and rapid technological change. Also, work sharing is more expensive than layoffs. In 1991, job sharing cost $160 million in UI benefits. Three factors account for most of the increased cost: the deferral of the two-week waiting period for UI, the fact that 30 percent of laid-off workers do not collect UI and may find new jobs, and the incidence of layoffs in the postprogram period. Despite the high cost of work sharing on UI, the program has positive social benefits for participants and their families.

Barriers to Health Outcomes in Labour Adjustment

Social GDP Indicators

Since the early 1940s, when gross domestic product (GDP) was introduced as a measure of production capacity, it has been used by economists, policy-makers, international agencies and the media to indicate economic progress. GDP tallies goods and services involving monetary transactions, but does not distinguish costs from benefits, or productive activities from destructive ones. It assumes that every market activity adds to well-being.

Recently, numerous observers have argued for a socially sensitive GDP. Cobb (1995), for example, challenged the use of the GDP as a measure of a nation's economic health and well-being. GDP ignores all activities outside of monetary exchange, regardless of their importance to the economy and society. Household and volunteer functions, such as child care, elder care, home-based activities and volunteer work in the community, are ignored. Other shortcomings of GDP as a measure of progress include the following:
- GDP treats crime, divorce and natural disasters as economic gain;
- GDP treats the depletion and degradation of natural resources as income;
- GDP increases with polluting activities, and again with cleanups;
- GDP does not account for income distribution;
- GDP ignores the hazards of living on foreign assets; and
- GDP ignores the social costs of underemployment.

As a result, the GDP says little about how the economy actually affects health and well-being. Cobb and colleagues argue for new indicators of progress, designed to measure the economy that actually exists.

As an alternative to GDP, the Genuine Progress Indicator (GPI) includes both market and nonmarket activity within a single, comprehensive frame-work. Like the GDP, the GPI begins with personal consumption, but unlike GDP, the GPI adjusts for income distribution, and adds and subtracts social and ecological costs and benefits. If policymakers are concerned with genuine economic progress, they must start asking some hard questions: What exactly is growing? What are the immediate and long-term implications of economic activity for human health and well-being? How do market activities affect the structure and natural habitat upon which the economy and human existence depends? National accounting, based on genuine progress indicators would prevent politicians and interest groups from hiding the effects of bad policy behind unrealistic progress indicators. Were a GPI to be used, the social costs of structural change and adjustment would probably become more transparent at the national and at the firm level. As Lavis (1996) has argued, if this form of national accounting, were widely reported and championed by labour adjustment policymakers, significant pressure would be created for national- and firm-level adjustment.

The Weak Institutional Role of Health

It is clear that labour market experience, particularly unemployment, can have negative health consequences (Jin et al. 1995; Hertzman et al. 1994; Grayson 1985, 1989, 1993). Notwithstanding this widely accepted relationship, public policies that affect the level of unemployment or the experiences of the unemployed are not designed with health considerations in mind (Lavis and Sullivan, forthcoming). Within a population, health outcomes are secondary objectives. Government decisions address the management of health services, not the health consequences of decision making in non-health sectors. We refer to this elsewhere as the "weak institutional role of health" in decision making (Lavis and Sullivan, forthcoming).

The explicit consideration of health in public policies is constrained as an intended consequence of well-intentioned and effective policies designed to increase access to and the quality of health care. Three main effects of policy legacies that hinder the population health approach can be identified (Lavis and Sullivan, forthcoming).

First, government officials and allied interest groups experienced in health administration tend to respond to health-related problems by developing or advocating more health-related programs. The new approach to improving health does not involve developing new Health Ministry programs per se, but establishing new perspectives in other ministries, such as Labour or Industry, where decisions with considerable health consequences are made.

Second, health care policies create resources and incentives for interest groups that focus on health. Professional groups (e.g., provincial medical associations) view investments in the population health measures as a divestment of health care obligations. The health care professions have reacted negatively to the population health approach, and have sometimes openly resisted it. Interest groups that focus on health, regardless of their good intentions, may not be best suited to undertaking population health measures alone. Resources and incentives may be better spent on groups with direct experience in developing or modifying health-related labour market policies.

Third, health care policies were designed to reflect government action, and may have been politically advantageous when health care was seen as a universal remedy and potential investments in it seemed unlimited. When they recognized the limitations of health care, politicians shifted their focus to a population health approach. However, health care policies are clearer than health-related labour market policies to interest groups and the public. Also, the health consequences of labour market policies may not be directly traceable to government action, which could discourage politicians from taking action to facilitate labour adjustment.

Past government efforts to improve health have created barriers to new health approaches, but they can be overcome (Lavis and Sullivan 1996). First, government decision makers and interest groups should abandon the notion that health care competes with population health. Population health can complement traditional public health activities as well as health care in the improvement of health, despite important differences between the models. While the public health approach focuses on reducing exposure to harmful aspects of the physical environment, the population health approach focuses specifically on the social environment. Further, while the primary objective of public health policy is health, the population health model involves the developing or modifying public policies of which health is a consequence, not the primary objective.

Because labour market policies can have either positive or negative health consequences, the state and employers should be able to reduce the social costs of public policy. The state could initiate changes in labour market policy that improve health—changes that affect the level of unemployment or the experiences of the unemployed. For example, the state could initiate or extend training and adjustment programs to help workers such as those described earlier in this paper, who have become unemployed through plant closures, layoffs, new skill requirements or technological changes.

In our view, three conditions favour political change: rethinking the place of population health; reformulating the concept of "health public policy"; and using multistakeholder advisory bodies close to decision makers to frame options and/or finding policy entrepreneurs to advance convincing social cost arguments for health in the labour adjustment field (Lavis and Sullivan, forthcoming).

Ministry of Health policymakers can contribute to the population health approach by offering technical support to other ministries (for example, Labour, Industry and Trade), both to develop and modify public policies, and to support policy evaluation. Researchers can contribute by researching the trade-offs faced by other ministries, and evaluating public policies developed or modified by other ministries to determine their health consequences. Population health advocates can contribute by continuing to lobby for it and by working with people in other areas to improve the articulation of public policy trade-offs.

CONCLUSIONS AND RECOMMENDATIONS

This paper has discussed and assessed labour adjustment policies and health. Recent increases in unemployment concern everyone in Canada, especially those who have lost their jobs or are at risk of losing them and the politicians that represent them. Despite the high-profile of unemployment as a national issue, the damage it can do to the physical and mental health of the population has generally received scant attention in public discourse and public policy.

Both the private and public sectors are faced with labour adjustment. In the private sector, the need to remain internationally competitive as well as profitable leads firms toward economic rationalization that frequently means layoffs, employment cutbacks, plant closures or relocation. In response to downward fiscal pressure associated with managing the public debt and sustaining a competitive tax environment, the public sector faces dramatic, rapid restructuring. Many governments and, through government, the broader public sector have embarked on massive layoffs. Since change caused by global forces seems inevitable, an active adjustment policy makes sense in a small economy such as Canada.

Living with Adjustment?

The political response of industrial countries to the new global context has varied. Katzenstein (1985) discerns three dominant political forms of contemporary political capitalism: liberalism in the United States and Britain; statism in Japan and France; and democratic corporatism in small European states and, to a lesser extent, in Germany. Liberal countries such as the United States rely on macroeconomic policies and market solutions. When the traditional market approach appears to fail, and selective intervention seems impossible, the United States tends to export the cost of change through various, limited, ad hoc protectionist policies. In contrast, statist countries such as Japan have the means and institutions to preempt the cost of change through policies that transform their economies. Exporting or preempting the cost of economic change are political options open to industrial states that are powerful enough to control either parts of their international environment or parts of their own societies. Canada, which has suffered significant job losses in recent years, cannot use either strategy.

In small corporatist-leaning states like Canada, economic change is imposed by major trading partners. Because they lack large domestic markets, small states must depend on global markets and cannot resort to protectionism. Because international markets force economic adjustments, small states devise economic and social policies to minimize the political and social costs of economic change. In short, they compensate for and live with change. The liberal and statist approaches to economic change differ markedly from the reactive, flexible, and incremental industrial adjustment of smaller states such as Canada. Canadian industry and governments must lead an active approach to labour market adjustment if they are to sustain competitive position and ensure optimal health for the population of Canada. Canada will also need a consolidated approach to income security for the long-term and chronically unemployed.

Like many other industrial countries, Canada is experiencing extensive structural economic change caused by globalization, technological change and liberalization of trade. The sources of structural changes in the global economy are diverse: new political developments in the international state system; major changes in the supply conditions and production structures of many countries; and continually falling communications and transport costs. Technological changes have made the world easier to navigate—goods, capital, people, and ideas travel faster and cheaper than ever before. But at no other time since 1945 have industrial countries been so concerned with economic competitiveness and security. The need to remain competitive and profitable has resulted in layoffs, plant closures and rising unemployment, with adverse impacts on population health and other social costs.

New Areas of Research

Globalization generates new labour force participation patterns, that might best be understood by studying labour market experiences and their associations with health. As Lavis (1996) has argued, the literature on the health consequences of unemployment experiences emerged after the Great Depression and subsequent recessions, not from a period of economic growth and change in employment strategies. Consequently, most of the research focuses almost exclusively on short-term and/or cyclical unemployment. Only a few studies examine the effects of long-term unemployment and job insecurity. There is little research on the health consequences of underemployment, structural unemployment (i.e., unemployment due to a mismatch between the skills or location of workers and the available work), worker discouragement, and employability insecurity (Lavis 1996). The four features of misuse of human potential (unemployment, discouragement of workers, underemployment, and fear of unemployment) and their long-term and structural considerations generate 10 unique misuse experiences (table 6), which may have health consequences. Health effects may also arise from overuse of the human potential of long-term employees (i.e., the over-employed), who are compelled by downsizing to assume added responsibilities and more work hours. These effects have also been understudied (Lavis 1996). The *Toronto Star* (Friday, April 12, 1996) quoting the *British Medical Journal* reported that British researchers associate higher workloads with increased disease and death rates. Recently, Brooker and colleagues (1996) demonstrated the sensitivity of work injuries to business cycle effects. The pace and duration of employment were considered important to injury cycles.

The categories in table 6 give us a taxonomy to explore the relationships between labour market experiences and health more systematically. We recommend that they be considered by Health Canada and Human Resources Development Canada in establishing a multiyear research program on the health consequences of these understudied labour market experiences.

National research organizations should also consider a multidisciplinary, multiyear plan of research, to investigate health inequities in Canada and study their origins and changing conditions. We suggest that the existing focus be concentrated and extended into a national health research strategy. The current research in this area has already affected provincial planning, and could be extended with a national research effort (Roos 1995).

Table 6

Features of human potential underuse and overuse

	Short-term and/or cyclical effects	Long-term and/or structural effects
Underuse		
Unemployment	Temporary layoff	Permanent job loss
Discouragement of workers	Lack of work	Lack of skills
Fear of unemployment	Job and employment insecurity	Insecurity of employability
Underemployment	Forced work sharing	Unwilling part-time employment
Overuse		
Overemployment	Temporary increase in work hours	Permanent increase in work hours

Source: Lavis, J., Unemployment, Work and Health: A Research Framework for a Changing World, 1996.

Multistakeholder Processes

The provincial and federal governments, where they are not already underway, should each consider using multistakeholder groups from outside the health care sector in the formulation of health policy. This is one way to ensure some focus on policies outside of the health care sector in health-related decision making.

There are both social and economic benefits to averting a decline in workforce skill levels. Skills must be upgraded and maintained through labour adjustment initiatives during restructuring. Such upgrading, in tandem with comprehensive income security, could do much to sustain Canada's competitive position and preserve the health of our population. Unlike the United States and Japan, Canada cannot export or preempt the cost of change. We must compensate for change and live with it.

Terrence Sullivan, *Ph.D., M.D., MPH, FHRPC, is president of the Institute for Work & Health. The Institute is a nonprofit corporation formally affiliated with the University of Toronto and the University of Waterloo. The Institute conducts innovative population-based health studies investigating the determinants of modern workplace health and the effective treatment and management of musculoskeletal injury. He is the workplace/workforce theme leader for the McMasterled National Centres of Excellence in Health Research, bringing together eighteen investigators involved in the study of workplace health matters.*

BIBLIOGRAPHY

ADAMS, O. B. 1981. *Health and Economic Activity: A Time-Series Analysis of Canadian Mortality and Unemployment Rates*. Ottawa (ON): Statistics Canada.

AKYEAMPONG, E.B. 1987. Persons on the margins of the labour force. *Labour Force* (Statistics Canada Cat. no. 71–001) April: 85–131.

_____. 1992. Discouraged workers: Where have they gone? *Perspectives on Labour and Income* (Statistics Canada Cat. no. 75–001) Autumn: 38–44.

AVISON, W. 1996. Unemployment and its health consequences. Working paper. London (ON): University of Western Ontario, Department of Psychiatry/Sociology. Unpublished.

BANTING, K. G. 1995. A house divided against itself: Internationalization and the welfare state. Unpublished.

BANTING, K. G., C. M. BEACH, and G. BETCHERMAN. 1995. Polarization and social policy reform: Evidence and issues. In *Labour Market Polarization and Social Policy Reform*, eds. K. G. BANTING, and C. M. BEACH. Kingston (ON): School of Policy Studies, Queen's University.

BETCHERMAN, G. 1996. Globalization, labour markets and public policy. In *States Against Markets*, eds. D. DRACHE, and P. BOYER. New York (NY): Routledge.

BRENNER, M. H. 1973. *Mental Illness and the Economy*. Cambridge (MA): Harvard University Press.

_____. 1987a. Economic change, alcohol consumption and heart disease in nine industrialized countries. *Social Science and Medicine* 25: 119–132.

_____. 1987b. Economic instability, unemployment rates, behavioural risks and mortality rates in Scotland, 1952–1983. *International Journal of Health Service* 17: 475–487.

_____. 1987c. Relation of economic change to Swedish health and social well-being. *Social Science and Medicine* 25: 183–195.

BROOKER, A.-S., J. W. FRANK, and V. S. TARASAK. 1996. Back pain claim rates and the business cycle: In contrast to acute claim rates. IWH Working Paper. Toronto: Institute for Work and Health.

BUNN, A. 1979. Ischaemic heart disease mortality and the business cycle in Australia. *American Journal of Public Health* 69: 772–781.

CAIRNS, E. D. CHRISTIANO, M. DAWSON, and M. GLASSFORD. 1993. A first step: Strategies for job retention in the health sector. HSTAP Discussion Paper (December). Toronto (ON): Health Sector Training and Adjustment Program. Unpublished.

CANADA. FEDERAL, PROVINCIAL AND TERRITORIAL ADVISORY COMMITTEE ON POPULATION HEALTH STRATEGIES FOR POPULATION HEALTH. 1994. *Strategies for Population Health: Investing in the Health of Canadians*. Federal, Provincial and Territorial Advisory Committee on Population Health. Ottawa (ON): Supply and Services Canada.

CANADA. STATISTICS CANADA. 1995. *Labour Force Annual Averages*. Ottawa (ON): Household Surveys Division, Statistics Canada.

_____. 1996. The labour market: Year-end review. *Perspectives on Labour and Income* (Statistics Canada Cat. no. 75–001). Ottawa (ON): Statistics Canada.

CANADIAN LABOUR FORCE DEVELOPMENT BOARD. 1995. CLFDB *Matters* 1(1).

CANADIAN LABOUR MARKET AND PRODUCTIVITY CONGRESS (CLMPC). 1992. The role of business-labour sectoral initiatives in economic restructuring. *Quarterly Labour Market and Productivity Review* 1–2: 26–38.

CATALANO, R. 1991. The health effects of economic insecurity. *American Journal of Public Health* 81: 1148–1152.

COBB, C. W. 1995. If the GDP is up, why is America down? *The Atlantic Monthly* (October): 59–78.

COSTA, G., and N. SEGMAN. 1987. Unemployment and mortality. *British Medical Journal* 294: 1550–1551.

COUTTS, J. 1996. Ontario hospitals face 20,000 layoffs. *Globe and Mail,* Saturday, February 24, A1, A10.

DAHLGREN, G., and F. DIDERICHSEN. 1986. Strategies for equality in health: Report from Sweden. *International Journal of Health Services* 16: 517–537.

D'ARCY, C. 1986. Unemployment and health: Data and implications. *Canadian Journal of Public Health* 77: 124–131.

D'ARCY, C., and C. M. SIDDIQUE.1985. Unemployment and health: An analysis of the Canada Health Survey. *International Journal of Health Service* 15(4): 609–635.

DENTON, F., and B. SPENCER. 1975. Health care costs when the population changes. *Canadian Journal of Economics* 12 (February): 34–48.

DEVERAUX, M. S. 1992. Alternative measures of unemployment. *Perspectives Labour Force* (Statistics Canada Cat. no. 75–001E), winter: 35–43.

DONNER, A., J. BERNARD, H. MASSE, A. DAGG, S. O'BRIEN, J. GRANT, R. WHITE, P. KUMAR, and A. YALNIZYAN. 1994. *Report of the Advisory Group on Working Time and the Distribution of Work.* Ottawa (ON): Supply and Services Canada.

DRACHE, D., and P. BOYER. 1996. *States Against Markets.* New York (NY): Routledge.

DRUCKER, P. F. 1993. *The Post-Capitalist Society.* New York (NY): Harper Business.

DUMAS, C. STATISTICS CANADA. Spring 1996. *Perspectives on Labour and Income.*

EVANS R. G. 1996. Going for gold: The redistributive agenda behind market-based health care reform. CIAR Working Paper no. 49. Toronto (ON): Canadian Institute for Advanced Research.

EVANS, R. G., BARER, M. L., and T. R. MARMOR. 1994. *Why Are Some People Healthy and Others Not? The Determinants of Population Health.* New York (NY): Aldine de Gruyter.

EYER, J. 1977. Does unemployment cause the death rate to peak in each business cycle? A multifactorial model of death rate change. *International Journal of Health Service* 7: 625–662.

FERRIE, J. E., M. J. SHIPLEY, M. G. MARMOT, S. STANSFIELD, and G. DAVEY SMITH. 1995. Health effects of anticipation of job change and non-employment: Longitudinal data from the Whitehall II study. *British Medical Journal* 311: 1264–1269.

FLEGG, A. 1982. Inequality of income, illiteracy and medical care as determinants of infant mortality in developing countries. *Population Studies* 36: 441–458.

FOGEL, R. W. 1993. New sources and new techniques for the study of secular trends in nutritional status, health, mortality, and the process of aging. *Historical Methods* 26 (1): 5–43.

FOOT, D. 1996. *Boom, Bust and Echo.* Toronto (ON): McFarlane, Walter & Ross.

FORTIN, D. 1984. Unemployment as an emotional experience: The process and the mediating factors. *Canada's Mental Health* (Sept.): 6–9.

FRANK, J., and J. F. MUSTARD. 1994. The determinants of health from an historical perspective. *Daedalus* 86 (3): 162–164.

GRAVELLE, H., G. HUTCHINSON, and J. STERN. 1981. Mortality and unemployment: A critique of Brenner's time-series analysis. *Lancet* (2): 675–679.

GRAVES, F. L., and T. DUGAS. 1993. *Work Sharing Evaluation.* A report prepared for the Insurance Programs Directorate, Program Evaluation Branch, Strategic Policy and Planning, Employment and Immigration Canada, Ottawa (ON).

GRAYSON, J.P. 1985. The closure of a factory and its impact on health. *International Journal of Health Services* 15: 69–93.

———. 1989. Reported illness after a CGE closure. *Canadian Journal of Public Health* 80: 16–19.

———. 1993. Health, physical activity level, and employment status in Canada. *International Journal of Health Services* 23 (4): 743–761.

GUNDERSON, M., and D. HYATT. 1996. *The Cost of Doing Nothing. Why an Active Labour Adjustment Strategy Makes Sense in Ontario's Health Sector.* Report to the Ontario Health Sector Training and Adjustment Program, Toronto (ON).

HAIVEN, L. 1995. Industrial relations in health care: Regulation, conflict and transition to the "wellness model". In *Public Sector Collective Bargaining in Canada*, eds. G. SWIMMER, and M. THOMPSON. Kingston (ON): IRC Press.

HAIVEN, L., and K. WETZEL. 1995. Labour adjustment and industrial relations amid structural reform in health care: A comparison of jurisdictions across Canada. Working Paper. Department of Labour Relations and Organizational Behaviour, University of Saskatchewan, Saskatoon. Unpublished.

HEALTH SECTOR TRAINING AND ADJUSTMENT PROGRAM. 1995. *Subsector Profiles: Appendix A* (November). Toronto (ON): Health Sector Training and Adjustment Program.

_____. 1995a. *Annual Report 1994–1995.* Toronto (ON): Health Sector Training and Adjustment Program.

_____. 1995b. *The Link* (September). Toronto (ON): Health Sector Training and Adjustment Program.

_____. 1995c. *Labour Adjustment Planning: Response to Metropolitan Toronto District Health Council* (October). Toronto (ON): Health Sector Training and Adjustment Program.

HEISZ, A. 1995. Changes in job tenure and job stability. Prepared for the Analytical Studies Branch, Statistics Canada, Ottawa (ON). Unpublished.

HERTZMAN, C., J. FRANK, and R. G. EVANS. 1994. Heterogeneities in health status and the determinants of population health. In *Why Are Some People Healthy and Others Not? Determinants of Health in Population*, eds. R. G. EVANS, M. L. BARER, and T. R. MARMOR. New York (NY): Aldine de Gruyter.

IVERSEN, L., O. ANDERSEN, and P. K. ANDERSEN 1987. Unemployment and mortality in Denmark, 1970–1980. *British Medical Journal* 295: 878–884.

JACKSON, G. 1993. Alternative concepts and measures of unemployment. *Labour Force* (Statistics Canada Cat. no. 71–001) February: 85–120.

JIN, R. L., C. P. SHAH, and T. J. SVOBODA. 1995. The impact of unemployment on health: A review of the evidence. *Canadian Medical Association Journal* 153(5): 529–540.

JOYCE, T. 1989. A time-series analysis of unemployment and health: The case of birth outcomes in New York City. *Journal of Health Economics* 8: 419–436.

KAPLAN, G. A., E. PAMUK, J. W. LYNCH, R. D. COHEN, and J. L. BALFOUR. 1996. Inequality in income and mortality in the United States: Analysis of mortality and potential pathways. *British Medical Journal* 312: 999–1003.

KASL, S. V., and S. COBB. 1970. Blood pressure changes in men undergoing job loss: A preliminary report. *Psychosomatic Medicine* 32: 19–38.

KASL, S. V., S. GORE, and S. COBB. 1975. The experience of losing a job: Reported changes in health, symptoms and illness behaviour. *Psychosomatic Medicine* 37: 106–122.

KATZENSTEIN, P. J. 1985. *Small States in World Markets.* Ithaca (NY): Cornell University Press.

KENNEDY, B. P., I. KAWACHI, and D. PROTHROW-STITH. 1996. Income distribution and mortality: Cross-sectional ecological study of the Robin Hood Index in the United States. *British Medical Journal* 312: 1004–1007.

LABOUR MONTHLY REVIEW. 1995. Annual data: Employment status of the working-age population, approximating U.S. concepts, 10 countries (November, p. 141). Washington (DC): U.S. Department of Labour.

LAVIS, J. 1996. Unemployment, work and health: A research framework for a changing world. Institute for Work and Health. Unpublished.

LAVIS, J., and T. SULLIVAN. Forthcoming. Health improvements and the state: Past policies, current constraints and the possibility of political change. In *Health Promotion: Linking Theory and Practice*, eds. L. GREEN, I. ROOTMAN, and B. POLAND. Newbury Park (CA): Sage Publications.

LE GRAND, J. 1987. Inequalities in health: Some international comparisons. *European Economic Review* 31: 182–191.

LEON, D., D. VAGERO, and P. OTTERBLAD OLAUSSON. 1992. Social class differences in infant mortality in Sweden: A comparison with England and Wales. *British Medical Journal* 305: 687–691.

LINN, M. W., R. S. SANDIFER, and S. STEIN. 1985. Effects of unemployment on mental and physical health. *American Journal of Public Health* 75: 502–506.

LUNDBERG, B. 1991. The LO Health Project: Trade Union Health Promotion in Sweden. Paper presented to the European Conference on Health Promotion in the Workplace (April), Barcelona, Spain.

MACKENBACH, J. 1994. Socioeconomic inequalities in health in the Netherlands: Impact of a five-year research program. *British Medical Journal* 309: 1487–1491.

MACKENBACH, J. 1996. Personal communication.

MARTIKAINEN, P. T. 1990. Unemployment and mortality among Finnish men, 1981–1985. *British Medical Journal* 301: 401–411.

MORISSETTE, R., J. MYLES, and G. PICOT. 1995. Earnings polarization in Canada, 1969–1991. In *Labour Market Polarization and Social Policy Reform*, eds. K .G. BANTIND, and C .M. BEACH. Kingston (ON): School of Policy Studies, Queen's University.

MORREL, S., R. TAYLOR, QUINE S., AND C. KERR. 1993. Suicide and unemployment in Australia. *Social Science and Medicine* 36: 749–756.

MOSER, K. A., A. J. FOX, and P. O. GOLDBLATT. 1986. Stress and heart disease: Evidence of association between unemployment and heart disease from the OPCS longitudinal study. *Postgraduate Medical Journal* 62: 797–790.

MOSER, K. A., P. O. GOLDBLATT, and A. J. FOX 1987. Unemployment and mortality: Comparison of the 1971 and 1981 longitudinal study census samples. *British Medical Journal* 294: 85–90.

O'GRADY, J. 1995. Incentives, fairness and social policy. Comment paper presented at the Workshop on Economic Growth and Income Equality. Laurentian University, Sudbury, Ontario (March 17–18).

ONTARIO TRAINING AND ADJUSTMENT BOARD. 1994. *Annual Report.* Toronto (ON): Ontario Training and Adjustment Board.

ORGANIZATION FOR ECONOMIC CO-OPERATION AND DEVELOPMENT (OECD). 1994. *The OECD Jobs Study.* Paris: OECD Publications Service.

———. 1995a. *The OECD Jobs Study, Part I: Labour Market Trends and Underlying Forces of Change.* Paris: OECD Publications Service.

———. 1995b. *The OECD Jobs Study, Part II: The Adjustment Potential of the Labour Market.* Paris: OECD Publications Service.

PREMIER'S COUNCIL ON HEALTH STRATEGY. 1991. *Nurturing Health: A Framework on the Determinants of Health.* Report of the Healthy Public Policy Committee. Toronto (ON): The Queen's Printer.

PONAK, A., and M. THOMPSON. 1994. Public sector collective bargaining. In *Union-Management Relations in Canada*, eds. M. GUNDERSON and A. PONAK. Toronto (ON): Addison-Wesley.

PLATT, S. 1984. Unemployment and suicidal behaviour: A review of the literature. *Social Science and Medicine* 19: 93–115.

PURCHASE, B. 1996. Health care and competitiveness. Proceedings of a National Health Care Policy Summit (March 18–19). Ottawa (ON): Canadian Medical Association.

REID, F. 1987. *Hours of Work and Overtime Policies to Reduce Unemployment. A report prepared for the Ontario Task Force on Hours of Work and Overtime.* Toronto (ON): Ontario Task Force on Hours of Work and Overtime.

———. 1995. *Working Less and Enjoying It More. A Paper for the National Forum on Family Security* (May). Ottawa (ON): National Forum on Family Security.

RIDDELL, W. 1986. *Adapting To Change: Labour Market Adjustment in Canada.* Toronto (ON): University of Toronto Press.

ROOS, N. 1995. From research to policy: What have we learned from designing the population health information system? *Medical Care* 33(12): 133–145.

SULLIVAN, T. 1996. Roundtable on the human face of regionalization. In *How Many Roads: Regionalisation and Health Care in Canada*, eds. J. DORLAND, and M. DAVIS. Kingston (ON): School of Policy Studies, Queen's University.

TORONTO STAR. 1996. Too much work can kill. Friday, April 12, p. A1.

WALDMANN, R. J. 1992. Income distribution and infant mortality. *Quarterly Journal of Economics* 107: 1283–1302.

WENNEMO, I. 1993. Infant mortality, public policy and inequality: A comparison of 18 industrialized countries. *Sociology of Health and Illness* 15: 429–446.

WHITE, J. 1990. *Hospital Strike.* Toronto (ON): Thompson Educational Publishing.

WHITEHEAD, M. 1995. Tackling inequalities: A review of policy initiatives. In *Tackling Inequalities in Health: An Agenda for Action*, eds. M. BENZEVAL, K. JUDGE, and M. WHITEHEAD. London: King's Fund.

WILKINSON, R. G. 1992. Income distribution and life expectancy. *British medical Journal* 304: 165–168.

_____. 1995. Commentary: A reply to Ken Judge: Mistaken criticisms ignore overwhelming evidence. *British Medical Journal* 311: 1285–1287.

WOLFSON, M. 1996. Three views on income equity. Robarts Centre Conference on Globalization, State Choices and Citizen Participation in Health Care Reform (April). York University, North York (ON). Unpublished.

WORLD DEVELOPMENT REPORT. 1995. Workers in an integrated world. *World Development Report.* New York (NY): Oxford University Press.

WORLD LABOUR REPORT. 1984. Employment incomes, social protection, new information technology. *World Labour Report.* Geneva, Switzerland: International Labour Office.

APPENDICES

APPENDIX 1

OECD sectoral employment trends, 1979–1990
Employment growth per capita
Annualized percentage change in employment divided
by the population aged 15–64

TOTAL	Agric.	Manuf.	Const.	Total priv. sector	General govt.	Total*
North America	−1.5	−1.5	0.7	0.7	0.2	0.6
Canada	−2.0	−1.4	0.6	0.7	0.3	0.6
United States	−1.4	−1.5	0.7	0.8	0.2	0.6
Japan	−3.3	0.1	−0.6	0.3	−0.7	0.2
European Comm.	−4.0	−1.8	−1.2	−0.5	0.6	−0.3
Belgium	−2.3	−1.9	−2.2	−0.3	0.3	−0.2
Denmark	−3.4	−0.1	−2.2	−0.4	1.1	0.0
France	−4.5	−2.5	−2.1	−1.0	0.7	−0.6
Germany	−3.9	−0.9	−1.6	−0.2	0.2	−0.2
Greece	−2.2	0.1	−2.8	−0.1	1.2	0.0
Ireland	−3.2	−1.5	−3.1	−0.8	−1.3	−0.9
Italy	−4.7	−1.7	−1.3	−0.3	0.6	−0.1
Luxembourg	−4.2	−2.0	1.2	1.0	1.4	1.0
Netherlands	−1.5	−1.5	−3.0	−0.6	−0.6	−0.6
Portugal	−4.3	−1.2	−0.9	−1.4	2.2	−1.0
Spain	−5.1	−1.8	−0.1	−1.1	3.4	−0.6
United Kingdom	−2.0	−3.2	0.8	0.1	0.1	0.1
EFTA**	−3.2	−1.4	0.3	−0.2	1.4	0.2
Finland	−3.5	−1.5	1.4	−0.2	2.2	0.3
Iceland	−1.9	−2.0	0.0	−0.1	1.9	0.4
Norway	−2.7	−2.8	−0.4	−0.6	1.8	0.0
Sweden	−3.4	−0.8	−0.1	0.0	0.9	0.3
Australia	−1.2	−1.9	0.3	0.5	0.4	0.5

Source: Excerpts from table 1.1, OECD Jobs Study 1995, p.4.

* This total does not include general government and other nongovernment services.

** European Free Trade Area.

APPENDIX 2

**Full-time and part-time employment by sex and age,
Canada and provinces**
Annual averages 1994

	Total thousands	Both sexes FT	PT	Males FT	PT	Females FT	PT
Canada	**13,292**	**11,038**	**2,254**	**6,599**	**690**	**4,438**	**1,564**
15–24 years	2,073	1,184	889	663	403	522	486
25–44 years	7,342	6,506	836	3,826	153	2,680	683
45 years and over	3,876	3,347	529	2,111	134	1,236	395
Newfoundland	**195**	**168**	**26**	**100**	**9**	**68**	**18**
15–24 years	32	21	11	11	5	10	6
25–44 years	110	100	10	57	–	42	8
45 years and over	53	48	5	32	–	16	4
Prince Edward Island	**56**	**47**	**9**	**27**	**–**	**20**	**6**
15–24 years	11	6	4	–	–	–	–
25–44 years	29	26	–	15	–	12	–
45 years and over	16	14	–	9	–	5	–
Nova Scotia	**380**	**309**	**71**	**185**	**22**	**124**	**48**
15–24 years	64	34	30	19	13	16	16
25–44 years	209	183	26	107	5	75	21
45 years and over	107	92	15	59	4	33	11
New Brunswick	**307**	**259**	**48**	**154**	**15**	**105**	**34**
15–24 years	52	33	19	18	9	15	10
25–44 years	169	151	18	88	–	63	15
45 years and over	86	75	11	48	–	27	8
Quebec	**3,156**	**2,681**	**475**	**1,602**	**155**	**1,079**	**320**
15–24 years	463	268	195	153	90	115	106
25–44 years	1,776	1,603	173	934	38	669	135
45 years and over	916	810	106	515	27	295	80
Ontario	**5,160**	**4,264**	**896**	**2,519**	**280**	**1,745**	**616**
15–24 years	781	411	370	224	171	187	199
25–44 years	2,849	2,533	316	1,477	58	1,057	257
45 years and over	1,530	1,320	210	819	51	501	159

Appendix 2 (cont.)

	Total thousands	Both sexes FT	Both sexes PT	Males FT	Males PT	Females FT	Females PT
Manitoba	511	416	95	255	27	161	68
15–24 years	90	54	36	31	16	23	20
25–44 years	269	233	36	140	5	93	31
45 years and over	152	129	23	84	6	45	17
Saskatchewan	457	376	81	231	23	145	57
15–24 years	76	46	30	27	14	19	15
25–44 years	238	209	30	126	4	83	26
45 years and over	143	121	21	78	6	43	16
Alberta	1,337	1,111	226	676	61	436	165
15–24 years	226	141	85	81	36	60	49
25–44 years	754	664	90	400	13	264	77
45 years and over	357	307	51	195	11	112	39
British Columbia	1,733	1,405	328	850	96	555	232
15–24 years	279	170	109	96	46	74	62
25–44 years	938	804	134	482	23	322	110
45 years and over	516	431	85	272	26	159	59

Source: Labour Force Annual Averages, 1989–1994, Household Surveys Division, Statistics Canada, 1995.

Note: Full-time employment consists of persons who usually work 30 hours or more per week, plus those who usually work less than 30 hours but consider themselves to be employed full-time (e.g., airline pilots); part-time employment consists of all other persons who usually work less than 30 hours per week.

APPENDIX 3

Employment shares in services, 1992
As a percentage of total employment

ISIC-1968 code	Wholesale and retail trade	Transport and communication	Finance, real estate and business services				Public admin.	Community, social and personal services					Recreation and cultural	Personal and household	Service sector total
			Total	Finance and insurance	Real estate and business	Total		Social, community and welfare services							
								Total	Education	Health	Welfare				
	6	7	8	81-82	83	9	91	93	931	933	934		94	95	6-9
North America	22,4	5,7	13,2	4,7	8,5	31,5	5,0	20,2	7,6	9,0	–		2,1	3,9	72,6
Canada	23,8	6,3	11,6	4,0	7,6	31,2	6,8	17,7	7,2	10,0	–		1,4	5,2	73,0
United States	22,2	5,6	13,3	4,8	8,5	31,5	4,8	20,5	7,7	8,9	1,4		2,2	3,7	72,6
Japan[1]	23,5	6,0	10,9	3,2	7,7	18,1	3,4	9,7	3,3	3,5	1,1		1,3	3,3	58,5
European Community	18,4	6,0	8,5	–	–	29,1	7,6	–	–	–	–		–	–	61,9
Belgium	17,3	7,0	9,3	5,3	4,0	35,8	6,3	18,4	8,1	6,0	4,1		1,5	8,5	69,3
Denmark[2]	14,6	7,0	9,2	3,6	5,5	34,9	5,2	24,2	–	–	–		2,1	2,2	65,6
France	16,1	6,2	9,5	3,3	6,2	32,9	9,4	17,6	7,3	6,2	–		1,6	4,2	64,7
Germany	16,9	5,8	8,8	4,2	4,6	27,0	7,8	14,5	–	–	–		1,3	2,1	58,5
Greece[2,3]	18,2	6,9	5,3	2,1	3,2	19,8	6,6	9,9	–	–	–		1,3	1,7	50,3
Ireland[2]	17,9	5,9	8,5	3,8	4,6	24,5	4,7	14,6	–	–	–		1,9	2,6	56,8
Italy	21,7	5,4	5,1	–	–	27,4	8,5	–	–	–	–		–	–	59,6
Netherlands	17,3	6,3	10,8	3,5	7,3	34,7	6,9	21,5	6,1	8,2	–		1,8	2,5	69,1
Portugal	19,8	4,8	6,5	3,2	3,3	24,5	7,2	–	7,2	4,3	–		–	–	55,6
Spain[4]	20,5	5,9	6,0	2,6	3,3	25,1	6,3	9,9	5,1	3,8	–		1,5	5,9	57,5
United Kingdom	18,8	6,2	11,2	3,6	7,6	30,9	6,8	17,4	6,8	6,0	2,4		3,1	67,1	–

Appendix 3 (cont.)

ISIC-1968 code	Wholesale and retail trade	Transport and communi-cation	Finance, real estate and business services				Community, social and personal services							Service sector total
			Total	Finance and insurance	Real estate and business	Total	Public admin.	Social, community and welfare services				Recreation and cultural	Personal and household	
								Total	Education	Health	Welfare			
	6	7	8	81-82	83	9	91	93	931	933	934	94	95	6-9
EFTA	17,1	6,9	10,1	-	-	31,1	5,3	-	-	-	-	-	-	65,3
Austria	18,9	6,6	7,5	3,8	3,7	23,7	7,5	12,1	-	-	-	1,0	0,8	56,6
Finland	13,4	7,6	8,8	3,5	5,3	33,6	5,1	20,3	7,1	7,3	6,0	4,0	2,7	63,3
Norway	17,9	8,0	7,8	2,8	4,9	37,0	5,6	26,0	7,9	10,6	6,0	1,9	2,7	70,7
Sweden	14,2	7,2	9,4	2,9	6,5	39,3	5,0	29,6	7,6	10,0	10,3	2,1	1,6	70,1
Switzerland	20,6	6,1	15,2	-	-	24,5	3,6	-	-	-	-	-	-	66,3
Oceania	24,5	6,3	11,6	4,2	7,3	27,8	4,7	19,0	-	-	-	1,9	2,1	70,2
Australia	25,2	6,4	11,7	4,3	7,4	27,7	4,5	19,4	7,5	7,5	-	1,9	1,9	71,0
New Zealand	21,0	6,1	10,8	3,7	7,1	28,4	6,0	16,7	-	-	-	2,0	2,8	66,2
Turkey	12,6	4,5	2,5	1,4	1,1	14,4	5,3	5,4	-	-	-	0,3	3,4	34,0
OECD	20,4	5,8	10,4	-	-	27,4	5,7	-	-	-	-	-	-	64,1

Sources: OECD. *Labour Force Statistics* and data provided by national statistical offices.
1. 1990 census results.
2. Data refer to 1991.
3. "Repair services" are included in manufacturing instead of "Personal and household services".
4. Education sector includes research and development activities.

Economic Policy Variables and Population Health

LARS OSBERG, PH.D.

Department of Economics
Dalhousie University

SUMMARY

Increasingly, medical specialists and society at large have begun to recognize that the health of individuals is heavily influenced by their psychological and social well-being. Since making a living is an inescapable preoccupation of most adults, the economy has a major influence on well-being, through its impacts on unemployment, insecurity/anxiety, individuals' sense of personal control, and economic inequality.

Controlling for age, education, occupation, level of physical activity and a host of other possible determinants of health status, the unemployed tend systematically to have poorer health outcomes than the employed. For most people, losing a job means much more than just losing income. Unemployment is often accompanied by social isolation, purposelessness, and a loss of occupational identity—as well as the stresses of low income and dependence on social transfers—all of which have adverse health implications. However, historically the jobs lost in declining firms and industries were replaced by new jobs in expanding sectors. The short-term unemployment which is created by job search and labour reallocation is likely to have much less impact on population health than long-term unemployment.

In the 1990s Canada has seen a long period of high unemployment and a substantial rise in long-term unemployment. Hence, for population health the crucial issue now is whether there are enough jobs of any type—i.e., whether there is enough aggregate demand in the economy. When there is not, firms are able to attract labour even if they offer only insecure, low-wage employment. In analyzing the determinants of population health, one must therefore add to the stress of unemployment the pressures of precarious employment. As well, unemployment indirectly influences population health through its impact on the divorce rate and family structure.

Economic insecurity has been a pervasive aspect of Canadian labour markets and Canadian societies in the 1990s. Increasing numbers of people are unsure whether their present options will be available to them in the future and are unable to form a concrete picture of an acceptable alternative. However, the issue underlying economic insecurity is not economic change, but the context of change. If there is strong aggregate demand for labour, replacement jobs are easily available for displaced workers. When public policies provide "social protection" to workers or when workers are protected by powerful unions or when private employers offer credible guarantees of continued employment, workers know that the essential aspects of their economic future are secure, even if their job duties may change. This context is important, since stress and anxiety have health implications. Furthermore, since some institutional arrangements can both facilitate change and enhance personal security, there is no simple "trade-off" between security and flexibility.

Medical researchers have noted that a sense of achievement, self-esteem, and personal control over life appears to affect health and well-being. Indeed, efficacy is a common denominator underlying income, education, and employment status—all of which are significant determinants of health. In the workplace, the structure of job hierarchies and the degree of devolution of authority influence workers' sense of control over day-to-day work outcomes. Within many companies, positive trends in job redesign can be seen.

A growing literature has documented the link between income inequality and variations in average life expectancy, and other health outcomes, among developed countries. In less developed countries, improvements in the average level of income are highly correlated with improvements in life expectancy, in large part because of the greater resistance to disease which accompanies improved nutrition. However, once most people have access to the basic material necessities of life, the causes of death shift from infectious diseases to degenerative cardiovascular diseases and cancers. The mortality and morbidity rates of the affluent are systematically lower than those of the poor, and among developed countries the average level of mortality is lower in countries with less overall income inequality. Economic policies to reduce inequality are therefore likely to improve population health, but because higher unemployment, greater insecurity, lessened efficacy, and greater economic inequality are all highly correlated, disentangling the pathways by which economic inequality influences the average health status of the population is a complex task.

Although unemployment, economic insecurity, a sense of loss of control over one's economic future, and heightened social inequality have impacts throughout society, three groups are particularly vulnerable: youth, the poorly educated, and displaced workers. In the depressed labour markets of the 1990s, youth unemployment has remained above 15 percent, and relative youth wages have fallen continuously since the early 1980s. Overwhelmingly, the jobs which have been created in the 1990s have required postsecondary education, and the poorly educated have been increasingly excluded from access to employment. Older workers who lose their jobs often find it extremely difficult to "start all over again" in the labour market.

In conclusion, because social expenditures on income transfers and on health care are hostage to the resumption of economic growth, because the level of unemployment has a strong direct impact on population health, and because high unemployment indirectly influences population health through its impacts on personal efficacy, economic insecurity and income inequality, macroeconomic policy has an important health dimension. In the late 1990s, the deficit and debt problems of Canadian governments largely preclude fiscal stimulus. However, monetary policy remains an extremely powerful policy lever. Hence, the main economic policy variable that can positively affect the health of Canadians is a monetary policy that emphasizes jobs and growth.

TABLE OF CONTENTS

INTRODUCTION

Increasingly, medical specialists and society at large have begun to recognize that "health," "illness" and "recovery" are not just simple issues of the medical treatment of disease or accidents. Both the objective prevalence of physical ailments and their subjective interpretation and impacts on life are influenced, in complex ways, by the social and psychological well-being of individuals. Since making a living is an inescapable preoccupation of most adults and since the rewards from and the ways in which people make their living affect many aspects of the rest of their lives, economics has a major influence on psychological and social well-being. Therefore, it makes sense to ask what the role economic policy variables might play in influencing the health of the population.

This paper starts with an examination of some of the economic determinants of health status. Unemployment, economic insecurity/anxiety, a sense of personal control over one's economic future and economic inequality are all interrelated aspects of the economic environment of individuals which can be expected to influence their health status. The paper then discusses the special problems of vulnerable groups within Canadian society and looks at directions for economic policy which could reasonably be expected to affect the health outcomes of Canadians, and which also have some degree of feasibility in the actual environment of Canada in the 1990s. The final section is a conclusion.

ECONOMIC DETERMINANTS OF HEALTH

Unemployment

As many studies in Canada and elsewhere have concluded, unemployment is bad for the health. Controlling for age, education, occupation, level of physical activity and a host of other possible determinants of health status, unemployed individuals tend, systematically, to have poorer health outcomes than employed individuals.[1] To understand why the experience of unemployment tends to produce ill health, it is useful to analyze why employment is important. As Jahoda (1979, 494) put it:

---

1. Schofield (1996, 3) provided a listing of some of the "large number of studies, both in Australia and overseas, which have established a relationship between unemployment and a range of measures of poor health." D'Arcy and Siddique (1987), D'Arcy (1986), Béland (1993), Ketso (1988) and Grayson (1993) represent some of the Canadian literature. Brenner (1971, 1973) and Brenner and Mooney (1983) are classic early articles on the subject.

There are latent consequences of employment as a social institution which meet human needs of an enduring kind. First among them is the fact that employment imposes a time structure on the waking day. Secondly, employment implies regularly shared experiences and contacts with people outside the family. Thirdly, employment links an individual to goals and purposes which transcend his own. Fourthly, employment defines aspects of status and identity. Finally, employment forces activity.

It is these "objective" consequences of work in complex industrialized societies which help us to understand the motivation to work beyond earning a living; to understand why work is psychologically supportive, even when conditions are bad; and, by the same token, to understand why unemployment is psychologically destructive.

As well as performing these important latent functions, employment also has the direct practical implication of enabling employed individuals to earn an income. And if a household is without employment, dependence on social transfers is unavoidable, with the stress of lower income, the loss of social respect and the anxiety about the future which that entails.

A major theme of this paper is the central importance of the level of unemployment as a determinant of health outcomes. However, to understand the relationship between unemployment and health, and the policy measures that might mitigate adverse health implications, it is also useful to distinguish among the types of unemployment experience which are likely to have (or not have) adverse implications for health. As many (e.g., Kelvin and Jarrett 1985) have noted, the psychological impacts of an unemployment spell can be expected to vary with its duration, since despondency and depression usually only begin to set in after a prolonged period of unemployment—the first few weeks of unemployment are often a period of relative optimism, activity and the productive use of time. There is also abundant evidence in labour economics that the reason for unemployment matters. Individuals who are laid off or who are dismissed have different patterns of labour market search and reemployment than those who quit their job voluntarily. (See Devine and Kiefer 1991.) It is, therefore, reasonable to expect that the health impacts of unemployment may also differ according to the initial cause of unemployment.

To analyze the health impacts of unemployment, and the policy measures that could be of assistance, one must therefore begin by asking "Why are people unemployed?" It is also necessary to recognize that being unemployed is not the same as being without a job. In the official labour force statistics, individuals without jobs can either be classified as "unemployed" (if they looked actively for work[2]) or "not in the labour force" (if they did not engage in job search). Within labour economics, the meaning and the ambiguities of the not in the labour force/unemployed distinction have often been debated, since observed behaviour (i.e., job search) may not be a reasonable guide to the reality of unemployment, when individuals who want employment withdraw from active job search, because they believe no jobs are available.

This ambiguity in the statistical measurement of unemployment points to the importance of the *subjective* interpretation of labour market events. Whether or not a spell of joblessness is interpreted as unemployment depends on both the labour market context within which an individual functions and whether or not a socially sanctioned alternative definition of their joblessness (e.g., as retired or housewife) is available. Similarly, the health implications of a spell of unemployment are likely to vary with both the social context and the social interpretation of joblessness, which varies over time, as social norms change.[3] Unemployment that is a normal part of an otherwise satisfying occupation (e.g., film crew, construction worker) or joblessness which can be easily relabelled as socially sanctioned labour force withdrawal (e.g., retirement) is unlikely to have the same health implications as the involuntary, long-duration unemployment of experienced workers which is the main focus of the literature on the psychological and health impacts of unemployment.

However, if all unemployment is assumed to be equivalent to leisure and if the amount of unemployment is seen as determined by the utility-maximizing choices of rational individuals, it is difficult to see why unemployment should have *any* adverse health impacts. Neoclassical labour economics starts from the perspective that individuals choose the number of hours they wish to supply to the labour market in order to maximize their utility. In the labour-leisure choice model, individuals can sell whatever number of hours they wish to employers, at a wage that is determined by their personal characteristics. Work is seen as a disutility, but individuals are seen as deriving utility from the income produced by employment and from "leisure". In the work-leisure dichotomy, all nonwork hours are defined

---

2. In addition, a fairly small number of jobless people are classed as unemployed without the requirement for an active job search, i.e., if they were on layoff, were available for work and were not looking because they expected to return to their previous job or if they had not actively looked for work but had a new job to start in four weeks or less.

3. Changing social norms, and the changing stresses of joblessness, can be illustrated by the very different social reactions married women can expect to receive in the 1990s to the statement "I am a housewife" compared to the reaction which could be expected in the 1970s, or the 1950s.

to be "leisure", and the distinction between leisure and unemployment, or between types of unemployment, is ignored. Variations over time, or across individuals, in total employment hours are explained by the labour-leisure choice model as arising in response to changing incentives. Variations among individuals in real wages and in the income available through social transfers, such as unemployment insurance, are considered to be the determining factors in unemployment.

Although the labour-leisure choice model has a long history in economics, the search perspective is more recent, dating from the early 1970s. This perspective starts from the truism that the probability of an unemployed individual getting a job is equal to the probability that the individual will receive a job offer times the probability that he will accept that offer. However, although in practice the job offer arrival rate is the most important determinant of unemployment duration (see Devine and Kiefer 1991, 140, 304), the search literature has focused on whether or not an individual will accept or reject available job offers. In other words, the focus is on the unemployed individual's choice of "reservation wage," (i.e. the lowest paid job offer that he will accept).

But if the unemployed are just choosing the weeks of leisure they prefer, or the reservation wage that makes them the best off in the long run, why do they tend to be sicker than employed individuals?[4] Supply-side interpretations of unemployment are, in general, hard to reconcile with the evidence on the adverse health implications of unemployment. The labour-leisure choice model of unemployment and the job search model of unemployment both appeal directly to the utility-maximizing choices of individuals as an explanation of unemployment, but one must also recognize that higher payroll taxes as a possible explanation of the higher unemployment of the 1990s (see Poloz 1994) are, ultimately, dependent on the voluntary supply-side choices of workers. As Allié (1994) made clear, in a neoclassical model, higher payroll taxes are predicted to decrease employment because workers want to supply less hours of work when their wages fall and employers can be expected to cut wages to compensate for the impacts of higher rates of payroll taxation on total labour costs. Only in the short

---

4. In addition, one can seriously question whether either the labour-leisure choice model or the voluntary job search choice model can reasonably explain the variation in aggregate unemployment over time, across countries or among individuals. In Canada, for example, the "choice" perspective on unemployment has often been used to assert that unemployment insurance system incentives are responsible for much of Canada's unemployment, but the empirical evidence is highly ambiguous. (See Osberg 1996, or Myatt 1996.) There is a good deal of evidence that the incentives of unemployment insurance are relatively unimportant, compared to the constraints imposed by the unavailability of employment. (See Phipps 1990, 1991; Osberg and Phipps 1993.)

term, before wage levels can adjust to an increase in indirect labour costs, will there be an increase in total labour costs and a demand side–based decrease in employment.

Although explanations of unemployment that view unemployment time as the result of voluntary, utility-maximizing individual choices cannot credibly be reconciled with the perspective that unemployment causes ill health, explanations of unemployment that emphasize the disappearance of jobs can be. There are two main candidates: the structural change argument and the deficient aggregate demand hypothesis.

Structural change has always been a conspicuous feature of capitalism. From the displacement of hand loom weavers by power loom technology in the eighteenth century to the replacement of bank tellers by automated teller machines (ATMs) in the 1990s, it has always been the case that workers have lost their jobs to technological and market changes. For more than two centuries, the jobs lost in declining sectors have been replaced by new jobs in expanding sectors. Although the popular press is replete with assertions that the technological and market changes of the 1990s are unprecedented, the popular press of previous decades was similarly impressed with the then unprecedented speed of change. And since qualitatively different types of structural change are inherently hard to compare (e.g., the rural-urban shift of the 1950s, compared to the computer revolution of the 1990s) it is not particularly easy to assess when change is "greater."[5]

Because the shedding of excess labour by declining firms is an inherent part of a dynamic capitalist system, one must also distinguish between demand deficient and structural unemployment. Strictly speaking, structural unemployment refers to the unemployment of those whose skills, location or other personal characteristics mean they cannot fill *available vacancies*. Unemployed workers with the wrong skills or who are in the wrong location to fill existing jobs can be said to be "structurally" unemployed. But if there are not enough jobs of any type, the cause of unemployment is more accurately assigned to deficiency of aggregate demand.

Structural change in a macroeconomic environment of strong aggregate demand generates some unemployment, but it is the frictional unemployment of job search which occurs when it takes time for the excess labour of declining sectors to locate jobs in expanding sectors. The Canadian labour market is normally characterized by a rather high level of geographic and interindustry mobility. For example, some 19 percent of Canadian workers changed their broad industry of employment between 1986 and 1987. (See Osberg et al. 1994, 59.)

---

5. Samson (1985) provided data on the coefficient of variation of change in employment levels by industry which indicated that, by this measure, the structural change of employment in Canada in the 1950s (a low unemployment decade) was *greater* than in the 1970s and 1980s.

From the point of view of unemployed individuals whose jobs have disappeared and who cannot get new ones, the distinction between structural and demand deficient unemployment may seem to be of secondary importance. If there are known to be jobs elsewhere or for other skills, unemployed individuals may hope that if they move, or retrain, they can take control of their own lives and become employed. Conversely, if it is clear that there is a generalized surplus of labour, the widespread realization that "there aren't jobs out there, so it's not my fault" may attenuate the stress of unemployment. But either way, there is no job. The psychological importance of the social isolation, boredom, lack of structure and identity implied by a lack of employment, and the financial impact of a lack of earnings, remains.

The distinction between demand deficient and structural unemployment is important for macroeconomic policymakers, who have to decide whether unemployment could be reduced by stimulating macroeconomic demand through lower interest rates, or whether an increase in aggregate demand would encounter the constraint of supply capacity, and thereby generate inflation. Indeed, macroeconomic decision makers may be highly uncertain as to the potential output capacity of the economy.[6] However, objective uncertainty about the rate of unemployment at which inflationary pressures might emerge may interact with the Bank of Canada's bureaucratic imperative of being seen to accomplish stated goals. If the sole priority of policy is to avoid inflation, this is not actually a difficult objective for a central bank to attain. It is always possible to maintain enough slack (i.e., excess unemployment) in the economic system to prevent any possibility of a resurgence of inflation, but only at the cost of perpetually high unemployment. As Fortin (1994) has argued convincingly, the Bank of Canada's estimates of the potential output capacity of the Canadian economy are systematically lower than those of other researchers, implying a systematic policy bias to excessive aggregate demand restraint and the achievement of inflation control targets.

From the point of view of population health, there is a further implication of high unemployment: when labour markets are persistently characterized by excess supply and a queue of available workers for any job opening, it makes sense for employers to alter their personnel policies. When employers can be sure that workers will be available, on an on-call basis, to meet any future surges in demand, they have less incentive to retain permanent employees in slack periods. In a depressed labour market, firms will often

---

6. As Setterfield et al. (1992) demonstrated, statistically reasonable estimates of the nonaccelerating inflation rate of unemployment (NAIRU) can be found which would place the NAIRU anywhere between 4.42 percent and 9.25 percent for adult male unemployment—a range which spans virtually the entire postwar historical experience of unemployment in Canada.

find it more profitable to shift to a strategy in which they employ a small group of permanent core workers, and hire casual employees on a just-in-time basis, to cope with any surges in output. As more firms shift from a permanent worker strategy to a core-casual strategy, the declining number of full-time jobs then produces an increase in aggregate unemployment and greater economic insecurity for the swelling pool of casual employees.[7]

When firms shift to a just-in-time labour strategy and call workers in to work only when they are needed, the financial risk of short-run fluctuations in sales is transferred to workers. Workers also have to cope, in their day-to-day lives, with unpredictability in their working time and scheduling. Given that individuals usually live in households and have to coordinate their schedules with others (e.g., to provide child care) the result is an increase in the stress of daily life.

High unemployment, therefore, has both direct and indirect impacts on the determinants of health. The direct impact is to deprive more unemployed people of their work environment—which means that they have to do without the social contacts and relationships of the workplace and the psychological supports emphasized earlier (Jahoda 1979). An indirect impact arises from the effects of high unemployment on the job structure as the easy availability of potential workers causes firms to adjust their employment strategies in ways which increase the stress levels of workers.

As well, high unemployment influences family structure. The literature on the determinants of health outcomes often emphasizes the importance of the social contacts and social support network available to individuals. The trend in Canada is for individuals to live in smaller households and to have fewer people available for social support. While the extended family has been replaced, in most instances, by the nuclear family for some decades now, the nuclear family is also shrinking in size. The long run decline in fertility rates means that adults today not only live with fewer children than their parents did, they also have fewer siblings available should they need help or social interaction. Increased numbers of never-married and divorced adults have also swollen the proportion of single-person households.

These trends are not entirely exogenous. As Orcutt et al. (1976), and others, have noted, the probability of divorce is significantly higher in households affected by unemployment. As a result, one implication of a long period of high unemployment is an increasing proportion of older single-person households. The stress of divorce can itself be expected to have health implications and, since middle-aged and older singles tend to have poorer health, an increase in divorces also tends to produce a shift in population demographics toward a demographic structure with a higher probability of

---

7. For a fuller model of this process, see Osberg (1995).

morbidity. (Although it is also true that high unemployment may mean the delayed departure or return to the parental household of adult children and, therefore, a decline in the number of young single-person households, the net impact of high unemployment on health, via demographics, will be negative, if the impact of single status is greater for older cohorts.) The bottom line is that although the social support of family ties can be an important buffer for individuals from the stresses of economic life, the family itself may disintegrate if the stresses of economic life become excessively high.

Economic Insecurity/Anxiety

Economic variables affect population health in part because of the stresses of economic life, one of the most important of which is economic insecurity. But what exactly is economic insecurity? Why does it happen?

The easiest way to define economic insecurity is to contrast it with economic security, which can be defined as an individual's expectation that at least one of the options that will be available to him in the future will generate a level of economic well-being which is comparable to, or greater than, that individual's present level of economic well-being. Greater economic insecurity corresponds to a decrease in an individual's expectation that at least one future option will be comparable to the present, and the best available option may be substantially worse than the present.[8]

In my opinion, economic insecurity is a pervasive aspect of Canadian labour markets and Canadian society in the 1990s. In my view, feelings of economic insecurity have increased quite dramatically over the last 20 years, and this has major ramifications. However, it must be recognized that "economic insecurity" is a term that is rarely heard in the discourse of economists, and there is no generally accepted definition or empirical measurement of the concept. Occasionally, data from polling firms (e.g., EKOS 1993) can be used to illustrate some dimensions of the issue, but there are no time series data available.

How can it be that economic insecurity is a major preoccupation of unions in their collective bargaining and of individuals in their daily lives, and yet economists give it so little attention? In part, the answer lies in a trained incapacity to perceive. The training of most economists starts from a "perfect competition" vision of the economy, in which individuals are

---

8. Clearly, feelings of insecurity are closely related to a sense of personal efficacy (which can be defined as the perception that an individual's actions can influence favourably their own future available options) and to feelings of pessimism or optimism about the future (which can be defined as an average expectation of the value of future options).

assumed to maximize their lifetime utility, subject only to the constraints of their resource endowment, the prices individuals face in competitive markets and the interest rate available in the capital market. In this vision of reality, individuals are presumed always to have market options available. And if the loss of a job creates the need to move to an available new job, and if it is presumed that individuals can borrow or lend in perfect capital markets to tide themselves over any fluctuations in income (due, perhaps, to the search time required to locate new employment), then there is little cost to job loss and little reason to feel insecure about such a prospect.

As well, it is convenient in much economic theorizing to assume "rational expectations." In its technical sense, this simply means that individuals are assumed, on average, to form an expectation of the future that is an accurate predictor (i.e., systematic excesses of optimism and pessimism are ruled out). More generally, individuals are presumed to be "rational" in the sense of weighing dispassionately the relative probabilities of different states of nature and the outcomes to be expected in each. In computing the expected value and possible dispersion of probability of outcomes, individuals are presumed to behave in a rather bloodless fashion: in economic models no one loses sleep, becomes depressed or lashes out in anger as he contemplates the future.

Although the perfect competition perspective can offer useful insights into some aggregate market behaviour, most individuals actually live in a microreality where the issues ignored by the perfect competition framework (e.g., "thin" markets, transaction costs and social institutions) have great practical importance. Labour market institutions determine the terms and conditions of employment of people and the degree of "tenure" an individual has in his current job, as well as the severance benefits available if the job is lost. Over time, the initial training and subsequent job experience of most workers effectively results in their labour being specialized to the point that they can only realistically compete for a small subset of all possible employment. And when individuals worry about job loss, and its possible implications, such as being unable to make the mortgage payments, their concerns reflect concrete social realities, such as the possible loss of social ties to the neighbourhood, and the disruption of their children's schooling, as well as the purely financial losses of a forced sale.

Economic insecurity is, then, partly about an environment in which increasing numbers of people are unsure whether their present options will be available to them in the future, and find themselves unable to form a concrete picture of an acceptable alternative. The questions "Where will I live? What will I do?" are key dimensions of a concrete vision of the future, yet an increasing number of Canadians can no longer be sure they know the answers.

In thinking about the connections among economic policy, insecurity and health, it is important to emphasize that the issue underlying economic insecurity is not just economic change, but also the *context* of change. As has already been noted, structural change has long been a prominent feature of capitalist economies, but whether the shedding of labour by declining firms and sectors generates significant economic insecurity, or not, depends on the institutional, social and economic context in which labour shedding occurs.

If labour markets are characterized by a strong aggregate demand for labour, such that replacement jobs are easily found, the availability of market options is, in itself, a source of security to both employed and unemployed individuals. However, in labour markets where jobs are hard to find, the prospect of being "on the market" produces insecurity. When public policies provide "social protection" to workers, either in the form of legal restrictions on layoffs, requirements for severance pay or generous transfer payments in the event of unemployment, the personal consequences to workers of labour shedding by their employers are less costly. If workers are protected by powerful unions or if private employers offer credible guarantees of continued employment (as in the Japanese Zaibatsu) then workers are assured that although their job duties may change, the essential aspects of their economic future are secure.

A variety of policies can, therefore, provide security for workers—either public sector or private sector institutions which protect employment rights *or* a macroeconomic context in which jobs are available to unemployed people. In designing policies that provide economic security to employees, governments have to be aware that in a dynamic, market-driven economy, employers need to be able to adapt to technological and market changes. But as Blank (1994) pointed out, when one looks in detail at the labour market institutions of advanced industrial nations, there is no simple trade-off between economic security for workers and labour market flexibility. In Canada, for example, the existence of publicly funded universal health insurance means that workers need not worry about inadequate health insurance coverage and the chance of catastrophic illness. Universal Medicare also means that Canadians do not experience the problem of the "job lock" that can occur in a private health insurance system when individuals may lose their coverage for existing ailments if they move to a new employer-paid health plan. Medicare in Canada, therefore, is an example of a program that provides increased economic security *and* increased labour market flexibility.

Other types of programs may have their main impact in pushing employers to particular *types* of adaptation to change. As Blank has pointed out, in many European countries, the cost of mandatory severance pay for laid-off workers creates an incentive for employers to react to a downturn in demand by decreasing the hours of work of all employees. On the other hand, the U.S.-style system of employer-paid benefits creates a fixed cost of employment *per worker*, which establishes an incentive to react to downturns in demand by laying off some workers entirely and concentrating remaining available hours of employment on the remaining employees.

In general, in a dynamic capitalist system one cannot expect anything other than continual pressure on firms to change and to adapt to change. For population health, the issue is whether the context of change—both in the institutional constraints on types of adaptation to change and the availability of alternative jobs—can leave workers with the economic security they need, while still enabling firms to find a viable type of adaptation.

Control/Efficacy

In October 1993, EKOS Research Associates asked a representative sample of Canadians whether they agreed or disagreed with the statement "I feel I have lost all control over my economic future." Fifty-two percent said they agreed. In a February 1994 repeat of the same question, 44 percent agreed. This sort of global sense that life is out of control and that one does not know, and is unable to influence, what the future may bring is likely to have significant health consequences. As Frank and Mustard (1994, 9) have noted:

> ...an individual's sense of achievement, self-esteem and control over his or her work and life appears to affect health and well being... How competence and coping skills relate to vulnerability to disease may be explained by improved understanding of the links between the brain and the endocrine pathways and the immune system.

In trying to understand the pathways by which social and economic events influence health, a sense of personal efficacy or control is a crucial intervening variable. Just as the decision to go skydiving has very different implications for stress levels and health than being thrown out of an airplane involuntarily, the stress created by the same social and economic events can be expected to have very different impacts, depending on the sense of control an individual has over the consequences of such events.

Indeed, it can be argued that efficacy is a common denominator underlying several significant socioeconomic determinants of health. As Béland (1993, 19) noted, income, education and employment status are a triptych which tends to predict health outcomes. As he puts it:

> ...income, education and unemployment are the very issues out of which health policy is made. It is thus legitimate for health policy measures to be preoccupied with schooling, income distribution and unemployment. Policies directed towards these sectors will not only influence health status and health risks, they will also affect needs for medical care.

By increasing an individual's sense of comprehending his environment, education provides an essential first step in managing one's life, and thereby affects each individual's sense of efficacy. Affluent people have choices to make, and a degree of control over their economic life, which is denied to poor individuals, whose resources are almost entirely consumed by non-discretionary expenditures. Unemployed persons have less money and more time available but, since they do not control whether a firm will offer them a job, they lose control over their future.

If personal efficacy is an important intervening variable in population health, one must also consider the locus within which a sense of personal control operates. At the workplace level, the structure of the job hierarchy and the degree of devolution of workplace authority influence the percentage of the population which feels some degree of control over day-to-day work outcomes. Conversely, the constraints which past company practice, collective bargaining or the law place on the arbitrary exercise of power by superiors also influence the prevalence of a sense of personal control. Within many companies today, there is a new emphasis on "delayering" and the "empowerment" of production workers. However, there is also a certain amount of shop floor cynicism that these buzz words of modern management, if not accompanied by some form of protection for the job security of employees, may simply mean an increase in responsibility, workload and workplace stress for the "empowered" workers who remain after "delayering."

At the broader social level, a sense of personal control over one's own life is imperiled when the basic assumptions of personal planning are called into question. Although it may be modern-day political wisdom to suppose that it is necessary to invoke a sense of imminent crisis to effect reforms, the drumbeat of dire (and misleading) predictions (e.g., that Canada is about to hit a "debt wall" or that the Canada Pension Plan [CPP] will go bankrupt or that Medicare is not sustainable) tends to create a societal anxiety level that cannot be healthy.

Inequality and Health

In recent years, several authors have argued that income inequality is the key determinant of variations in average life expectancy at birth among developed countries.[9] Wilkinson (1994, 1995b) argued that during earlier historic epochs in developed countries, and in much of the less-developed world today, a large proportion of the population has suffered from chronic

---

9. Judge (1995) took aim at Wilkinson's conclusions in a critical review. Wilkinson's reply (1995a) emphasized the robustness of his results to data choices and the corroborating work of others such as Waldmann (1992), Duleep (1995), McIsaac and Wilkinson (1995).

hunger and the reduced resistance to infectious disease which that implies. In these conditions, improvements in the average level of income are highly correlated with improvements in life expectancy. Indeed, the historical record in developed countries is quite clear that major declines in mortality due to specific diseases (e.g., tuberculosis) occurred well before the development of medical science or improvements in public health. However, once the vast majority of the population gains reliable access to the basic material necessities of life, there appears to be an epidemiological transition: the main causes of death shift from infectious diseases to degenerative cardio-vascular diseases and cancers (Wilkinson 1994, 65).

In affluent countries, poor people have a greater prevalence of many of the risk factors, such as obesity or smoking, which tend to be rich people's problems in poor countries. Even when controlling for the prevalence of such risk factors, there is an important influence of income on the prevalence of health problems. Waldmann's (1992) study of infant mortality indicated that the issue is not the absolute level of resources available to poor people in each country. When the absolute level of income of poor people was controlled, infant mortality was higher in countries where the share of rich people was greater. As Wilkinson (1994) argued, even though rich people in every country tend to live longer than poor people, the gradient in life expectancy is smaller in countries with a more equal income distribution, implying that not only relatively poor individuals, but also relatively affluent individuals, tend to live longer in countries with greater income equality.

The argument that variations in economic inequality are now the main determinant of variations in the health status of developed countries has gained wide currency.[10] However, economic inequality is a very complex idea, with a host of alternative plausible measures,[11] and the measurement of health status can be similarly problematic. In fact, the inequality or health status of a population is the result of the large number of complex processes,

---

10. Judge (1995) provides an extensive listing of the citations to Wilkinson's work.

11. The alternative statistical measures of inequality (e.g., the Gini ratio, the Theil index or the coefficient of variation) differ in their sensitivity to different parts of the income distribution. (See Jenkins 1991.) As Burkhauser et al. (1996) pointed out, the household equivalence scales in use in developed countries differ substantially in their implications for the perceived prevalence of poverty among younger and older cohorts. It also can be argued that wealth inequality is a better indicator of economic inequality than inequality in annual incomes, but a number of alternative definitions of wealth exist. (See Wolff 1991.) And so on.

whose impacts are aggregated over a number of diverse subpopulations.[12] What is it about inequality that adversely affects health? Do we expect that it is the *fact* of inequality that has impacts on population health or is it something about the *processes* which differentiate incomes that produce adverse health outcomes?[13]

Why does economic inequality affect health? Most studies have been highly aggregative. Using data on inequality, the industrial composition of output and the death rate of men aged 50 to 54, Duleep (1995), for example, argued that the relationship between inequality and mortality arises because the relationship between individual income and individual health is non-linear. If the health-income relationship is nonlinear, then a society with a more polarized income distribution, i.e., a society which has more people at the extremes of the income distribution, will have higher than average mortality because the mortality gains of the more affluent are outnumbered by the mortality losses of the poor. In looking at overall mortality and emphasizing the link between individual mortality and individual incomes, this perspective differs somewhat from Marmot (1994) or Frank and Mustard (1994), who emphasized *relative* income, and the position of individuals in the social hierarchy, as predictive of stress, despair and feelings of helplessness—all of which are associated with adverse health outcomes. Such a perspective would tend to emphasize health gradients throughout the population, but McIsaac and Wilkinson (1995) focused on the bottom end of the income distribution (i.e., the *share* of total income received by the bottom 30 percent of households) and estimated the correlation of that income share with mortality from infectious diseases, neoplasms, ischaemic heart disease, other circulatory and respiratory disorders, liver disease, traffic accidents, and other causes.

Different authors have emphasized different aspects of economic inequality, and different possible causes for the inequality-mortality relationship. Furthermore, in looking at different causes of death (e.g., traffic accidents or cancer), it is clear that there must be quite different pathways of influence, which likely impinge differently on specific segments of the population.

---

12. For example, in Canada in the 1980s the distribution of male earnings became increasingly unequal, but the distribution of female earnings became somewhat more equal (MacPhail 1996).

13. It might be protested that one cannot have economic inequality without some process of income and wealth generation, but it is conceivable that decisions made in the past (e.g., land reform or inheritance taxation) can have important impacts on the distribution of endowments which now condition the distribution of income, whatever the nature of current processes of income generation.

The issue of unemployment also illustrates the difficulties surrounding any attempt to disentangle the relative importance of economic processes and outcomes on population health. As argued earlier, unemployment has direct impacts on several crucial dimensions of individual pychosocial well-being, including the fact that the experience of unemployment deprives individuals of a major part of their social support network. The prevalence of unem-ployement also increases feeling of insecurity and anxiety for both employed and unemployed individuals. Those who do not know whether their current job will continue or whether alternatives are available lose their sense of control over their own future. And since the probability of unemployment is significantly higher among the poorer paid, an increase in unemployment produces an increase in income inequality.[14] Although there is good reason to think that insecurity/anxiety, efficacy/control and the level of inequality are all factors which independently play a role in the determination of health outcomes, each is also highly correlated with trends in unemployment.

VULNERABLE GROUPS

Although such macroeconomic trends as changes in the rate of unemploy-ment or the level of inequality have impacts throughout society, three groups are likely to be particularly affected: youth, poorly educated individuals and displaced older workers.

When the unemployment rate rises and falls, most people are not directly affected. The direct experience of unemployment is highly concentrated in the labour force, since many senior workers are protected from layoff by the seniority provisions of collective agreements or by their established value to the firm—due to the firm-specific knowledge they have acquired over their working career. As well, short-term contracts or on-call working arrange-ments can be more easily imposed on new employees than on continuing employees. As a consequence, the impact of slack labour markets is felt more acutely by new entrants to the labour force than by established workers.

In the depressed labour markets of the 1990s, youth unemployment has remained above 15 percent. The trend to falling youth wages detected in the 1980s has accelerated, and workers under 30 have been particularly affected by involuntary part-time employment. The trend to part-time work has meant that young workers may have to piece together two (or more) part-time jobs to generate an income. Without the benefit of years of prior earnings from which to acquire savings, young workers are more dependent on social transfers to tide themselves over any spell of unemployment and

---

14. See Erksoy (1994), Johnson (1995) or Beach and Slotsve (1996).

are, therefore, particularly exposed to the impact of reductions in unemployment insurance and social assistance generosity.

The objective reality of the youth labour market in Canada in the 1990s has been pretty depressing, but from the point of view of both physical and mental health, the subjective impact of economic events is also important. Since average individual earnings after inflation have been flat since the late 1970s and since the national unemployment rate has been relatively high since 1981, Canadians under 30 have never really seen a period of extended prosperity such as earlier generations experienced from 1946 to 1977.[15] But they have seen two extremely severe recessions, a great deal of downsizing and continual cutbacks to the welfare state. The repeated message of media commentary, and of life events, is the necessity of reducing aspirations and living within (lessened) means. As a consequence, the life experience of Canadians under 30 does not produce the same level of hope for better days that came naturally to earlier generations. And although the pathways between the psychological state of individuals and their physical ailments are not well mapped, it does seem clear that despair is not good for the health.

All this adds up to substantially increased levels of economic stress for Canadians under 30. And since most parents of very young children are in this age range, those children are indirectly vulnerable to the stresses of time, money, insecurity and despair that their parents experience. Although young children do not participate in the labour market, they are clearly important victims of the family violence and family breakup that is produced by the high-stress labour market their parents inhabit.

In addition to the long-standing connection between health and education, poorly educated individuals have been particularly vulnerable to the economic trends of the 1990s. Employment creation since the 1980s has been concentrated in jobs which require postsecondary education, to the detriment of the relative wages and employment prospects of poorly educated persons. Although Canada has not seen the same degree of widening of the earnings differential between high school and university graduates as has been observed in the United States (due to the greater increase in the supply of university graduates in Canada), it is now increasingly difficult for the poorly educated to find a place in the Canadian workforce. The health deficit of the poorly educated is deepened by the increasing impacts of unemployment and poverty.

In thinking about the health impacts of economic events, it is also important to recognize that the stress of unemployment can be particularly acute for displaced older workers, who may have decades of habituation to an accustomed work role, neighbourhood, lifestyle and occupational identity.

---

15. The brief exception being the Toronto–Southern Ontario labour market in 1988–1989, with a counterbalancing severe contraction in 1990–1992.

Plant closings or corporate downsizing in small towns or rural areas may leave individuals with very few realistic options in the local area. Even in major metropolitan labour markets, the duration of unemployment is particularly long for displaced older workers, and the probability of experiencing a large wage drop in subsequent employment is relatively high. Psychologically, the impact of having to "start all over again," and the feeling that a lifetime of contribution to society has no recognized value, can also be extremely stressful. The stress of adjustment is particularly great for those who dropped out of school before graduation 30 to 40 years ago (when such a decision was very common) and who have to start back to school at a level that may be below that of their children. And since older workers have lived much of their lives during times when there was much less emphasis on the health implications of risk factors such as smoking or lack of exercise, the health deficit of such behaviours may well magnify the impacts of the stress of job displacement.

POLICY DIRECTIONS

A Macroeconomy of Jobs and Hope

Any discussion of economic policy has to start from a perception of what is possible and then proceed to an assessment of priorities. In my view, it is possible to use macroeconomic policy to stimulate aggregate demand in the Canadian economy, so total output will grow faster and the labour market will generate more jobs, less unemployment, less economic insecurity and less inequality. Faster economic growth would create a macroeconomic environment in which individuals have real labour market options, can begin to feel some sense of control over their own lives and have some hope for the future. A healthy demand for labour in the Canadian economy is, arguably, both a direct contributor to population health and an essential precondition for the success of other framework policies.

In thinking about how to create jobs in Canada, there is no avoiding the crucial role of the level of aggregate demand for goods and services. In a market economy, jobs in the private sector exist because employers perceive, when they hire labour, that they will be able to sell the goods and services which their workers will produce, at a profit. The demand for labour is a derived demand, which depends ultimately on the demand for goods and services.

The two main avenues available to government to stimulate aggregate demand for goods and services in the economy are fiscal and monetary policy. Stimulating the Canadian economy by fiscal policy would involve either reducing taxation or increasing program expenditures (or both). By increasing the net spending of the public sector, governments could stimulate aggregate demand for goods and services, and thereby stimulate employment creation. Unfortunately, this would be at the cost of increasing the deficit and swelling the net debt of the public sector.

At current levels of national debt, further additions to the debt would run the risk of creating such a high debt-to-Gross Domestic Product (GDP) ratio that the ratio might become unstable, and debt-servicing costs might escalate dramatically. In this author's view, the debt and deficit problems of Canadian governments are, in 1996, very real and very pressing, and foreclose the option of stimulative fiscal policy on any appreciable scale.[16]

However, in a small open economy with a flexible exchange rate, monetary policy remains a very powerful policy lever with which to influence the macroeconomy. And it is worth emphasizing that there is no disagreement about the power of the Bank of Canada to influence aggregate demand in the Canadian economy from day to day. As the present governor (Thiessen 1995, 2, 8, 9) of the Bank has argued:

> When central banks take monetary policy actions, they set in motion a series of consequences that starts with an influence on financial markets, works through changes in spending, production and employment, and ends with an effect on the price level or, more specifically, the rate of inflation in the price level. Economists call this chain of developments the "transmission mechanism."

> Changes in interest rates affect aggregate demand through a number of channels—the cost of capital, the incentive to save rather than to spend, and the effects on wealth and cash flow. The main components of demand that are affected are housing, consumer spending on durables, business investment in fixed capital and inventory investment. The extent of the response of spending will depend in part on how long the changed level of interest rates is expected to persist. This will be an important factor for those entities that borrow at the shorter end of the market.

> The way in which the exchange rate affects demand is also relatively straightforward. A change in the value of the Canadian dollar will initially change the prices of those goods and services produced in Canada that are traded internationally and whose prices are set in world markets, vis-à-vis

---

16. As the contributors to Osberg and Fortin (1996) noted, the main reason for the current deficit and debt problems of Canadian governments is the very restrictive monetary policy pursued by the Bank of Canada since 1988. By the latter part of the 1980s, all Canadian governments had, by a mixture of taxation increases and expenditure reductions, begun to run surpluses of taxation over program expenditure and were beginning to reduce their debt-to-GDP ratios. These debt reduction plans were derailed by the surge in real interest rates engineered by the Bank of Canada as it attempted to bring "price stability" to Canada. (See Fortin 1996 or Kneebone 1996.)

those whose prices are not, or at least not entirely, determined in world markets. These changes in relative prices will set in train a series of demand and supply responses that will affect the output of Canadian-produced goods, largely through their impact on exports and imports.

The final link in the long chain is from movements in aggregate demand to the rate of inflation. In our view, underlying inflation is affected primarily by the level of slack in the economy and by the expected rate of inflation. The driving force behind inflation over time is, thus, the cumulative effect of the pressure of aggregate demand on capacity.

There is no real disagreement that monetary policy is a very powerful tool to regulate the level of aggregate demand in Canada, but there is disagreement over how that power should be used. In the view of the Bank of Canada, the *sole* objective of monetary policy should be the maintenance of "price stability."[17] The Bank of Canada has a very pessimistic appraisal of the potential output capacity of the Canadian economy[18] and a desire to err on the side of caution in preventing any chance of inflation resurgence. As a consequence, the Bank steps in to restrain aggregate demand whenever the economy approaches its (pessimistic) estimate of potential output, thereby guaranteeing perpetually high unemployment.

Since high unemployment has so many channels of influence to health outcomes, it is crucial for the Bank of Canada to begin to balance its concern for inflation with a concern for full employment—as its legal mandate in fact requires.[19]

Social Transfers

In the 1980s in Canada, unemployment was higher than in the 1970s, and there was a trend to greater inequality in the distribution of earned income, but transfer payments often compensated. The distribution of total income

---

17. In practical terms price stability is now interpreted as keeping the core rate of inflation in the consumer price index (i.e., excluding fuel, indirect taxes and food) between 1% and 3% per annum.

18. This pessimism is guaranteed by methodological assumption, since the Bank uses the Hodrick-Prescott filter to construct its measure of potential output. Since this is essentially a weighted moving average of past output, poor macro-economic performance in the recent past heavily influences the estimate of maximum productive potential in the present.

19. The legal mandate of the Bank of Canada is to "mitigate by its influence fluctuations in the general level of production, trade, prices and unemployment, so far as may be possible in the scope of monetary action and generally to promote the economic and financial welfare of Canada." But, since 1988, the Bank has redefined its objectives to a focus on "price stability" alone.

(including transfer payments) among Canadian households therefore remained relatively stable. In comparison to other Organization for Economic Cooperation and Development (OECD) nations (except the United States), Canada does not spend a high percentage of GDP on transfer payments. However, in Canada unemployment insurance has been a much more important component of transfers than in many other countries.

Partly because unemployment insurance payments go immediately to those who are affected by unemployment, and such people tend to be relatively poor, unemployment insurance payments in the 1980s filled part of the hole created by higher unemployment and increased inequality in the distribution of working hours. (See Osberg et al. 1996.)

When most of the unemployed receive unemployment insurance benefits and the potential duration of benefits is long enough that relatively few exhaust their UI benefits before locating employment, fewer have to rely on social assistance. However, by 1995, a series of reforms to unemployment insurance in Canada had reduced UI generosity to a level comparable to that of 1957 or 1970. In fact, by 1995 Canadian UI had become less generous than the UI system in place in New York State. (See Sargent 1995.)

In 1996, the system was revised again, to cut another $1.2 billion from its expenditures.[20] Even before the latest revisions, a steadily falling percentage of unemployed persons had been able to claim benefits, due to the disqualification from entitlement of people who voluntarily quit or were fired, increased entrance requirements and decreased benefit duration. By June 1997, claimants were only about 34 percent of unemployed persons. And although all these revisions might be expected to place greater stress on the social assistance program, there have been simultaneous cuts to social assistance benefit levels and tightened eligibility requirements in many provinces (most notably Ontario).

If cuts to unemployment insurance and social assistance were occurring in a context where employment opportunities were easily available, they would have relatively little impact on economic inequality, or economic insecurity, or on individuals' sense of control over their own lives, because the alternative of a job would be available. Hence, one could expect any health implications to be substantially mitigated. However, this is not the case. In the 1990s, social transfers are being substantially reduced at a time when the measured unemployment rate remains high (9.0 percent in September 1997). Furthermore, it must be stressed that the unemployment rate would be substantially higher, were it not for the fact that the labour force participation rate remains depressed (by about three percentage points)

---

20. Aggregate UI benefits are anticipated to fall by $2 billion, but since expenditure on employment assistance measures is to rise by $800 million, the net cut is $1.2 billion.

because so many Canadians have withdrawn from an active job search. In short, current trends in the weakening of Canada's social safety net seem certain to exacerbate the insecurity, inequality and stress of economic life which also tends to produce adverse health outcomes. If there is a change in monetary policy to encourage economic growth and job creation, these cuts to the social safety net will be of less importance. In the current context they are likely to be very important.

Indeed, since the stated cause of the cuts to social programs in Canada in recent years has been the concern of Canadian governments to reduce their deficits, and since the cause of the deficit problems of Canadian governments in the 1990s was the high interest rates of the 1988 to 1992 period and the collapse in output which that produced,[21] social programs are, in a very real sense, hostage to monetary policy.

Social Protection Legislation

Capitalism is an economic system in which jobs are continually being lost at some firms and created at others. As Davis et al. (1996) noted, developed market economies are all characterized by fairly high rates of job reallocation, with a range from approximately 16 percent to 30 percent per annum.[22] If such change occurs in the context of reasonably rapid growth, the potentially adverse impacts of job reallocation in insecurity and unemployment are greatly mitigated. When structural change occurs in the context of slack labour markets, there is often "no place to go" for job losers. Long-term unemployment for job losers and continual anxiety for job keepers is the result. Furthermore, as the unemployment rate increases and new jobs become hard to find, the *type* of entrant into the pool of unemployed also changes, since the number of people who voluntarily quit falls and the number of involuntary dismissals rises when labour markets turn soft. The

---

21. As Osberg and Fortin (1996) noted, when the debt-GDP ratio is at the level it was in the mid-1980s, it is the difference between interest rates and the growth rate which is crucial to debt stability. In fact, Canadian governments had begun to run surpluses of taxation over program expenditure by 1988, but their deficit reduction plans were derailed by the escalation of interest rates engineered by the Bank of Canada.

22. At 20.7 percent per annum in manufacturing, the rate of job reallocation in Canada was similar to that in the United States (19.4 percent) and in Italy (19.9 percent). The fact that there is no necessary trade-off between labour market flexibility and a highly developed welfare state is indicated by the fact that the rate of job reallocation in Sweden (23.5percent) and in France (23.3 percent) is somewhat higher. Germany had relatively low job reallocation (16.0 percent) while Australia and Denmark were on the high side (at 29.3 percent and 29.8 percent respectively). (See Davis et al. 1996, 21.)

labour market *context* is, therefore, crucial both for individual behaviour and for the practical impacts of social protection legislation.

When voluntary quits are high (because attractive new jobs are opening up elsewhere) the cost to firms of social protections for existing workers is relatively low because voluntary attrition can fairly quickly achieve any desired reduction in the labour force. When there is a high rate of voluntary turnover, constraints on arbitrary layoffs by firms or the requirement that they provide adequate severance payments provide some peace of mind to workers, but the impact on firms is limited because they do not have to be as frequently invoked. In this context, the marginal value to workers of job security protections may be small, but so is the cost to employers of providing them.

In times when jobs are scarce (as now), job security is both felt to be needed by workers and most likely to be costly to firms. Voluntary quits have a strong cyclical pattern and, when few people are leaving voluntarily (because new jobs are hard to find), employers have to resort more often to layoffs to achieve any desired downsizing. Unfortunately, it is also at times like the present that employers seem to have the political power to prevent any expansions of social protection legislation. In the current context, it seems to be unrealistic to urge new legislation to protect workers from arbitrary dismissal, to entrench job security after a probationary period or to increase severance pay requirements. More limited objectives, such as improved procedures for the advanced notification of layoffs, are likely the most that can be hoped for on the regulatory front.

Although social protection legislation is, like the transfer system, hostage to the health of the macroeconomy and the conduct of monetary policy, there are some structural reforms which may be possible. There are a number of price-type incentives in the structure of tax and social welfare legislation that may be inappropriate from the perspective of a population health concern with worker security. Reference has already been made to the impact of employer-paid health insurance, which has a lump-sum cost per worker to employers and, therefore, creates an incentive to minimize the number of employees and react to downturns in demand by reducing the number of employees (but working them for as long, or longer hours) rather than by spreading the same decline in labour demand over the workforce as a whole, by instituting work weeks with fewer hours. To the extent that coverage under Medicare in Canada is eroded and private (employer paid) health insurance fills the gap, this incentive to layoffs, rather than work sharing, will increase. Similarly, caps on UI coverage of earnings, or CPP employer-paid premiums, also establish fixed, per-employee costs, and provide an incentive to emphasize layoffs rather than work sharing. However, since payroll taxes in Canada are relatively low, compared to their level in other developed countries,[23] the actual impact on employment structure of these cost features is not likely to be as important as elsewhere.

---

23. See Lin et al. (1996).

This paper has discussed the role of insecurity, inequality and a lack of a sense of personal efficacy in increasing the probability of ill health, so it is worthwhile mentioning that collective bargaining influences all three. As the industrial relations literature argues, providing workplace security is a major objective of unions. Individual security is enhanced by seniority rights, disciplinary grievance and appeal rights, layoff restrictions and the fact that terms and conditions of employment cannot be unilaterally altered—unlike the "employment at will" situation. By providing an avenue by which individuals can, if they become active in the union, influence their terms and conditions of employment, it can be argued that unionization increases the sense of personal control and efficacy that individuals feel. And since lower-paid individuals have the greatest wage gains from unionization and since unions tend to equalize wages within workplaces, unionization tends to reduce inequality—both within firms and in society as a whole. (See Lemieux 1993.) Hence, since there is good reason to think that collective bargaining affects positively some of the dimensions of economic life which have positive impacts on health, legislation which affects the ease or difficulty of union organizing can be seen as an economic policy variable affecting health.

CONCLUSION

By a number of routes, this paper has kept returning to the importance of full employment for population health and the desirability of a shift in monetary policy to enable economic growth and job creation. In part, this emphasis on the importance of reducing unemployment arises from the close connection between unemployment and the other economic determinants of ill health (insecurity, lack of efficacy and inequality) that have been identified in the literature. As well, persistently high unemployment can be expected to produce changes in the institutional structure of labour markets and the demographic structure of the population which increase the stress levels individuals are subject to and which erode the social institutions which help to buffer them from stress. High unemployment and excessively tight monetary policy are also important because the financial constraints of an underperforming macroeconomy and excessively high interest charges on the national debt are forcing cuts in the social safety net. In the 1980s, social transfers were extremely important in mitigating in Canada the rise in inequality and insecurity that was observed in the United States and the United Kingdom, but the 1990s have seen major cuts.

In short, because high unemployment has a strong impact on population health, both directly and indirectly, and because the other economic and social policies that might assist health policy are held hostage to a resumption of economic growth and job creation, the main economic policy variable that can positively affect the health of Canadians is a monetary policy that emphasizes jobs and growth.

Lars Osberg *has an honours B.A. in economics and politics from Queen's University and a Ph.D in economics from Yale University. He is McCulloch professor of economics at Dalhousie University. He is the author of numerous refereed articles, book chapters, reviews and reports, and coauthor or editor of eight books, most recently* Vanishing Jobs: Canada's Changing Workplaces *(1995),* Unnecessary Debts *(1996) and* The Unemployment Crisis: All for Naught *(1996). His major fields of research interest have been the determinants of poverty and economic inequality, with particular emphasis in recent years on the impact of unemployment, structural change in labour markets and social policy.*

BIBLIOGRAPHY

ALLIÉ, E. 1994. Impacts of changes in UI contributions and maximum insurable earnings: A general equilibrium model. Paper presented at the Canadian Employment Research Forum Conference on the Evaluation of Unemployment Insurance, October 15, 1994. Strategic Research, Human Resources Development Canada, mimeo.

BEACH, C. M., and G. A. SLOTSVE. 1996. *Are We Becoming Two Societies? Income Polarization and the Myth of the Declining Middle Class in Canada.* Toronto (ON): C. D. Howe Institute.

BÉLAND, F. 1993. Expenditure on ambulatory medical care over the long term in the Quebec Medicare System. Discussion paper prepared for the Ninth Meeting of Consultative Committee on Social Policy, Health Canada, Mont-Tremblant, Quebec, December 12–14, 1993.

BLANK, R. 1994. *Social Protection Versus Economic Flexibility: Is There a Trade-off?* National Bureau of Economic Research. Chicago and London: University of Chicago Press.

BRENNER, M. H. 1971. Economic changes and heart disease mortality. *American Journal of Public Health* 61: 606–611.

BRENNER, M.H. 1973. *Mental Illness and the Economy.* Cambridge (MA): Harvard University Press.

BRENNER, M. H., and A. MOONEY. 1983. Unemployment and health in the context of economic change. *Social Science and Medicine* 17: 1125–1138.

BURKAUSER, R. V., T. M. SMEEDING, and J. MERZ. 1996. Relative inequality and poverty in Germany and the United States using alternative equivalence scales. *The Review of Income and Wealth* 4: 381–400.

D'ARCY, C. 1986. Unemployment and health: Data and implications. *Canadian Journal of Public Health* 77(supp. 1, May/June): 125–131.

D'ARCY, C. and C. M. SIDDIQUE. 1987. Health and unemployment: Findings from a national survey. In *Health and Canadian Society: Sociological Perspectives,* 2nd ed., eds. D. COBURN et al. Toronto (ON): Fittshenry and Whiteside. pp. 239–261.

DAVIS, S. J., J. C. HALTIWANGER, and S. SCHUH. 1996. *Job Creation and Destruction.* Cambridge (MA): MIT Press.

DEVINE, T. J., and N. M. KIEFER. 1991. *Empirical Labour Economics: The Search Approach.* Oxford: Oxford University Press.

DULEEP, H. O. 1995. Mortality and Income Inequality among Economically Developed Countries. *Social Security Bulletin.* Social Security Administration, Office of Research and Statistics, 58 (summer): 34–50.

EKOS Research Associates. 1993. *A Mid-Campaign Report: The EKOS Election 1993 Analysis.* Ottawa (ON): EKOS Research Associates, October 1.

_____. 1994. *"Rethinking Government 94–1" Phase 1 Final Report.* Ottawa, July 26.

ERKSOY, S. 1994. The effects of higher unemployment on the distribution of income in Canada: 1981–1987. *Canadian Public Policy* 20 (September): 318–328.

FORTIN, P. 1994. A diversified strategy for deficit control: Combining faster growth with fiscal discipline. Department of Economics, University of Quebec at Montreal, mimeo.

FORTIN, P. 1996. The Canadian fiscal problem: The macroeconomic connection. In *Unnecessary Debts,* eds. L. OSBERG and P. FORTIN. Toronto (ON): James Lorimer & Company. pp. 26–38.

FRANK, J. W., and J. F. MUSTARD. 1994. The determinants of health from a historical perspective. *Daedalus: Journal of the American Academy of Arts and Sciences, Health and Wealth* 123 (fall): 1–19.

GRAYSON, J.P. 1993. Health, physical activity level, and employment status in Canada. *International Journal of Health Services* 23(4): 743–761.

JAHODA, M. 1979. The psychological meanings of unemployment. *New Society*, September 6, pp. 422–425.

JENKINS, S. 1991. The measurement of income inequality. In *Economic Inequality and Poverty: International Perspectives*, ed. L. OSBERG. Armonk (NY): M. E. Sharpe. pp. 3–38.

JOHNSON, S. 1995. More evidence on the effect of higher unemployment on the Canadian size distribution of income. *Canadian Public Policy* 21 (December): 423–428.

JUDGE, K. 1995. Income distribution and life expectancy: A critical appraisal. *British Medical Journal* 311 (November): 1282–1285.

KELVIN, P., and J. JARRETT. 1985. *Unemployment: Its Social Psychological Effects.* Cambridge: Cambridge University Press.

KETSO, V. 1988. Work and the welfare costs of unemployment. Ph.D. thesis,. Halifax (NS): Department of Economics, Dalhousie University.

KNEEBONE, R. D. 1996. Four Decades of Deficits and Debt. In *Unnecessary Debts*, eds. L. OSBERG, and P. FORTIN. Toronto (ON): James Lorimer & Company. pp. 39–70.

LEMIEUX, T. 1993. Unions and wage inequality in Canada and the United States. In *Small Differences That Matter: Labour Markets and Income Maintenance in Canada and the United States*, eds. D. CARD, and R. FREEMAN. Chicago (IL): National Bureau of Economic Research, University of Chicago Press. pp. 69–108.

LIN, Z., C. BEACH, and G. PICOT. 1996. *Payroll Taxes in Canada.* Mines Analytical Studies Branch, Statistics Canada, Ottawa (ON).

MACLEAN, B., and L. OSBERG. Eds. 1996. *The Unemployment Crisis: All For Naught?* Montreal (QC) and Kingston (ON): McGill-Queen's University Press.

MACPHAIL, F. 1996. Three essays on trends in poverty and inequality in Canada. Ph.D. thesis. Halifax (NS): Department of Economics, Dalhousie University.

MARMOT, M. G. 1994. Social differentials in health within and between populations. *Daedalus: Journal of the American Academy of Arts and Sciences, Health and Wealth* 123 (Fall): 197–216.

MCISAAC, S. J., and R. G. WILKINSON. 1995. Cause of death, income distribution and problems response rates. Working paper no. 136. Luxembourg Income Study, Maxwell School of Citizenship and Public Affairs, Syracuse University, Syracuse, New York, December 1995.

MYATT, T. 1996. Why do we know so little about unemployment determination and the effects of unemployment insurance? In *The Unemployment Crisis: All For Naught?*, eds. B. K. MACLEAN, and L. OSBERG. Montreal (QC) and Kingston (ON): McGill-Queen's University Press. pp. 107–128.

ORCUTT, C., S. CALDWELL, and R. WERTHEIMER. 1976. *Policy Exploration through Micro-Analytic Simulation.* Washington (DC): The Urban Institute.

OSBERG, L. 1995. Concepts of unemployment and the structure of employment. *Economie Appliquée* 48(1): 157–181.

———. 1996. Unemployment insurance and unemployment—revisited. In *The Unemployment Crisis: All For Naught?*, eds. B. K. MACLEAN, and L. OSBERG. Montreal (QC) and Kingston (ON): McGill-Queen's University Press. pp. 75–106.

OSBERG, L., and P. FORTIN. 1996. *Unnecessary Debts.* Toronto (ON): James Lorimer & Company.

OSBERG, L., and S. PHIPPS. 1993. Labour supply with quantity constraints: Estimates from a large sample of Canadian workers. *Oxford Economic Papers* 5(2): 269–291.

———. 1994. The distributional implications of unemployment insurance—A micro-simulation analysis. Department of Economics, Dalhousie University, February 1994, mimeo.

OSBERG, L., S. ERKSOY, and S. PHIPPS. 1996. Unemployment, unemployment insurance and the distribution of income in Canada in the 1980s. In *The Distribution of the Economic Well-Being in the 1980s—An International Perspective*, eds. P. GOTTSCHALK, B. GUSTAFSSON, and E. PALMER. Cambridge University Press.

OSBERG, L., D. GORDON and Z. LIN. 1994. Inter-regional migration and inter-industry labour mobility in Canada: A simultaneous approach. *Canadian Journal of Economics* 27 (February): 58–79.

PHIPPS, S. 1990. Quantity constrained household responses to UI Reform. *Economic Journal* 100: 124–140.

_____. 1991. Behavioural response to UI Reform in constrained and unconstrained models of labour supply. *Canadian Journal of Economics* 14(1): 34–54.

POLOZ, S. S. 1994. The causes of unemployment in Canada: A review of the evidence. Working paper no. 94–11, Research Department, Bank of Canada, Ottawa, November 1994.

SAMSON, L. 1985. A study of the impact of sectoral shifts on aggregate unemployment in Canada. *Canadian Journal of Economics* 18(3): 518–530.

SARGENT, T. C. 1995. An index of unemployment insurance disincentives. Working paper no. 95–10, Economics Studies and Policy Analysis Division, Department of Finance, Ottawa (ON).

SCHOFIELD, D. 1996. The impact of employment and hours of work on health status and health service use. Discussion paper no. 11, National Centre for Social and Economic Modelling, University of Canberra, March 1996.

SETTERFIELD, M. A., D. V. GORDON, and L. OSBERG. 1992. Searching for a Will o' the wisp: An empirical study of the NAIRU in Canada. *European Economic Review* 36: 119–136.

THIESSEN, G. 1995. Uncertainty in the transmission of monetary policy in Canada. The Hermes-Glendon Lecture, York University, Toronto, March 30, 1995, mimeo.

WALDMANN, R. J. 1992. Income distribution and infant mortality. *Quarterly Journal of Economics* November: 1283–1302.

WILKINSON, R. G. 1994. The epidemiological transition: From material scarcity to socially disadvantaged? *Daedalus, Journal of the American Academy of Arts and Sciences, Health and Wealth* 133 (Fall): 61–77.

_____. 1995a. Commentary: Mistaken criticisms ignore overwhelming evidence. *British Medical Journal* 311 (November): 1285–1287.

_____. 1995b. Health, redistribution and growth. In *Paying for Inequality: The Economic Cost of Social Injustice*, eds. A. GLYN, and D. MILIBAND. London: IPPAR/Rivers Oram Press.

WOLFF, E. N. 1991. The inequality of wealth. In *Economic Inequality and Poverty: International Perspectives*, ed. L. OSBERG. Armonk (NY): M. E. Sharpe Publishers. pp. 92–133.

Series
Canada Health Action: Building on the Legacy
Papers Commissioned by the National Forum on Health

Volume 1
Determinants of Health

Children and Youth

Jane Bertrand
Enriching the Preschool Experiences of Children

Paul D. Steinhauer
Developing Resiliency in Children from Disadvantaged Populations

David A. Wolfe
Prevention of Child Abuse and Neglect

Christopher Bagley and Wilfreda E. Thurston
Decreasing Child Sexual Abuse

Barbara A. Morrongiello
Preventing Unintentional Injuries among Children

Benjamin H. Gottlieb
Strategies to Promote the Optimal Development of Canada's Youth

Paul Anisef
Making the Transition from School to Employment

Pamela C. Fralick and Brian Hyndman
Youth, Substance Abuse and the Determinants of Health

Gaston Godin and Francine Michaud
STD and AIDS Prevention among Young People

Tullio Caputo and Katharine Kelly
Improving the Health of Street/Homeless Youth

Series
Canada Health Action: Building on the Legacy
Papers Commissioned by the National Forum on Health

Volume 2

Determinants of Health

Adults and Seniors

William R. Avison
The Health Consequences of Unemployment

Mary J. Breen
Promoting Literacy, Improving Health

Neena L. Chappell
Maintaining and Enhancing Independence and Well-Being in Old Age

Sandra O'Brien Cousins
Promoting Active Living and Healthy Eating among Older Canadians

Victor W. Marshall and Philippa J. Clarke
Facilitating the Transition from Employment to Retirement

Dr. Robyn Tamblyn and Dr. Robert Perreault
Encouraging the Wise Use of Prescription Medication by Older Adults

Daphne Nahmiash
Preventing, Reducing and Stopping the Abuse and Neglect of Older Canadian Adults in Canadian Communities

Series
Canada Health Action: Building on the Legacy
Papers Commissioned by the National Forum on Health

Volume 3
Determinants of Health
Settings and Issues

Series
Canada Health Action: Building on the Legacy
Papers Commissioned by the National Forum on Health

Volume 4

Striking a Balance

Health Care Systems in Canada and Elsewhere

Geoffroy Scott
International Comparison of the Hospital Sector

Astrid Brousselle
Controlling Health Expenditures: What Matters

Wendy Kennedy
Managing Pharmaceutical Expenditures: How Canada Compares

Centre for International Statistics
Health Spending and Health Status: An International Comparison

Damien Contandriopoulos
How Canada's Health Care System Compares with that of Other Countries: An Overview

Delphine Arweiler
International Comparisons of Health Expenditures

Marc-André Fournier
The Impact of Health Care Infrastructures and Human Resources on Health Expenditures

Ellen Leibovich, Howard Bergman and François Béland
Health Care Expenditures and the Aging Population in Canada

Raisa Deber and Bill Swan
Puzzling Issues in Health Care Financing

Terrence Sullivan
Commentary on Health Care Expenditures, Social Spending and Health Status

Allan M. Maslove
National Goals and the Federal Role in Health Care

Raiser Deber, Lutchmie Narine, Pat Baranek et al.
The Public-Private Mix in Health Care

John Marriott and Ann L. Mable
Integrated Models: International Trends and Implications for Canada

Steven G. Morgan
Issues for Canadian Pharmaceutical Policy

Series
Canada Health Action: Building on the Legacy
Papers Commissioned by the National Forum on Health

Volume 5

Making Decisions

Evidence and Information

Joan E. Tranmer, S. Squires, K. Brazil, J. Gerlach, J. Johnson, D. Muisner, B. Swan, Dr. R. Wilson
Using Evidence-Based Decision Making: What Works, What Doesn't

Paul Fisher, Marcus J. Hollander, Thomas MacKenzie, Peter Kleinstiver, Irina Sladecek, Gail Peterson
Decision Support Tools in Health Care

Charlyn Black
Building a National Health Information Network

Robert Butcher
Foundations for Evidence-Based Decision Making

Carol Kushner and Michael Rachlis
Consumer Involvement in Health Policy Development

Frank L. Graves and Patrick Beauchamp (EKOS Research Associates Inc.), and David Herle (Earnscliffe Research and Communications)
Research on Canadian Values in Relation to Health and the Health Care System

Thérèse Leroux, Sonia Le Bris, Bartha Maria Knoppers, with the collaboration of Louis-Nicolas Fortin and Julie Montreuil
The Feasibility of a National Canadian Advisory Committee on Ethics: Points to Consider

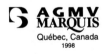

AGMV
MARQUIS
Québec, Canada
1998